Practical Guide to Transcranial Direct Current Stimulation

Helena Knotkova • Michael A. Nitsche
Marom Bikson • Adam J. Woods
Editors

Practical Guide to Transcranial Direct Current Stimulation

Principles, Procedures and Applications

Springer

Editors
Helena Knotkova
MJHS Institute for Innovation
in Palliative Care
New York, NY
USA

Department of Family and Social Medicine
Albert Einstein College of Medicine
Bronx, NY
USA

Marom Bikson
Department of Biomedical Engineering
The City College of New York
New York, NY
USA

Michael A. Nitsche
Department of Psychology and
Neurosciences
Leibniz Research Centre for Working
Environment and Human Factors
Dortmund
Germany

University Medical Hospital Bergmannsheil
Bochum
Germany

Adam J. Woods
Center for Cognitive Aging and Memory
(CAM), McKnight Brain Institute
Department of Clinical and Health
Psychology, College of Public Health and
Health Professions, University of Florida
Gainesville, FL
USA

ISBN 978-3-319-95947-4 ISBN 978-3-319-95948-1 (eBook)
https://doi.org/10.1007/978-3-319-95948-1

Library of Congress Control Number: 2018955563

This Springer imprint is published by the registered company Springer Nature Switzerland AG
The registered company address is: Gewerbestrasse 11, 6330 Cham, Switzerland

Foreword

This is the most comprehensive book on the subject of transcranial direct current stimulation (tDCS) yet written. Its editors and authors are some of the most accomplished scientists in their fields. They are intelligent, hardworking, and passionate about their research in a way that helps them to succeed where others fail. Few of them started their careers focused on tDCS, but came to it through a variety of avenues: engineering, electronics, psychology, neuroscience, medicine, and others. All have found through the course of their professions that brain stimulation, and tDCS in particular, might fill a niche that has been lacking until now.

Over the last decade, brain stimulation has undergone extraordinary growth for the study of the healthy human brain and for the study and treatment of brain and mental illness. In terms of brain stimulation, tDCS is becoming the most widespread method. Many advantages of tDCS have helped to fuel this growth. Its most basic requirements are a source of controlled current and electrodes that can be temporarily fixed to the body. Compared with most other methods of stimulation, and pharmaceuticals, this makes tDCS technically simpler and much less expensive to administer. Also, as we can find in this book, it appears to be safe. This combination of low cost, simplicity, and safety has generated a lot of interest in tDCS. The many potential advantages of tDCS have driven efforts to increase its efficacy, without which tDCS is useless. These ongoing attempts are described here with great detail.

The increasing use of tDCS has allowed for the testing of hypotheses regarding the brain basis of cognition and behavior that could not be studied in healthy humans until its development. One of these is how changes in behavior are associated with changes in activity of specific brain regions and networks. If a brain region supports a specific behavior, or patterns of behavior, then increasing or decreasing activity in that region should influence that behavior. tDCS applied to a brain region may facilitate brain states that improve (or suppress) different forms of cognition, such as learning, memory, attention, or perception. Many studies described in this book have shown alterations in these forms of cognition using tDCS applied to brain areas suspected of being involved in these forms of cognition and others that have failed. tDCS offers another line of evidence as to how brain areas are involved in these cognitive processes. In addition, once identified, tDCS-based methods could be used to enhance cognition for real-world purposes. Effective and reliable methods for cognitive enhancement based on tDCS could lead to many benefits in neuroergonomics, which is the use of our understanding of the mind and brain to enhance work and technology, along with a variety of other endeavors including education, science, sports, music, and art. Indeed, all areas of human endeavor could benefit from a reliable method of altering cognition.

In addition, it offers hope for new forms of treatment that could reduce suffering for the many millions of patients with clinical disorders who are currently not helped or are even being hindered by available medical treatments. Those suffering from disorders such as addiction, depression, anxiety, psychosis, chronic pain, traumatic brain injury, stroke, dementia, and many others have a need for medical solutions that are safer, more effective, and more economical than what is currently available. The huge physical, emotional, and economic drain on society makes it imperative that we leave no stone unturned in looking for answers. tDCS offers us at least a chance to reduce this suffering. Many of the latest advances using tDCS to reduce the impact of these disorders are described in this book. There is definite progress in improving the ability of tDCS to help fight these disorders.

At the same time, tDCS has suffered many problems often associated with new technologies. Early successes lead to exuberance and high expectations for the technology's future potential. Eventually though, some early results cannot be replicated in subsequent studies, inexperienced users make mistakes that complicate the literature, and the hype associated with a few early successes does not play out. This can turn into indifference and even resentment on the part of the media and broader scientific community, stifling funding and publications needed for potentially important and useful research. In addition, if one considers the vast number of ways that tDCS can be applied, and the even larger number of ways that electric current can be modulated in time, it can be concluded that a nearly infinite variety of methods for applying TES are available. A single unsuccessful attempt is often described as a "failure of tDCS." However, one failed attempt leaves many millions of alternatives yet untried, with those that succeed still waiting to be discovered.

Finding new successes for tDCS is a large focus of this book. Methods to optimize tDCS effects described here include modeling of current pathways combined with neuroimaging of individual differences in brain structure and organization, leading to individualized electrode montages. Optimization of more general experimental procedures across laboratories is also called for. A large variety of methods, which vary in current intensity, density, and duration, electrode types, methods of electrode placement, sham control, and blinding procedures, can be found in the studies described throughout this book. While beneficial in terms of discovery (e.g., one method may result in a new discovery, while another equally valid method does not for some reason), this makes it very difficult to compare across studies and laboratories. Such problems contribute to the perceived lack of replication in the field, but this may result from procedural differences across studies, with few "true" replications actually being performed.

While this book has much to say about the success stories of tDCS, and hope for its future, this is not hype. It relates the hard science of what tDCS is about and its limitations. Its main points regarding the technical and experimental underpinnings of tDCS research are meant to inform, not inflame, and to give the reader a sense of the underlying reality of this method, at least as it is understood today. The reader will undoubtedly come away with a much better grasp of the current status of this dynamic and still expanding field, along with many questions. One of these is: What is the full description of the effects of tDCS at each level of the nervous system? tDCS interacts with the nervous system at every level, from the molecular up through to the systems and gross anatomical levels, with both neurons and glia, all to different degrees depending on their physical properties and the exact tDCS protocol used. Some of these interactions may also vary minute by minute as tDCS progresses. As with pharmaceuticals, it is impossible to know for sure if we have captured every point of interaction between a treatment and the human body and every aspect of this very complex process. Chances are good that we are missing something with an important influence on brain and behavior. Only further study can help to answer these questions.

From its beginning, tDCS has pointed out many flaws and inadequacies in our understanding of the nervous system. How could this low a level of current cross the skull and enter the brain? When action potential threshold is 10–20 mV above resting potential for a typical neuron, how could a change of 0.5 mV or less have any effect? Uncertainty regarding mechanisms such as these leaves many other details of tDCS uncertain. What is the spatial resolution of tDCS? That is, how far can an electrode be moved while still producing similar results within an individual? Most importantly, what is the tDCS electrode size and placement and stimulation polarity, amplitude, and duration that will produce the best results for a given application?

As with most areas of science, there is no real end to this process of discovery. Along the way, we may find a few nuggets of truth that stand up to further study, and many more questions will arise. With so many people around the world lacking safe and effective medical care, the hope is that this work will lead to new forms of treatment that will help to reduce their suffering. The ultimate goal of all science is to increase our understanding of the world around us and to use this in order to help give people a better quality of life that is less burdened by suffering and despair. This effort, and the hope behind it, is what shines through this book most of all.

Albuquerque, NM, USA Vincent P. Clark

Preface

The field of brain stimulation has enormously expanded over the past decades. Technological progress in biomedical and engineering sciences facilitated advances in understanding physiological and pathological neural dynamics in the central nervous system that represent functional targets for brain stimulation and mechanisms that underlie the brain stimulation effects.

Among specific techniques of noninvasive stimulation, transcranial direct current stimulation (tDCS) has gained steadily growing interest by scientists, clinicians, and the public. This is not surprising, as tDCS research can facilitate insight into neurophysiological mechanisms underlying the development and maintenance of difficult-to-treat disorders and symptoms, as well as provide insight into the linkage between neurophysiological characteristics of neural networks and functional and behavioral outcomes. Further, aiming for enduring alterations of neuronal activity, tDCS bears enormous clinical potential in a broad range of medical disciplines, such as neurology, psychiatry, pain management, or neurorehabilitation, because pathological changes in neural activity are common in many diseases and neurostimulation techniques can be employed to attempt functional normalization of the neural circuitry.

Hand in hand with growing interest in tDCS, new questions and challenges have emerged, and a need for tDCS professional education and training has tremendously expanded. This *Practical Guide to Transcranial Direct Current Stimulation* is the first comprehensive textbook for tDCS; it provides an overview and in-depth discussion of principles, mechanisms, procedures, and applications of tDCS, as well as methodological considerations, ethics, and professional conduct pertaining to this technique. We hope that this book helps bridge the existing gap in tDCS instructional materials for those who engage in research or clinical applications of this promising technique.

New York, NY, USA — Helena Knotkova
Dortmund, Germany — Michael A. Nitsche
New York, NY, USA — Marom Bikson
Gainesville, FL, USA — Adam J. Woods

Abbreviations

ABD	Abduction
ACC	Anterior cingulate cortex
ACh	Acetylcholine
AC-PC	Anterior commissure-posterior commissure
AD	Alzheimer's disease
ADAS-Cog	Alzheimer's Disease Assessment Scale-Cognitive subscale
Add	Adduction
ADHD	Attention deficit hyperactivity disorder
AE	Adverse event
ADL	Activities of daily living
ADM	Abductor digiti minimi muscle
AEP	Auditory evoked potential
AH	Auditory hallucinations
AHRQ	Agency for Healthcare Research and Quality
AHRS	Auditory Hallucination Rating Scale
AMPA	α-Amino-3-hydroxy-5-methyl-4-isoxazolepropionic acid
AMPAR	α-Amino-3-hydroxy-5-methyl-4-isoxazolepropionic acid receptor
AMT	Active motor threshold
AN	Anorexia nervosa
AP	Anteroposterior
AR	Augmented reality
ARAT	Action Research Arm Test
ARS	Autoregressive
ASL	Arterial spin labeling
a-tDCS	Anodal-tDCS
AV	Atrioventricular
BART	Balloon Analog Risk Task
BBT	Box and Block Test
BD	Bipolar disorder
BDNF	Brain-derived neurotrophic factor
BMI	Body mass index

BN	Bulimia nervosa
BOLD	Blood oxygen level dependent
BPA	Brachial plexus avulsion
BP_{ND}	Nondisplaceable binding potential
BOLD-fMRI	Blood oxygen level dependent functional magnetic resonance imaging
bvFTD	Behavioral variant frontotemporal dementia
CAD	Computer-aided design
CCT	Cognitive control therapy
CCQB	Cocaine Craving Questionnaire Brief
CPP	Conditioned place preference
CABG	Coronary artery bypass grafting
CATIE	Clinical Antipsychotic Trials of Intervention Effectiveness
CBLP	Chronic leg and back pain
CBP	Chronic back pain
CBS	Corticobasal syndrome
CBT	Cognitive behavioral therapy
CDSS	Calgary Depression Scale in Schizophrenia
CES	Cranial electrotherapy stimulation
CET	Cranial electrostimulation therapy
CFR	Code of Federal Regulations
CGMP	Current good marketing practice
CM	Corticomotoneuronal or chronic migraine
CM-PF	Center median-parafascicular
CN-NINM	Cranial nerve noninvasive neuromodulation
CNS	Central nervous system
COMT	Catechol-*o*-methyltransferase
CONSORT	Consolidated Standards of Reporting Trials
COP	Center of pressure
CPSP	Central post-stroke pain
CRPS	Complex regional pain syndrome
CSF	Cerebrospinal fluid
CT	Computed tomography
c-tDCS	Cathodal-tDCS
CUtLASS	Cost Utility of the Latest Antipsychotic Drugs in Schizophrenia Study
CVS	Caloric vestibular stimulation
CW	Continuous wave
CSD	Cortical spreading depression
dACC	Dorsal anterior cingulate cortex
DALY	Disability-adjusted life year
DAT	Dementia–Alzheimer's type
DBS	Deep brain stimulation
DC	Direct current
DCN	Dorsal cochlear nucleus

DCS	Direct current stimulation
DeoxyHb	Deoxygenated hemoglobin
DIY	Do-it-yourself
DLB	Dementia with Lewy bodies
DLF	Dorsolateral funiculus
DLPFC	Dorsolateral prefrontal cortex
dPMC	Dorsal premotor cortex
DPNS	Direct peripheral nerve stimulation
DRG	Dorsal root ganglion
DSM-III-R	Diagnostic and Statistical Manual of Mental Disorders, Third Edition Revised
DTI	Diffusion tensor imaging
DTNS	Direct trigeminal nerve stimulation
DW	Diffusion weighted
DWI	Diffusion weighted imaging
EA	Electroanesthesia
ECT	Electroconvulsive therapy
ED	Eating disorder
EEG	Electroencephalography
E-field	Electrical field
EMG	Electromyography
EOG	Electrooculogram
EN	Electronarcosis
ERCP	Endoscopic retrograde cholangiopancreatography
ERN	Error-related negativity
ERP	Event-related potential
ES	Electrosleep
EST	Electroshock therapy
EU	European Union
FBBS	Failed back surgery syndrome
FCS	Fronto-cingulo-striatal
FD	Frequency domain
FDI	First dorsal interosseous muscle
FDA	US Food and Drug Administration
FE	Finite element
FEA	Finite element analysis
FEM	Finite element method
FEAST	Focal electrically administered seizure therapy
FES	Functional electrical stimulation
FISSFO	Fade in, short stimulation, fade out
FM	Fibromyalgia
FMA	Fugl-Meyer Assessment
fMRI	Functional magnetic resonance imaging
fNIRS	Functional near-infrared spectroscopy
FTD	Frontotemporal dementia

GABA	Gamma-aminobutyric acid
GBD	Global Burden of Disease
GMI	Graded motor imagery
GUI	Graphical user interface
GVS	Galvanic vestibular stimulation
HC	Healthy controls
HD	High definition
HD-tDCS	High-definition transcranial direct current stimulation
HFO	High-frequency oscillation
HHb	Deoxy-hemoglobin
HRV	Heart rate variability
IASP	International Association for the Study of Pain
IBS	Irritable bowel syndrome
IC	Informed consent
ICA	Independent component analysis
ICD	Implantable cardioverter defibrillator
iCNES	Invasive cranial nerve electrical stimulation
ICS	Invasive cortical stimulation
IDE	Investigational device exemption
IF	Integrate-and-fire
IHI	Interhemispheric inhibition
IPG	Internal pulse generator
IS	Interferential stimulation
IVR	Immersive virtual reality
IEC	International Electrotechnical Commission
IPG	Implantable pulse generator
IRB	Institutional review board
JTT	Jebsen Taylor test
KVIQ	Kinesthetic and Visual Imagery Questionnaire
KVIQ10	Kinesthetic and Visual Imagery Questionnaire – short version
LDLPFC	Left dorsolateral prefrontal cortex
LEP	Laser evoked potential
LIF	Leaky integrate-and-fire
LFMS	Low-field magnetic stimulation
LFO	Low-frequency oscillations
LLP	Late positive potential
lLLP	Later part of LLP
LPFC	Lateral prefrontal cortex
LM	Lateromedial
LTD	Long-term depression
LTP	Long-term potentiation
L-VGCC	L-type voltage-gated calcium channel
mBLL	Modified Beer-Lambert law
MC	Monte-Carlo
MCBB	MATRICS Consensus Cognitive Battery

MCI	Mild cognitive impairment
MCS	Motor cortex stimulation
MDD	Medical Devices Directive
MEP	Motor evoked potential
MER	Microelectrode recording
MET	Microcurrent electrical therapy
MFC	Medial-frontal cortex
MHC	Multilayer hydrogel composite
MI	Motor imagery
MIDAS	Migraine Disability Assessment
MIQ	Movement Imagery Questionnaire
MIQ-R	Movement Imagery Questionnaire-Revised
MIQ-RS	Movement Imagery Questionnaire-Revised, Second Edition
MIT	Melodic intonation therapy
MNI	Montreal Neurological Institute
MMN	Mismatch negativity
mPFC	Medial prefrontal cortex
MR	Magnetic resonance
MRC	Medical Research Council
MRI	Magnetic resonance imaging
MRS	Magnetic resonance spectroscopy
MRSI	Magnetic resonance spectroscopic imaging
MS	Multiple sclerosis
MSO	Maximal stimulator output
MST	Magnetic seizure therapy
MUNE	Motor unit number estimation
NAc	Nucleus accumbens
NE	Noradrenergic
NET	Neuroelectric therapy
NFT	Neurofibrillary tangles
NHS	National Health System
NIBS	Noninvasive brain stimulation
NIMH	National Institute of Mental Health
NIR	Near-infrared
NIRS	Near-infrared spectroscopy
NMDA	*N*-Methyl-D-aspartate
NMDAR	*N*-Methyl-D-aspartate receptor
NOS	Nitric oxide synthase
NPS	Neuropathic Pain Scale
NRS	Numerical rating scale
NSAID	Nonsteroidal anti-inflammatory drug
NVC	Neurovascular coupling
NVU	Neurovascular unit
O2Hb	Oxy-hemoglobin
OCD	Obsessive-compulsive disorder

ONS	Optic nerve stimulation
OR	Operating room
OT	Occupational therapy
o-tDCS	Oscillating-tDCS
PA	Prism adaptation
PACU	Postanesthesia care unit
PAG	Periaqueductal grey
PCA	Patient-controlled analgesia
PD	Parkinson's disease
PANSS	Positive and Negative Syndrome Scale
PENS	Percutaneous electrical nerve stimulation
PET	Positron emission tomography
PGE2	Prostaglandin E2
PI	Principal investigator
PLP	Phantom limb pain
PMR	Percutaneous laser myocardial revascularization
PNS	Peripheral nerve stimulation
PNFS	Peripheral nerve field stimulation
PPA	Primary progressive aphasia
PPC	Posterior parietal cortex
POMS	Profile of Mood States
PPF	Paired-pulse facilitation
PROCESS	Prospective Randomized Controlled Multicenter Trial on the Effectiveness of Spinal Cord Stimulation
PSN	Primary sensory neurons
PSP	Post-stroke pain
PSTH	Peristimulus time histogram
PSYRATS	Psychotic Symptom Rating Scales
preSMA	Pre-supplementary motor area
PT	Physical therapy
PVA	Polyvinyl alcohol
PVG	Periventricular grey
RAGT	Robot-assisted gait training
rCBF	Regional cerebral blood flow
RCT	Randomized controlled trial
RF	Radiofrequency
rIFC	Right inferior frontal cortex
rIFG	Right inferior frontal gyrus
RM	Receptor-mediated neurotransmission
ROI	Region of interest
RS	Remotely supervised
rsfMRI	Resting state functional magnetic resonance imaging
RSN	Resting state network
rTMS	Repetitive transcranial magnetic stimulation
Rx	Receivers

S1	Somatosensory
SAI	Short-latency afferent inhibition
SEP	Somatosensory evoked potential
SAE	Serious adverse event
SANS	Scale for the Assessment of Negative Symptoms
SCS	Spinal cord stimulation
SD	Source-detector
SDMT	Symbol Digit Modalities Test
SE	Standard error
SEF	Somatosensory evoked magnetic field
SEM	Standard error of means
SERT	Serotonin reuptake transporter
SFS	Simple finger sequence
SICI	Short-interval intracortical inhibition
SLM	Left superior temporal gyrus
SMA	Supplementary motor area
SNRI	selective norepinephrine reuptake inhibitors
so-tDCS	Slow oscillating-tDCS
SPA	Stimulation-produced analgesia
SPECT	Single photon emission computed tomography
SRT	Simple reaction time
SST	Stop-signal task
SSRI	Selective serotonin reuptake inhibitors
STAR*-D	Sequenced Treatment Alternatives to Relieve Depression
STN	Subthalamic nucleus
SUNCT	Short-lasting unilateral neuralgiform headache with conjunctival injection and tearing
T	Tesla
TD	Time domain
ts-DCS	Transspinal direct current stimulation
TDMI	Time-Dependent Motor Imagery Screening Test
TEM	Treatment-emergent (hypo)mania
TKA	Total knee arthroplasty
TRD	Treatment-resistant depression
tSMS	Transcranial static magnetic stimulation
tACS	Transcranial alternating current stimulation
TBS	Theta burst stimulation
TCES	Transcutaneous cranial electrical stimulation
TCET	Transcerebral electrotherapy
TCMP	Transcranial micropolarization
$tcPO_2$	Transcutaneous oxygen pressure
tDCS	Transcranial direct current stimulation
TEM	Treatment-emergent hypomania/mania
tES	Transcranial electrical stimulation
TENS	Transcutaneous electrical nerve stimulation

TMS	Transcranial magnetic stimulation
TNP	Trigeminal neuropathic pain
TNS	Trigeminal nerve stimulation
tPCS	Transcranial pulsed current stimulation
tRNS	Transcranial random noise stimulation
TSCS	Transcutaneous spinal cord stimulation
TUS	Transcranial ultrasound
Tx	Transmitters
UNODC	United Nations Office on Drugs and Crime
UPDRS	Unified Parkinson's Disease Rating Scale
VAS	Visual Analogue Scale
vmPFC	Ventro-medial prefrontal cortex
VEP	Visual-evoked potential
VDCC	Voltage dependent calcium channel
VGNC	Voltage gated sodium channel
VOI	Volume of interest
VMIQ	Vividness of Movement Imagery Questionnaire
VPM	Ventroposteromedial
VMR	Vasomotor reactivity
VNS	Vagus nerve stimulation
VPL	Ventroposterolateral
VR	Virtual reality
VTA	Ventral tegmental area
WDR	Wide dynamic range
WECS	Within Electrode Current Steering
WHO	World Health Organization
WM	White matter
3D	Three-dimensional
YLD	Years lived with disability

Contents

Part I Basic Aspects: Principles, Mechanisms, Approaches

1 **Transcranial Direct Current Stimulation Among Technologies for Low-Intensity Transcranial Electrical Stimulation: Classification, History, and Terminology** 3
Nigel Gebodh, Zeinab Esmaeilpour, Devin Adair, Pedro Schestattsky, Felipe Fregni, and Marom Bikson

2 **Principles of Transcranial Direct Current Stimulation (tDCS): Introduction to the Biophysics of tDCS** 45
Davide Reato, Ricardo Salvador, Marom Bikson, Alexander Opitz, Jacek Dmochowski, and Pedro C. Miranda

3 **Mechanisms of Acute and After Effects of Transcranial Direct Current Stimulation** 81
Marom Bikson, Walter Paulus, Zeinab Esmaeilpour, Greg Kronberg, and Michael A. Nitsche

4 **Current Methods and Approaches of Noninvasive Direct Current–Based Neuromodulation Techniques** 115
Walter Paulus and Alberto Priori

5 **Transcranial Direct Current Stimulation Modulation of Neurophysiological Functional Outcomes: Neurophysiological Principles and Rationale** 133
Helena Knotkova, Michael A. Nitsche, and Rafael Polania

6 **Safety of Transcranial Direct Current Stimulation** 167
Pnina Grossman, Adam J. Woods, Helena Knotkova, and Marom Bikson

Part II Transcranial Direct Current Stimulation Step-By-Step Practicum

7 Methodological Considerations for Selection of Transcranial Direct Current Stimulation Approach, Protocols and Devices 199
Shapour Jaberzadeh, Donel Martin, Helena Knotkova, and Adam J. Woods

8 Stimulation Parameters and Their Reporting 225
Adam J. Woods, Helena Knotkova, Alexa Riggs, Dennis Q. Truong, and Marom Bikson

9 Role of Computational Modeling for Dose Determination 233
Ricardo Salvador, Dennis Q. Truong, Marom Bikson, Alexander Opitz, Jacek Dmochowski, and Pedro C. Miranda

10 Transcranial Direct Current Stimulation Electrodes 263
Niranjan Khadka, Adam J. Woods, and Marom Bikson

11 Transcranial Direct Current Stimulation Integration with Magnetic Resonance Imaging, Magnetic Resonance Spectroscopy, Near Infrared Spectroscopy Imaging, and Electroencephalography 293
Adam J. Woods, Marom Bikson, Kenneth Chelette, Jacek Dmochowski, Anirban Dutta, Zeinab Esmaeilpour, Nigel Gebodh, Michael A. Nitsche, and Charlotte Stagg

12 Methodological Considerations for Transcranial Direct Current Stimulation in Clinical Trials 347
Roy H. Hamilton, Sudha K. Kessler, Laura Castillo-Saavedra, Felipe Fregni, Donel Martin, Colleen Loo, Helena Knotkova, and Adam J. Woods

13 Home-Based Patient-Delivered Remotely Supervised Transcranial Direct Current Stimulation 379
Helena Knotkova, Ashley Clayton, Michael Stevens, Alexa Riggs, Leigh E. Charvet, and Marom Bikson

14 Transcranial Direct Current Stimulation Ethics and Professional Conduct 407
Andrea Antal, Adam J. Woods, and Helena Knotkova

Part III Clinical Potential and Applications

15 Transcranial Direct Current Stimulation in Psychiatry: Mood Disorders, Schizophrenia and Other Psychiatric Diseases 431
Andre Russowsky Brunoni and Ulrich Palm

16 The Use and Efficacy of Transcranial Direct Current Stimulation in Individuals with Neurodegenerative Dementias 473
Annalise Rahman-Filipiak, Jaclyn M. Reckow, Adam J. Woods, Michael A. Nitsche, and Benjamin M. Hampstead

17 Transcranial Direct Current Stimulation in Stroke Rehabilitation: Present and Future 509
Oluwole O. Awosika and Leonardo G. Cohen

18 Transcranial Direct Current Stimulation Potential for Pain Management 541
Helena Knotkova, Jeffrey J. Borckardt, Alexa Riggs, and Alexandre F. DaSilva

19 Transcranial Direct Current Stimulation in Aging Research 569
Adam J. Woods, Daria Antonenko, Agnes Flöel, Benjamin M. Hampstead, David Clark, and Helena Knotkova

20 Transcranial Direct Current Stimulation in Cognitive Neuroscience 597
Priyanka P. Shah-Basak, Roy H. Hamilton, Michael A. Nitsche, and Adam J. Woods

21 Challenges, Open Questions and Future Direction in Transcranial Direct Current Stimulation Research and Applications 627
Michael A. Nitsche, Helena Knotkova, Adam J. Woods, and Marom Bikson

Index 641

Contributors

Devin Adair, BA The Graduate Center of the City University of New York, Department of Psychology, New York, NY, USA

Andrea Antal, PhD Department of Clinical Neurophysiology, University Medical Center, Georg-August University Göttingen, Göttingen, Germany

Daria Antonenko, MD Department of Neurology, NeuroCure Clinical Research Center, Charité – Universitätsmedizin, Berlin, Germany

Oluwole O. Awosika, MD Human Cortical Physiology and Stroke Neurorehabilitation Section, National Institutes of Health, Bethesda, MD, USA

Department of Neurology and Rehabilitation Medicine, University of Cincinnati College of Medicine, Cincinnati, OH, USA

Marom Bikson, PhD Department of Biomedical Engineering, The City College of New York, New York, NY, USA

Jeffrey J. Borckardt, PhD Departments of Psychiatry, Anesthesia, and Stomatology, Medical University of South Carolina, Charleston, SC, USA

Andre Russowsky Brunoni, HC-FMUSP Service of Interdisciplinary Neuromodulation, Laboratory of Neurosciences (LIM-27), Department and Institute of Psychiatry, University of São Paulo, São Paulo, Brazil

Department of Psychiatry and Psychotherapy, Ludwig-Maximilian University Munich, Munich, Germany

Laura Castillo-Saavedra, MD Spaulding Neuromodulation Center, Department of Physical Medicine and Rehabilitation, Spaulding Rehabilitation Hospital, Harvard Medical School, Boston, MA, USA

Leigh E. Charvet, PhD Department of Neurology, New York University Langone Medical Center, New York, NY, USA

Kenneth Chelette ANT Neuro North America, Philadelphia, PA, USA

David Clark, ScD Department of Aging and Geriatric Research, Brain Rehabilitation Research Center, Malcom Randall VA Medical Center, Gainesville, FL, USA

Vincent P. Clark, PhD University of New Mexico, Mind Research Network, Albuquerque, NM, USA

Ashley Clayton, MA Department of Neurology, New York University Langone Medical Center, New York, NY, USA

Leonardo G. Cohen, MD Human Cortical Physiology and Stroke Neurorehabilitation Section, National Institutes of Health, Bethesda, MD, USA

Alexandre F. DaSilva, DDS, DMedSc The Molecular & Behavioral Neuroscience Institute (MBNI), Ann Arbor, MI, USA

Biologic & Materials Sciences, School of Dentistry, Ann Arbor, MI, USA

Jacek Dmochowski, PhD Neural Engineering Laboratory, Department of Biomedical Engineering, Grove School of Engineering, The City College of the City University of New York, New York, NY, USA

Anirban Dutta, PhD Neuroengineering and Informatics for Rehabilitation Laboratory, Jacobs School of Medicine & Biomedical Sciences, Department of Biomedical Engineering, University at Buffalo SUNY, Buffalo, NY, USA

Zeinab Esmaeilpour, MS Department of Biomedical Engineering, The City College of the City University of New York, New York, NY, USA

Agnes Flöel, MD Department of Neurology, University Medical Hospital Greifswald, Greifswald, Germany

Felipe Fregni, MD, PhD, MPH, MMSc, ME Spaulding Neuromodulation Center, Department of Physical Medicine and Rehabilitation, Spaulding Rehabilitation Hospital, Harvard Medical School, Boston, MA, USA

Nigel Gebodh, MS, BE Department of Biomedical Engineering, The City College of the City University of New York, New York, NY, USA

Pnina Grossman Department of Biomedical Engineering, The City College of the City University of New York, Grove School of Engineering, New York, NY, USA

Roy H. Hamilton, MD, MS Department of Neurology, University of Pennsylvania, Philadelphia, PA, USA

Department of Physical Medicine and Rehabilitation, University of Pennsylvania, Philadelphia, PA, USA

Goddard Laboratories, Room 518, University of Pennsylvania, Philadelphia, PA, USA

Benjamin M. Hampstead, PhD Department of Mental Health Services, Veterans Affairs Ann Arbor Healthcare Systems, Ann Arbor, MI, USA

Department of Psychiatry, University of Michigan, Ann Arbor, MI, USA

Shapour Jaberzadeh, PhD Department of Physiotherapy, School of Primary Health Care, Faculty of Medicine Nursing and Health Sciences, Monash University, Melbourne, Australia

Sudha K. Kessler, MD, MSCE Departments of Neurology and Pediatrics, Perelman School of Medicine at the University of Pennsylvania, Philadelphia, PA, USA

Children's Hospital of Philadelphia, Philadelphia, PA, USA

Niranjan Khadka Department of Biomedical Engineering, The City College of New York, CUNY, City College Center for Discovery and Innovation, New York, NY, USA

Helena Knotkova, PhD MJHS Institute for Innovation in Palliative Care, New York, NY, USA

Department of Family and Social Medicine, Albert Einstein College of Medicine, Bronx, NY, USA

Greg Kronberg, MS Department of Biomedical Engineering, The City College of the City University of New York, New York, NY, USA

Colleen Loo, MD School of Psychiatry, Black Dog Institute, The University of New South Wales, Sydney, NSW, Australia

Donel Martin, PhD, MClinNeuro Black Dog Institute, The University of New South Wales, Sydney, NSW, Australia

Pedro C. Miranda, PhD Instituto de Biofisica e Engenharia Biomedica, Faculdade de Ciencias, Universidade de Lisboa, Lisbon, Portugal

Michael A. Nitsche, MD Department of Psychology and Neurosciences, Leibniz Research Centre for Working Environment and Human Factors, Dortmund, Germany

University Medical Hospital Bergmannsheil, Bochum, Germany

Alexander Opitz, PhD Department of Biomedical Engineering, University of Minnesota, Minneapolis, MN, USA

Ulrich Palm, MD Department of Psychiatry and Psychotherapy, Ludwig-Maximilian University Munich, Munich, Germany

Walter Paulus, MD Department of Clinical Neurophysiology, University Medical Center Göttingen, Göttingen, Germany

Rafael Polania, PhD ETH Zurich, Decision Neuroscience Lab, Department of Health Sciences and Technology, Zurich, Switzerland

Alberto Priori, MD, PhD "Aldo Ravelli" Research Center for Neurotechnology and Experimental Brain Therapeutics, University of Milan Medical School, Milan, Italy

Annalise Rahman-Filipiak, PhD Department of Mental Health Services, Veterans Affairs Ann Arbor Healthcare Systems, Ann Arbor, MI, USA

Department of Psychiatry, University of Michigan, Ann Arbor, MI, USA

Davide Reato, PhD Champalimaud Centre for the Unknown, Neuroscience Programme, Lisbon, Portugal

Jaclyn M. Reckow, PhD Department of Mental Health Services, Veterans Affairs Ann Arbor Healthcare Systems, Ann Arbor, MI, USA

Department of Psychiatry, University of Michigan, Ann Arbor, MI, USA

Alexa Riggs, MPH MJHS Institute for Innovation in Palliative Care, New York, NY, USA

Ricardo Salvador, PhD Neuroelectrics, Barcelona, Spain

Pedro Schestattsky, PhD Neurology Service, Hospital de Clínicas de Porto Alegre, Department of Internal Medicine, UFRGS, Porto Alegre, Brazil

Hospital Moinhos de Vento, Porto Alegre, Brazil

Priyanka P. Shah-Basak, PhD Rotman Research Institute, Baycrest Health Sciences, Toronto, ON, Canada

Charlotte Stagg, MRCP DPhil Oxford Centre for fMRI of the Brain, Nuffield Department of Clinical Neurosciences, University of Oxford, Oxford, UK

Oxford Centre for Human Brain Activity, Department of Psychiatry, University of Oxford, Oxford, UK

Michael Stevens, PhD Department of Psychiatry, Yale University School of Medicine, New Haven, CT, USA

Dennis Q. Truong, MS Department of Biomedical Engineering, The City College of the City University of New York, New York, NY, USA

Adam J. Woods, PhD Center for Cognitive Aging and Memory (CAM), McKnight Brain Institute, Department of Clinical and Health Psychology, College of Public Health and Health Professions, University of Florida, Gainesville, FL, USA

Part I
Basic Aspects: Principles, Mechanisms, Approaches

Chapter 1
Transcranial Direct Current Stimulation Among Technologies for Low-Intensity Transcranial Electrical Stimulation: Classification, History, and Terminology

Nigel Gebodh, Zeinab Esmaeilpour, Devin Adair, Pedro Schestattsky, Felipe Fregni, and Marom Bikson

Classification of tDCS Among Other Brain Stimulation Techniques

Classification of tDCS Among Techniques

The field of brain stimulation dates to the discovery of electrical phenomena, which is not surprising given that human and animal responses to electrical shock are among the earliest evidence for the existence of electricity (Bischoff 1801; Galvani and Aldini 1792; Volta 1800). Research and human trials on electrical brain stimulation, and underling bioelectric phenomena, has been continuous. Modern brain stimulation as a field has branched and evolved into many different categories of devices and tech-

N. Gebodh · Z. Esmaeilpour
Department of Biomedical Engineering, The City College of the City University of New York, New York, NY, USA

D. Adair
The Graduate Center of the City University of New York, Department of Psychology, New York, NY, USA

P. Schestattsky
Neurology Service, Hospital de Clínicas de Porto Alegre, Department of Internal Medicine, UFRGS, Porto Alegre, Brazil

Hospital Moinhos de Vento, Porto Alegre, Brazil

F. Fregni
Spaulding Neuromodulation Center, Department of Physical Medicine and Rehabilitation, Spaulding Rehabilitation Hospital, Harvard Medical School, Boston, MA, USA

M. Bikson (✉)
Department of Biomedical Engineering, The City College of New York, New York, NY, USA
e-mail: bikson@ccny.cuny.edu

H. Knotkova et al. (eds.), *Practical Guide to Transcranial Direct Current Stimulation*, https://doi.org/10.1007/978-3-319-95948-1_1

niques, but whose commonality remains to alter brain or specific nervous system functions by introducing electrical currents through electricity or magnetism. The contemporary landscape of stimulation techniques covers a vast expanse of applications and nomenclatures, many with overlapping aspects. An introduction to tDCS should therefore place it among this landscape of brain stimulation techniques. This includes presenting a simplified mapping and categorization of selected historical and contemporary stimulation techniques and showing how they are categorically interrelated. This by no means should be taken as a complete assortment of stimulation techniques (Guleyupoglu et al. 2013), but rather to clarify the unique features and historical role of tDCS in modern neuromodulation.

When it comes to the categorizing methods of stimulation, several different approaches can be taken. A first simple arrangement is to group stimulation methods into invasive and non-invasive procedures (Fig. 1.1). At this level of division, the obvious distinction lies in the placement of stimulating electrodes. Invasive brain stimulation techniques involve patients undergoing anesthesia or receiving analgesics and having stimulating electrodes surgical implanted in specified regions of the brain, spinal cord, subcutaneously, or around nerves. These implanted electrodes are then activated and used to deliver electrical stimulation to specific regions of the brain, the spinal cord, or specific nerves. Primary stimulation targets are considered local and adjacent to implanted electrodes (McIntyre et al. 2004). Non-invasive techniques, on the other hand, involves the external placement of electrodes (or magnetic coils) without breaking the skin or entering the body cavity, and do not require surgical procedures for application. These noninvasive electrodes or stimulation apparatuses are placed on areas like the scalp, forehead, or shoulders, though which electricity or magnetism is then delivered. Regions that are influenced by stimulation depend on both the electrode montage and individual anatomy (Dmochowski et al. 2011).

Both invasive and noninvasive categorizations can be further divided into techniques intended to either stimulate the brain (transcranial or intracranial) and those techniques targeting extra-cranial structures (non-transcranial or non-intracranial). For non-invasive brain stimulation (NIBS), transcranial encompasses stimulation techniques that intend to pass electricity, magnetism, or sound through the skull and have specific sub-cranial brain (cortical) targets, whereas non-transcranial encompasses delivering current to extra-cranial targets and thus having non-cortical targets. For invasive brain stimulation (IBS), intracranial techniques include deep brain stimulation (DBS), which targets but is not exclusive to specific limbic, basal ganglia, and thalamic brain areas. Non-intracranial IBS techniques include implants such spinal cord stimulation (SCS) – used to treat chronic pain – (Cameron 2004) and direct peripheral nerve stimulation (DPNS) that involves the implantation of an electrode on a nerve (Oh et al. 2004). Other examples of non-intracranial IBS techniques include invasive cranial nerve electrical stimulation (iCNES) techniques. Some iCNES techniques include vestibular prostheses (VP; Golub et al. 2014); optic nerve stimulation (ONS), used for the restoration of vision (Brelen et al. 2010); vagus nerve stimulation (VNS), first approved by the FDA to treat epilepsy (Beekwilder and Beems 2010); and direct trigeminal nerve stimulation (DTNS), which involves implanting electrode cuffs or arrays directly on a nerve (Slavin et al. 2006). In terms

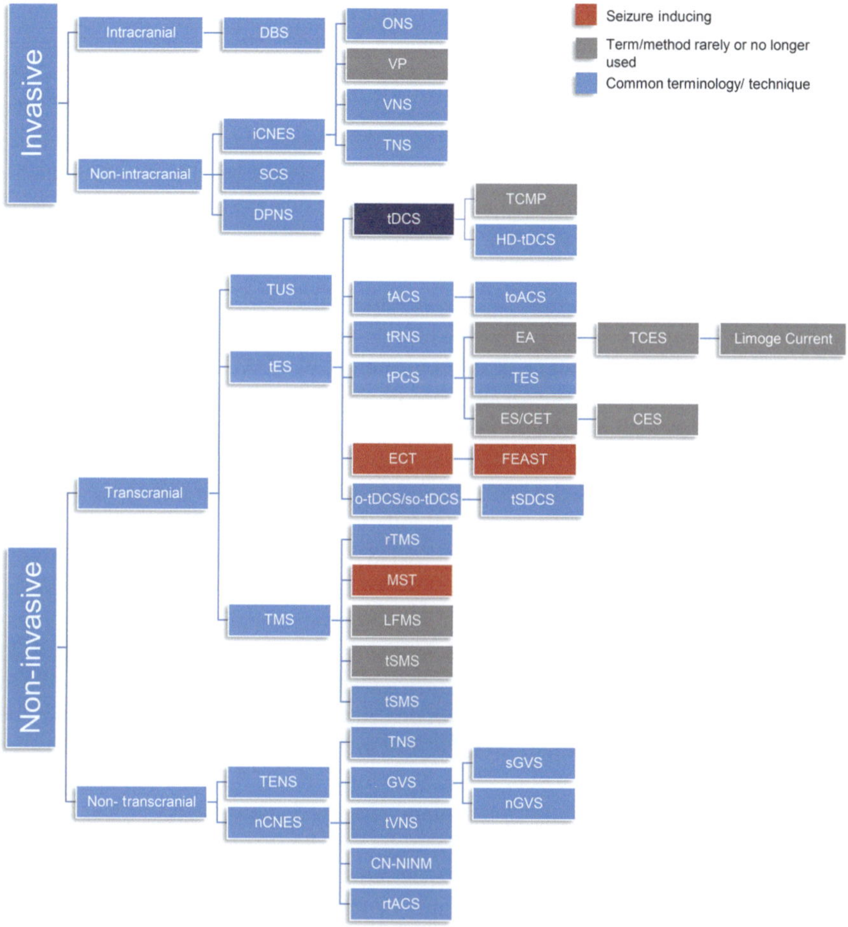

Fig. 1.1 Arrangement of stimulation techniques with common terminology (light blue), terms and methods that are rarely or no longer used (gray), and highlights of seizure-inducing techniques (red). tDCS is highlighted (dark blue) to show its place among the selected techniques

of noninvasive brain stimulation (NIBS) that targets sub-cranial regions, techniques can involve the use of electrical stimulation through electrodes on the scalp, magnetic stimulation with a coil near the scalp, or stimulation with ultrasonic sound through an ultrasound transducer placed on the scalp. Thus, NIBS with transcranial targets is divided into the broad categories of transcranial magnetic stimulation (TMS), transcranial electrical stimulation (tES), and the emerging field of transcranial ultrasound (TUS) modulation (Fig. 1.1; Legon et al. 2014).

Non-transcranial electrical stimulation techniques include transcutaneous electrical nerve stimulation (TENS; Robertson et al. 2006), and noninvasive cranial nerve electrical stimulation (nCNES); both of which utilize electrical currents to stimulate nerves. TENS targets all peripheral nerves, whereas nCNES techniques specifically target cranial nerves. nCNES can be subdivided into repetitive transorbital alternative current stimulation (rtACS; Gall et al. 2010; Bola et al. 2014), trigeminal nerve stimulation (TNS; DeGiorgio et al. 2011; Schoenen et al. 2013), galvanic vestibular stimulation (GVS; Fitzpatrick and Day 2004), transcutaneous vagus nerve stimulation (tVNS; Frangos et al. 2015; Hein et al. 2013; Kraus et al. 2013), and cranial nerve noninvasive neuromodulation (CN-NINM; Danilov et al. 2014). As the name implies, GVS is historically applied using direct current, however with different vestibular targets emerging, the technique has expanded to include stochastic/noisy GVS (Samoudi et al. 2012; Yamamoto et al. 2005) and sinusoidal GVS (Coats 1972).

TMS techniques' main distinction from tES is the use magnetic coils to induce electrical current in the brain (George and Aston-Jones 2010). TMS can be sub-categorized to include repetitive TMS (rTMS; Lefaucheur et al. 2014), seizure-inducing magnetic seizure therapy (MST; Kayser et al. 2015; Lisanby et al. 2003), and the relatively new transcranial static magnetic stimulation (tSMS; Gonzalez-Rosa et al. 2015) and low-field magnetic stimulation (LFMS; Rohan et al. 2004).

Transcranial electrical stimulation approaches pass electrical current directly to the brain via electrodes on the head (Paulus et al. 2013). These techniques include tDCS, transcranial alternating current stimulation (tACS; Antal and Paulus 2013), transcranial random noise stimulation (tRNS; Terney et al. 2008), transcranial pulsed current stimulation (tPCS; Morales-Quezada et al. 2015; Fitzgerald 2014), oscillating tDCS (o-tDCS D'Atri et al. 2015) or sinusoidal oscillating tDCS (so-tDCS; Eggert et al. 2013), and seizure-inducing electroconvulsive therapy (ECT) with the subset, focal electrically administered seizure therapy (FEAST; Spellman et al. 2009). The o-tDCS /so-tdcs technique can further be broken down to include transcranial sinusoidal stimulation (tSDCS). On the other hand, tPCS can be further broken down into "TES", a supra threshold form of tPCS (Kalkman et al. 1992; Zentner et al. 1989); transcutaneous cranial electrical stimulation (TCES; Limoge et al. 1999), a derivative of electroanesthesia (EA; Smith et al. 1967; Wilson et al. 1968) which can include high frequency currents (Limoge et al. 1999); and cranial electrotherapy stimulation (CES; Schmitt et al. 1986), which was derived from electrosleep (ES; Dimitrov and Ralev 2015) and later called cranial electrostimulation therapy (CET; Knutson et al. 1956). Though ECT can also involve the use of pulsed waveforms, it involves unique stimulation schemes, and is not a tPCS sub-category here.

tDCS, like other techniques, is associated with derivative nomenclature and variants. These variants are rooted in the same principles of tDCS (delivering direct current across the head); however, they both take different approaches to how direct current is delivered. For instance, High Definition-tDCS (HD-tDCS) aims to focalize current distribution across the brain so that specific regions are better targeted. There are numerous montage variations of HD-tDCS (Borckardt et al. 2012; Dmochowski et al. 2011; Kuo et al. 2013; Nikolin et al. 2015) including the most common 4 × 1 HD-tDCS montage (Alam et al. 2016; Datta et al. 2009; Hill et al. 2017; Shekhawat et al. 2015; Shen et al. 2016). Another tDCS derivative is transcranial micropolarization (TCMP), which aims to deliver current intensities (700–1000 μA) on that are much less than conventional tDCS (Ilyukhina et al. 2005; Shelyakin et al. 1998). Other terminology associated with tDCS exists, such as "anodal/cathodal tDCS" or "lateralized" montages, however these are descriptive of the intended outcome of stimulation and not necessarily distinct technique categories (see below).

The fundamental distinction between tDCS and other categorizations of tES is the waveform delivered to the brain during stimulation (Fig. 1.2). tDCS is the only class of neuromodulation technique that delivers a sustained direct current (DC). Almost all other techniques (and essentially all invasive and magnetic techniques) use pulsed stimulation (such as tPCS) while other non-invasive variants include AC waveforms (such as tACS) or random noise (such as tRNS). Thus, the use of a sustained direct current is a characteristic feature of tDCS, and one that should be kept in mind when considering any unique neurophysiologic, cognitive, or behavioral outcomes.

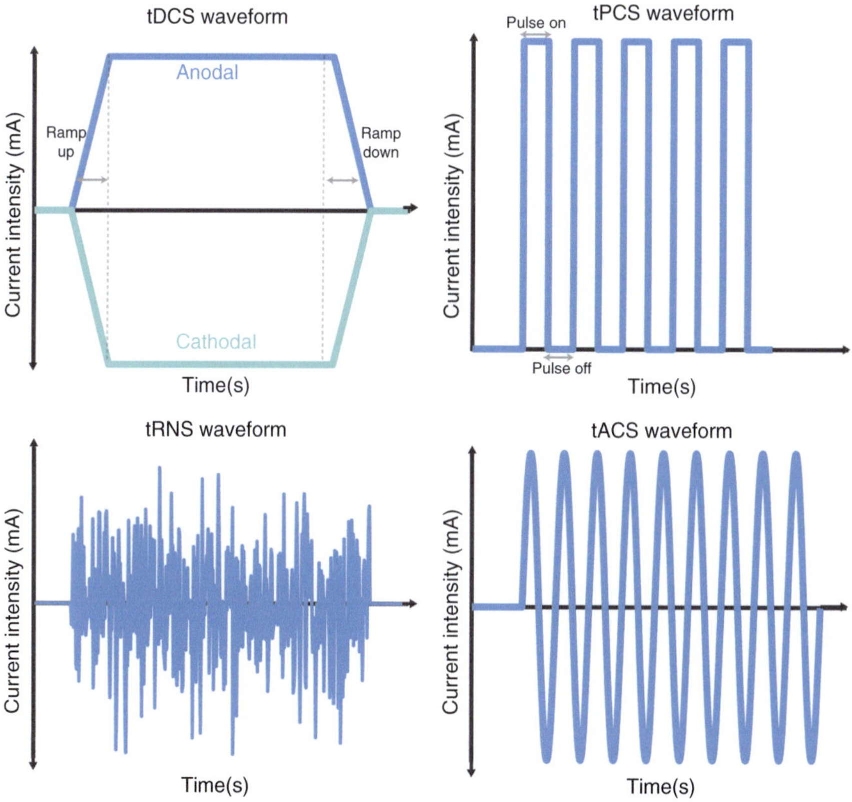

Fig. 1.2 Waveforms of different tES techniques. The tDCS waveform is shown for anodal (blue) and cathodal (light blue) electrodes, which must always be active concurrently. Typically, the current is increased to or ramped up to the desired current intensity and when said intensity is reached the current intensity is held at that level for the duration of stimulation. The tACS waveform shows a typical oscillatory current delivery between electrodes. The tRNS waveform shows a generalized random noise current intensity being delivered during stimulation. The tPCS waveform shows a generalized pulse train of current. Here the duration of pulse on and pulse off time can vary depending on the type of tPCS being done

The Case for Simplicity of tDCS

Direct current represents the most simplistic waveform – though this does not preclude tDCS from producing unique and profound neuromodulatory effects that arise from a sustained current. Nonetheless, regarding the development and adoption of tDCS, we propose that this simplicity underpins the unique role of tDCS in the emergence of modern non-invasive neuromodulation and its grounding in science. Decades of modern work have firmly established that direct current stimulation (DCS) changes neuronal excitability and plasticity. To explain the unique role of tDCS in modern neuromodulation, some historical context is necessary.

Direct current was the first form of brain stimulation generated using a device (as opposed to electric fish or static electricity) since it was the simplest to build – connecting a "voltaic pile" (early battery) to the body. Thus, this approach was the earliest example of electrical stimulation in humans and animals (leading to early theories of the role of electricity in physiology). Later, the first demonstration of long term potentiation was made using direct current (Bindman et al. 1964; Gartside 1968; Gartside and Lippold 1967), preceding the well cited studies of Bliss and Lomo (1973). Monophasic pulse stimulation later integrated mechanical methods to rapidly connect and disconnect the DC battery.

The emergence of other stimulation waveforms (e.g. complex pulsed patterns) paralleled development in electronics (Guleyupoglu et al. 2013). For example, the emergence of the microcontroller allowed for the generation of any arbitrary waveform. Enabled by this flexibility, the twentieth century saw the emergence of numerous variations in waveforms, most of which were claimed to be unique and proprietary. The purported uniqueness facilitated marketing of devices but also resulted in reduced transparency of performance. For example, at the end of the twentieth century, devices FDA-cleared for CES each promised a unique waveform (Fig. 1.3). In a sense this uniqueness (exclusivity) impeded clinical research which benefits from uniformity across labs (reproducibility) and transparency. At the turn of the century though, even career researchers in neuromodulation often could not explain the difference in nomenclature (e.g. does electro-sleep use direct current? is CES and CET the same? Guleyupoglu et al. 2013).

In this context, the early work on tDCS that emerged circa 2000 was characterized by (1) high transparency in a simple and reproducible waveform (e.g. 1 mA sustained for 10 min); and (2) a foundation based, not on clinical experience, but on neurophysiological data (e.g. modulation of TMS evoked responses; Fig. 1.4). These two fundamental characteristics, followed by dozens of rigorous human neurophysiology trials (including multiple independent replications) and animal electrophysiology (steming from our own group; Bikson et al. 2004) established the scientific foundation of tDCS. Work on tDCS, in turn, supported a new era in modern NIBS research. For example, modern tACS approaches mimicked tDCS montages, similarly used a basic and well-defined waveform (single sinusoid), and identical neurophysiology markers of response prior to clinical trials. Clinical trials that used tDCS (starting from our group; Fregni 2005; Fregni et al. 2006b) were

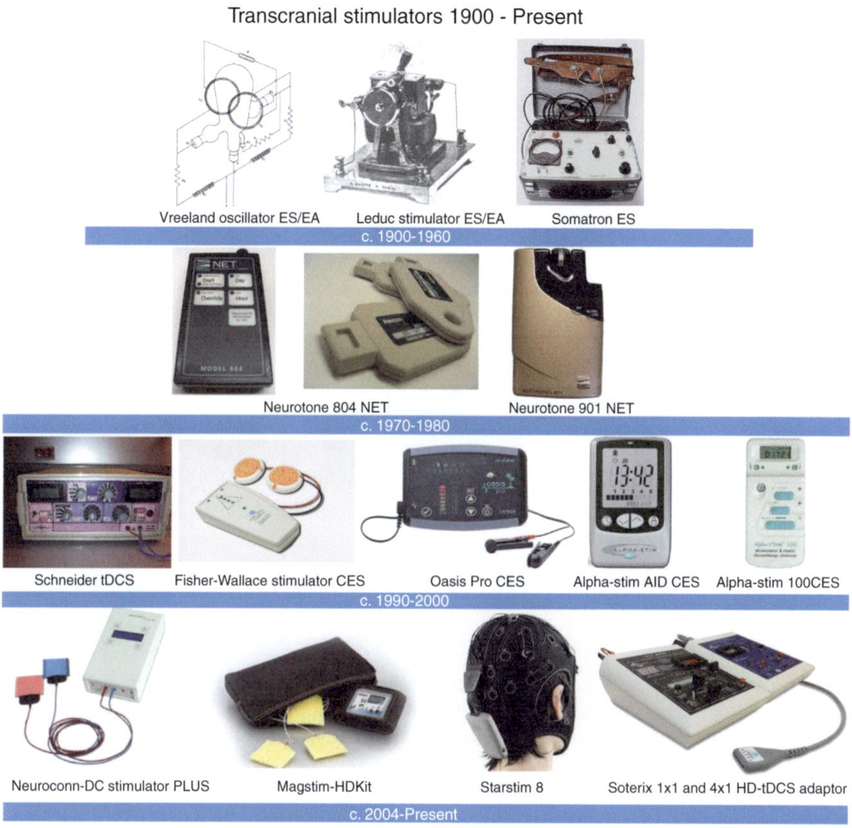

Fig. 1.3 The evolution of transcranial stimulators spanning 1900 to present day. Early ES/EA devices were developed between 1900 and 1960. These early devices were followed NeuroElectric Therapy (NET) devices between 1970 and 1980. Later more established tDCS, tACS, and iontophoresis devices were developed, some of which are still used today. During the early aughts, more advanced and modern stimulation techniques were developed starting from 2004 to present day

rationalized based on these human and animal neurophysiology studies. In the past 15 years, hundreds of studies on tDCS mechanisms have shown that the effects of tDCS are – not surprisingly – more complex than initially hypothesized. But this ongoing work should be understood as building on the broad scientific base of tDCS, rather than somehow challenging it. In this regard, work on tDCS mechanisms continues to be a touching stone for other neuromodulation techniques (Brunoni et al. 2012b; Fertonani and Miniussi 2016; Giordano et al. 2017; Jackson et al. 2016; Paulus et al. 2013).

An unintended consequence of the perceived "simplicity" of tDCS is that new groups adopting the technique may assume that precision and careful control in technology, training, and protocols is not critical for rigor. In fact, reproducibility requires the selection of only appropriate equipment and accessories, certification

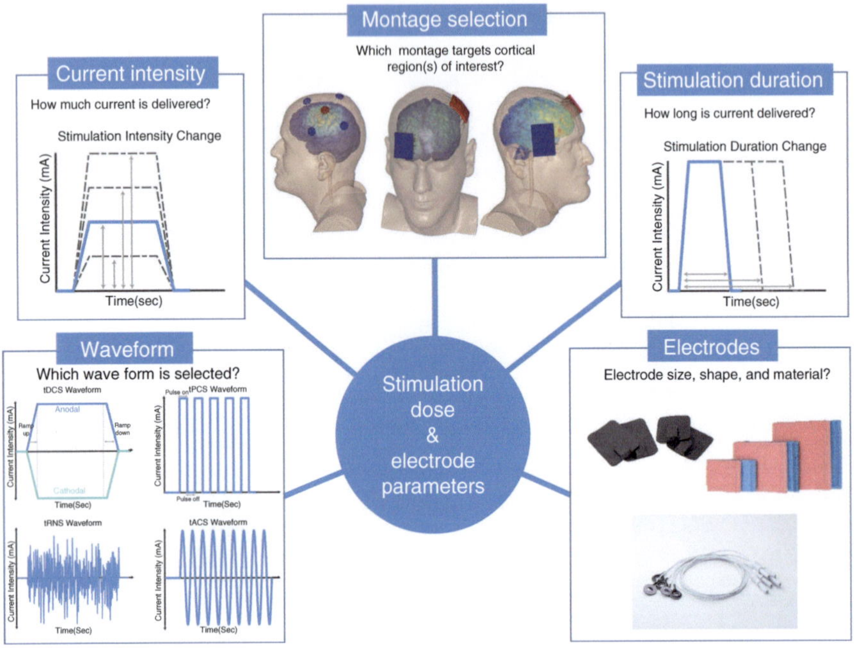

Fig. 1.4 Stimulation dose and electrode parameters include the selection of the stimulation waveform, the current intensity, the montage, stimulation duration, and electrodes. With waveform selection several different waves can be selected, ranging from a direct current waveform to alternating current, pulsed current, or random noise current. In the case of intensity, the amount of current to be delivered is defined. With montage, the placement of electrodes on the scalp are selected. In the case of duration, the amount of time that current is introduced to the body is defined. With electrodes, the size and type of electrodes are selected. Each parameter is an essential part to defining and reporting dose in tES

of staff on experimental equipment, and adherence to well established protocols (Woods et al. 2016). Failure to do so leads to variable and potentially inconsequential results that have little or no relevance to the tDCS field.

tDCS Terminology Including Components and Stimulation Parameters

The broad landscape of stimulation approaches – in many cases with subtle variations in waveform – make the need for standardized nomenclature critical. Such standardization help to foster proper understanding of tDCS techniques, aid in clinical trial development, break down the barrier to adoption, and encourage higher scientific validation. Better understanding and definitive nomenclature would in turn allow patients and healthcare providers to make improved and informed decisions when it comes to various tDCS technique options. Here, we present some key terminology used in the tDCS literature, and as relevant, broader tES terms which help position (distinguish) tDCS.

Our approach was to define terms as used conventionally in the tDCS field – and we do not propose new or altered terminology. Nonetheless, inconsistent, and at times confusing use of terminology, required us to constrain definitions. In defining tDCS itself there is a compromise between broad definitions – which allows for needed dose exploration and optimization such as higher currents – and more restrictive definitions that create the least possible ambiguity – such as limited current levels that have been extensively tested. In our approach, we adopted broader definitions, even including dose ranges yet to be tested, while also defining "conventional" practices that are limited to the most common conventions. This approach to taxonomy is intended neither to imply safety nor efficacy.

We note that following conventions of use in the field, tES classifications are not simply literal – meaning a classification is rarely the literal amalgamation of each word in the technique name. Rather, the classifications provided here are proper names. Compared to a definition based strictly on semantics, tES classifications are typically more restrictive based on both dose and intent. The use of lower case "t" emphasizes classifications are proper names.

Dose

The classification of a brain stimulation technique is itself based on the definition of dose. Following the method of Peterchev et al. (2012), tES dose is defined "by all parameters of the stimulation device that affect the electromagnetic field generated in the body." Dose thus includes stimulation waveform (e.g. AC/DC), intensity, and duration; as well as the number of electrodes and their shape (Peterchev et al. 2012).

Each class classification of tES (e.g. tDCS, tACS, CES) is restricted in part by dose and intended outcomes. For example, tDCS is understood to be a modulatory technique which may exclude approaches intended to directly induce neuronal firing. While dose is defined by describing *all* relevant parameters of stimulation (Fig. 1.5), classification may relate to only a selection of these parameters (i.e. tDCS is defined by the waveform irrespective of electrode montage). We emphasize, the classification of a study does not reduce the need to fully report the complete dose applied to allow interpretation and reproduction of methods (Peterchev et al. 2012). Every tDCS trial must fully document dose. The method used to select the dose (e.g. subject titration, prior experience) and summary metrics (e.g. electrode current density or total charge) are important, but does not diminish the need to fully report the final dose applied.

Furthermore, though not always part of "dose", complete details of the electrode assembly including electrode material, coupling medium, electrode size (area), electrode thickness, and any relevant details on electrode age/prior-use must be

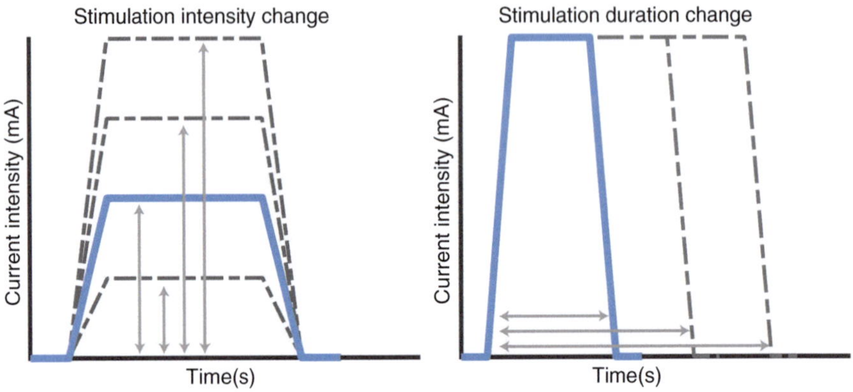

Fig. 1.5 Stimulation intensity changes alters the amount of current that is delivered. Current intesites in tDCS can range from (but are not limited to) 0.5–2 mA. Stimulation duration changes alteres the time over which current is delivered. With tDCS current delivery times can range from (but are not limited to) 10–30 min, with ramp up and ramp down times between 10 and 30 s

provided or referenced for reproducibility. To this end, our definition attempts to disambiguate how terms of tDCS technology are used and defined.

tES

The term *transcranial electrical stimulation* (tES) is the preferred nomenclature for any non-invasive medical device intended to directly change brain function by passing low- or high-amplitude electrical currents, of any waveform, through at least one electrode on the scalp.

Though variants of tES as a global classification have been proposed, a review of relevant historical (Guleyupoglu et al. 2013) and modern literature confirms tES is the most conventional terminology. Non-Invasive brain electrical stimulation and transcranial current stimulation (first used in only 2008; Datta et al. 2008) are comparatively rare. Upper-case first letter “TES” is not preferred because of association with supra-threshold single pulse waveforms (Merton and Morton 1980).

The intended outcome of tES includes direct actions on the central nervous system (even if peripheral actions such a cranial nerve stimulation, peripheral vascular and muscle actions, etc. cannot be excluded). Specific intended outcomes often appear in definitions of tES classifications. Devices that use any implanted electrodes, including intracranial or subcutaneous, should not be included in tES – regardless of whether such techniques result in current passage across the cranium.

Non-invasive medical procedures are typically defined as not breaking the skin or entering the body cavity. Non-invasive medical devices do not involve an invasive medical procedure. tES is thus non-invasive. While the current delivered by tES crosses into the body and produces physiologic responses (including changing skin properties), this does not meet the standard for an invasive medical procedure/device, any more than a stone used for massage (which transfers physical force into the body) or a heating blanket (transferring heat into the body).

Session

A session of tDCS refers to a set program of stimulation, provided over a limited (fixed) time. Repetitive, when used in the context of tDCS, typically refers to multiple sessions.

tDCS

Transcranial direct current stimulation (tDCS) is a tES technique in which the dose waveform is a sustained direct current (DC) applied to the head (at least one cephalic electrode) to produce a direct change in brain function. The intensity of tDCS is limited with the intention of modulating excitability and/or ongoing activity rather than triggering action potentials (as the brain is active, tDCS will change the ongoing firing rate of neurons; Reato et al. 2013). The sustained waveform of tDCS reflects this intention. Thus, our definition of tDCS includes both a dose component (specifically a waveform characterized by a sustained current) and the intended mechanisms of action (specifically sustained polarization and neuromodulation).

Conventional tDCS

Conventional tDCS would include protocols (e.g. waveform intensities and durations) that are commonly used in current human and clinical exploratory studies, as well as formal trials. Conventional current intensities span 0.1 (used often in sham) to 3.0 mA; with most efforts between 1.0 and 2.5 mA (Fig. 1.6). Conventional durations span 4 s (used only for transient changes; Nitsche and Paulus 2000) to several minutes (typically 10–40 used for durable changes; Ohn et al. 2008). However, tDCS intensity and current is not restricted per our general definition above. Conventional intensities are limited to a few milliamps relating to tolerability of skin using existing electrode technologies (Minhas et al. 2010). Stimulation is applied over skin which is not compromised by a pre-existing burn or injury (e.g. open wound) and is thus largely homogenous. However, acne or non-injurious spots are typically not exclusions for electrode placement locations. Skin preparation typically excludes significant abrasion (intend to remove epidermis; Shiozawa et al. 2013), though cleaning of the skin/hair with saline or alcohol is sometimes used

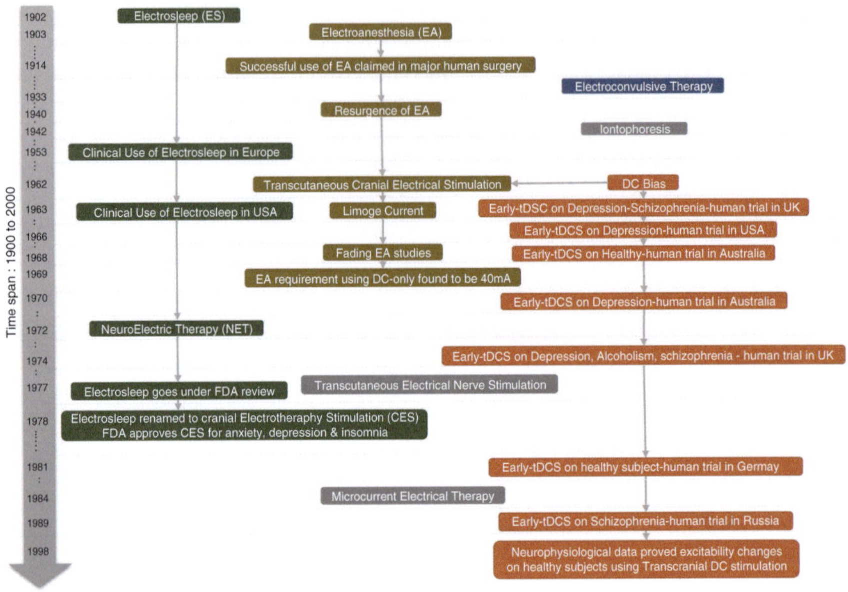

Fig. 1.6 A brief history of tES stimulation spanning 1902 to 1998. Cranial stimulation methods used in twentieth century are categorized in five lines including methods with direct current

(DaSilva et al. 2011). Any advancement in the development of electrodes used for conventional tDCS may permit current amplitudes to exceed 3 mA, assuming improvements in skin tolerability, which in turn would expand intensity limits for conventional tDCS with potential impacts on outcomes. In any given session, conventional tDCS uses a single current amplitude with minimal variation during stimulation, except for one ramp up and ramp down period (typically a 10–30 s linear ramp).

Conventional tDCS uses electrode assemblies of 5 × 5 cm to 5 × 7 cm to interface with skin-electrolyte contact areas, though both smaller and larger electrode assemblies have been explored (Nitsche et al. 2007). Conventional tDCS electrode assemblies use either a metal or conductive rubber electrodes (Kronberg and Bikson 2012). Electrolytes or more commonly isotonic saline (saturated in a sponge) gels and/or creams have also been used. The details of electrode assembly (see definition) design is considered important for tolerability. Conventional tDCS commonly uses two electrodes, though three or four electrode montages are conceivable. tDCS limits on the number of electrodes is related to the conventional size of electrodes, since using larger electrodes limits the number that can be positioned on the scalp (see also HD-tDCS).

A single tDCS session is defined as the period from initiation of current flow (start of ramp up) to end of current flow (end of ramp down). However, conventionally the "duration" of a tDCS session is exclusive of the ramp up or ramp down period and thus refers to the period when tDCS is sustained at the target current (e.g. 2 mA).

tDCS must involve at least one electrode on the scalp. The anode is defined as any electrode where current (positive charge) enters the body and the cathode is defined as any electrode where the current (positive charge) exits the body. tDCS must have at least one anode and at least one cathode.

Anode/Cathode

The anode (also called Anode Electrode) is the electrode where positive current enters the body. For two electrodes in tDCS, the anode has a positive voltage relative to the cathode. The cathode (also called Cathode Electrode) is the electrode from which positive current exits the body.

In other approaches, such as tACS, when the current controlled waveform is applied to any given electrode, changes polarity of each electrode is seen (e.g., a biphasic sinusoid applied such that the current direction to any given electrode changes in direction) where the electrodes switch from being an anode to a cathode during stimulation based on the frequency of stimulation. For this reason, an "anode" is not used in biphasic stimulation. However, for tDCS as defined here, polarity should not change within a session and so electrodes that are the anode and the cathode remain fixed as such.

"Anodal-tDCS" (a-tDCS), "Cathodal-tDCS" (c-tDCS)

While semantically transcranial direct current stimulation could include any waveform that does not change polarity (e.g. even a monophasic triangle wave), tDCS as used across current human trials involves only sustained direct current. The lower-case "t" in tDCS is thus important to emphasize a proper name. As tDCS dose is defined as a waveform of a sustained direct current, only the intensity (in milliamps), duration (in seconds or minutes), and ramp up/down details, are needed to specify the waveform to each electrode. Fundamentally, the mechanisms of tDCS are speculated to derive from the sustained polarization of neuronal assemblies (Bikson et al. 2004; Bindman et al. 1964; Nitsche and Paulus 2000), which in turn results from sustained current delivery. Use of waveforms that are speculated to produce physiologic changes – even in part – based on the change in current, are thus not strictly tDCS as defined here. Hence trains of monophasic pulses are not tDCS as defined here, rather they are classified as tPCS, even when a DC offset is included. Similarly, an oscillating transcranial direct current stimulation (a monophasic square waveform), or a rectified or monophasic sinusoidal waveform are not included in tDCS as defined here, but they can be considered as variants of tDCS (e.g. see transcranial oscillating direct current stimulation, toDCS).

The terminology "anodal-tDCS" (a-tDCS) and "cathodal-tDCS" (c-tDCS), though common, should be used with caution. All tDCS methods involve at least one anode and one cathode (to complete a minimal circuit), and all current entering the cortex must exit (and pass through intermediary brain regions). There is no pure unipolar tDCS (effects exerted under one electrode only), as may be implied by the terms anodal-tDCS or cathodal-tDCS in describing an intervention. Anodal-tDCS or cathodal-tDCS in this context, thus reflect the *intended* outcome of stimulation by the specific electrode that is assumed to be more relevant, and thus these terms are understood as only an expected outcome (or hypothesis). However, the extent to which anodal and cathodal sources produce net effects on excitation and inhibition, especially in the context of brain processing and behavior, are complex and unresolved. The preferred language should be "the anodal-tDCS *over* brain region X" (Clemens et al. 2014) or "anode at scalp coordinate X defined by EEG 10-10" rather than "anodal tDCS *of* brain region X" since the latter incorrectly implies that current is delivered to just that brain region (Datta et al. 2009) and moreover over-simplistic intended outcomes. Still more precise semantics would consist of stating "anodal-*electrode over* brain region X".

Just because there are well established, montage specific effects on bio-markers (e.g. TMS MEPs) or behaviors associated with brain regions nominally targeted by tDCS, this does not imply that current was restricted to or solely influential by the brain area "under" the electrode.

"Active", "Stimulating", "Return" or "Reference" Electrode

The terms "return" or "reference" electrode is typically used to describe an electrode with presumed "physiological inertness" or perceived lack of importance – (e.g. not being in proximity to the brain regions of interest). However, all electrodes are functional – even when they are not related to the hypothesis tested – in the engineering sense that they are used to carry current. The physiological activity of "return" electrodes can be theoretically reduced for example by increasing electrode size or using a ring of electrodes (Datta et al. 2008; Nitsche et al. 2007); nonetheless, the configuration of these electrodes needs to be explicit and their polarity and configuration must be indicated. The configuration and position of the "return" electrode has a profound effect on current flow near the "active" electrode and use of an extra-cephalic electrode evidently does not cancel the role of this electrode in brain current flow (Bikson et al. 2010; Truong et al. 2014).

Analogous to how anodal-tDCS and cathodal-tDCS are descriptive, the terms "active" or "stimulating" electrode refers to those electrodes presumed to be physiologically active – or more specifically that a physiological/behavioral outcome of interest is due to current passed through these electrodes. The terms "active", "stimulating", "return", and "reference" are thus terms that typically relate to the "intent" of stimulation and if they are used it should be (i) with the recognition that despite intent, the physiological actions of stimulation may be unexpected (ii) the complete stimulation dose is documented (e.g. it is never appropriate to exclude details of reference electrode size, placement, and materials). The term "reference" may also be used in the mathematical context of defining polarity (e.g. 5 V relative to the reference electrode), without presumptions of "intent", which is sound.

Electrode Assembly, Electrode, and Electrolyte

The electrode assembly refers to all components that carry current between the device lead wire and the scalp (such as metal electrode, conducting rubber electrode, electrolyte, sponge) and/or materials used to shape these components or otherwise direct current flow (casing, sponge, rivets). The headgear used to position the electrodes on the body or scalp is not included in the electrode assembly. The headgear must include some components that do not conduct current flow.

Technically the electrode in an electrode assembly refers only to the material (or surface) where charge carried by electrons is converted to charge carried by electrodes. For tES, this is limited to the metal and/or conductive rubber in contact with the electrolyte (such a saline or gel). In electrochemistry literature (Merrill et al. 2005), electrode refers only to the one element in the electrode assembly that is conductive and, in almost all applications of tES, does not touch the skin. However, in the tDCS (and broader tES) literature electrode has been used to refer to the entire electrode assembly. Ambiguity in this regard limits reproducibility. For example, it should be made clear if provided dimensions (e.g. 5 × 5 cm) refer to the electrode (e.g. the conductive rubber or metal) or rather the overall electrode assembly or sponge (the skin contact area).

It is conventional to discuss montage and waveform in terms of electrode (rather than electrode assembly). For example, delivery of 1 mA to an electrode implies delivery of 1 mA through the electrode assembly. Use of an electrode as an "anode" is correct and implied the electrode assembly functions as an anode. The conventions in the literature describing montage and waveform referencing "electrode" are typically appropriate if (i) the distinction between electrode and electrode assembly is clear to the writer and readers and (ii) details of the electrode assembly, including the electrode design, are explicit.

The electrolyte is the component of the electrode assembly where charge is carried by ions. It is in contact with both the electrode and the skin and completes a circuit of electricity flow. The electrolyte may be saline or other salt containing solution (Dundas et al. 2007) or the electrolyte may be a salt-containing hydrogel or fatty (oily) cream. To prevent spread, the electrolyte may be suspended in a porous material like a sponge and/or contained by a holding vessel like a cup. In some cases, such as with fatty creams, the electrolyte may be sufficiently viscous not to require a suspension. Notably though, oily creams or fats may change the impedance properties of the skin stressing the importance of attending to the resistivity of preparations. Regardless, the electrolyte is always a barrier between the electrode and the skin. The minimum path distance between the electrode and the skin that passes through the electrolyte is the minimum electrode-skin distance. This minimum distance may be determined by a physical non-conductive (e.g. plastic) separator or holder, by sponge thickness, or by the thickness of the paste (where special care must be taken to ensure the electrode does not approach skin).

Some studies have used water to saturate tES electrodes and in such cases the water presumably either contains some ions or absorbs it from the skin. "Salt-free" gels and creams have also been evaluated for tES (Minhas et al. 2010), but often have other chemical substitutes for supporting charge transfer and should not be used without validation.

Headgear

All components that are used to position and hold the electrode to the body are part of the head-gear. As defined here the headgear is primarily fabricated using non-conductive components (e.g. elastic or fabric). However, some conductive components like the electrode assembly and the lead (wires) may be integrated into the headgear. The head-gear serves to hold these components in place, position them relative to the scalp, and/or facilitate set-up.

Resistance (Impedance)

Resistance is a ubiquitous term in tDCS and is considered important in pre-testing and monitoring of stimulation, though clarification on its usage is useful. As tDCS is current controlled, the voltage output (across two electrode and tissue) of the stimulator is adjusted to maintain a controlled current application. When the term "resistance" is used in the context of tDCS what is generally being referred to is the voltage at the output of the current source divided by the current applied – through the application of Ohm's law. Typically, prior to stimulation, as the stimulator probes resistance, a small imperceptible test current is applied and the resulting voltage noted; here again, division of the voltage by the test current is similarly used to calculate resistance. However, neither before nor during stimulation, is the electrode and tissue simply resistive (e.g. explained only by ohms law). For example, prior to stimulation, the "resistance" calculated will depend on the current test applied (Hahn et al. 2013). The term "impedance" refers to the broader relation between current applied and the voltage need to maintain this current flow. Linear impedance includes frequency specific responses (e.g. the response to sinusoids of varied frequency). The electrode and tissue are complex non-linear impedance. For example, the impedance may change over time.

What does all this subtlety mean for the simple and consistent use of "resistance" in tDCS? It is accepted that during tDCS a significantly increased voltage (at the current source output) is associated with an overall impedance increase, which would indicate non-optimal conditions at the electrode or electrolyte-skin interface. This is biophysically justified since maintaining a low electrode "over-potential" voltage – a voltage that occurs specifically across the electrode interface as a result of electrochemical conditions (for detailed discussion, see Merrill et al. 2005) – and high conductivity (e.g. good gel/saline contact with the electrode and skin) are associated with minimized chemical reactions and good contact. These factors, in turn, promote but do no guarantee tolerable stimulation. Variability in the outcomes of tDCS methods can come about due to differences in the resistance – or more properly the impedance – of the skin. While "resistance" may be reported, investigators should recognize the impedance value is not a fixed property of the system but reflects how the measurement is obtained. The pre-stimulation "resistance" reported is a function of the device used while the "resistance" during stimulation is a global measure integrating several factors. In this qualified sense, "resistance" may be used interchangeably with "impedance" in conventional tDCS. To compensate for these issues some devices adopt "quality units" which may also be reported as a substitute for resistance, but only when noting the type of device.

High-Definition Transcranial Direct Current Stimulation (HD-tDCS)

HD-tDCS is defined as any tDCS montage using electrodes with a compact (e.g. < 5 cm^2) skin-electrolyte that is defined by a rigid holder (e.g. comparable to EEG designs). In some cases, the increased current density necessitates use of specially designed electrodes (Minhas et al. 2010) that are called High-density electrodes.

Two or more electrodes may be used for HD-tDCS. A feature of smaller electrodes is the potential to use a higher number of electrodes and/or electrodes in closer proximity; this in turn provides increased flexibility in montage design (Dmochowski et al. 2013) as well as facilitates simultaneous recording of EEG during tDCS (Roy et al. 2014).

HD-tDCS may use a varied number of electrodes, including 2, 5, or more depending on the stimulation objectives and device constraints (Dmochowski et al. 2011, 2013). HD-tDCS may be optimized for focality (sparring non-targeted brain regions) or for overall intensity (with diffuse brain current flow).

4 × 1 HD-tDCS Montage

The 4 × 1 Montage is a deployment of HD-tDCS where one center electrode is surrounded by four electrodes of the opposite polarity (Datta et al. 2009; Kuo et al. 2013) – thus forming a ring around the center electrode. If the center is an anode, the four surround electrodes are cathodes. If the center is a cathode the four surround electrodes are anodes. The 4 × 1 HD-tDCS montage is intended to restrict current predominantly to the cortex circumscribed by the ring (Edwards et al. 2013) and can produce more unidirectional stimulation since the role of the polarity of the four return electrodes is distinct and so presumed diminished. Whereas 4 × 1 refers to a particular electrode configuration, HD-tDCS indicates any montage with small ("HD") electrodes.

(Slow) Oscillating Transcranial Direct Current Stimulation, Transcranial Sinusoidal Direct Current Stimulation (tSDCS)

Oscillatory tDCS (o-tDCS) is a form of tDCS using direct current stimulation where the intensity of stimulation is regularly modulated but which remains monophasic such that the polarity of stimulation is never inverted. The stimulation waveform is typically a monophasic square or a monophasic sinusoidal wave. o-tDCS and its variants conventionally use electrode montages adapted from tDCS.

Slow oscillatory tDCS (so-tDCS) conventionally refers to a signal with a frequency below 1 Hz (e.g. 0.75 Hz; Groppa et al. 2010). Often, so-tDCS is applied between a supra-orbital electrode and an electrode on the mastoid. Transcranial sinusoidal direct current stimulation (ts-DCS) is a form of o-tDCS where the waveform is a monophasic (biased) sinusoid. so-tDCS may also be used to describe protocols with sinusoidal waveforms and low frequency (Eggert et al. 2013; Groppa et al. 2010). ts-DCS frequencies and intensities span those used in tACS (Antal et al. 2008).

The duty cycle of o-tDCS and its derivatives may be varied (e.g. 5 intervals with 1 min gap; Eggert et al. 2013). The distinction between o-tDCS and forms of tDCS which is applied intermittently and repeatedly (repetitive tDCS; e.g. 15 s on tDCS, 15 s off tDCS, repeated; Marshall et al. 2004) is, as defined here, one of intended outcome – where o-tDCS is expected to produce changes in part through the change in current (namely the neurophysiologic intended outcomes are assumed to reflect the non-static nature of current flow), while tDCS is assumed to produce its outcome primarily during the sustained phase (namely the neurophysiologic outcomes are assume to reflect actions when the current is sustained, even if interactions across tDCS sessions are expected). Evidently, this distinction of intention is subtle (and subject to change/interpretation) and we emphasize that all studies would report the dose applied regardless of terminology used.

Early and Modern History of tDCS, Alongside Historical tES Developments

Early History of tDCS and tES (Before 1900)

Early uses of electrical stimulation to modify brain function predates the invention of man-made electricity. Observations from 43–48 A.C. showed that placing a live torpedo fish induced a strong discharge over scalp that resulted in pain relief in headache. Later in the eleventh century, this method was used in patients with epilepsy by Ibn-Sidah. He suggested that stimulation of frontal bone could be used as a treatment for epileptic patients (Priori 2003). Thus, studies with electric fish included the initial attempts of brain stimulation which continued until voltaic piles were invented. In the late eighteenth century, Luigi Galvani invented the voltaic cell and together with his experiments involving animal electricity, he conducted foundational bioelectrical (electrophysiology) studies. As early as 1755, Charles Le Roy conducted experiments in a blind man with the purpose of restoring sight. In this experiment wires were placed around the subject's head and leg. Although he perceived phosphenes and the experiment was repeated several times, the subject remained blind. In terms of early stimulation techniques for treatment, Giovanni Aldini (Zaghi et al. 2009) recommended galvanism for patients with deafness, amaurosis, and "insanity"; reporting good results with this technique especially when it was used in patients with "melancholia". Aldini also treated patients with personality disorders and reported complete rehabilitation following transcranial administration of electrical currents (Parent 2004). These early studies used rudimentary batteries and were inherently constant voltage stimulation, where the resulting current depended on the variable body resistance. During the nineteenth century several studies utilized electrical stimulations in various parts of the world. The variability among such studies made drawing concise conclusion about their findings extremely difficult. In addition, these studies failed to report crucial information including patients' diagnosis, stimulation parameters as well as lack of scientific rigor in study design. These studies also made no attempt to estimate the amount of electricity each case received (Newth 1873). The potential value of electrical therapy was recognized and remarked upon by Dr. Alexander Robertson in the late nineteenth century, when he advised the following:

> *...The therapeutic value of electricity in mental disease is not by any means hypothetical only; it has been repeatedly proved to be of real value by numerous observers in this country (UK), in America, and especially on the continent. So long ago as 1804, Galvani's nephew, Aldini, is reported as having cured two cases of melancholia by galvanism to the satisfaction of several disinterested physicians who watched the cases. Galvanism is not a remedy to be used indiscriminately, or in a hazard way. It is not a toy, but a very potent means of doing good or harm, and must be used very cautiously and scientifically...*

Late History of tDCS and tES (1900–2000)

Over the course of the twentieth century, direct voltage continued to be intermittently tested, but electro-medicine involved pulsed stimulation became dominant. Early efforts began with simple circuits and basic devices, where a crank intermittently connected the mechanical connection between the battery and the subject; and later evolved into to modern current control circuits. The increasingly complex waveforms that were made possible by this advance in electrical engineering including Cranial Electrotherapy Stimulation and its variants (Guleyupoglu et al. 2013). We categorized tES in the twentieth century into fives streams (Fig. 1.6), four of which spans decades plus one additional stream of contemporary approaches. These streams are: (1) CES that descended from ES or CET; (2) EA, which went through several periods of waning interested and resurgence when new waveform variations were proposed including TCES, and Limoge Current; (3) Polarization or direct current stimulation, which includes tDCS, TCMP, and HD-tDCS; (4) ECT, initially called Electroshock Therapy; and (5) Contemporary approaches that have been explored intensively over last decades such as tACS, tSDCS, and tRNS. As discussed above, many contemporary approaches developed following the emergence and methodology of tDCS.

Electrosleep (ES), the method of stimulating brain to produce a sleep-like state, was initiated in 1902 (Robinovitch 1914). Most of the work related to this topic was conducted mainly in Russia, until 1953 when clinical usage of this method began in Europe (Smith 2006). In 1977 ES and its derivatives went under review by FDA and in 1978 it was classified as a class III device for treatment of insomnia, anxiety, and depression. Modern CES is thus a historical descendant of ES with continuous use and development over the century.

In parallel with initiation of ES, EA which induced anesthesia using high frequency stimulation, was first described in 1903 (Leduc and Rouxeau 1903). One of the first published claims of EA's success during surgeries was made in the 1914 by Leduc (1914), however safety and tolerability concerns, as well as the development of early chemical anesthetics may have contributed to quelling of interest in EA. In the 1940s research on EA focused on chemical primers being used in conjunction with EA and soon after its use appeared to largely halt due to side effects. Although side effects were discovered, research into variants of EA continued and the term TCES was adopted around 1960–1963 with the intended use to potentiate some drug effects with the goal of drastic reduction in pharmacologic anesthetic agents. Circa 1965, interferential stimulation (IS) was proposed by Russian scientists who had two pairs of electrodes that could apply sinusoidal waves with slightly different frequencies. The intention of this approach was that through pulsation, higher frequencies would create a lower frequency where the two frequencies intersect. This was clinically desired as low frequencies were presumed more efficacious in inducing EA whereas higher frequencies were more desirable for tolerability. Historical EA and TCES used current intensities that were typically well above those used in contemporary tES.

Direct current stimulation has been used intermittently as a component in both ES and EA. In 1957, a DC bias was added to ES. In 1964, Redfearn and Lippold investigated polarizing current for treatment of neuropsychiatric diseases; their use of prolonged stimulation was motivated by animal studies showing that prolonged direct current stimulation could produce lasting changes in excitability (Bindman et al. 1964). The majority of studies after Lippold were relatively small and used comparable dose (Table 1.1). Commonly used current intensities from 1964 to 1998 raged from 0.5 to 0.1 mA; though Redfearn and his colleagues used up to 3 mA in one patient. The most common electrode montage was active electrode(s) above eyebrow (supra-orbital) and reference electrode in an extra-cephalic position (e.g., leg, hand). In alternative montages, the active electrodes could be placed on occipital and temporal areas of the scalp. Apart from the leg and arm, the return electrodes were also placed on the mastoid bone or collarbone. Active electrode size was 0.1 to 0.2 cm^2 (mean 1.26 cm^2). The reference electrode area was often larger than the active ones (Baker 1970; Lifshitz and Harper 1968), but in some cases they were the same size (Elbert et al. 1981).

Table 1.1 tDCS studies published between 1960 and 1998

Study	N	Disease	Design	Electrode montage	Intensity (mA)	Duration Of stimulation	Electrode	Findings	Side effects
Lippold et al. (1964), UK	32	Depression/ Schizophrenia	Uncontrolled double-blind	Anodes over each eyebrows and cathode over right knee	0.1–3[a]	0.5–5[b] h (duration of stimulation varied in subjects based on their condition and improvement).	1.26 cm^2 Chloride silver discs covered with saline-soaked gauze	In scalp-positive polarization patients became more alert and more involved with the environment; in scalp-negative polarization quietness and withdrawal was seen. They have often found an effect at 0.25 mA for each anode whereas there had repeatedly been no effect at 0.15 mA scalp positive stimulation[c].	Tremor during scalp-positive, nausea, sleepiness
Costain et al. (1964), UK	24	Depression	Controlled double-blind, crossover	Anodes over each eyebrows and cathode over one knee	0.25 for each anode %current was started from 0.1 for each eyebrow and gradually increased	8 h per day for 12 days	1.26 cm^2 Silver discs covered with saline-soaked gauze	Improvement of anxiety, agitation and somatic symptoms.	Faint, blue flashes, skin sensitivity, mild headaches
Redfearn et al. (1964),UK	29	Refractory depression	Open label	Anodes over each eyebrows and cathode over one knee	0.1–0.25 for each anode	0.5–11[b] h (duration for each person was based on side effects), 5 times a week for 6 months.	1.26 cm^2 Chlorided silver discs covered with saline-soaked gauze	13 cases showed clinical improvement that lasted only 1-2 days It has been suggested that a dosage of 0.4 mA in each lead for period on 8 hours per day was more effective in many patients.	Mild headache, skin sensitivity

(continued)

Table 1.1 (continued)

Study	N	Disease	Design	Electrode montage	Intensity (mA)	Duration Of stimulation	Electrode	Findings	Side effects
Ramsay et al. (1966), USA	20	Depression	Open label	Anodes over each eyebrows and cathode over one knee	0.15–0.3 for each anode	4–6[b] h per day. Total stimulation time varies.	–	14 definitely improved, 4 equivocal improved, 2 did not improve	Few side effects reported (does not mention which)
Herjanic et al. (1967), Unknown location	20	Depression/ Schizophrenia	Uncontrolled Open label	–	0.1–0.5	–	–	All patients improved their depressive symptoms	None reported
Lifshitz and Harper (1968), USA	5	Schizophrenia	Controlled double-blind crossover	Anodes over eyebrows and cathodes over homolateral thighs.	0.33 for each channel of stimulation	6 h per day for 2 weeks only on week days followed by 2 week rest period.	Pure silver electrodes covered by surgical gauze soaked with normal saline. Anode = 1 × 2.5 cm and cathode = 2 × 4 cm	No significant effects either for scalp positive or scalp negative stimulation.	Skin irritation was fairly marked for 3 patients. Skin lesion consisted of erythema, papules and pustules which principally appeared under negative electrode.
Sheffield et al. (1968), Australia	6	Healthy	Controlled double-blind	Anodes over eyebrows and cathode over one leg	0.25 for each lead% current started from 0.03 mA and gradually increased in 90 min	3 h, each person was stimulated twice (positive and negative) in different days.	Chlorided silver discs covered with saline soaked lint pads. Anode= 0.5 inch diameter, cathode= 0.75 inch diameter.	Happier and more alert with scalp-positive polarization but results don't show significant changes in mood in subjects compared to control.	Moody and sleepy with scalp-negative polarization

Carney et al. (1970), Australia	119	Depression	Open label, uncontrolled	–	0.25	–	–	Improvement in excited behavior and mood; relapse on stopping treatment and improvement on recommencing.	None reported
Arfai et al. (1970), USA	19	Depression	Controlled double-blind clinical trial	Anodes over eyebrows and cathodes over thighs	0.25 for each independent channel	8 h per day during 6 days each week (totally 12 applications)	Chlorided silver discs	No significant effects	None reported
Hall et al. (1970), USA	18	Healthy	Controlled double-blind	Anodes over each eyebrows and cathode over knee	0.15 and 0.3 for each lead	2 h, each person was stimulated 3 times (scalp positive, scalp negative and sham) in different days.	Metallic mesh electrodes. Skin was rubbed by alcohol and local anesthetic was used.	No significant effect.	None reported
Baker (1970), Rhodesia	107	Depression	Random group of patients treated with brain polarization.	Anodes over each eyebrows and cathode over upper arm or forearm	0.4 for each lead$_{\%}$ current started with 0.2 mA and gradually reached 0.4 in half an hour	5[b] h per day for 6–8 sessions.	Silver plates covered with lint soaked in saline and gel was used for skin Anode= 10 cm^2 and cathode= 20 cm^2.	84% reported sustained improvement. Anxiety was not relieved.	Skin sensitivity, tachycardia and migraine
Nias and Shapiro (1974), UK	1	Schizophrenia with Depression	Controlled double-blind clinical trial	Anodes over each eyebrows and two cathodes attached to right knee	0.4 for each lead	3–4 h per day for 14–120 sessions.	–	Improvement with negative and worsening with positive stimulation	Tingling on the forehead.
	1	Alcoholism with Depression			0.5 for each lead			Improvement with positive stimulation	

(continued)

Table 1.1 (continued)

Study	N	Disease	Design	Electrode montage	Intensity (mA)	Duration Of stimulation	Electrode	Findings	Side effects
Elbert et al. (1981), Germany	48	Healthy	Single-blinded	Anode over vertex and cathodes over earlobes	0.26	1 h in a session (half of task was done in cathodal and the rest was done in anodal stimulation).	1.5 cm diameter Silver discs	Vertex positive current tends to develop faster reaction times and higher skin conductance responses than vertex-negative currents.	None reported
Elbert et al. (1981), Germany	32	Healthy	Single-blinded	Anode over vertex and cathode over collarbone to both sides which were linked	0.25	1 h in a session (half of it was anodal and the other half was cathodal stimulation).	1.5 cm diameter Silver discs	Results suggest that subjects reacted after a shorter interval when negative pole was applied compared to positive stimulation.	None reported
Korsakov (1989), Russia	48	Schizophrenia	Open label clinical trial	Anode over Occipital cortex OR anode over frontal CORTEX cathode=mastoid	0.05–0.2	–	Silver cup electrodes	Cathodal on occipital cortex increased visual sensitivity (discrimination of the brightness of a pair of light flashes), anodal decreased.	None reported

[a]Just for one person 3 mA was used and it was applied while putting local anesthetic under electrode
[b]Device was portable and patients could go about their normal hospital business and returning to the lab at pre-arranged times
[c]They has two other failed trials before the present study. The essential difference between this trial and two others were electrodes placed over eyebrows, currents were lower and they were passed for much longer time

These early studies employed several sessions of stimulation, with a median of 14 sessions (ranging from 1 to 120 sessions). The median of the total duration of stimulation was 30 h. Redfearn et al. conducted among the highest total dose studies, with 960 h total time of stimulation across sessions (Redfearn et al. 1964). The median duration of sessions was 4.5 h, with a maximum of 11 h (Redfearn et al. 1964). Reflecting the long duration of stimulation in many studies, the devices were often portable and patient could move around the hospital or go home. In most studies from this era, stimulation apparatus was made of low voltage dry batteries in a pack with a potentiometer to produce constant current. In one early study (Elbert et al. 1981), an optocoupled system driven by the analog output provided constant current which had a ramp up period of 6 s to increase current from zero to 0.25 mA. In all the studies, electrodes were metallic, either pure silver or silver chloride disks.

We note that in direct current stimulation methods before the modern period (before 1998), the active electrode's mean size was smaller, current was lower, and session durations were higher. As discussed next, approaches used in the modern era was heavily derived from canonical neurophysiological studies (circa 2000), which were in fact not intended to optimize clinical benefit. It is thus interesting that contemporary efforts to enhance clinical efficacy now consider using longer duration sessions along with more sessions which benefit from home-use devices (Charvet et al. 2015), and are thus closer to these early clinical efforts.

Modern tDCS 2000+

The Canonical Methodological Paradigm

While research using low-intensity currents continued throughout the twentieth century, the modern resurgence in the investigation of weak direct and alternating currents is linked to seminal neurophysiology work circa 2000 (Nitsche and Paulus 2000). This work and subsequent neurophysiologic studies (Clark et al. 2012; Leite et al. 2013) established the foundations of modern tDCS as evidenced through the establishment of certain canonical dose paradigms. These include use of currents in the 1 mA range, use of large sponge based electrodes (in the 30 cm^2 range), use of long duration stimulation (tens of minutes), and intention to produce polarity specific modulation with the anode/cathode placed over the region to be excited/inhibited (often with the other electrodes in a forehead/SO position). While the understanding of brain response to a given tDCS dose have continued to evolve through rigorous investigations (Monte-Silva et al. 2010; Ohn et al. 2008; Reis et al. 2015) and new techniques have been invented (Nikolin et al. 2015), the basic rational for tDCS design has continued to dominate the design of trials. Namely aspects like 1–2 mA, 10–20 min of "anodal/cathodal" tDCS to "increase/decrease" function using a large sponge electrode placed on the scalp over the target with the functional role of the other electrode assumed unimportant. In both neurophysiological studies and clinical trials, there has been only a conservative escalation of both dose and sessions.

Brief Overview of Current Understanding of Neurophysiological Mechanisms

While passage of current through surface electrodes results in some shunting of current at the scalp as well as cerebrospinal fluid (CSF), a portion of current will penetrate to the brain, producing a peak electric field of approximately 0.3 V/m per 1 mA applied (Datta et al. 2009; Huang et al. 2017). While the resulting electric fields are low intensity (for comparison, TMS produces an almost 100 V/m electric field), the sustained "DC" electric field produced during tDCS will polarize the transmembrane neuronal potential (Jackson et al. 2016). This polarization, in turn, can influence "excitability" including the responsiveness to synaptic input (Rahman et al. 2013), modulate the firing rate of individual neurons (Miranda et al. 2006; Wagner et al. 2007), and change information processing by cells (Huang et al. 2017) and networks (Reato et al. 2013).

Importantly, when sustained for several minutes and present during ongoing LTP, direct currents can modulate plasticity (Jackson et al. 2016). tDCS-modulated neuro-plastic changes may be associated with alteration of neuronal ionic channels, such as the L-type voltage gated calcium channel (L-VGCC), and N-methyl-D-aspartate (NMDA) receptors (Paulus 2011; Stagg and Nitsche 2011). Mechanisms analogous to long-term potentiation (LTP) or long-term depression (LTD) have thus been attributed to tDCS effects on plasticity. Notably, since the current used in tDCS is subthreshold, it does not induce action potentials (Bikson et al. 2004); instead it modulates spontaneous neuronal activity (evoked, ongoing/endogenous activity) in a polarity-dependent fashion. Since tDCS does not necessarily produce, but instead modulates activity, it has the feature of being "functionally selective" where only paired plasticity (e.g. the training matched with stimulation) is boosted (Bikson and Rahman 2013).

The effects of tDCS are stimulation polarity dependent. Surface anodal stimulation will typically produce inward current flow at the cortex, which is expected to produce somatic depolarization of pyramidal cortical neurons and apical dendrite hyperpolarization, while surface cathodal stimulation will typically produce outward current flow at the cortex and is expected to result in somatic hyperpolarization of pyramidal cortical neurons and apical dendrite depolarization (Radman et al. 2009; Zaghi et al. 2010). Changes in brain excitability were classically assumed to track somatic polarization, at least for moderate stimulation intensities (e.g. 1 mA) and durations (e.g. 15 min). However, ongoing and rigorous investigation of tDCS cellular targets and dose response indicate a more nuanced mechanism. For example, the cellular targets of tDCS may include axons (Rahman et al. 2013), dendrites (Kronberg et al. 2017), glia (Monai et al. 2016), or endothelial cells (Lopez-Quintero et al. 2010). New cellular targets, in turn, suggest varied and more nuanced dependence on tDCS stimulation polarity (Rahman et al. 2013). The dose response to increasing tDCS intensity may be nonlinear with increasing current, duration, or brain activity (Jamil et al. 2017).

There is also increasing sophistication about the anatomical targets of tDCS and montage design. While the nominal targets of tDCS are often simplistically assumed to be under the electrodes, the current flow produced using conventional tDCS in fact spans all cortical regions between and around the electrodes (Datta et al, 2009; Huang et al. 2017; Jog et al. 2016). It is therefore important to take care to distinguish between stimulating with an electrode "over" a region and specifically targeting "of" that region. Moreover, current flow with conventional montages is expected to reach deep structures (Bikson et al. 2010; Brunoni et al. 2012a; DaSilva et al. 2012; Keeser et al. 2011; Miranda et al. 2006; Salvador et al. 2010; Zaghi et al. 2010). In addition to tDCS having effects on brain regions distant from the electrode due to physical diffusion of current flow, tDCS may also modulate distant networks which are functionally connected to directly stimulated regions (Nitsche et al. 2005). For example, tDCS has been found to modulate resting-state functional connectivity after prefrontal stimulation (Keeser et al. 2011). As noted, to counteract diffusivity, tDCS may be "functionally" focalized by timing stimulation with specific tasks (Cano et al. 2013; Cohen Kadosh et al. 2010) – this combination with training is relevant for clinical applications as discussed next.

There are arguably no neuromodulation techniques that have been subject to as extensive neurophysiological investigation at the animal and human level as tDCS. In just the last decade, there have been dozens of human trials addressing nuance in dose response (Giordano et al. 2017; Jamil et al. 2017; Woods et al. 2016), which are supported by animal trials indicating the effects of tDCS are pathway and state specific (Bikson and Rahman 2013). While challenges remain, including in addressing individual dose response, it is important that the basic rationale for using direct current to alter brain function is exhaustively tested.

Brief Overview of Rationale for Various Clinical Applications

Due to the neuromodulatory effects of tDCS, including its effects on excitability-measures and rate of learning (Buch et al. 2017; Kim et al. 2017; Kronberg et al. 2017) tDCS has been tested as a treatment for several neuropsychiatric disorders and to accelerate neuro-rehabilitation (Brunoni et al. 2012b) Since plasticity/excitability/activity is pathologically altered in many neurological and psychiatric diseases, tDCS is most often used to "re-adjust" or re-balance the system; examples here include epilepsy, pain, and depression, amongst others. A second rationale for testing of tDCS is the relevance of plasticity, and cortical activity/excitability alterations, for learning and memory formation; and therefore, potential conjunctive application of tDCS during rehabilitation/training: examples include motor rehabilitation, visual restauration, dystonia (Furuya et al. 2014), and Alzheimer´s disease. Evidently the (individual) etiology of disease as well as the brain response is complex, the ability of tDCS to alter excitability and plasticity is a starting point to rationalize clinical trials (Lefaucheur et al. 2017; Naro et al. 2016).

For instance, tDCS has been used for motor learning enhancement in stroke rehabilitation (Schlaug et al. 2008), for behavioral performance enhancement with Alzheimer's patients (Boggio et al. 2009b; Ferrucci et al. 2009; see also Chap. 12), for modulation of emotional affective neural circuits in depression patients (Boggio et al. 2009b; see also Chap. 13; Bueno et al. 2011; Kalu et al. 2012), and for patients with chronic pain (Boggio et al. 2008; Fenton et al. 2009; Fregni et al. 2006c; Gabis et al. 2009; Zaghi et al. 2011). In stroke neurorehabilitation, tDCS has shown benefits when used together with other interventions such as rehabilitation training (see Chap. 11) or occupational therapy in humans (Nair et al. 2011; Zhu and Schlaug 2011). In terms of pain, tDCS has been applied to cases of chronic pain refractory to pharmacologic interventions (Lefaucheur et al. 2008; Nizard et al. 2012) and for a number of different pain conditions such as fibromyalgia, pelvic pain, and neuropathic pain (DaSilva et al. 2012; Fenton et al. 2009; Fregni et al. 2006a).

Indirect support for clinical interventions also come from experiments in healthy volunteers on cognitive function. Numerous studies have also examined the effects of tDCS on learning in healthy subjects, suggesting improvement in implicit learning (Kincses et al. 2004), motor memory (Galea and Celnik 2009), working memory (Mulquiney et al. 2011; Ohn et al. 2008), and memory retrieval (Boggio et al. 2007; see also Chap. 9; Boggio et al. 2009a; Chi et al. 2010).

The clinical effectiveness of tDCS for any given indication depends from many factors, with adoption ultimate dependent on efficacy, safety, as well as a range of regularly, commercial, and payer issues. Regarding safety, the broad consensus of researchers and clinicians is there is no evidence for a serious adverse event being caused by tDCS (Russo et al. 2017) – which is made evident, in a sense, by the routine testing of tDCS on healthy subjects (e.g. up to 6 weeks in college students; Paneri et al. 2016). Regarding efficacy, clinical trials for a broad range indications are at varied phases, through for many treatments encouraging results often support ongoing clinical trials. For some indications, notable chronic pain and depression the consensus among researcher and clinicians is for moderate evidence for efficacy (Aparicio et al. 2016; Bikson et al. 2016; Lefaucheur et al. 2017; Spagnolo and Goldman 2017; Zhu et al. 2017), which also correspond to indications for which tDCS has been approved for treatment in some regions (e.g. the EU). It should also be noted that many tDCS trials include relatively small sample sizes and clinically homogeneous populations, and often use surrogate outcomes. Moreover, clinical trials vary in dose and inclusions/exclusion (e.g. concurrent use of medication) – which can profoundly affect outcomes and there is variation in outcome measures themselves, which makes it important to draw conclusions with care. Noting ongoing progress in addressing the mechanisms of tDCS (above), many questions remain especially in the context of treating the damages of pathophysiological brain. There is thus broad support for ongoing research especially aimed at optimization of dose (since the limited permutations tested so far could not be optimal), resolve individual responsiveness (recognizing that at useful treatment does not need to be effective for every patient), and incorporation of new technology – discussed next.

Emerging Technologies and Models

The field of tDCS is advancing, with new approaches and methodologies of tDCS recently developed. Many of these developments focus on improved method to deliver current to the brain. One such development is "High-Definition" tDCS (HD-tDCS), which utilizes an array of smaller gel-based electrodes, in contrast to the two large sponge-based electrode used in conventional tDCS. The position and current at each HD electrode can be optimized for a variety of desired outcomes, such as intensity or targeting (Dmochowski et al. 2011). One HD-tDCS configuration, the "4 × 1 ring" electrode montage, has been shown to be a more focused method of stimulation compared to conventional tDCS (Fig. 2.7; Datta et al. 2009; Edwards et al. 2013). The 4 × 1 HD-tDCS configuration has been shown to be a reliable method of targeting specific cortical areas, can produce plasticity changes that may outlast conventional tDCS (Kuo et al. 2013). Clinical application of 4 × 1 HD-tDCS are expanding, for example showing reduced perception on pain in fibromyalgia patients (Castillo-Saavedra et al. 2016; Villamar et al. 2013a, b) and in experimental pain (Borckardt et al. 2012).

A further important area of development for targeting of tDCS is use of EEG. Especially using HD-tDCS which can be integrated with EEG systems, there is compelling case for using clinical sub-population or subject-specific EEG to deliver a customized tDCS distribution. The notion of recording and HD-tDCS with the same or adjacent scalp electrodes is loosely based on the concept of reciprocity, which has only recently been formalized for non-invasive electrical stimulation (Dmochowski et al. 2013). Prior this this formalization, there have been varied empirical proposal to guide tDCS from EEG ranging from simple (Cancelli et al. 2016), to complex (Fernandez-Corazza et al. 2016; Wagner et al. 2016). EEG has also been suggested as useful to classify responders to tDCS (Al-Kaysi et al. 2016; Castillo-Saavedra et al. 2016) and broadly as a tool to diagnose the effects of tDCS (Cosmo et al. 2015; D'Atri et al. 2016; Mancini et al. 2016). The integration with EEG thus is an important frontier for tDCS optimization, but alongside this promise it is critical to consider technical concerns in implementation (Noury et al. 2016; Chap. 11).

There is a long-standing interest to use functional mapping information from fMRI to identify targets for tDCS (Clark et al. 2012; Teichmann et al. 2016) and access outcomes (Jang et al. 2009; see Chap. 11; Clark et al. 2011; Lin et al. 2017; Cabral-Calderin et al. 2016; Cavaliere et al. 2016). However, there is a push for more sophisticated and numerically formalized methods to systematically combine spatial imaging with spatial targeting of (HD)-tDCS (Dunlop et al. 2016; Hunter et al. 2013). For example, it possible to co-register current flow and imaging data in analysis (Halko et al. 2011). A further interesting development is the use of MRI to image current flow produced by tDCS (Antal et al. 2014; Jog et al. 2016).

There have been various proposals on customized tDCS to a subject's anatomy. This is motivated by individual differences in anatomy leading to different brain current flow patterns for the same dose (Bikson et al. 2012b; Datta et al. 2012; Kim et al. 2013; Truong et al. 2013). One approach using individual MRI derived models of current flow to customize dose (Bikson et al. 2012a; Ruffini et al. 2013; Opitz et al. 2015; see Chap. 9). This approach was first suggested in stroke where individual brain lesions distort brain current flow patterns (Datta et al. 2011; Otal et al. 2016) leading to pilot clinical trials in customized tDCS in rehabilitation (Dmochowski et al. 2013). An alternative line of proposed personalization of the stimulation is by adapting the electrode shape (rather than position and current at electrodes) to fit the structural and functional features of individual subjects (Cancelli et al. 2015). Approaches used shaped concentric ring electrodes, to approximate the 4 × 1 HD-tDCS montage, are also proposed (Bortoletto et al. 2016).

One of the most promising features of tDCS is the ability to deploy to a wide range of environments, including home use. But there has been a dearth of studies using tDCS at home compared to the at the clinic/academic center, which in part reflected the need to establish efficacy in controlled environment but also the lack of availability until recently, of suitable equipment and protocols. Providing a patient with a device certified for use by an expert creates significant risk of misuse (Cabrera et al. 2014). Remote-Supervised tDCS is thus a key development to provide rigorous protocols and equipment for home-based use, including rules to maintain reproducibility and tolerability from clinic to home (Charvet et al. 2015; Knotkova et al. 2017a, Chapter 13). Efforts to develop better tDCS electrodes are often guided by simplicity and replicability for home (remote supervised) use, including single-use pre-saturated snap electrodes with single-position head-gear (Chap. 10). The need for remote based tDCS is emphasized by evidence that the effect of transcranial direct current stimulation (tDCS) is cumulative – thus treatment protocols typically require multiple consecutive sessions spanning weeks or months. The desire for remote based tDCS must be critically balanced with the development of subject/trial specific telemedicine interventions (Kasschau et al. 2015; Charvet et al. 2015; Knotkova et al. 2017b).

In the coming years, significant advances in tDCS are expected including new technology for customized stimulation in the form of more specific brain targeting (e.g. HD-tDCS), patient specific image-guided dosage parameters, and technology more easily deployable in clinical and home environments.

References

Al-Kaysi, A. M., Al-Ani, A., Loo, C. K., Powell, T. Y., Martin, D. M., Breakspear, M., & Boonstra, T. W. (2016). Predicting tDCS treatment outcomes of patients with major depressive disorder using automated EEG classification. *Journal of Affective Disorders*.

Alam, M., Truong, D. Q., Khadka, N., & Bikson, M. (2016). Spatial and polarity precision of concentric high-definition transcranial direct current stimulation (HD-tDCS). *Physics in Medicine and Biology, 61*(12), 4506–4521.

Antal, A., Bikson, M., Datta, A., Lafon, B., Dechent, P., Parra, L. C., & Paulus, W. (2014). Imaging artifacts induced by electrical stimulation during conventional fMRI of the brain. *NeuroImage, 85*(Pt 3), 1040–1047.

Antal, A., Boros, K., Poreisz, C., Chaieb, L., Terney, D., & Paulus, W. (2008). Comparatively weak after-effects of transcranial alternating current stimulation (tACS) on cortical excitability in humans. *Brain Stimulation, 1*(2), 97–105.

Antal, A., & Paulus, W. (2013). Transcranial alternating current stimulation (tACS). *Frontiers in Human Neuroscience, 7*:317.

Aparicio, L. V., Guarienti, F., Razza, L. B., Carvalho, A. F., Fregni, F., & Brunoni, A. R. (2016). A systematic review on the acceptability and tolerability of transcranial direct current stimulation treatment in neuropsychiatry trials. *Brain Stimulation, 9*(5), 671–681.

Baker, A. (1970). Brain stem polarization in the treatment of depression. *South African Medical Journal, 44*(16), 473–475.

Beekwilder, J., & Beems, T. (2010). Overview of the clinical applications of vagus nerve stimulation. *Journal of Clinical Neurophysiology, 27*(2), 130–138.

Bikson, M., Datta, A., Rahman, A., & Scaturro, J. (2010). Electrode montages for tDCS and weak transcranial electrical stimulation: role of "return" electrode's position and size. *Clinical Neurophysiology: Official Journal of the International Federation of Clinical Neurophysiology, 121*(12), 1976.

Bikson, M., Grossman, P., Thomas, C., Zannou, A. L., Jiang, J., Adnan, T., … Woods, A. J. (2016). Safety of transcranial direct current stimulation: Evidence based update 2016. *Brain Stimulation, 9*(5), 641–661.

Bikson, M., Inoue, M., Akiyama, H., Deans, J. K., Fox, J. E., Miyakawa, H., & Jefferys, J. G. (2004). Effects of uniform extracellular DC electric fields on excitability in rat hippocampal slices in vitro. *The Journal of Physiology, 557*(Pt 1), 175–190.

Bikson, M., & Rahman, A. (2013). Origins of specificity during tDCS: Anatomical, activity-selective, and input-bias mechanisms. *Frontiers in Human Neuroscience, 7*, 688.

Bikson, M., Rahman, A., & Datta, A. (2012a). Computational models of transcranial direct current stimulation. *Clinical EEG and Neuroscience, 43*(3), 176–183.

Bikson, M., Rahman, A., Datta, A., Fregni, F., & Merabet, L. (2012b). High-resolution modeling assisted design of customized and individualized transcranial direct current stimulation protocols. *Neuromodulation, 15*(4), 306–315.

Bindman, L. J., Lippold, O., & Redfearn, J. (1964). The action of brief polarizing currents on the cerebral cortex of the rat (1) during current flow and (2) in the production of long-lasting after-effects. *The Journal of Physiology, 172*(3), 369.

Bischoff, C. H. E. (1801). *Commentatio de usu galvanismi in arte medica speciatim vero in morbis nervorum paralyticis: additis tab. aeneis II, Ienae, In BibliopolioAcademico.*

Bliss, T. V., & Lomo, T. (1973). Long-lasting potentiation of synaptic transmission in the dentate area of the anaesthetized rabbit following stimulation of the perforant path. *The Journal of Physiology, 232*(2), 331–356.

Boggio, P. S., Fregni, F., Valasek, C., Ellwood, S., Chi, R., Gallate, J., … Snyder, A. (2009a). Temporal lobe cortical electrical stimulation during the encoding and retrieval phase reduces false memories. *PLoS One, 4*(3), e4959.

Boggio, P. S., Khoury, L. P., Martins, D. C., Martins, O. E., De Macedo, E., & Fregni, F. (2009b). Temporal cortex direct current stimulation enhances performance on a visual recognition memory task in Alzheimer disease. *Journal of Neurology, Neurosurgery, and Psychiatry, 80*(4), 444–447.

Boggio, P. S., Nunes, A., Rigonatti, S. P., Nitsche, M. A., Pascual-Leone, A., & Fregni, F. (2007). Repeated sessions of noninvasive brain DC stimulation is associated with motor function improvement in stroke patients. *Restorative Neurology and Neuroscience, 25*(2), 123–129.

Boggio, P. S., Zaghi, S., Lopes, M., & Fregni, F. (2008). Modulatory effects of anodal transcranial direct current stimulation on perception and pain thresholds in healthy volunteers. *European Journal of Neurology, 15*(10), 1124–1130.

Bola, M., Gall, C., Moewes, C., Fedorov, A., Hinrichs, H., & Sabel, B. A. (2014). Brain functional connectivity network breakdown and restoration in blindness. *Neurology, 83*(6), 542–551.

Borckardt, J. J., Bikson, M., Frohman, H., Reeves, S. T., Datta, A., Bansal, V., … George, M. S. (2012). A pilot study of the tolerability and effects of high-definition transcranial direct current stimulation (HD-tDCS) on pain perception. *The Journal of Pain, 13*(2), 112–120.

Bortoletto, M., Rodella, C., Salvador, R., Miranda, P. C., & Miniussi, C. (2016). Reduced current spread by concentric electrodes in transcranial electrical stimulation (tES). *Brain Stimulation, 9*(4), 525–528.

Brelen, M. E., Vince, V., Gerard, B., Veraart, C., & Delbeke, J. (2010). Measurement of evoked potentials after electrical stimulation of the human optic nerve. *Investigative Ophthalmology & Visual Science, 51*(10), 5351–5355.

Brunoni, A. R., Ferrucci, R., Fregni, F., Boggio, P. S., & Priori, A. (2012a). Transcranial direct current stimulation for the treatment of major depressive disorder: A summary of preclinical, clinical and translational findings. *Progress in Neuro-Psychopharmacology & Biological Psychiatry, 39*(1), 9–16.

Brunoni, A. R., Nitsche, M. A., Bolognini, N., Bikson, M., Wagner, T., Merabet, L., … Fregni, F. (2012b). Clinical research with transcranial direct current stimulation (tDCS): Challenges and future directions. *Brain Stimulation, 5*(3), 175–195.

Buch, E. R., Santarnecchi, E., Antal, A., Born, J., Celnik, P. A., Classen, J., … Cohen, L. G. (2017). Effects of tDCS on motor learning and memory formation: A consensus and critical position paper. *Clinical Neurophysiology, 128*(4), 589–603.

Bueno, V. F., Brunoni, A. R., Boggio, P. S., Bensenor, I. M., & Fregni, F. (2011). Mood and cognitive effects of transcranial direct current stimulation in post-stroke depression. *Neurocase, 17*(4), 318–322.

Cabral-Calderin, Y., Anne Weinrich, C., Schmidt-Samoa, C., Poland, E., Dechent, P., Bahr, M., & Wilke, M. (2016). Transcranial alternating current stimulation affects the BOLD signal in a frequency and task-dependent manner. *Human Brain Mapping, 37*(1), 94–121.

Cabrera, L. Y., Evans, E. L., & Hamilton, R. H. (2014). Ethics of the electrified mind: Defining issues and perspectives on the principled use of brain stimulation in medical research and clinical care. *Brain Topography, 27*(1), 10.1007/s10548-10013-10296-10548.

Cameron, T. (2004). Safety and efficacy of spinal cord stimulation for the treatment of chronic pain: A 20-year literature review. *Journal of Neurosurgery. Spine, 100*(3), 254–267.

Cancelli, A., Cottone, C., Parazzini, M., Fiocchi, S., Truong, D., Bikson, M., … Parazzini, M. (2015). Transcranial direct current stimulation: Personalizing the neuromodulation. *Conference Proceedings: Annual International Conference of the IEEE Engineering in Medicine and Biology Society, 2015*, 234–237.

Cancelli, A., Cottone, C., Tecchio, F., Truong, D. Q., Dmochowski, J., & Bikson, M. (2016). A simple method for EEG guided transcranial electrical stimulation without models. *Journal of Neural Engineering, 13*(3), 036022.

Cano, T., Morales-Quezada, J. L., Bikson, M., & Fregni, F. (2013). Methods to focalize noninvasive electrical brain stimulation: Principles and future clinical development for the treatment of pain. *Expert Review of Neurotherapeutics, 13*(5), 465–467.

Castillo-Saavedra, L., Gebodh, N., Bikson, M., Diaz-Cruz, C., Brandao, R., Coutinho, L., … Weiss, M. (2016). Clinically effective treatment of fibromyalgia pain with high-definition transcranial direct current stimulation: Phase II open-label dose optimization. *The Journal of Pain, 17*(1), 14–26.

Cavaliere, C., Aiello, M., Di Perri, C., Amico, E., Martial, C., Thibaut, A., ... Soddu, A. (2016). Functional connectivity substrates for tDCS response in minimally conscious state patients. *Frontiers in Cellular Neuroscience, 10*, 257.

Charvet, L. E., Kasschau, M., Datta, A., Knotkova, H., Stevens, M. C., Alonzo, A., ... Bikson, M. (2015). Remotely-supervised transcranial direct current stimulation (tDCS) for clinical trials: Guidelines for technology and protocols. *Frontiers in Systems Neuroscience, 9*, 26.

Chi, R. P., Fregni, F., & Snyder, A. W. (2010). Visual memory improved by non-invasive brain stimulation. *Brain Research, 1353*, 168–175.

Clark, V. P., Coffman, B. A., Mayer, A. R., Weisend, M. P., Lane, T. D., Calhoun, V. D., ... Wassermann, E. M. (2012). TDCS guided using fMRI significantly accelerates learning to identify concealed objects. *NeuroImage, 59*(1), 117–128.

Clark, V. P., Coffman, B. A., Trumbo, M. C., & Gasparovic, C. (2011). Transcranial direct current stimulation (tDCS) produces localized and specific alterations in neurochemistry: A (1) H magnetic resonance spectroscopy study. *Neuroscience Letters, 500*(1), 67–71.

Clemens, B., Jung, S., Mingoia, G., Weyer, D., Domahs, F., & Willmes, K. (2014). Influence of anodal transcranial direct current stimulation (tDCS) over the right angular gyrus on brain activity during rest. *PLoS One, 9*(4), e95984.

Coats, A. (1972). The sinusoidal galvanic body-sway response. *Acta Oto-Laryngologica, 74*(1-6), 155–162.

Cosmo, C., Ferreira, C., Miranda, J. G., do Rosario, R. S., Baptista, A. F., Montoya, P., & de Sena, E. P. (2015). Spreading effect of tDCS in individuals with attention-deficit/hyperactivity disorder as shown by functional cortical networks: A randomized, double-blind, sham-controlled trial. *Frontiers in Psychiatry, 6*, 111.

D'Atri, A., De Simoni, E., Gorgoni, M., Ferrara, M., Ferlazzo, F., Rossini, P. M., & De Gennaro, L. (2015). Frequency-dependent effects of oscillatory-tDCS on EEG oscillations: A study with Better OSCillation detection method (BOSC). *Archives Italiennes de Biologie, 153*(2-3), 124–134.

D'Atri, A., De Simoni, E., Gorgoni, M., Ferrara, M., Ferlazzo, F., Rossini, P. M., & De Gennaro, L. (2016). Electrical stimulation of the frontal cortex enhances slow-frequency EEG activity and sleepiness. *Neuroscience, 324*, 119–130.

Danilov, Y. P., Tyler, M. E., Kaczmarek, K. A., & Skinner, K. L. (2014). New approach to neurorehabilitation: cranial nerve noninvasive neuromodulation (CN-NINM) technology. In *SPIE sensing technology+ applications* (p. 91120L-91120L-91110). International Society for Optics and Photonics, Baltimore, Maryland, United States.

DaSilva, A. F., Mendonca, M. E., Zaghi, S., Lopes, M., DosSantos, M. F., Spierings, E. L., ... Fregni, F. (2012). tDCS-induced analgesia and electrical fields in pain-related neural networks in chronic migraine. *Headache: The Journal of Head and Face Pain, 52*(8), 1283–1295.

DaSilva, A. F., Volz, M. S., Bikson, M., & Fregni, F. (2011). Electrode positioning and montage in transcranial direct current stimulation. *Journal of Visualized Experiments: JoVE, 51*.

Datta, A., Baker, J. M., Bikson, M., & Fridriksson, J. (2011). Individualized model predicts brain current flow during transcranial direct-current stimulation treatment in responsive stroke patient. *Brain Stimulation, 4*(3), 169–174.

Datta, A., Bansal, V., Diaz, J., Patel, J., Reato, D., & Bikson, M. (2009). Gyri-precise head model of transcranial direct current stimulation: Improved spatial focality using a ring electrode versus conventional rectangular pad. *Brain Stimulation, 2*(4), 201–207.e201.

Datta, A., Elwassif, M., Battaglia, F., & Bikson, M. (2008). Transcranial current stimulation focality using disc and ring electrode configurations: FEM analysis. *Journal of Neural Engineering, 5*(2), 163–174.

Datta, A., Truong, D., Minhas, P., Parra, L. C., & Bikson, M. (2012). Inter-individual variation during transcranial direct current stimulation and normalization of dose using MRI-derived computational models. *Frontiers in Psychiatry, 3*, 91.

DeGiorgio, C. M., Fanselow, E. E., Schrader, L. M., & Cook, I. A. (2011). Trigeminal nerve stimulation: Seminal animal and human studies for epilepsy and depression. *Neurosurgery Clinics of North America, 22*(4), 449–456.

Dimitrov, D. T., & Ralev, N. (2015). Signals and systems for electrosleep. *Elektronika ir Elektrotechnika, 93*(5), 95–98.

Dmochowski, J. P., Datta, A., Bikson, M., Su, Y., & Parra, L. C. (2011). Optimized multi-electrode stimulation increases focality and intensity at target. *Journal of Neural Engineering, 8*(4), 046011.

Dmochowski, J. P., Datta, A., Huang, Y., Richardson, J. D., Bikson, M., Fridriksson, J., & Parra, L. C. (2013). Targeted transcranial direct current stimulation for rehabilitation after stroke. *NeuroImage, 75*, 12–19.

Dundas, J. E., Thickbroom, G. W., & Mastaglia, F. L. (2007). Perception of comfort during transcranial DC stimulation: Effect of NaCl solution concentration applied to sponge electrodes. *Clinical Neurophysiology, 118*(5), 1166–1170.

Dunlop, K. A., Woodside, B., & Downar, J. (2016). Targeting neural endophenotypes of eating disorders with non-invasive brain stimulation. *Frontiers in Neuroscience, 10*, 30.

Edwards, D., Cortes, M., Datta, A., Minhas, P., Wassermann, E. M., & Bikson, M. (2013). Physiological and modeling evidence for focal transcranial electrical brain stimulation in humans: A basis for high-definition tDCS. *NeuroImage, 74*, 266–275.

Eggert, T., Dorn, H., Sauter, C., Nitsche, M. A., Bajbouj, M., & Danker-Hopfe, H. (2013). No effects of slow oscillatory transcranial direct current stimulation (tDCS) on sleep-dependent memory consolidation in healthy elderly subjects. *Brain Stimulation, 6*(6), 938–945.

Elbert, T., Lutzenberger, W., Rockstroh, B., & Birbaumer, N. (1981). The influence of low-level transcortical DC-currents on response speed in humans. *International Journal of Neuroscience, 14*(1-2), 101–114.

Fenton, B. W., Palmieri, P. A., Boggio, P., Fanning, J., & Fregni, F. (2009). A preliminary study of transcranial direct current stimulation for the treatment of refractory chronic pelvic pain. *Brain Stimulation, 2*(2), 103–107.

Fernandez-Corazza, M., Turovets, S., Luu, P., Anderson, E., & Tucker, D. (2016). Transcranial electrical neuromodulation based on the reciprocity principle. *Frontiers in Psychiatry, 7*, 87.

Ferrucci, R., Bortolomasi, M., Vergari, M., Tadini, L., Salvoro, B., Giacopuzzi, M., … Priori, A. (2009). Transcranial direct current stimulation in severe, drug-resistant major depression. *Journal of Affective Disorders, 118*(1), 215–219.

Fertonani, A., & Miniussi, C. (2016). Transcranial electrical stimulation: What we know and do not know about mechanisms. *The Neuroscientist.*

Fitzgerald, P. B. (2014). Transcranial pulsed current stimulation: A new way forward? *Clinical Neurophysiology, 125*(2), 217–219.

Fitzpatrick, R. C., & Day, B. L. (2004). Probing the human vestibular system with galvanic stimulation. *Journal of Applied Physiology, 96*(6), 2301–2316.

Frangos, E., Ellrich, J., & Komisaruk, B. R. (2015). Non-invasive access to the vagus nerve central projections via electrical stimulation of the external ear: fMRI evidence in humans. *Brain Stimulation, 8*(3), 624–636.

Fregni, F. (2005). Transcranial direct current stimulation of the unaffected hemisphere in stroke patients. *Neuroreport, 16*(14), 1551.

Fregni, F., Boggio, P. S., Lima, M. C., Ferreira, M. J., Wagner, T., Rigonatti, S. P., … Freedman, S. D. (2006a). A sham-controlled, phase II trial of transcranial direct current stimulation for the treatment of central pain in traumatic spinal cord injury. *Pain, 122*(1), 197–209.

Fregni, F., Boggio, P. S., Nitsche, M. A., Marcolin, M. A., Rigonatti, S. P., & Pascual-Leone, A. (2006b). Treatment of major depression with transcranial direct current stimulation. *Bipolar Disorders, 8*(2), 203–204.

Fregni, F., Marcondes, R., Boggio, P., Marcolin, M., Rigonatti, S., Te, S., … Pascual-Leone, A. (2006c). Transient tinnitus suppression induced by repetitive transcranial magnetic stimulation and transcranial direct current stimulation. *European Journal of Neurology, 13*(9), 996–1001.

Furuya, S., Nitsche, M. A., Paulus, W., & Altenmuller, E. (2014). Surmounting retraining limits in musicians' dystonia by transcranial stimulation. *Annals of Neurology, 75*(5), 700–707.

Gabis, L., Shklar, B., Kesner Baruch, Y., Raz, R., Gabis, E., & Geva, D. (2009). Pain reduction using transcranial electrostimulation: A double-blind. *Journal of Rehabilitation Medicine, 41*(4), 256–261.

Galea, J. M., & Celnik, P. (2009). Brain polarization enhances the formation and retention of motor memories. *Journal of Neurophysiology, 102*(1), 294–301.

Gall, C., Fedorov, A. B., Ernst, L., Borrmann, A., & Sabel, B. A. (2010). Repetitive transorbital alternating current stimulation in optic neuropathy. *NeuroRehabilitation, 27*(4), 335–341.

Galvani, L., & Aldini, G. (1792). Aloysii Galvani … De Viribus Electricitatis In Motu Musculari Comentarius. Cum Joannis Aldini Dissertatione Et Notis. *Accesserunt Epistolae ad animalis electricitatis theoriam pertinentes*. Mutinæ: Apud Societatem Typographicam.

Gartside, I. B. (1968). Mechanisms of sustained increases of firing rate of neurones in the rat cerebral cortex after polarization: Role of protein synthesis. *Nature, 220*(5165), 383–384.

Gartside, I. B., & Lippold, O. C. (1967). The production of persistent changes in the level of neuronal activity by brief local cooling of the cerebral cortex of the rat. *The Journal of Physiology, 189*(3), 475–487.

George, M. S., & Aston-Jones, G. (2010). Noninvasive techniques for probing neurocircuitry and treating illness: Vagus nerve stimulation (VNS), transcranial magnetic stimulation (TMS) and transcranial direct current stimulation (tDCS). *Neuropsychopharmacology, 35*(1), 301–316.

Giordano, J., Bikson, M., Kappenman, E. S., Clark, V. P., Coslett, H. B., Hamblin, M. R., … Calabrese, E. (2017). Mechanisms and effects of transcranial direct current stimulation. *Dose-Response, 15*(1), 1559325816685467.

Golub, J. S., Ling, L., Nie, K., Nowack, A., Shepherd, S. J., Bierer, S. M., … Rubinstein, J. T. (2014). Prosthetic implantation of the human vestibular system. *Otology & Neurotology: Official Publication of the American Otological Society, American Neurotology Society [and] European Academy of Otology and Neurotology, 35*(1), 136–147.

Gonzalez-Rosa, J. J., Soto-Leon, V., Real, P., Carrasco-Lopez, C., Foffani, G., Strange, B. A., & Oliviero, A. (2015). Static magnetic field stimulation over the visual cortex increases alpha oscillations and slows visual search in humans. *The Journal of Neuroscience, 35*(24), 9182–9193.

Groppa, S., Bergmann, T. O., Siems, C., Molle, M., Marshall, L., & Siebner, H. R. (2010). Slow-oscillatory transcranial direct current stimulation can induce bidirectional shifts in motor cortical excitability in awake humans. *Neuroscience, 166*(4), 1219–1225.

Guleyupoglu, B., Schestatsky, P., Edwards, D., Fregni, F., & Bikson, M. (2013). Classification of methods in transcranial electrical stimulation (tES) and evolving strategy from historical approaches to contemporary innovations. *Journal of Neuroscience Methods, 219*(2), 297–311.

Hahn, C., Rice, J., Macuff, S., Minhas, P., Rahman, A., & Bikson, M. (2013). Methods for extra-low voltage transcranial direct current stimulation: Current and time dependent impedance decreases. *Clinical Neurophysiology, 124*(3), 551–556.

Halko, M. A., Datta, A., Plow, E. B., Scaturro, J., Bikson, M., & Merabet, L. B. (2011). Neuroplastic changes following rehabilitative training correlate with regional electrical field induced with tDCS. *NeuroImage, 57*(3), 885–891.

Hein, E., Nowak, M., Kiess, O., Biermann, T., Bayerlein, K., Kornhuber, J., & Kraus, T. (2013). Auricular transcutaneous electrical nerve stimulation in depressed patients: A randomized controlled pilot study. *Journal of Neural Transmission, 120*(5), 821–827.

Hill, A. T., Rogasch, N. C., Fitzgerald, P. B., & Hoy, K. E. (2017). Effects of prefrontal bipolar and high-definition transcranial direct current stimulation on cortical reactivity and working memory in healthy adults. *NeuroImage, 152*, 142–157.

Huang, Y., Liu, A. A., Lafon, B., Friedman, D., Dayan, M., Wang, X., … Parra, L. C. (2017). Measurements and models of electric fields in the in vivo human brain during transcranial electric stimulation. *eLife, 6*.

Hunter, M. A., Coffman, B. A., Trumbo, M. C., & Clark, V. P. (2013). Tracking the neuroplastic changes associated with transcranial direct current stimulation: A push for multimodal imaging. *Frontiers in Human Neuroscience, 7*, 495.

Ilyukhina, V. A., Kozhushko, N. Y., Matveev, Y. K., Ponomareva, E. A., Chernysheva, E. M., & Shaptilei, M. A. (2005). Transcranial micropolarization in the combined therapy of speech and general psychomotor retardation in children of late preschool age. *Neuroscience and Behavioral Physiology, 35*(9), 969–976.

Jackson, M. P., Rahman, A., Lafon, B., Kronberg, G., Ling, D., Parra, L. C., & Bikson, M. (2016). Animal models of transcranial direct current stimulation: Methods and mechanisms. *Clinical Neurophysiology, 127*(11), 3425–3454.

Jamil, A., Batsikadze, G., Kuo, H. I., Labruna, L., Hasan, A., Paulus, W., & Nitsche, M. A. (2017). Systematic evaluation of the impact of stimulation intensity on neuroplastic after-effects induced by transcranial direct current stimulation. *The Journal of Physiology, 595*(4), 1273–1288.

Jang, S. H., Ahn, S. H., Byun, W. M., Kim, C. S., Lee, M. Y., & Kwon, Y. H. (2009). The effect of transcranial direct current stimulation on the cortical activation by motor task in the human brain: An fMRI study. *Neuroscience Letters, 460*(2), 117–120.

Jog, M. V., Smith, R. X., Jann, K., Dunn, W., Lafon, B., Truong, D., … Wang, D. J. (2016). In-vivo imaging of magnetic fields induced by transcranial direct current stimulation (tdcs) in human brain using mri. *Scientific Reports, 6*, 34385.

Kalkman, C. J., Drummond, J. C., Kennelly, N. A., Patel, P. M., & Partridge, B. L. (1992). Intraoperative monitoring of tibialis anterior muscle motor evoked responses to transcranial electrical stimulation during partial neuromuscular blockade. *Anesthesia and Analgesia, 75*(4), 584-589.

Kalu, U., Sexton, C., Loo, C., & Ebmeier, K. (2012). Transcranial direct current stimulation in the treatment of major depression: A meta-analysis. *Psychological Medicine, 42*(09), 1791–1800.

Kasschau, M., Sherman, K., Haider, L., Frontario, A., Shaw, M., Datta, A., … Charvet, L. (2015). A protocol for the use of remotely-supervised transcranial direct current stimulation (tDCS) in multiple sclerosis (MS). *Journal of Visualized Experiments : JoVE, 106*, e53542.

Kayser, S., Bewernick, B., Matusch, A., Hurlemann, R., Soehle, M., & Schlaepfer, T. E. (2015). Magnetic seizure therapy in treatment-resistant depression: Clinical, neuropsychological and metabolic effects. *Psychological Medicine, 45*(05), 1073–1092.

Keeser, D., Meindl, T., Bor, J., Palm, U., Pogarell, O., Mulert, C., … Padberg, F. (2011). Prefrontal transcranial direct current stimulation changes connectivity of resting-state networks during fMRI. *The Journal of Neuroscience, 31*(43), 15284–15293.

Kim, J. H., Kim, D. W., Chang, W. H., Kim, Y. H., & Im, C. H. (2013). Inconsistent outcomes of transcranial direct current stimulation (tDCS) may be originated from the anatomical differences among individuals: A simulation study using individual MRI data. *Conference Proceedings: Annual International Conference of the IEEE Engineering in Medicine and Biology Society, 2013*, 823–825.

Kim, M. S., Koo, H., Han, S. W., Paulus, W., Nitsche, M. A., Kim, Y. H., … Shin, Y. I. (2017). Repeated anodal transcranial direct current stimulation induces neural plasticity-associated gene expression in the rat cortex and hippocampus. *Restorative Neurology and Neuroscience*.

Kincses, T. Z., Antal, A., Nitsche, M. A., Bártfai, O., & Paulus, W. (2004). Facilitation of probabilistic classification learning by transcranial direct current stimulation of the prefrontal cortex in the human. *Neuropsychologia, 42*(1), 113–117.

Knotkova, H., Riggs, A., Patel, V., Troung, D., Arce, D., Bernstein, H., … Bikson, M. (2017a). Processing #24 a novel approach to determining M1 tDCS montage without neuronavigational measurements, suitable for patients in home settings. *Brain Stimulation: Basic, Translational, and Clinical Research in Neuromodulation, 10*(4), e78–e80.

Knotkova, H., Riggs, A., & Portenoy, R. K. (2017b). Proceedings #23 a patient-tailored protocol of tDCS stimulation paired with telehealth support for at-home symptom management in seriously ill patients with multiple chronic symptoms. *Brain Stimulation: Basic, Translational, and Clinical Research in Neuromodulation, 10*(4), e77–e78.

Knutson, R. C., Tichy, F. Y., & Reitman, J. H. (1956). The use of electrical current as an anesthetic agent. *The Journal of the American Society of Anesthesiologists, 17*(6), 815–825.

Kraus, T., Kiess, O., Hösl, K., Terekhin, P., Kornhuber, J., & Forster, C. (2013). CNS BOLD fMRI effects of sham-controlled transcutaneous electrical nerve stimulation in the left outer auditory canal – a pilot study. *Brain Stimulation, 6*(5), 798–804.

Kronberg, G., & Bikson, M. (2012). Electrode assembly design for transcranial direct current stimulation: A FEM modeling study. *Conference Proceedings: Annual International Conference of the IEEE Engineering in Medicine and Biology Society, 2012*, 891–895.

Kronberg, G., Bridi, M., Abel, T., Bikson, M., & Parra, L. C. (2017). direct current stimulation modulates LTP and LTD: Activity dependence and dendritic effects. *Brain Stimulation, 10*(1), 51–58.

Kuo, H.-I., Bikson, M., Datta, A., Minhas, P., Paulus, W., Kuo, M.-F., & Nitsche, M. A. (2013). Comparing cortical plasticity induced by conventional and high-definition 4× 1 ring tDCS: A neurophysiological study. *Brain Stimulation, 6*(4), 644–648.

Leduc, S. (1914). Cerebral electrization. *Archives of the Roentgen Ray, 19*(5), 160–162.

Leduc, S., & Rouxeau, A. (1903). Influence du rythme et de la period sur la production de l'inhibition par les courants intermittents de basse tension. *CR Seances Soc Biology, 55*, 899–901.

Lefaucheur, J.-P., André-Obadia, N., Antal, A., Ayache, S. S., Baeken, C., Benninger, D. H., … Garcia-Larrea, L. (2014). Evidence-based guidelines on the therapeutic use of repetitive transcranial magnetic stimulation (rTMS). *Clinical Neurophysiology, 125*(11), 2150–2206.

Lefaucheur, J. P., Antal, A., Ahdab, R., Ciampi de Andrade, D., Fregni, F., Khedr, E. M., … Paulus, W. (2008). The use of repetitive transcranial magnetic stimulation (rTMS) and transcranial direct current stimulation (tDCS) to relieve pain. *Brain Stimulation, 1*(4), 337–344.

Lefaucheur, J. P., Antal, A., Ayache, S. S., Benninger, D. H., Brunelin, J., Cogiamanian, F., … Paulus, W. (2017). Evidence-based guidelines on the therapeutic use of transcranial direct current stimulation (tDCS). *Clinical Neurophysiology, 128*(1), 56–92.

Legon, W., Sato, T. F., Opitz, A., Mueller, J., Barbour, A., Williams, A., & Tyler, W. J. (2014). Transcranial focused ultrasound modulates the activity of primary somatosensory cortex in humans. *Nature Neuroscience, 17*(2), 322–329.

Leite, J., Carvalho, S., Fregni, F., Boggio, P. S., & Goncalves OF. (2013). The effects of cross-hemispheric dorsolateral prefrontal cortex transcranial direct current stimulation (tDCS) on task switching. *Brain Stimulation, 6*(4), 660–667.

Lifshitz, K., & Harper, P. (1968). A trial of transcranial polarization in chronic schizophrenics. *The British Journal of Psychiatry: the Journal of Mental Science, 114*(510), 635.

Limoge, A., Robert, C., & Stanley, T. H. (1999). Transcutaneous cranial electrical stimulation (TCES): A review 1998. *Neuroscience and Biobehavioral Reviews, 23*(4), 529–538.

Lin, R. L., Douaud, G., Filippini, N., Okell, T. W., Stagg, C. J., & Tracey, I. (2017). Structural connectivity variances underlie functional and behavioral changes during pain relief induced by neuromodulation. *Scientific Reports, 7*, 41603.

Lisanby, S. H., Luber, B., Schlaepfer, T. E., & Sackeim, H. A. (2003). Safety and feasibility of magnetic seizure therapy (MST) in major depression: Randomized within-subject comparison with electroconvulsive therapy. *Neuropsychopharmacology, 28*(10), 1852.

Lopez-Quintero, S. V., Datta, A., Amaya, R., Elwassif, M., Bikson, M., & Tarbell, J. M. (2010). DBS-relevant electric fields increase hydraulic conductivity of in vitro endothelial monolayers. *Journal of Neural Engineering, 7*(1), 16005.

Mancini, M., Brignani, D., Conforto, S., Mauri, P., Miniussi, C., & Pellicciari, M. C. (2016). Assessing cortical synchronization during transcranial direct current stimulation: A graph-theoretical analysis. *NeuroImage, 140*, 57–65.

Marshall, L., Molle, M., Hallschmid, M., & Born, J. (2004). Transcranial direct current stimulation during sleep improves declarative memory. *The Journal of Neuroscience, 24*(44), 9985–9992.

McIntyre, C. C., Grill, W. M., Sherman, D. L., & Thakor, N. V. (2004). Cellular effects of deep brain stimulation: Model-based analysis of activation and inhibition. *Journal of Neurophysiology, 91*(4), 1457–1469.

Merrill, D. R., Bikson, M., & Jefferys, J. G. (2005). Electrical stimulation of excitable tissue: Design of efficacious and safe protocols. *Journal of Neuroscience Methods, 141*(2), 171–198.

Merton, P., & Morton, H. (1980). Stimulation of the cerebral cortex in the intact human subject. *Nature, 285*(5762), 227–227.

Minhas, P., Bansal, V., Patel, J., Ho, J. S., Diaz, J., Datta, A., & Bikson, M. (2010). Electrodes for high-definition transcutaneous DC stimulation for applications in drug delivery and electrotherapy, including tDCS. *Journal of Neuroscience Methods, 190*(2), 188–197.

Miranda, P. C., Lomarev, M., & Hallett, M. (2006). Modeling the current distribution during transcranial direct current stimulation. *Clinical Neurophysiology, 117*(7), 1623–1629.

Monai, H., Ohkura, M., Tanaka, M., Oe, Y., Konno, A., Hirai, H., … Hirase, H. (2016). Calcium imaging reveals glial involvement in transcranial direct current stimulation-induced plasticity in mouse brain. *Nature Communications, 7*, 11100.

Monte-Silva, K., Kuo, M.-F., Liebetanz, D., Paulus, W., & Nitsche, M. A. (2010). Shaping the optimal repetition interval for cathodal transcranial direct current stimulation (tDCS). *Journal of Neurophysiology, 103*(4), 1735–1740.

Morales-Quezada, L., Cosmo, C., Carvalho, S., Leite, J., Castillo-Saavedra, L., Rozisky, J., & Fregni, F. (2015). Cognitive effects and autonomic responses to transcranial pulsed current stimulation. *Experimental Brain Research, 233*(3), 701–709.

Mulquiney, P. G., Hoy, K. E., Daskalakis, Z. J., & Fitzgerald, P. B. (2011). Improving working memory: Exploring the effect of transcranial random noise stimulation and transcranial direct current stimulation on the dorsolateral prefrontal cortex. *Clinical Neurophysiology, 122*(12), 2384–2389.

Nair, D. G., Renga, V., Lindenberg, R., Zhu, L., & Schlaug, G. (2011). Optimizing recovery potential through simultaneous occupational therapy and non-invasive brain-stimulation using tDCS. *Restorative Neurology and Neuroscience, 29*(6), 411–420.

Naro, A., Milardi, D., Russo, M., Terranova, C., Rizzo, V., Cacciola, A., … Quartarone, A. (2016). Non-invasive brain stimulation, a tool to revert maladaptive plasticity in neuropathic pain. *Frontiers in Human Neuroscience, 10*, 376.

Newth, A. (1873). The galvanic current applied in the treatment of insanity. *The Journal of Mental Science, 1874*(19), 79–86.

Nikolin, S., Loo, C. K., Bai, S., Dokos, S., & Martin, D. M. (2015). Focalised stimulation using high definition transcranial direct current stimulation (HD-tDCS) to investigate declarative verbal learning and memory functioning. *NeuroImage, 117*, 11–19.

Nitsche, M., & Paulus, W. (2000). Excitability changes induced in the human motor cortex by weak transcranial direct current stimulation. *The Journal of Physiology, 527*(3), 633–639.

Nitsche, M. A., Doemkes, S., Karakose, T., Antal, A., Liebetanz, D., Lang, N., … Paulus, W. (2007). Shaping the effects of transcranial direct current stimulation of the human motor cortex. *Journal of Neurophysiology, 97*(4), 3109–3117.

Nitsche, M. A., Seeber, A., Frommann, K., Klein, C. C., Rochford, C., Nitsche, M. S., … Tergau, F. (2005). Modulating parameters of excitability during and after transcranial direct current stimulation of the human motor cortex. *The Journal of Physiology, 568*(Pt 1), 291–303.

Nizard, J., Lefaucheur, J.-P., Helbert, M., de Chauvigny, E., & Nguyen, J.-P. (2012). Non-invasive stimulation therapies for the treatment of refractory pain. *Discovery Medicine, 14*(74), 21–31.

Noury, N., Hipp, J. F., & Siegel, M. (2016). Physiological processes non-linearly affect electrophysiological recordings during transcranial electric stimulation. *NeuroImage, 140*, 99–109.

Oh, M. Y., Ortega, J., Bellotte, J. B., Whiting, D. M., & Aló, K. (2004). Peripheral nerve stimulation for the treatment of occipital neuralgia and transformed migraine using a C1-2-3 subcutaneous paddle style electrode: A technical report. *Neuromodulation: Technology at the Neural Interface, 7*(2), 103–112.

Ohn, S. H., Park, C.-I., Yoo, W.-K., Ko, M.-H., Choi, K. P., Kim, G.-M., … Kim, Y.-H. (2008). Time-dependent effect of transcranial direct current stimulation on the enhancement of working memory. *Neuroreport, 19*(1), 43–47.

Opitz, A., Paulus, W., Will, S., Antunes, A., & Thielscher, A. (2015). Determinants of the electric field during transcranial direct current stimulation. *NeuroImage, 109*, 140–150.

Otal, B., Dutta, A., Foerster, A., Ripolles, O., Kuceyeski, A., Miranda, P. C., … Ruffini, G. (2016). Opportunities for guided multichannel non-invasive transcranial current stimulation in poststroke rehabilitation. *Frontiers in Neurology, 7*, 21.

Paneri, B., Adair, D., Thomas, C., Khadka, N., Patel, V., Tyler, W. J., … Bikson, M. (2016). Tolerability of repeated application of transcranial electrical stimulation with limited outputs to healthy subjects. *Brain Stimulation, 9*(5), 740–754.

Parent, A. (2004). Giovanni Aldini: from animal electricity to human brain stimulation. *The Canadian Journal of Neurological Sciences, 31*(04), 576–584.

Paulus, W. (2011). Transcranial electrical stimulation (tES–tDCS; tRNS, tACS) methods. *Neuropsychological Rehabilitation, 21*(5), 602–617.

Paulus, W., Peterchev, A. V., & Ridding, M. (2013). Transcranial electric and magnetic stimulation: Technique and paradigms. *Handb Clinical Neurology, 116*, 329–342.

Peterchev, A. V., Wagner, T. A., Miranda, P. C., Nitsche, M. A., Paulus, W., Lisanby, S. H., … Bikson, M. (2012). Fundamentals of transcranial electric and magnetic stimulation dose: Definition, selection, and reporting practices. *Brain Stimulation, 5*(4), 435–453.

Priori, A. (2003). Brain polarization in humans: A reappraisal of an old tool for prolonged non-invasive modulation of brain excitability. *Clinical Neurophysiology, 114*(4), 589–595.

Radman, T., Ramos, R. L., Brumberg, J. C., & Bikson, M. (2009). Role of cortical cell type and morphology in subthreshold and suprathreshold uniform electric field stimulation in vitro. *Brain Stimulation, 2*(4), 215–228.e213.

Rahman, A., Reato, D., Arlotti, M., Gasca, F., Datta, A., Parra, L. C., & Bikson, M. (2013). Cellular effects of acute direct current stimulation: Somatic and synaptic terminal effects. *The Journal of Physiology, 591*(10), 2563–2578.

Reato, D., Rahman, A., Bikson, M., & Parra, L. C. (2013). Effects of weak transcranial alternating current stimulation on brain activity-a review of known mechanisms from animal studies. *Frontiers in Human Neuroscience, 7*, 687.

Redfearn, J., Lippold, O., & Costain, R. (1964). Preliminary account of the clinical effects of polarizing the brain in certain psychiatric disorders. *The British Journal of Psychiatry, 110*(469), 773–785.

Reis, J., Fischer, J. T., Prichard, G., Weiller, C., Cohen, L. G., & Fritsch, B. (2015). Time- but not sleep-dependent consolidation of tdcs-enhanced visuomotor skills. *Cerebral Cortex, 25*(1), 109–117.

Robertson, V. J., Low, J., Ward, A., & Reed, A. (2006). *Electrotherapy explained: Principles and practice*. Elsevier Health Sciences.

Robinovitch, L. (1914). *Electrical analgesia, sleep and resuscitation. Anesthesia*. New York, NY: Appleton.

Rohan, M., Parow, A., Stoll, A. L., Demopulos, C., Friedman, S., Dager, S., … Renshaw, P. F. (2004). Low-field magnetic stimulation in bipolar depression using an MRI-based stimulator. *The American Journal of Psychiatry, 161*(1), 93–98.

Roy, A., Baxter, B., & He, B. (2014). High-definition transcranial direct current stimulation induces both acute and persistent changes in broadband cortical synchronization: A simultaneous tDCS-EEG study. *IEEE Transactions on Biomedical Engineering, 61*(7), 1967–1978.

Ruffini, G., Wendling, F., Merlet, I., Molaee-Ardekani, B., Mekonnen, A., Salvador, R., … Miranda, P. C. (2013). Transcranial current brain stimulation (tCS): Models and technologies. *IEEE Transactions on Neural Systems and Rehabilitation Engineering, 21*(3), 333–345.

Russo, C., Souza Carneiro, M. I., Bolognini, N., & Fregni, F. (2017). Safety review of transcranial direct current stimulation in stroke. *Neuromodulation*.

Salvador, R., Mekonnen, A., Ruffini, G., & Miranda, P. C. (2010). Modeling the electric field induced in a high resolution realistic head model during transcranial current stimulation. *Conference Proceedings: Annual International Conference of the IEEE Engineering in Medicine and Biology Society, 2010*, 2073–2076.

Samoudi, G., Nissbrandt, H., Dutia, M. B., & Bergquist, F. (2012). Noisy galvanic vestibular stimulation promotes GABA release in the substantia nigra and improves locomotion in hemiparkinsonian rats. *PLoS One, 7*(1), e29308.

Schlaug, G., Renga, V., & Nair, D. (2008). Transcranial direct current stimulation in stroke recovery. *Archives of Neurology, 65*(12), 1571–1576.

Schmitt, R., Capo, T., & Boyd, E. (1986). Cranial electrotherapy stimulation as a treatment for anxiety in chemically dependent persons. *Alcoholism: Clinical and Experimental Research, 10*(2), 158–160.

Schoenen, J., Vandersmissen, B., Jeangette, S., Herroelen, L., Vandenheede, M., Gérard, P., & Magis, D. (2013). Migraine prevention with a supraorbital transcutaneous stimulator A randomized controlled trial. *Neurology, 80*(8), 697–704.

Shekhawat, G. S., Sundram, F., Bikson, M., Truong, D., De Ridder, D., Stinear, C. M., … Searchfield, G. D. (2015). Intensity, duration, and location of high-definition transcranial direct current stimulation for tinnitus relief. *Neurorehabilitation and Neural Repair, 30*(4), 349–359.

Shelyakin, A., Preobrazhenskaya, I., Pisar'kova, E., Pakhomova, Z. M., & Bogdanov, O. (1998). Effects of transcranial micropolarization of the frontal cortex on the state of motor and cognitive functions in extrapyramidal pathology. *Neuroscience and Behavioral Physiology, 28*(4), 468–471.

Shen, B., Yin, Y., Wang, J., Zhou, X., McClure, S. M., & Li, J. (2016). High-definition tDCS alters impulsivity in a baseline-dependent manner. *NeuroImage, 143*, 343–352.

Shiozawa, P., da Silva, M. E., Raza, R., Uchida, R. R., Cordeiro, Q., Fregni, F., & Brunoni, A. R. (2013). Safety of repeated transcranial direct current stimulation in impaired skin: A case report. *The Journal of ECT, 29*(2), 147–148.

Slavin, K. V., Colpan, M. E., Munawar, N., Wess, C., & Nersesyan, H. (2006). Trigeminal and occipital peripheral nerve stimulation for craniofacial pain: A single-institution experience and review of the literature. *Neurosurgical Focus, 21*(6), 1–5.

Smith, R., Tatsuno, J., & Zouhar, R. (1967). Electroanesthesia: A review-1966. *Anesthesia and Analgesia, 46*(1), 109.

Smith, R. B. (2006). *Cranial electrotherapy stimulation: Its first fifty years, plus three*. Washington DC: A Monograph.

Spagnolo, P. A., & Goldman, D. (2017). Neuromodulation interventions for addictive disorders: Challenges, promise, and roadmap for future research. *Brain*.

Spellman, T., Peterchev, A. V., & Lisanby, S. H. (2009). Focal electrically administered seizure therapy: A novel form of ECT illustrates the roles of current directionality, polarity, and electrode configuration in seizure induction. *Neuropsychopharmacology, 34*(8), 2002–2010.

Stagg, C. J., & Nitsche, M. A. (2011). Physiological basis of transcranial direct current stimulation. *The Neuroscientist, 17*(1), 37–53.

Teichmann, M., Lesoil, C., Godard, J., Vernet, M., Bertrand, A., Levy, R., … Valero-Cabre, A. (2016). Direct current stimulation over the anterior temporal areas boosts semantic processing in primary progressive aphasia. *Annals of Neurology, 80*(5), 693–707.

Terney, D., Chaieb, L., Moliadze, V., Antal, A., & Paulus, W. (2008). Increasing human brain excitability by transcranial high-frequency random noise stimulation. *The Journal of Neuroscience, 28*(52), 14147–14155.

Truong, D. Q., Huber, M., Xie, X., Datta, A., Rahman, A., Parra, L. C., … Bikson, M. (2014). Clinician accessible tools for GUI computational models of transcranial electrical stimulation: BONSAI and SPHERES. *Brain Stimulation, 7*(4), 521–524.

Truong, D. Q., Magerowski, G., Blackburn, G. L., Bikson, M., & Alonso-Alonso, M. (2013). Computational modeling of transcranial direct current stimulation (tDCS) in obesity: Impact of head fat and dose guidelines. *NeuroImage Clinical, 2*, 759–766.

Villamar, M. F., Volz, M. S., Bikson, M., Datta, A., DaSilva, A. F., & Fregni, F. (2013a). Technique and considerations in the use of 4x1 ring high-definition transcranial direct current stimulation (HD-tDCS). *JoVE: Journal of Visualized Experiments*, (77), e50309–e50309.

Villamar, M. F., Wivatvongvana, P., Patumanond, J., Bikson, M., Truong, D. Q., Datta, A., & Fregni, F. (2013b). Focal modulation of the primary motor cortex in fibromyalgia using 4x1-ring high-definition transcranial direct current stimulation (HD-tDCS): Immediate and delayed analgesic effects of cathodal and anodal stimulation. *The Journal of Pain, 14*(4), 371–383.

Volta, A. (1800). On the electricity excited by the mere contact of conducting substances of different kinds. In a letter from Mr. Alexander Volta, FRS Professor of Natural Philosophy in the University of Pavia, to the Rt. Hon. Sir Joseph Banks, Bart. KBPRS. *Philosophical Transactions of the Royal Society of London*, 403–431.

Wagner, S., Lucka, F., Vorwerk, J., Herrmann, C. S., Nolte, G., Burger, M., & Wolters, C. H. (2016). Using reciprocity for relating the simulation of transcranial current stimulation to the EEG forward problem. *NeuroImage, 140*, 163–173.

Wagner, T., Fregni, F., Fecteau, S., Grodzinsky, A., Zahn, M., & Pascual-Leone, A. (2007). Transcranial direct current stimulation: A computer-based human model study. *NeuroImage, 35*(3), 1113–1124.

Wilson, A. S., Sances, A., & Larson, S. J. (1968). Effect of electroanesthesia on timing behavior. *Anesthesia and Analgesia, 47*(6), 663-667.

Woods, A. J., Antal, A., Bikson, M., Boggio, P. S., Brunoni, A. R., Celnik, P., ... Nitsche, M. A. (2016). A technical guide to tDCS, and related non-invasive brain stimulation tools. *Clinical Neurophysiology, 127*(2), 1031–1048.

Yamamoto, Y., Struzik, Z. R., Soma, R., Ohashi, K., & Kwak, S. (2005). Noisy vestibular stimulation improves autonomic and motor responsiveness in central neurodegenerative disorders. *Annals of Neurology, 58*(2), 175–181.

Zaghi, S., Acar, M., Hultgren, B., Boggio, P. S., & Fregni, F. (2009). Noninvasive brain stimulation with low-intensity electrical currents: Putative mechanisms of action for direct and alternating current stimulation. *The Neuroscientist, 16*(3), 285–307.

Zaghi, S., Acar, M., Hultgren, B., Boggio, P. S., & Fregni, F. (2010). Noninvasive brain stimulation with low-intensity electrical currents: Putative mechanisms of action for direct and alternating current stimulation. *The Neuroscientist, 16*(3), 285–307.

Zaghi, S., Thiele, B., Pimentel, D., Pimentel, T., & Fregni, F. (2011). Assessment and treatment of pain with non-invasive cortical stimulation. *Restorative Neurology and Neuroscience, 29*(6), 439–451.

Zentner, J., Kiss, I., & Ebner, A. (1989). Influence of anesthetics-nitrous oxide in particular-on electromyographic response evoked by transcranial electrical stimulation of the cortex. *Neurosurgery, 24*(2), 253–256.

Zhu, C. E., Yu, B., Zhang, W., Chen, W. H., Qi, Q., & Miao, Y. (2017). Effiectiveness and safety of transcranial direct current stimulation in fibromyalgia: A systematic review and meta-analysis. *Journal of Rehabilitation Medicine, 49*(1), 2–9.

Chapter 2
Principles of Transcranial Direct Current Stimulation (tDCS): Introduction to the Biophysics of tDCS

Davide Reato, Ricardo Salvador, Marom Bikson, Alexander Opitz, Jacek Dmochowski, and Pedro C. Miranda

Human research on transcranial electrical stimulation provides direct evidence that weak electric currents can affect brain function in health and disease. However, limitations on both the control of stimulation delivery (including, e.g., dose/repetition and anatomical variations), factors known to influence modulation (e.g., brain state) and variability of outcome measures make it difficult to delineate a general framework to explain the effects of the stimulation based solely on human research. In this regard, computational models of tDCS and animal studies, either in vivo or in vitro, can help to develop a specific biophysical framework while being informed by results from humans.

The biophysics of tDCS, and more broadly neuromodulation, is based on specific and quantitative (equation-based) models of brain stimulation with explicit parameters (preferably based on measurable physical quantities such as field strength, membrane potential) and well-defined brain signals whose neuronal substrates are known. This is required to guarantee testable and refutable hypothesis.

D. Reato (✉)
Champalimaud Centre for the Unknown, Neuroscience Programme, Lisbon, Portugal
e-mail: davide.reato@neuro.fchampalimaud.org

R. Salvador
Neuroelectrics, Barcelona, Spain

M. Bikson
Department of Biomedical Engineering, The City College of New York, New York, NY, USA

A. Opitz
Department of Biomedical Engineering, University of Minnesota, Minneapolis, MN, USA

J. Dmochowski
Neural Engineering Laboratory, Department of Biomedical Engineering, Grove School of Engineering, The City College of the City University of New York, New York, NY, USA

P. C. Miranda
Instituto de Biofísica e Engenharia Biomédica, Faculdade de Ciências, Universidade de Lisboa, Lisbon, Portugal

H. Knotkova et al. (eds.), *Practical Guide to Transcranial Direct Current Stimulation*, https://doi.org/10.1007/978-3-319-95948-1_2

Each biophysical model of tDCS must support an incremental establishment of a comprehensive theory for tDCS. This is in contrast to more heuristic or qualitative descriptions of tDCS (e.g. "anodal stimulation makes the brain more excitable which increases function.") – such theories are typically a priori used to justify trials (e.g. "anode over dorsolateral prefrontal cortex [dLPFC] to boost mood") rather than test refutable mechanistic hypothesis.

In this chapter we describe the biophysics of tDCS. In the first section we review the basic physical principles that describe how computational models relate the electric current applied at the electrodes to electric field generated inside the brain. In the second part, we illustrate how such electric fields affect neuronal activity, focusing on results from animal studies because they allow a direct link between stimulation parameters and neuronal substrate.

Physical Principles

Transcranial direct current stimulation (tDCS) is a non-invasive technique which has been shown to modulate cortical excitability (Nitsche and Paulus 2000, 2001) and is currently envisioned as a promising tool in several neurological and psychiatric disorders, as well as stroke recovery and chronic pain (Fregni et al. 2006; Nitsche et al. 2009; Nitsche and Paulus 2009; Schlaug et al. 2008). The neuromodulatory effects elicited by tDCS depend on the electric field (E-field, measured in *Volts per meter*, *V/m*) induced in the nervous system. This field is induced by two or more electrodes placed in contact with the scalp and connected to a stimulation device. The electrodes consist of conductive materials, such as metal or conductive rubber, connected to stimulator leads. This material is in contact with a conductive solution, the electrolyte, which is usually a conductive fluid or a gel. Examples of the latter include large (25 or 35 cm^2) "sponge-sock" electrodes soaked in physiological saline solution, with a conductive rubber pad, which is connected to the stimulator wires, located inside (Minhas et al. 2010; Nitsche et al. 2008; Ruffini et al. 2013; Saturnino et al. 2015). Smaller electrodes usually use gel as an electrolyte (Ruffini et al. 2014; Sehm et al. 2013). In modern current-controlled stimulators, the current (*I* measured in *Amperes*, *A*) that enters the volume (via the electrodes) is controlled during the stimulation (Peterchev et al. 2012). In these stimulators, the voltage difference between the electrodes is controlled by the device so that the current reaches the intensity specified by the user regardless of the time-varying impedance at the electrode-skin interface. The current flows from the anode to the cathode and the voltage difference between these two electrodes is always positive in tDCS (although not constant [Minhas et al. 2010]).

A weak, 1–2 mA, and long lasting, 1–30 min, current is usually chosen in tDCS (Nitsche et al. 2008). The current is kept constant throughout the protocol, except at the beginning/end, where it increases/decreases linearly in time: ramp-up/down period. The duration of these ramp periods is usually 10 s (Minhas et al. 2010;

Nitsche et al. 2008). For purely resistive tissues, a valid approximation for DC signals (as discussed below), the E-field induced in the head during tDCS is proportional to the applied current (Peterchev et al. 2012). The spatial distribution of the E-field and its direction depend on several other parameters, like the shape and positions of the electrodes (Saturnino et al. 2015), the current injected by each electrode, the geometry of the head tissues (Opitz et al. 2015) and their electrical conductivity properties (Datta et al. 2009; Miranda et al. 2006; Miranda et al. 2013). The way neurons are affected by the E-field depends on its magnitude and direction, as will be discussed in more detail later in this chapter, as well as on the duration of stimulation. The calculation of the E-field in the head volume for a given electrode montage is deemed the "forward problem" in tDCS. The mathematical formulation of the forward problem in tDCS is well known from electrostatics: the E-field induced in the head can be obtained from the gradient of a scalar function (the electric potential, V measured in *Volts*) which is a solution of the Laplace equation (Rush and Driscoll 1968, 1969). However, analytical solutions of the resulting equations can usually only be obtained in simple approximations for the head geometry (such as a spherical geometry (Dmochowski et al. 2012) and hence numerical methods are commonly employed to obtain the E-field (Datta et al. 2009; Miranda et al. 2013).

Electric Properties of Tissues

In general, for electrical stimulation using arbitrary waveforms, the current induced in the head can be divided into an ohmic (resistive) component and a displacement (capacitive) current. The first component arises from the movement of the free ions that exist in the intra and extracellular fluids of the head tissues. The property of materials that describes how well they can conduct electricity by means of free charges is called electrical conductivity (σ in *Siemens per meter, S/m*). The second component of the current results from the polarization of localized charge distributions in the cellular membrane (Pethig and Kell 1987). The permittivity (ε in *Farads per meter, F/m*) of a medium is a measure of how easy this polarization is induced by an applied E-field. The values of these dielectric properties (σ and ε) depend on the frequency of the currents: permittivity values decrease with frequency, whereas conductivity values increase with it (Pethig and Kell 1987).

For purely ohmic materials, the waveform of the E-field follows that of the current. When capacitive currents exist, this is no longer the case and strong distortions of the current's waveform can occur (Wagner et al. 2014a). The latter exist only when the current varies with time. Since, the current in tDCS is mostly constant during stimulation, the displacement current can be considered zero. Even during the ramp-up/down period, when the current changes in time, the relatively low rate of change with time will not give rise to a strong displacement current (Opitz et al. 2016).

Knowledge about the conductivity of biological tissues is therefore crucial in tDCS. Several studies have appeared reporting measurements of these properties in biological tissues in a wide range of frequencies (Baumann et al. 1997; Gabriel et al. 1996a, b; Geddes and Baker 1967; Koessler et al. 2016; Logothetis et al. 2007; Oostendorp et al. 2000). The disparity between recording methods, tissue preparation and types (*in vivo* vs *ex vivo*) however, has led to the appearance of inconsistent data among studies (Gabriel et al. 1996a; Wagner et al. 2014a). This is especially true in the DC to low frequency range because measuring the dielectric properties in that region is technically more challenging (Schwan 1966; Wagner et al. 2014a). These uncertainties are a major cause for concern regarding computational predictions of E-field distributions during tDCS since changes in tissue conductivity values have been shown to significantly affect the E-field peak values and distribution (Laakso et al. 2015; Salvador et al. 2012).

Another important aspect concerning the conductivity and permittivity values is the fact that they are anisotropic in some tissues, i.e. the dielectric properties of the tissues are different depending on direction. This is typically due to the presence of structures that limit the flow of ions along specific directions. In the white matter (WM) the limiting structures are the axons of the neurons that constitute this tissue. These typically constrain the movement of ions in a direction parallel to the fiber (Geddes and Baker 1967). In the skull, anisotropy results from the presence of three layers of different tissues: a layer of cancellous bone between two layers of more insulating compact bone in the top part of the skull (Akhtari et al. 2002). This arrangement results in a higher effective conductivity in a direction tangential to the skull surface compared to the effective conductivity perpendicular to it (e.g. Opitz et al. 2015; Rampersad et al. 2011; Wagner et al. 2014b).

For anisotropic media, the conductivity is described as a symmetric tensor. In the WM, the conductivity tensor can be estimated via diffusion tensor imaging (DTI) (Basser et al. 1994). DTI allows for the estimation of the water molecules' diffusion tensor by acquiring diffusion weighted images (DWI) along several directions (Huisman 2010). Since the flow of ions and water molecules is thought to be constrained by the same structures, the conductivity tensor can then be obtained from the diffusion tensor (Tuch et al. 2001). This method, however, is limited by the fact that the scaling of the diffusion tensor components can be done in a variety of image processing ways and each produce very different conductivity values which highly affects the E-field calculations (Opitz et al. 2011; Tuch et al. 2001).

The Spatial Distribution of the Electric Field: Insights from Modelling Studies

The E-field induced in the head during tDCS is a vector whose magnitude and direction changes from tissue to tissue but also within each individual tissue. Since most computational studies model the tissues as connected volumes bounded by smooth surfaces (Datta et al. 2009; Miranda et al. 2006, 2013), discontinuities arise in the E-field's magnitude and direction at these surfaces, provided the two tissues that are separated by them have different conductivities (Miranda et al. 2003). The discontinuities are such that the magnitude of the E-field's component in the direction perpendicular to the surface (the normal component) is always higher in the side of the surface belonging to the tissue with the lowest conductivity. This discontinuity is proportional to the ratio between the difference and the sum of the conductivities of the two tissues (Miranda et al. 2003). No such effect occurs for the component of the E-field parallel to the surface (the tangential component), which is continuous across these interfaces (Tofts 1990). This also means that the E-field's principal direction tends to be perpendicular to the interfaces in the tissues with very low bulk conductivities (like the skull) and parallel to them in tissues with comparatively high conductivities (like the cerebrospinal fluid). In many modelling studies, the current density (J in *Ampere per squared meter*, A/m^2) is reported instead of the E-field (Sadleir et al. 2010). The latter is also a vector which, in isotropic media, is proportional to the E-field: J is the product of the electric conductivity and the E-field. For anisotropic media, since the conductivity can no longer be described by a scalar but by a matrix instead (conductivity tensor), the current's density direction is no longer the same as that of the E-field (Miranda et al. 2003).

Most of what is presently known about the E-field distribution comes from computational modelling studies. The results obtained in these models can sometimes be counterintuitive. An example of one of such result is the fact that the E-field magnitude on the scalp under each electrode is not homogeneous. This can be seen in Fig. 2.1a, where the maxima of the E-field's magnitude are seen to be located at the electrode's edges. This also shows that the metric reported in many different studies, the ratio of the current to the electrode's area, cannot be used to estimate the current density under the electrode since the latter, like the E-field, is not uniformly distributed under the electrodes (see also Miranda et al. 2009). The maxima on the scalp are also much higher than those attained in the brain.

Another counterintuitive aspect of the E-field's distribution in tDCS arises when one analyses it in the brain. The E-field shown in Fig. 2.1b, e displays properties in line with results from spherical head models (Datta et al. 2008; Miranda et al. 2006): a stronger field at the top of the gyri beneath the electrodes and with a direction perpendicular to the local cortical sheet and tangential to it in the region in between the electrodes. These results, however, were obtained for a fully homogeneous model (all tissues represented with the same conductivity value). A more realistic model for the conductivities of the tissues results in the E-field distributions shown in Fig. 2.1d, g. These results, which have been shown in a number of modelling studies (Datta et al. 2009; Miranda et al. 2013), arise from the effects of the low conductivity of the skull, which reduce the magnitude of the E-field in the brain (compare Fig. 2.1b with c). Another contribution comes from the combination of the high conductivity of the CSF, and the convoluted geometry of the corti-

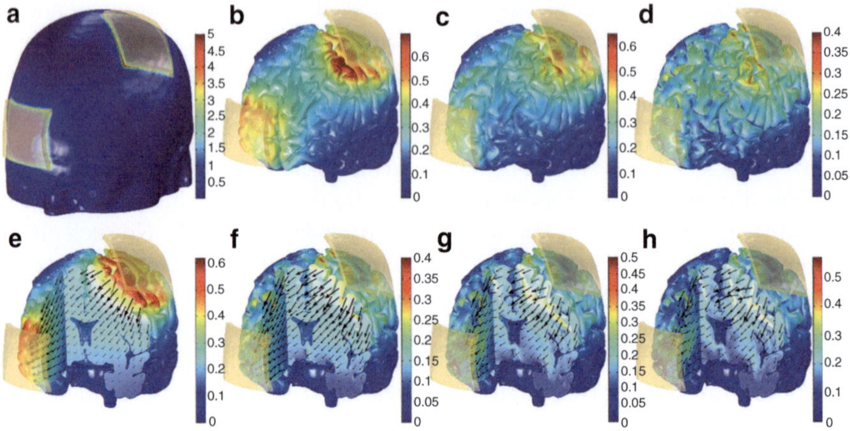

Fig. 2.1 Impact of the electrical conductivities of the tissues in E-field distribution in a realistic head model. The model contains two homogeneous electrodes ($\sigma_{electrodes} = 2\ S/m$) located over the left hemisphere's hand-knob region (anode) and the right supra-orbital region (cathode). A current of 1 *mA* was injected at the anode. (**a, b**) E-fields distribution in the scalp (**a**) and the brain (**b**) in a homogeneous model where all tissues have an isotropic conductivity of 0.33 *S/m*. (**c**) Same as *B* but with the skull's conductivity set to 0.008 *S/m*. (**d**) Same as *C* but with the CSF's conductivity set to 1.79 *S/m*. (**e**) Same as *B* but now showing the direction of the E-field and its magnitude in a sagittal slice passing through the middle of the cathode and a coronal one passing through the middle of the anode. (**f**) Same as *E* but with the skull's and CSF's conductivities set to 0.008 *S/m* and 1.79 *S/m*, respectively. (**g**) Same as *F* but with the WM's conductivity set to 0.15 *S/m*. (**h**) Same as *G* but for an anisotropic conductivity for the GM and WM. False color: electric field (V/m)

cal surface. This reduces the E-field's magnitude in the brain, due to the shunting effect of the CSF, but creates localized maxima at the bottom of the sulci under the electrodes. The latter arise because the shunted current enters the GM perpendicularly at the bottom of the sulci (Miranda et al. 2013). The presence of the CSF therefore boosts the field at the bottom of the sulci in a direction perpendicular to the GM's outer surface, as shown in Fig. 2.1f. Finally, the inclusion of the WM as a tissue with different conductivities than the GM (Fig. 2.1g), introduces a discontinuity at the GM-WM interface which tends to increase the E-field in the WM (which has a lower isotropic conductivity) as compared to the one induced in a homogenous brain model (Fig. 2.1f). The inclusion of an anisotropic WM produces subtler changes in the results (compare Fig. 2.1g with h). In this case, the E-field tends to decrease along the main direction of the fibers since the latter corresponds to higher conductivity values compared to those of the isotropic case. The E-field in the direction perpendicular to the fibers tends to increase its value since the conductivity is much smaller than the ones in the isotropic model (see also Opitz et al. 2011).

Comparisons with Other Brain Stimulation Techniques

There are several other techniques which are used to induce an E-field in the brain non-invasively and thus affect the state of neurons. Two of them are closely related to tDCS because they use the same method to induce the E-field: transcranial alternating current stimulation (tACS) and random noise current stimulation (tRNS). tACS has been shown to interfere with ongoing brain waves or rhythms (Herrmann et al. 2013; Kanai et al. 2008; Zaehle et al. 2010), whereas high frequency tRNS has been shown to increase cortical excitability in the motor cortex (Moliadze et al. 2010; Terney et al. 2008). The difference is essentially related to the waveform of the current. The current remains constant in tDCS (apart from the ramp-up/down periods at the beginning and the end), whereas in tACS it varies sinusoidally in time with a low frequency (1–45 Hz) and in tRNS it follows a white-noise band-limited waveform (0.1 – 640 *Hz*). For these low frequencies, the capacitive component of the current in the tissues is still much smaller than the resistive current, so the E-field waveform is in phase with that of the current as well (Plonsey and Heppner 1967). Since the current varies between a negative and a positive maximum value, the direction of the E-field will change in time, which does not occur in tDCS.

Another technique of interest is transcranial magnetic stimulation (TMS), which has been shown to be able to elicit motor responses when used over the primary motor cortex (Barker and Jalinous 1985; Hallett 2007). TMS produces a time-varying magnetic field which will induce a time-varying E-field, a processed described by Faraday's law of electromagnetic induction (Eaton 1992). The magnetic field is generated by the passage of a very high magnitude (~1 – 3 *kA*) and short lasting (<1 *ms*) time-varying current through a coil located close to the target region in the head. The current is generated by a high-powered stimulator device connected to the coil (Peterchev et al. 2008). The E-field induced in the head depends not only on the coil's geometry and its position but also on the head geometry. Besides, it has very different properties than the one induced in tDCS, as shown in Fig. 2.2 for the field induced by a figure-8 coil in an orientation traditionally used to achieve stimulation of the motor cortex (Di Lazzaro et al. 1998). See also (Salvador et al. 2015) for a more detailed description. One of these differences is the induced E-field's magnitude, which is much higher in TMS (~100 *V*/*m*) than in tDCS (~0.4 *V*/*m*). The orientation of the field and the location of the maxima is also substantially different (compare Fig. 2.2c with d). The maxima in TMS are predominantly located at the top of the gyri under the coil and the E-field there is oriented tangentially to the cortical surface. In tDCS the orientation of the field is predominantly radial to this surface at the top of the gyri, and local maxima also appear at the bottom of the sulci where the E-field induced in TMS is already very low. The temporal variation of the induced E-field in TMS follows that of the rate of change of the current in the coil (Roth et al. 1991) which depends on stimulator

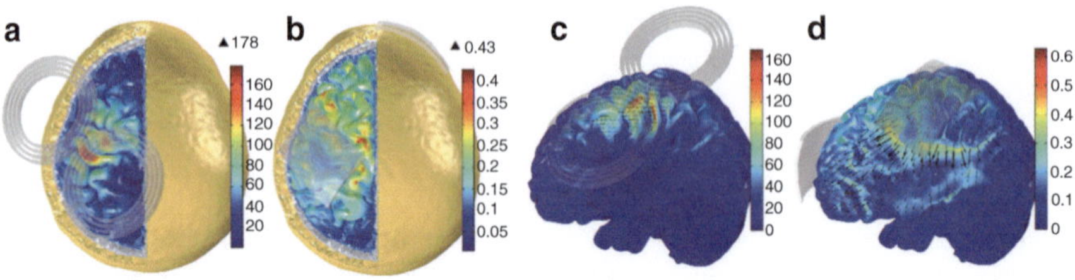

Fig. 2.2 E-field distribution in TMS (**a**, **c**) and tDCS (**b**, **d**). The first two figures show the geometry and position of the figure-8 coil (**a**) and 7 × 5 cm^2electrodes (**b**). (**c**, **d**) show the E-field distribution in a sagittal slice passing through the hand-knob cortical representation for TMS and tDCS respectively. The field induced in TMS was obtained for a value of dI/dt of 67 $A/\mu s$, whereas the current injected by the tDCS electrodes was set to 1 mA. The tissues in the head were given isotropic electrical conductivities based on values found in the literature, except the WM and GM which were modelled as anisotropic (for more details see Salvador et al. (2015). False color: electric field (V/m)

type (Peterchev et al. 2008). This has been disputed by recent studies which seem to indicate that at the frequency of variation of the E-field in TMS, the capacitive component of the induced current might be significant which could alter significantly the E-field waveform (Wagner et al. 2014a).

Effects of Weak Direct Current Stimulation on Neuronal Activity in Animal Models

The main advantage of using animal models is the possibility of directly measuring the effects of weak currents at multiple scales, from distinct compartments of single cells all the way to full populations responsible for measurable behaviors. At the same time, the stimulation parameters can be controlled usually with higher precision than human studies, pharmacological and genetic manipulations can be easily applied (in a manner dangerous or impossible in humans) and electrophysiology and imaging can be performed routinely (including small network, synapse, and single cell measurements).This section provides a review of the current experimental evidence on the effects of weak electrical direct current (DC) on neuronal activity and highlights the biophysical models that emerge from this data. Human literature on this matter, mainly coming from pharmacological interventions, is not explicitly considered here since this has been already discussed elsewhere in this book and in previous reviews (for example see Stagg and Nitsche 2011; Woods et al. 2016).

Animal research on the biophysics of DC stimulation started over a century ago. While studying the origin of voltage gradients in the brain, Fritsch and Hitzig in

1870 noticed that anodal stimulation increased the excitability of the brain while cathodal decreased it (Fritsch and Hitzig 1870). However, a first wave of quantitative research on the use of transcranial electrical stimulation to study brain function did not begin until the second half of the twentieth century. Studies using different animal preparations characterized in great details the effects of weak electric fields, such as those induced by transcranial stimulation, on neuronal activity. In the majority of these studies, however, the stimulation was used more as a tool to understand the origin of electric events/oscillations in the brain, not with the aim to validate a tool for neuromodulation (Bindman et al. 1964; Creutzfeldt et al. 1962; Terzuolo and Bullock 1956). A second wave of basic animal research on transcranial electrical stimulation started after seminal papers in humans showed that weak currents could modulate cortical excitability (Priori et al. 1998) and these changes could persist after the stimulation period (Nitsche and Paulus 2000). This second wave of animal research, that is still very active, does not aim at simply reproducing the results of human studies in animal models but, more importantly, at finding generic principles that explain how weak electric currents affect neurons and neuronal circuits.

The previous section of this chapter illustrated how computational current-flow models of transcranial electrical stimulation provide precise estimations of current densities (and electric fields) generated inside the brain. These estimates provide the numbers needed in animal studies to set the stimulation amplitudes and directions. However, knowing current flow by itself is not enough to predict the effects of such currents on neurons. Ultimately, the way a weak current affect brain function is determined by its interaction with neurons.

Brain function is evidently complex and determined by the concerted activity of large number of neurons and interconnected brain areas. These areas are composed of neuronal circuits made of different types of neurons and other non-neuronal cell types. To properly estimate the effects of weak electric currents on the brain it is therefore necessary to consider different scales: single neurons, how they are connected and interact, how they communicate with other neuronal and non-neuronal populations and how these populations ultimately support behavior usually in concert with other brain areas. As previously mentioned, animal research allows this type of multi-scale approach to study the temporal and spatial effects the stimulation.

This section describes the literature on the effects of weak direct currents on neuronal activity at these different scales in animal models. Building on prior reviews that addressed a selection of these aspects (Bikson et al. 2012; Krause et al. 2013; Márquez-Ruiz et al. 2014; Pelletier and Cicchetti 2015; Reato et al. 2013b; Woods et al. 2016), here the emphasis is on the different scales at which electric currents can affect neuronal activity. Moreover, apart for reviewing the known literature on this topic, new frontiers in this field of research and open questions are highlighted. The hope is that this may help guiding future research and that the list of open questions will look obsolete in a few years from now.

Effects of Weak Direct Current Stimulation on Membrane Potential, Firing Rate and Spike Timing

Whether neurons are passive or active affects how weak electrical stimulation affects their function. "Passive" here refers to those neurons whose membrane voltage is not close to the threshold for action potential generation (10–20 mV over resting membrane potential). In the literature, the effects of weak electric fields on this neuron would be called sub-threshold. "Active" neurons are those that receive massive synaptic inputs and are so depolarized that they occasionally (or often) generate action potentials.

Passive Neurons

The most widely accepted notion regarding the effects of DC currents on brain activity is that neurons under the anode are excited while neurons under the cathode are inhibited. This simple explanation of tDCS effects (anode: excitatory, cathode: inhibitory) is supported by seminal work of Jefferys (Jefferys 1981). By stimulating electrically granule cells in quiescent guinea-pig hippocampal slices, Jefferys showed that extracellular voltage fluctuations across a cell are able to modulate the membrane potential. This induced polarization is depolarizing (higher membrane potential) for the soma during anodal stimulation and hyperpolarizing (lower membrane potential) for cathodal, whenever neurons are aligned with their apical dendrite pointing towards the electrode. The membrane polarization at the soma affects the size of monosynaptic evoked potentials, with anodal stimulation increasing the response size while cathodal decreasing. Interestingly, Jefferys also found that the induced extracellular voltages are not uniform across neurons but changed depending on the cellular compartment. Similar results were found by Chan et al. for Purkinje cells in turtle cerebellar slices (Chan et al. 1988).

A later study by Bikson et al. (2004) further characterized Jefferys' hippocampal preparation by directly measuring the membrane polarization of hippocampal CA1 neurons and determining that the membrane potential at the soma changes linearly with the electric field magnitude in a polarity specific manner. The deflection of the membrane voltage at the soma is in the order of 0.1 mV of polarization per V/m electric field applied for pyramidal CA1 neurons. Moreover, using voltage sensitive dyes, the authors found that the polarization of neurons is compartment specific: soma depolarizing fields (anodal) hyperpolarize the dendrites and, vice-versa, soma hyperpolarizing fields (cathodal) depolarize the dendrites (Fig. 2.3a, b). These results were all consistent with the earlier findings of Jefferys (1981) and Chan et al. (1988). In addition, Bikson et al. showed that weak electric fields perpendicular to the main orientation of a neuron do not polarize the somatic membrane significantly (though may still influence function).

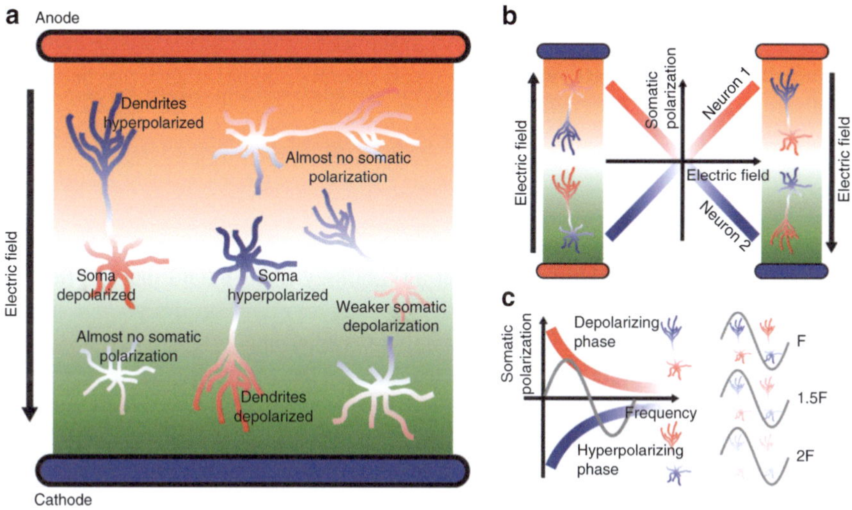

Fig. 2.3 Weak electric fields applied extracellularly polarize neuronal membrane. (**a**) Induced polarization is polarity- and compartment-specific and strongly depends on neuronal orientation relative to the electric field applied and morphology. (**b**) Somatic polarization depends linearly on the electric field amplitude. (**c**) Polarization decreases exponentiallthe equation is called the ay with the frequency of the field applied. (**a** and **b** are based on data from Jefferys (1981), Chan et al. (1988) and Radman et al. (2009). **c** is based on data from Deans et al. (2007))

The sensitivity of neurons to extracellular electric fields as measured in Bikson et al. is called the coupling constant (how many millivolts the somatic voltage of a neuron changes per V/m electric field applied). The estimation provided by Bikson et al. (0.1–0.2 mV/V/m) was confirmed for pyramidal cortical neurons in ferret slices by Fröhlich and McCormick (Frohlich and Mccormick 2010) and for CA3 pyramidal neurons in hippocampus by Deans et al. (2007). In the latter study, the coupling constant was directly measured varying the frequency of the field applied. Because of the membrane capacitative and resistive properties, the response of a neuron to an electric field is low-pass filtered: high frequency stimulation induces a small polarization compared to low frequencies. Therefore, the study by Deans et al. confirmed that the coupling constant depends on the frequency of the stimulation applied (Fig. 2.3c). A couple of years later, Radman et al. added another key element to consider when evaluating the effects of electric fields on neurons (Radman et al. 2009). By performing a morphologic reconstruction of biocytin-filled neurons, the authors found that the coupling constant strongly depends on neuronal morphology. Neurons with a symmetric dendritic arbor, like fast spiking interneurons, were polarized by external electric fields much less than neurons with a more asymmetric morphology, such as pyramidal neurons. Similar results were also reported in another study for hippocampal neurons (Berzhanskaya et al. 2013).

To summarize, the biophysical model that emerges from these studies is that the voltage fluctuations (*ΔV*, units: V or mV) at the soma induced by spatially uniform DC electric fields (*E*, units: V/m or mV/mm) oriented along the primary dendritic axis can be described by.

$$\Delta V = c_E\left(M\right)E,$$

where c_E is the coupling constant (units: m or mm). The coupling constant is in general a complex function of neuronal morphology (*M*). A field that is oriented perpendicularly to the primary dendritic axis has no effect on the voltage at the soma, while its effect is maximum for parallel orientations.

The effect of an external applied electric field on the membrane potential can be determined by a formulation known as cable theory (for a recent review see (Rahman et al. 2015)). The generic equation that describes how the membrane potential of a neuron (V_m) is linked to the extracellular potential (V_e) as a function of time (*t*) and space (*x*) is the following:

$$\frac{\partial V_m}{\partial t} + \frac{\partial^2 V_m\left(x\right)}{\partial x^2} - V_m = \lambda^2 \frac{\partial^2 V_e\left(x\right)}{\partial x^2},$$

where the right side of the equation is called the activating function. Here, λ is the membrane length constant, which depends only on the electrophysiological properties of the membrane. This relatively complex equation can be simplified in particular conditions and solved analytically. In general, however, numerical methods can be used to solve it for multi-compartment neuronal models. There is a large amount of theoretical work in which cable theory was used to estimate polarization profiles of neurons subjected to an extracellular electric field (V_e) (Basser and Roth 2000; Chan and Nicholson 1986; Hause 1975; Joucla and Yvert 2009; Mcintyre and Grill 1999; Miranda et al. 2007; Plonsey and Barr 1998; Rahman et al. 2013; Ranck 1975; Svirskis et al. 1997; Tranchina and Nicholson 1986). However, one inevitable outcome of this classic theory is that the polarization profile produced by extracellular fields is not simple, even for tDCS. In the specific case in which a neuron compartment can be approximated as a very long (>5λ) straight cylindrical segment, as in the case of long dendrite or axon (terminal) processes of cortical or hippocampal neurons, the coupling constant c_E can be expressed directly as a function of the polarization length and the angle between the main neuronal axis and the electric field (*θ*):

$$c_E = \lambda \cos\theta$$

While the estimation of somatic membrane polarization is robust across brain regions and species, a sophisticated analysis of tDCS effects must account for the distributed profile of polarization (Fig. 2.3a). Though it is correct that an "anodal" direct field will depolarize the soma of cortical pyramidal neurons in a hippocampal slice, it will inevitable hyper-polarize their dendrites (Bikson et al. 2004), which can change dendritic processing (Fig. 2.3b). In addition, in tDCS, cortical folding will cause local changes in the orientation of neurons relative to the electric field such that neurons in adjacent cortical regions may be polarized in opposite direction (Rahman et al. 2013; Reato et al. 2013a). This was also anticipated by Terzuolo and Bullock as early as 1956, who wrote "*Finally, current flowing along the surface of the grey matter (tangential directed flow as opposed to inward/outward radial flow) may influence brain function by polarizing structures oriented along the surface, namely afferent axons.*" (Terzuolo and Bullock 1956).

The effects of stimulation on neuronal physiology can be understood by using computational models of single neurons. These models are based on a set of equations that describes how the membrane potential of a compartment of a neuron, V, evolves in time. The best-known is the Hodgkin-Huxley model (Hodgkin and Huxley 1952). The general formulation of a Hodgkin-Huxley-like model is:

$$C\frac{dV}{dt} = -\sum_x I_x + I,$$

where C is the membrane capacitance, I an applied current and I_x describes in general all the possible currents, either ionic, synaptic, due to input currents from other compartments, etc.

In their original formulation, Hodgkin and Huxley considered current contributions from sodium, potassium and a leakage current, such that the equation is:

$$C\frac{dV}{dt} = -g_{Na}m^3h\left(V - E_{Na}\right) - g_K n^4\left(V - E_K\right) - g_L\left(V - E_L\right) + I,$$

where $g_{Na,K,L}$ are the maximum conductances for sodium and potassium and leakage currents, m and h describe the probability that sodium channels are open or inactivated, n the probability that potassium channels are open and $E_{Na,K,L}$ the reversal potential for sodium, potassium and leakage channels respectively, and I is an applied current. Importantly for tDCS, the driving force terms $(V - E_X)$ are directly affected by changes in membrane potential, such that, for example if an externally applied electric field increases the voltage by ΔV (i.e. polarizes the membrane), then the driving force for all the conductances will be altered to $(V + \Delta V - E_X)$. Additionally, all the probabilities for channels to be open or inactivated are also time and voltage dependent. Therefore, changes in membrane potential affect directly ionic currents in two ways.

Synaptic conductances are also voltage dependent because their magnitude can be expressed as:

$$I_{syn} = g_{syn}\left(V - E_{syn}\right),$$

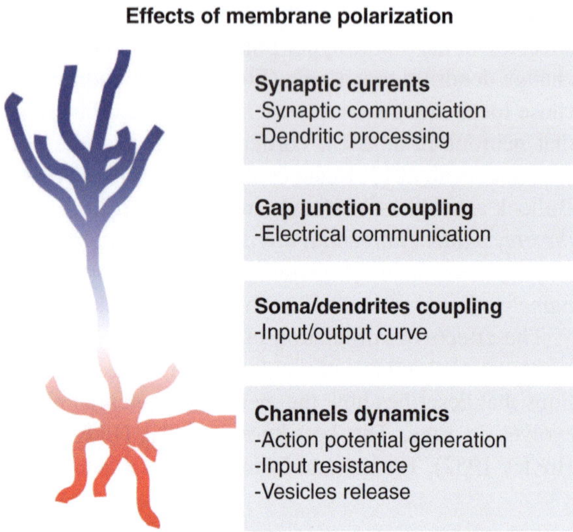

Fig. 2.4 Summary of the multiple potential effects of membrane polarization on the electrical and synaptic activity of neurons

where the values of the parameters depends on the type of synaptic current (AMPA, NMDA, GABAa, GABAb, etc.). Current through gap-junctions connecting neurons or electrotonic coupling of neuronal compartments also depend on voltage differences. Finally the release on synaptic vesicles depends also on voltage changes.

In summary, any effect on membrane voltage affects potentially every aspect of neuronal, electrical and synaptic activity (Fig. 2.4). Therefore, the notion that tDCS affects neuronal function by inducing a membrane polarization must be extended by considering how that voltage fluctuation modulates the neuronal activity of interest. For example, depolarization of the somatic compartment is usually associated with hyperpolarization of the dendrites. Depolarization of the soma increases the excitability of the neuron and hyperpolarization of the dendrites increases the driving force for excitatory synaptic inputs, while reducing the one for inhibitory inputs. How this dichotomy may be solved is an intense area of research (see next sections).

Active Neurons

Assuming no synaptic inputs (as in many in vitro models) the polarization induced by electric fields generated during tDCS is too small (0.1–0.5 mV) to increase the membrane voltage of a neuron from rest sufficiently to generate an action potential (10–20 mV over resting membrane voltage). How does tDCS therefore affect neuronal activity at all?

In contrast to typical in vitro conditions, neurons in the brain are often spontaneously active even when animals do not receive any specific sensory stimulus or are engaged in any specific task. The general level of activity depends strongly on the behavioral state of the animal and specific patterns of neuronal firing are determined by intrinsic cellular and network properties (ion channel expression, number, type and strength of synaptic inputs, etc.). When animals are explicitly engaged in a task, neurons are usually highly depolarized, exhibit spiking activity and are in a high conductance state (Destexhe et al. 2003). Therefore, when a neuron is already active, it seems more appropriate to consider the effects of the stimulation on the firing activity. This intuitive idea was already proposed and demonstrated a long time ago. In fact, Terzuolo and Bullock in 1956 (Terzuolo and Bullock 1956) already pushed forward ideas that are nowadays at the core of our understanding of the biophysics of transcranial electrical stimulation. In their study, they used crayfish and lobsters to test the effects of weak currents applied extracellularly on neurons while keeping the synaptic inputs under tight control. They used electric fields of the order of 1 V/m, a value completely reasonable for transcranial electrical stimulation applied with common stimulation protocols. Interestingly, some of the sentences from that paper contain already the majority of key concepts for describing the effects of electric fields on neurons. Here we report a few of those. *"We have not seen in the literature, however, a quantitative evaluation of the sensitivity of nerve cells to electric fields in terms of voltage gradient across some appropriate dimension of the neuron. We have undertaken to estimate the threshold value as being the unique value of greatest interest and have found this to be far lower for modulation of the frequency of an already active neuron than for the excitation of a silent one."* Already then, it was recognized that: *"it will be realized that there will be no characteristic value for this membrane potential change, since in an equatorial region of the cell, with respect to the axis of polarization, the potential across the membrane will not be changed at all during polarization, and on one side of this line it will be increased and on the other side decreased."* Finally, *"These values of voltage gradient were all obtained in the best axis of polarization of the neuron. When the field was rotated, a significant increase of the applied current was necessary in order to reproduce the same effect as that obtained in the axono-dendritic axis"* It is quite astonishing that as early as 60 years ago the biophysics of DCS was already quite understood. The findings of Terzuolo and Bullock were then confirmed in vivo in anesthetized rats and in cat encéphale isolé. Bindman et al. (1964) applied electrical stimulation transcranially and found that firing rates are increased/decreased by anodal/cathodal stimulation (Fig. 2.5a). They also found that evoked potentials are similarly affected in a polarity-specific manner by the stimulation. Importantly, the authors found that stimulation applied for longer than 5 min induces long-lasting changes in firing rates. Purpura and Mcmurtry (1965) also reported changes in firing rates induced in a polarity specific-manner and linked the results to the orientation of neurons and induced polarization (even if the currents applied were high enough to directly generate action potentials). Similar results were also found a few years before by Creutzfeldt et al. (1962) by recording from motor and visual cortex of cat encéphale isolé while applying currents of the order of 1 mA transcortically. In particular, they also found that the relationship between firing rate changes and current applied is approximately linear. Consistently with previous studies, they also found that electrically evoked activity is modulated by weak electrical stimulation.

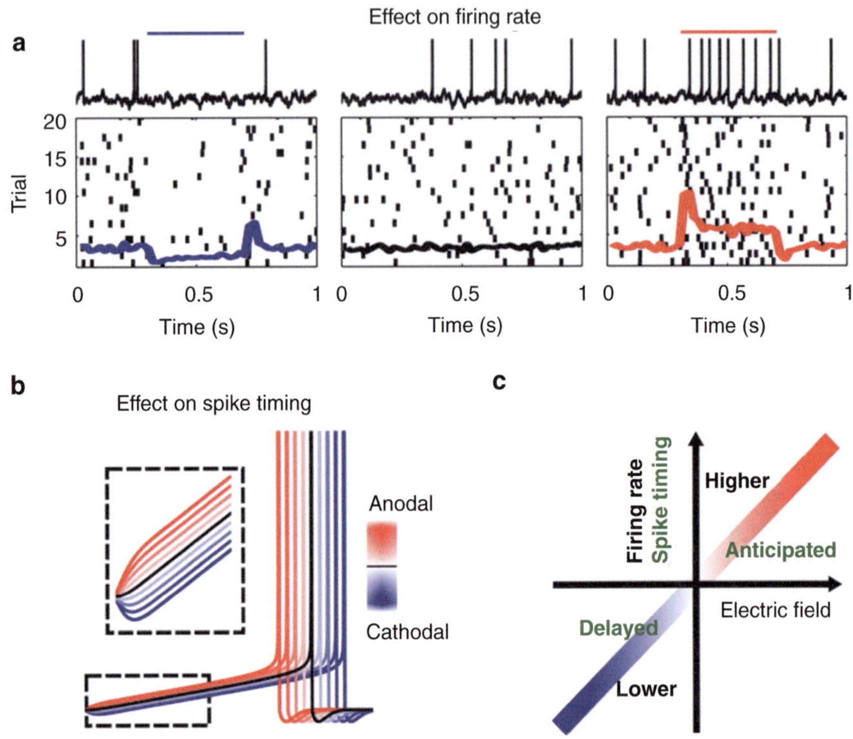

Fig. 2.5 Schematics of the effects of weak DC currents on active neurons. (**a**) Anodal/cathodal (blue/red) stimulation increases/decreases firing rate compared to control conditions (black). Top row: membrane voltage during the application of the stimulation. Bottom row: raster plot (each line represents an action potential) and average firing rate change across trials during stimulation or control conditions. (**b**) Anodal stimulation anticipates action potential generation while cathodal delays it. Control condition in black. (**c**) The effects on both firing rate and spike timing are linear with electric field amplitude. (**a** is based on data from Bindman et al. (1964) and Reato et al. (2010). **b** is based on data from Radman et al. (2007); **c** is based on data from all the previous)

The work of Gartside added more key elements to the after-stimulation effects of electric fields on neuronal firing (Gartside 1968). After inducing lasting effects as in Bindman's work, the author cooled the whole body of rats to completely abolish neuronal activity. After the temperature was left free to rise again to normal levels, the changes in firing rate induced by the electrical stimulation were still present. The author therefore suggested that these persisting changes are not driven by reverberation of the activity but *"The underlying mechanism must involve some type of synaptic modification."*

Years later, Chan and Nicholson (1986) found that the firing rate of Purkinje cells in the cerebellum is very sensitive to weak electric fields (even though the stimulation was alternating current). Firing rate increases by about 6 spikes per second per millivolt depolarization applied, a value that is consistent with results in cat visual cortex (but no electrical stimulation was applied (Carandini and Ferster 2000) and rat hippocampal slices (Reato et al. 2010)).

Apart from changes in firing rate, weak electric fields can also affect spike timing. Changes in spike timing do not necessary imply changes in rate, such that even if the average rate is the same, the timing of these events can be altered by electrical stimulation. A clear evidence of this phenomenon was provided by Radman et al. (2007). They patched hippocampal neurons and then linearly drove the membrane towards the threshold for action potential generation. In some trials, they applied a spatially uniform electric field on the top of that depolarization. They found that somatic anodal stimulation sped up the threshold crossing, while cathodal slowed it down (Fig. 2.5b, c). Furthermore, Radman et al. also showed that AC stimulation can entrain the spiking activity of single neurons, a key result for explaining how weak electric currents can entrain full neuronal populations (Deans et al. 2007; Frohlich and Mccormick 2010; Ozen et al. 2010; Reato et al. 2010).

Changes in firing rate and spike timing produced by weak electric stimulation have been modeled throughout the years often using single-neuron descriptions that are simplified compared to the Hodgkin-Huxley formalism. These models assume that neurons can be described as a single compartment (the soma) and are particularly suited for implementation in large populations of synaptically connected neurons.

Parra and Bikson (Parra and Bikson 2004) used an integrate-and-fire (IF) neuron model to show that the spike coherence in a neuronal population increased when small polarizations where applied to the whole network. Their model was described by:

$$\tau \frac{dV}{dt} = -V + RI,$$

where R is the membrane resistance, τ the time constant, V the membrane voltage, and the term I includes both the synaptic currents from other neurons and the contribution from an external electric field. We can refer to this as "RI" formalism, with direct analogy to how compartment-based biophysical models of electrical stimulation incorporate the effects of electric fields as equivalent intracellular current injection (Lafon et al. 2016; Park et al. 2005). Expanding on this formalism to describe the effects of weak electric fields, Reato et al. (2010) implemented Izhikevich's single neuron model (Izhikevich 2003, 2007) to reproduce the effects of electric fields on a network of excitatory and inhibitory neurons (see following section). The differential equation that describes the voltage is

$$\frac{dV}{dt} = f(V) - u(V) + I_{syn} + I_E$$

where I_{syn} is the sum of the synaptic inputs from other neurons, $u(V)$ an adaptation variable and $f(V)$ is a combination of a linear and quadratic function of the voltage that also give rise to the action potential generation (a reset of the voltage is then necessary). Electrical stimulation can be implemented as a current term I_E, such that

$$I_E = k_E E,$$

where k_E is the conversion factor that must be set to reproduce the correct polarization levels expected by the application of the electric field. In other words, if the value of the somatic membrane potential is V without stimulation and $V + \Delta V$ when the electric field is applied, the parameter k_E must be tuned such that the current I_E induces a change equal to ΔV. This type of simple modeling formalism has been broadly adopted including in simulate the effects of gamma oscillations in vitro (Reato et al. 2010, 2015) as well as slow-waves in humans (Reato et al. 2013a) and in ferrets (Ali et al. 2013).

A similar simplified approach has been recently used to simulate the effects of electric fields on neuronal populations underlying decision-making processes (Bonaiuto and Bestmann 2015; Hammerer et al. 2016). Bonaiuto and colleagues used the exponential leaky integrate-and-fire (LIF) (Brette and Gerstner 2005), where the voltage dynamics is described by:

$$C\frac{dV}{dt} = g(V) + I_{syn} + I_E$$

The function $g(V)$ is a combination of linear and exponential functions. Similarly to Reato et al.'s approach using Izhikevich's model, the effects of electric fields can be implemented by directly adding an external current input I_E.

The use of simplified single-neuron models allows for the simulation of large neuronal populations. However, when full populations of neurons are stimulated, the average synaptic inputs in the network must be considered to estimate or predict the effects of weak currents on single neurons. In fact, as suggested in a recent review (Paulus and Rothwell 2016), if a neuron receives multiple synaptic inputs, the membrane becomes leakier. This translates to lower input resistance and therefore a smaller direct polarization induced by electric fields. Thus, while population activity can amplify the small effects of weak currents on neurons (Reato et al. 2010), strong synaptic tone decreases the polarization induced on single neurons. None-the-less, since active neurons are often near firing threshold, active systems are expected to be significantly more sensitive to polarization. This is turn leads to the notion of "functional targeting" discussed in the next sections.

Summary of the Effects of Weak Direct Current Stimulation on Membrane Potential, Firing Rate and Spike Timing and Open Questions

The summarized literature delineates a precise view on the effects of weak electric fields, such those induced by tDCS, on single neurons. When neurons are not active, weak stimulation induces a small polarization of the membrane. When neurons are active, the effects of fields are on firing rate and spike timing. Somatic anodal stimulation increases firing rate and shorten the time required to reach the threshold for action potential generation. Somatic cathodal stimulation has the opposite effect. However, many open questions and debates remain on the effects of tDCS on single neurons:

1. The dichotomy anodal/excitatory vs cathodal/inhibitory is not precise. Modulation of membrane potential does not directly translate to increased/decreased excitability, since these concepts are linked to the desired effect of the stimulation. For example, depolarization of the soma may lead to easier generation of action potential, an effect that may be considered excitatory. Depolarization of the dendrites however may not be beneficial for post-synaptic neurons. An increase in membrane potential decreases the synaptic response of post-synaptic neurons because it reduces the driving force. Considering that neurons constantly experience compartment-specific polarizations, it cannot be assumed that electric fields always have a net excitatory or inhibitory effect.
2. The polarization of dendrites and axons has been predicted by modelling studies but never measured experimentally. A common assumption, for example, is that stimulation does not affect morphologically symmetric neurons. However, this assumption is mainly based on somatic polarization (the so-called somatic doctrine [Bikson et al. 2012]). It cannot be excluded that polarization of axons and dendrites may be very effective in modulating cellular functions ([Rahman et al. 2013], see next paragraph).
3. The coupling constant has not been measured directly in vivo. This experiment is quite critical to assure that the results from the in vitro literature can really be used to guide and support human research. Moreover, whether brain state and therefore high or low conductance neuronal states affect coupling constant is not known.
4. Effects of weak electric fields on non-neuronal type of cells have not been exhaustively studied yet (Monai et al. 2016). For example, coupling constant for glial cells has never been measured before. These types of cells are critical for neuronal function and seem to mediate some of the lasting effects of electric fields (see next section).

Effects of Weak Direct Current Stimulation on Synapses and Neuronal Populations

Ultimately, to affect brain function weak electric fields must exert significant effects on whole neuronal populations. A priori, the effects of stimulation on single neurons could be altered, amplified or damped (or completely disappear) at the population level. It is therefore not surprising that many studies on the biophysics of tDCS have now focused on neuronal populations and the effects of weak electric fields on synapses. The majority of animal studies in vitro on this topic involved the use of evoked responses or analyzed the effects of the stimulation on neuronal oscillations. In some of these studies, plastic effects were reported. In vivo studies on the other hand, provide great opportunities to study the effects of electrical stimulation on behavior.

Evoked Responses In Vitro

The most commonly studied animal model of transcranial stimulation is the modulation by applied electric fields of evoked population responses, which, to a first approximation, provide a measurement of synaptic currents on post-synaptic neurons. A stimulating electrode, usually bipolar, is placed close to fibers tract in vitro or in vivo. A very short (<1 ms) current pulse is then applied to generate action potentials in axons. An extracellular recording electrode is used to record the population response (local field potential, LFP) around the dendrites or somas of the post-synaptic neurons. A weak electric field is then applied to modulate the population response. Many of the studies mentioned in the previous paragraph reported modulation of evoked responses by weak electric currents. In particular, electric fields whose orientation is parallel to the somatodendritic axis of a neuron and pointing towards the soma (anodal stimulation for cortical cells) increase the evoked response, while fields with opposite orientation (cathodal for cortical cells) decrease the response (Fig. 2.6a). These results were found consistently for cortical (Bindman et al. 1964; Creutzfeldt et al. 1962; Purpura and Mcmurtry 1965) and hippocampal CA1 neurons (Bikson et al. 2004; Jefferys 1981). In recent years, new studies helped deepening our understanding on the effects of weak currents in this preparation.

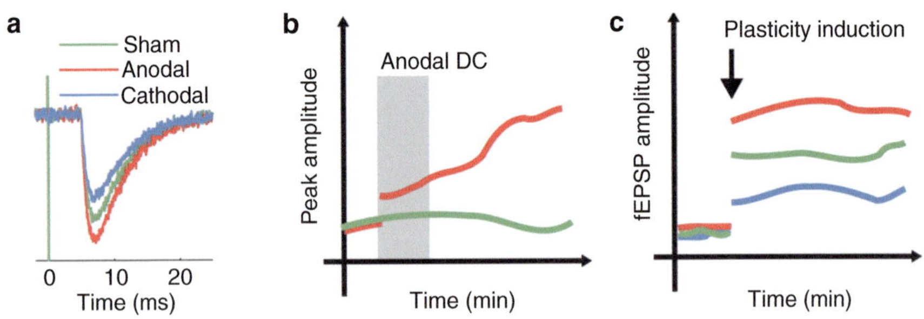

Fig. 2.6 Schematics of the effects of weak DC currents on evoked responses. (**a**) Anodal/cathodal (blue/red) stimulation increases/decreases the amplitude of evoked responses (green). (**b**) When evoked responses are combined with prolonged DC stimulation (~10 min), the amplitude of the response increases and this change outlasts the stimulation period. (**c**) When DC stimulation is applied during plasticity induction (LTP), the amount of potentiation is modulated bi-directionally by weak DC stimulation (fEPSP: field excitatory post-synaptic potential). The green line represents the control condition, red anodal stimulation and blue cathodal. (**a** is based on data from Creutzfeldt et al. 1962; Bindman et al. 1964; Purpura and Mcmurtry 1965; Jefferys 1981; Bikson et al. 2004; Rahman et al. 2013. **b** is based on data from Fritsch et al. 2010; **c** is based on data from Ranieri et al. 2012)

Rahman and colleagues used evoked responses in rat motor cortex to test the effects of weak DC stimulation (Rahman et al. 2013). The authors stimulated different cortical pathways and applied electric fields of different polarities, amplitudes and orientations relative to the stimulated neurons. They confirmed that when electric fields are oriented parallel to the dendrosomatic axis, the response is modulated in the same way as for hippocampal slices. They then tried to stimulate pathways perpendicular to the applied field. From what was previously known, such fields should induce no net polarization at the soma and therefore no effects on evoked responses. However, the authors reported a modulation of the responses comparable in magnitude to that found for the pathways parallel to the electric field. To understand this surprising result, Rahman et al. used a computational model of a single neuron in a spatially uniform electric field and found that terminal polarization could explain the experimental results. While these findings were not tested experimentally, they suggest that, at least in some cases, somatic polarization does not fully explain the effects of weak electrical stimulation. Importantly, these findings are consistent with a previous study in hippocampus (Kabakov et al. 2012).

Additional animal studies aimed at understanding how weak electrical stimulation can induce lasting effects on neuronal excitability as found in human studies. Fritsch and colleagues (Fritsch et al. 2010) combined electrophysiology, pharmacology and genetic tools to elucidate the cellular mechanisms underlying the lasting effects induced by tDCS. They evoked population responses in mouse motor cortex slices and applied weak DC stimulation extracellularly. They found that application of prolonged stimulation (15 min) induces a potentiation of the response (Fig. 2.6b). The change starts minutes after the stimulation onset and the magnitude of the responses continues to increase even after the cessation of the stimulation. Importantly, the effects are NMDA-dependent, and the lasting changes critically depend on whether or not synaptic co-activation is applied (and its frequency), suggesting that the state of the cortical network may dictate the susceptibility to the stimulation. Finally, by using genetic tools, the authors found that DC stimulation enhances the release of BDNF and that BDNF receptors are required for plasticity induction. In fact, when the authors repeated the same experiments using mice where these receptors were knocked down, they found that the effects of DC stimulation vanished.

Ranieri and colleagues, using evoked responses in hippocampal slices, critically improved our understanding on tDCS lasting effects (Ranieri et al. 2012). They applied a standard stimulation protocol to induce plasticity at the CA3 to CA1 synapse (Schaffer collateral) and found that anodal stimulation increased long-term potentiation (LTP) while cathodal decreased it. They further showed evidence that these effects may be due to an increased expression of zif268 protein (an early gene). The findings of this work suggested that weak electrical stimulation, while not inducing plasticity per se, may strongly modulate ongoing plasticity in a bi-directional manner (Fig. 2.6c).

Confirming and expanding this hypothesis, a study by Kronberg et al. (2016) showed that weak DC stimulation effectively modulates LTP and depression (LTD). Kronberg et al. used a typical experimental model of hippocampal plasticity in brain slices (as in Ranieri et al. study, (2012) in which stimulation of axonal afferents (Schaffer collaterals) can lead to post-synaptic potentiation or depression depending on the frequency of pre-synaptic activation (Cooper and Bear 2012). The authors found that DC stimulation biases plasticity towards potentiation, such that LTP is enhanced and LTD is reduced. Importantly, the authors found that similar effects could be induced using either anodal or cathodal stimulation, but with the effects localized in different dendritic compartments (apical/basal dendrites). Finally, Kronberg et al. clearly showed that DC stimulation alone or applied when plasticity was blocked did not lead to any synaptic changes.

Taken together, these studies on the lasting effects induced by weak electric currents suggest that stimulation alone does not produce significant persisting synaptic effects if not paired with activity or ongoing plasticity. This underlies the concept of "functional targeting", in which stimulation paradigms can be targeted to specific neuronal populations depending on their activity and plasticity-permissive states (Jackson et al. 2016).

Finally, in the previous section we pointed out the possible issue that arises from compartment-specific polarization of the neuronal membrane. The polarity of somatic polarization (depolarization/hyperpolarization) is opposite than dendritic. A study by Lafon et al. (2016) shed light on this issue. By combining electrophysiology in hippocampal rat brain slices and computational models based on previous research (Park et al. 2005; Prescott et al. 2008; Yi et al. 2014), Lafon et al. found that weak constant electric fields affect neuronal input/output function, i.e. the relationship between strength of synaptic inputs and the firing they induce on the post-synaptic neuron. Moreover, the authors found that somatic and dendritic polarization may have a synergistic effect for anodal stimulation: soma-depolarizing electric fields increase the likelihood of neuronal firing while also increasing the driving force for synaptic input at the dendrites. However, the effects of electric fields of opposite polarity (cathodal) tend to cancel out. This result suggests how an asymmetry between the effects of anodal and cathodal stimulation may arise directly at the single neuron level.

Oscillations In Vitro

Another in vitro experimental model commonly used to study the effects of weak electric fields is pharmacologically-induced oscillations or seizure-like population activity. However, in almost all the studies in the field, alternating currents (Ali et al. 2013; Berenyi et al. 2012; Deans et al. 2007; Frohlich and Mccormick 2010; Ozen et al. 2010; Reato et al. 2010) or Gaussian waveforms (Francis et al. 2003) were applied. Reviews on tACS are already present in the literature (Herrmann et al. 2013; Reato et al. 2013b) and so here the focus is just on DC stimulation studies.

Using high extracellular concentration of potassium in hippocampal slices to generate seizure-like activity, Gluckman and colleagues (Gluckman et al. 1996) tested whether relatively weak electric fields could reduce epileptic activity. They found that when fields were hyperpolarizing for the soma (cathodal stimulation), the seizure was temporarily stopped.

Pharmacologically induced beta/gamma oscillations in the hippocampus have been used to study the effects of AC stimulation (Deans et al. 2007). However, Reato and colleagues characterized in more detail the effects of the stimulation (Reato et al. 2010). By using many frequencies (AC) and amplitudes in brain slices and a computational model they found that the effects of stimulation on the oscillations presumably depend on the interplay between excitation and inhibition (Fig. 2.7a), whose balance is a critical feature of this type of rhythm (Atallah and Scanziani 2009). In particular, when using DC stimulation, Reato et al. found that soma depolarizing (anodal) stimulation increases the power of the oscillations while

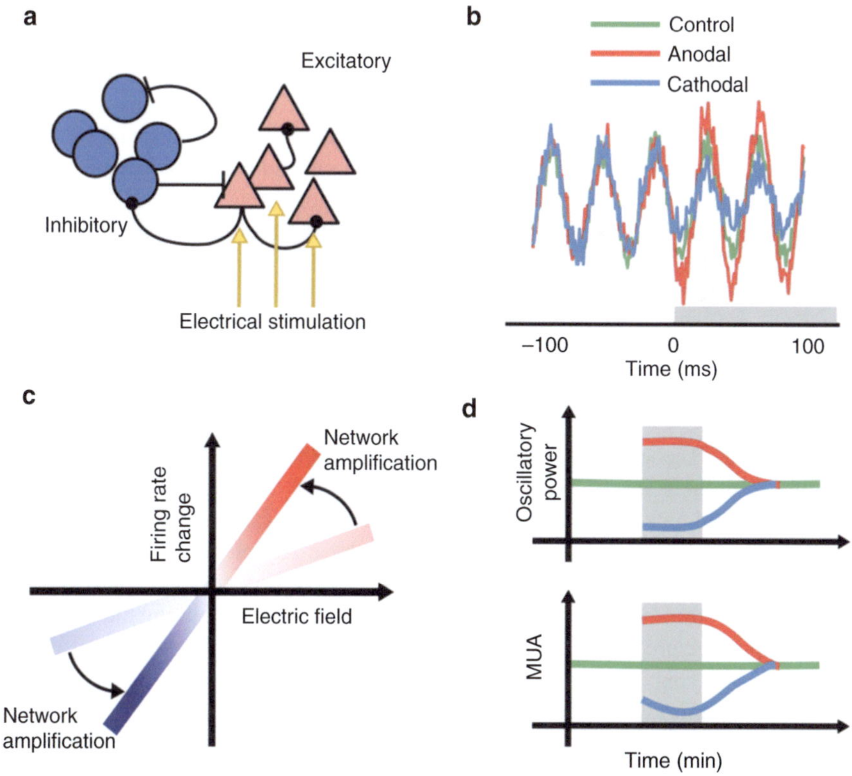

Fig. 2.7 Schematics of the effects of weak DC stimulation on gamma oscillations induced in vitro. (**a**) Gamma oscillations in vitro are generated by the interplay between excitatory and inhibitory neurons. (**b**) Anodal/cathodal (blue/red) stimulation increases/decreases the power of the oscillations compared to control experiments (green). (**c**) The modulation of the firing activity of single neurons by weak DC stimulation is amplified by the population. (**d**) When stimulation is applied for a prolonged time (10 min) the power of the oscillations and multi-unit activity modulation outlast the stimulation period for about 10 min. (**a**–**c** are based on data from Reato et al. 2010. **d** is based on Reato et al. 2015)

cathodal decreases it (Fig. 2.7b). They explained the results as evidence of altered excitation and inhibition. When the firing rate of excitatory neurons is increased, inhibition compensates. Because the inhibition is fed by excitation and sets the tone of the oscillations, the result at the population level is an increase in oscillatory power. The opposite is true for cathodal stimulation. Lower firing rates of excitatory neurons lead to lower balanced inhibition and decreased gamma power. Using a computational model (see previous section), the authors showed that the weak effects of DC stimulation on single neurons (for example firing rate modulation) are amplified by the population dynamics (Fig. 2.7c). Importantly, the same authors found a similar amplification at the population level when implementing a computational model of slow-wave activity (Reato et al. 2013a).

The same group used the same in vitro preparation in a later study in which DC stimulation was applied not just for few seconds but for 10 min (Reato et al. 2015). Monitoring power and frequency of the oscillations as well as multi-unit activity (a proxy for population firing rate), they found that the stimulation induces lasting effects on the neuronal population in a polarity-dependent manner (Fig. 2.7d). Anodal stimulation increases the power of the oscillations and multi-unit activity, while cathodal decreases both. Based on the hypothesis of balanced excitation and inhibition during gamma oscillations and the same computational model they used in their previous study, the authors suggested that the results could be explained by balanced synaptic changes of both excitatory and inhibitory synapses. While intriguing, however, this hypothesis has not been directly tested experimentally.

Plasticity and Behavioral Effects In Vivo

A decade ago, Liebetanz et al. found that tDCS applied in rats is able to modulate pathological states. In a first study, cortical spreading depression (CSD) was induced in anesthetized rats using a high potassium chloride solution (Liebetanz et al. 2006a). Neither sham nor cathodal stimulation have any effect of the CSD while anodal stimulation significantly increases the propagation speed of the CSD. In another study, the authors showed that tDCS is effective in modulating the threshold for epileptic seizure generation (Liebetanz et al. 2006b). The threshold was determined by applying a biphasic pulse train to the cortex to induce seizures. When anodal stimulation was applied, there were no changes on the threshold. However, cathodal stimulation applied for 60 min or 30 min at double intensity decreased the threshold for more than 2 h (Fig. 2.8a).

Another group also found that prolonged DC stimulation over the motor cortex of anesthetized mice induces an increase (anodal) or decrease (cathodal) of motor evoked responses (MEPs) that outlasts the stimulation period (Cambiaghi et al. 2010). The same group also later found, using anesthetized mice, that the amplitude of visually evoked potentials can be modulated with DC stimulation in a polarity-dependent manner (Cambiaghi et al. 2011). Anodal stimulation increases the amplitude of the evoked potential and cathodal decreases. The effects of the

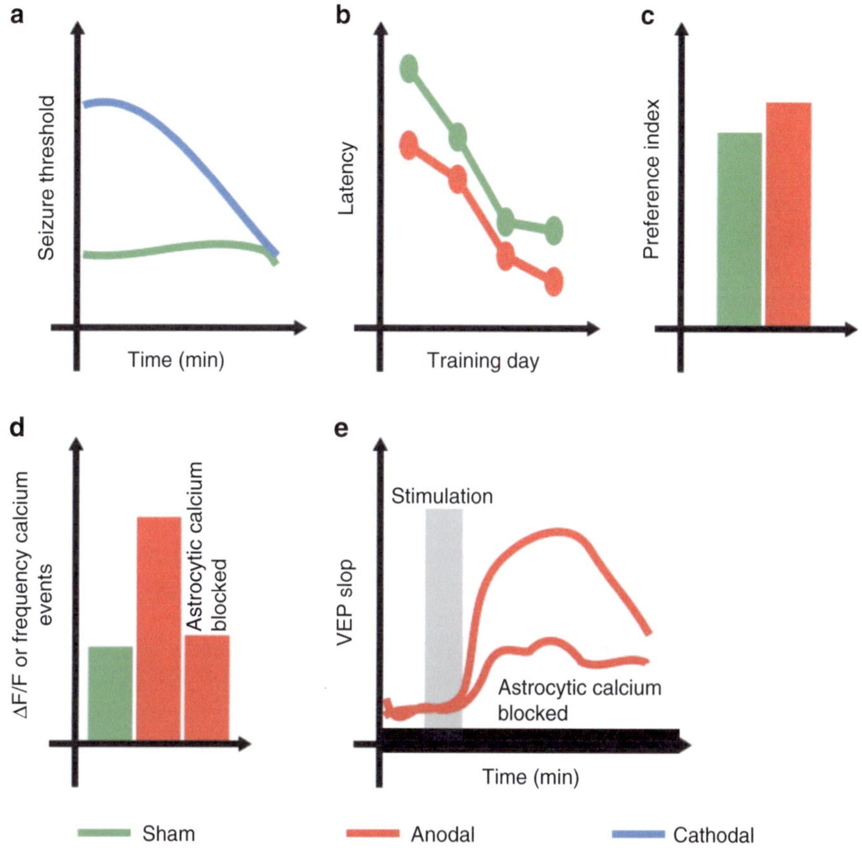

Fig. 2.8 Schematics of the effects of weak DC stimulation on in vivo animal models. (**a**) Cathodal stimulation increases the threshold for seizure generation (anticonvulsant effect). (**b**) Anodal tDCS improves performances in a Morris water maze test (lower latency) compared to non-stimulated animals. (**c**) Anodal tDCS improves performances in a novel object recognition task. (**d**) Anodal tDCS induces high amplitude and frequency calcium events in cortical populations that are driven by astrocytic calcium. (**e**) The lasting increase of visually evoked responses after tDCS is strongly limited when calcium transients in astrocytes are blocked. (**a** is based on data from Liebetanz et al. 2006a. **b** and **c** are based on data from Podda et al. 2016). **d** and **e** are based on data from Monai et al. 2016)

stimulation also persist for the 10 min following the termination of the current application.

An important study on tDCS effects on neuronal population in vivo came from Marquez-Ruiz and colleagues (Marquez-Ruiz et al. 2012). Instead of using electrically evoked responses (as usually done in in vitro models), the authors induced sensory responses in awake rabbits by delivering air puff to the whisker pad. When DC stimulation was applied over the somatosensory cortex, the LFP induced by the sensory stimulus was increased in magnitude during anodal and decreased during cathodal stimulation. The effect of cathodal stimulation persists after the cessation of the stimulation and the effects were abolished after blocking adenosine A1 receptors. Importantly, stimulation was able to directionally modulate eye blink conditioning. Using paired-pulse stimuli, the authors further found that the effects of tDCS are mediated by the modulation of thalamo-cortical synapses at presynaptic sites.

Two recent studies reported effects of tDCS on hippocampal plasticity. Application of anodal tDCS in freely moving mice boosts the amount of LTP that can be induced in slices ex-vivo by stimulating the Shaffer collateral pathway (Rohan et al. 2015). The authors also reported an increase in pair-pulse facilitation (PPF). The effects are NMDA receptor-dependent for LTP but not for PPF. The modulation depends on the stimulation amplitude and significant LTP enhancement can be found also 1 week after the stimulation. Interestingly, there authors did not find any effects on evoked responses before LTP induction. Using a similar approach, a different group stimulated mice with tDCS for 20 min (Podda et al. 2016). They confirmed that anodal stimulation leads to stronger LTP induction while cathodal decreases the amount of LTP without affecting basal synaptic transmission. To test whether the stimulation had an effect on hippocampal learning, mice were then tested on two different behavioral tasks (Morris water maze test and novel object recognition test) a day after receiving anodal stimulation. In both cases, mice performed better than mice subjected to sham stimulation (Fig. 2.8b, c). To confirm the lasting effects of the stimulation, the same tests were then performed a week after the stimulation. The authors reported very similar effects on electrophysiological tests and behavior. The authors then tried to elucidate the molecular pathway by which tDCS affected hippocampal plasticity. They found that tDCS induces differential regulation of exon-specific BDNF mRNAs and BDNF expression is higher after tDCS due to increased histone acetylation promoting BDNF transcription.

While the results of all the previous studies are broadly consistent with each other, a new study just expanded the view on how tDCS may affect brain function. Using a transgenic mouse line expressing G-CaMP7 in astrocytes and a subpopulation of excitatory neurons, Monai and colleagues (Monai et al. 2016) found that DC stimulation over the visual cortex induces large calcium transients across the whole cortex (Fig. 2.8d). The transients are larger and longer than the spontaneous ones. Notably, the effects vanish when mice that lack the receptor responsible for calcium elevations in astrocytes (IP_3R2) are used (Fig. 2.8e). When the authors used a cranial to image the target area at single-cell resolution, they found that the modulation of transients is due to effects mainly on astrocytes. With further experiments, the authors found that the effects on calcium surges are mediated by noradrenergic activation of adenosine A1 receptors. The authors further reported that lasting enhancements of sensory responses (either visual or somatosensory) by transcranial stimulation vanish when calcium transients are blocked in astrocytes.

Summary of the Effects of Weak Direct Current Stimulation on Synapses and Neuronal Populations and Open Questions

While the effects of weak electric fields on single neurons are well characterized, both experimentally and theoretically, a general framework for neuronal populations is still lacking. Evoked responses can be modulated bi-directionally by weak electric fields both in vitro and in vivo. The effects appear to depend not just on somatic but possibly also on terminal polarization. DC stimulation increases or decreases the power of gamma oscillations presumably by affecting firing rate of single neurons. When applying stimulation on large neuronal populations, the effects on single neurons seem to be amplified by the network endogenous dynamics.

Until a few years ago, it was not clear how weak currents could induce lasting effects on neuronal activity. The literature presented here clarified the mechanisms. BDNF has been consistently linked to the lasting effects of DC stimulation, and NMDA receptors also play a major role in plasticity induction. Glial cells may also mediate the lasting effects of DC stimulation. Electrical stimulation can induce behavioral effects, including boosting learning and modulating sensory responses and pathological states. However, many questions remain open:

1. Experimental and modeling results suggest that the weak effects of electric fields on single neurons are amplified by the network. Under which conditions this is true is not clear. Does it apply for all or only specific types of oscillations? What is the role of brain state in determining the effects of the DC stimulation? (for AC stimulation, see Alagapan et al. 2016).
2. The modulation of gamma oscillations seems to depend on the interplay between excitatory and inhibitory neurons. A common assumption is that the effects on inhibition are indirect, through modulations of the excitatory population. What are the direct effects on inhibitory neurons at the population level? If inhibitory neurons are affected by DC stimulation, do the effects outlast the stimulation period?
3. Current flow during tDCS is such that neurons are depolarized or hyperpolarized depending on their orientation relative to the electric field. The mixed effects across a population pose a critical problem to understand tDCS effects: do the effects just cancel out such that there is no net effect on brain activity? Human studies show that this is not the case. Supported by a computational model, it was previously hypothesized that population activity may rectify the effects of mixed polarizations in the case of slow-wave oscillations and monophasic quasi-DC stimulation (Reato et al. 2013a). However, the results may be specific to the specific oscillatory rhythm and may not apply to others. Understanding how to interfere with neuronal population dynamic with specific stimulation parameters is crucial to improve the specificity of the stimulation.
4. The brain is always spontaneously active but often without showing any clear oscillatory activity. There is a full line of research on the dynamics of neuronal

networks and the computations they can perform even without synchronous activity (Renart et al. 2010; Vogels et al. 2005). How DC stimulation may affect non-oscillatory brain activity remains unknown.

5. Until now, all the animal research on tDCS has focused almost exclusively on the temporal aspects of the stimulation (but see Xu et al. 2014) without considering in detail the possible spatial aspects. For example, oscillatory activity can be generated in localized positions in a brain area and so the general effects of DC stimulation may depend on the distribution of fields across the brain relative to the pools of neurons that generate the activity within the network.
6. Cortical and hippocampal networks have been the main subject of studies on the effects of weak electric fields on neuronal populations. However, many networks in the brain do not show the same architecture. For example, the cerebellum, an area that can be easily stimulated transcranially (Galea et al. 2009; Grimaldi et al. 2016; Jayaram et al. 2012), has a very different neuronal organization. The lack of recurrent connections across Purkinje cells, presumably the most polarizable cells in the cerebellar cortex, implies that weak electric fields may easily regulate the output of the cerebellar cortex without unexpected non-linearities.
7. Glial cells and neurons form what has been called a tri-partite synapse (Araque et al. 1999). Their role in synaptic transmission and plasticity is now well-established (Di Castro et al. 2011; Panatier et al. 2011). Glial cells are electrotonically connected through gap-junctions and can feedback into neuronal activity through calcium-dependent glutamate release (Haydon and Carmignoto 2006). This feedback can strongly affect the dynamics of neuronal activity, including in pathological conditions like epileptic seizures (Gomez-Gonzalo et al. 2010; Reato et al. 2012). The effects of weak electric fields on the glial cells' potassium buffering activity has been studied in only one work (Gardner-Medwin and Nicholson 1983). It is certain that any direct effect of stimulation on glial cells may affect the dynamics of neuronal populations.
8. What is the relationship between BDNF and glial cells-mediated lasting effects of transcranial electrical stimulation? Are there many plasticity mechanisms that are induced/affected by DC stimulation?

Emerging Framework: Functional Targeting by tDCS

In the last few years, our understanding of the mechanisms of interaction between electric fields and cells in the brain has been boosted by detailed animal studies. The body of literature reviewed in this chapter converges to suggest that tDCS may functionally target neuronal function (Jackson et al. 2016) (Rahman et al. 2017) – the cellular concept of "functional targeting" provide an important substrate for how tDCS may boost specific tasks/learning. For acute effects, DCS modulations depend on the specific targeted neuronal population and its own ongoing dynamics, usually determined by the interplay between different cell types. At the same time, lasting effects of DCS are also mediated by modulation of ongoing neuronal activity and plasticity. In this view, it seems that the effects of tDCS alone are not sufficient to generate lasting changes if not coupled with ongoing activity and/or plasticity. Thus, the cellular framework of "functional targeting" may provide the foundation for explaining at the single neuron/population/synapse levels why tDCS seems to be effective in humans mainly when applied during tasks/training paradigms.

However, to better define this framework and take full advantage of its predictive power, it is necessary to define a clear link between functional targeting and basic biophysical principles. Ideally, the notion of functional targeting should emerge spontaneously by basic biophysical principles. If this was the case, findings about specific tDCS studies could become more easily generalizable to other stimulation applications. In the future, a single multi-scale biophysical model could be used to guide human research by providing the best stimulation parameters (electrode montage, applied current, waveform, etc.) to stimulate specific neuronal activity in brain areas of interest. This model should take into consideration not only single cells but also how they work together as populations to support behavior. The computational neurostimulation approach (Bestmann et al. 2015) aims exactly at providing a multi-scale approach that bridges effects on single neurons directly to behavioral consequences of stimulation. This may represent a first step to fully unravel how tDCS affects brain function and take full advantage of this powerful technique.

References

Akhtari, M., Bryant, H. C., Mamelak, A. N., Flynn, E. R., Heller, L., Shih, J. J., … Sutherling, W. W. (2002). Conductivities of three-layer live human skull. *Brain Topography, 14*(3), 151–167.

Alagapan, S., Schmidt, S. L., Lefebvre, J., Hadar, E., Shin, H. W., & Frhlich, F. (2016). Modulation of cortical oscillations by low-frequency direct cortical stimulation is state-dependent. *PLoS Biology, 14*(3), e1002424.

Ali, M. M., Sellers, K. K., & Frohlich, F. (2013). Transcranial alternating current stimulation modulates large-scale cortical network activity by network resonance. *The Journal of Neuroscience: The Official Journal of the Society for Neuroscience, 33*(27), 11262–11275.

Araque, A., Parpura, V., Sanzgiri, R. P., & Haydon, P. G. (1999). Tripartite synapses: Glia, the unacknowledged partner. *Trends in Neurosciences, 22*(5), 208–215.

Atallah, B. V., & Scanziani, M. (2009). Instantaneous modulation of gamma oscillation frequency by balancing excitation with inhibition. *Neuron, 62*(4), 566–577.

Barker, A. T., & Jalinous, R. (1985). Non-invasive magnetic stimulation of human motor cortex. *Lancet, 1*(8437), 1106–1107.

Basser, P. J., Mattiello, J., & Lebihan, D. (1994). MR diffusion tensor spectroscopy and imaging. *Biophysical Journal, 66*(1), 259–267.

Basser, P. J., & Roth, B. J. (2000). New currents in electrical stimulation of excitable tissues. *Annual Review of Biomedical Engineering, 2*, 377–397.

Baumann, S. B., Wozny, D. R., Kelly, S. K., & Meno, F. M. (1997). The electrical conductivity of human cerebrospinal fluid at body temperature. *IEEE Transactions on Bio-medical Engineering, 44*(3), 220–223.

Berenyi, A., Belluscio, M., Mao, D., & Buzsaki, G. (2012). Closed-loop control of epilepsy by transcranial electrical stimulation. *Science, 337*(6095), 735–737.

Berzhanskaya, J., Chernyy, N., Gluckman, B. J., Schiff, S. J., & Ascoli, G. A. (2013). Modulation of hippocampal rhythms by subthreshold electric fields and network topology. *Journal of Computational Neuroscience, 34*(3), 369–389.

Bestmann, S., de Berker, A. O., & Bonaiuto, J. (2015). Understanding the behavioural consequences of noninvasive brain stimulation. *Trends in Cognitive Sciences, 19*(1), 13–20.

Bikson, M., Inoue, M., Akiyama, H., Deans, J. K., Fox, J. E., Miyakawa, H., & Jefferys, J. G. (2004). Effects of uniform extracellular DC electric fields on excitability in rat hippocampal slices in vitro. *The Journal of Physiology, 557*. (Pt 1, 175–190.

Bikson, M., Reato, D., & Rahman, A. (2012). Cellular and network effects of transcranial direct current stimulation. In P. M. Rossini (Ed.), *Transcranial brain stimulation*. CRC Press (pp. 55–91).

Bindman, L. J., Lippold, O. C., & Redfearn, J. W. (1964). The action of brief polarizing currents on the cerebral cortex of the rat (1) during current flow and (2) in the production of long-lasting after-effects. *The Journal of Physiology, 172*, 369–382.

Bonaiuto, J. J., & Bestmann, S. (2015). Understanding the nonlinear physiological and behavioral effects of tDCS through computational neurostimulation. *Progress in Brain Research, 222*, 75–103.

Brette, R., & Gerstner, W. (2005). Adaptive exponential integrate-and-fire model as an effective description of neuronal activity. *Journal of Neurophysiology, 94*(5), 3637–3642.

Cambiaghi, M., Teneud, L., Velikova, S., Gonzalez-Rosa, J. J., Cursi, M., Comi, G., & Leocani, L. (2011). Flash visual evoked potentials in mice can be modulated by transcranial direct current stimulation. *Neuroscience, 185*, 161–165.

Cambiaghi, M., Velikova, S., Gonzalez-Rosa, J. J., Cursi, M., Comi, G., & Leocani, L. (2010). Brain transcranial direct current stimulation modulates motor excitability in mice. *The European Journal of Neuroscience, 31*(4), 704–709.

Carandini, M., & Ferster, D. (2000). Membrane potential and firing rate in cat primary visual cortex. *The Journal of neuroscience : the official journal of the Society for Neuroscience, 20*(1), 470–484.

Chan, C. Y., Hounsgaard, J., & Nicholson, C. (1988). Effects of electric fields on transmembrane potential and excitability of turtle cerebellar Purkinje cells in vitro. *The Journal of Physiology, 402*, 751–771.

Chan, C. Y., & Nicholson, C. (1986). Modulation by applied electric fields of Purkinje and stellate cell activity in the isolated turtle cerebellum. *The Journal of Physiology, 371*, 89–114.

Cooper, L. N., & Bear, M. F. (2012). The BCM theory of synapse modification at 30: Interaction of theory with experiment. *Nature Reviews Neuroscience, 13*(11), 798–810.

Creutzfeldt, O. D., Fromm, G. H., & Kapp, H. (1962). Influence of transcortical d-c currents on cortical neuronal activity. *Experimental Neurology, 5*, 436–452.

Datta, A., Bansal, V., Diaz, J., Patel, J., Reato, D., & Bikson, M. (2009). Gyri-precise head model of transcranial direct current stimulation: Improved spatial focality using a ring electrode versus conventional rectangular pad. *Brain Stimulation, 2*(4), 201–207.

Datta, A., Elwassif, M., Battaglia, F., & Bikson, M. (2008). Transcranial current stimulation focality using disc and ring electrode configurations: FEM analysis. *Journal of Neural Engineering, 5*(2), 163–174.

Deans, J. K., Powell, A. D., & Jefferys, J. G. (2007). Sensitivity of coherent oscillations in rat hippocampus to AC electric fields. *The Journal of Physiology, 583*(Pt 2), 555–565.

Destexhe, A., Rudolph, M., & Pare, D. (2003). The high-conductance state of neocortical neurons in vivo. *Nature Reviews Neuroscience, 4*(9), 739–751.

Di Castro, M. A., Chuquet, J., Liaudet, N., Bhaukaurally, K., Santello, M., Bouvier, D., … Volterra, A. (2011). Local Ca2+ detection and modulation of synaptic release by astrocytes. *Nature Neuroscience, 14*(10), 1276–1284.

Di Lazzaro, V., Oliviero, A., Profice, P., Saturno, E., Pilato, F., Insola, A., … Rothwell, J. C. (1998). Comparison of descending volleys evoked by transcranial magnetic and electric stimulation in conscious humans. *Electromyography and Motor Control-Electroencephalography and Clinical Neurophysiology, 109*(5), 397–401.

Dmochowski, J. P., Fau, B. M., Parra, L. C., & Parra, L. C. (2012). The point spread function of the human head and its implications for transcranial current stimulation. (1361-6560 (electronic)). D – NLM: NIHMS409753. *Physics in Medicine and Biology, 57*(20), 6459.

Eaton, H. (1992). Electric field induced in a spherical volume conductor from arbitrary coils: Application to magnetic stimulation and MEG. *Medical & Biological Engineering & Computing, 30*(4), 433–440.

Francis, J. T., Gluckman, B. J., & Schiff, S. J. (2003). Sensitivity of neurons to weak electric fields. *The Journal of Neuroscience: The Official Journal of the Society for Neuroscience, 23*(19), 7255–7261.

Fregni, F., Gimenes, R., Valle, A. C., Ferreira, M. J. L., Rocha, R. R., Natalle, L., … Boggio, P. S. (2006). A randomized, sham-controlled, proof of principle study of transcranial direct current stimulation for the treatment of pain in fibromyalgia. *Arthritis and Rheumatism, 54*(12), 3988–3998.

Fritsch, B., Reis, J., Martinowich, K., Schambra, H. M., Ji, Y., Cohen, L. G., & Lu, B. (2010). Direct current stimulation promotes BDNF-dependent synaptic plasticity: Potential implications for motor learning. *Neuron, 66*(2), 198–204.

Fritsch, G., & Hitzig, E. (1870). Über die elektrische Erregbarkeit des Grosshirns. *Archives Anatomy Physiololy Wissen, 37*, 300–332.

Frohlich, F., & Mccormick, D. A. (2010). Endogenous electric fields may guide neocortical network activity. *Neuron, 67*(1), 129–143.

Gabriel, C., Gabriel, S., & Corthout, E. (1996a). The dielectric properties of biological tissues: I. Literature survey. *Physics in Medicine and Biology, 41*(11), 2231–2249.

Gabriel, S., Lau, R. W., & Gabriel, C. (1996b). The dielectric properties of biological tissues. 2. Measurements in the frequency range 10 Hz to 20 GHz. *Physics in Medicine and Biology, 41*(11), 2251–2269.

Galea, J. M., Jayaram, G., Ajagbe, L., & Celnik, P. (2009). Modulation of cerebellar excitability by polarity-specific noninvasive direct current stimulation. *The Journal of Neuroscience, 29*(28), 9115–9122.

Gardner-Medwin, A. R., & Nicholson, C. (1983). Changes of extracellular potassium activity induced by electric current through brain tissue in the rat. *The Journal of Physiology, 335*, 375–392.

Gartside, I. B. (1968). Mechanisms of sustained increases of firing rate of neurons in the rat cerebral cortex after polarization: Reverberating circuits or modification of synaptic conductance? *Nature, 220*(5165), 382–383.

Geddes, L. A., & Baker, L. E. (1967). The specific resistance of biological material--a compendium of data for the biomedical engineer and physiologist. *Medical & Biological Engineering, 5*(3), 271–293.

Gluckman, B. J., Neel, E. J., Netoff, T. I., Ditto, W. L., Spano, M. L., & Schiff, S. J. (1996). Electric field suppression of epileptiform activity in hippocampal slices. *Journal of Neurophysiology, 76*(6), 4202–4205.

Gomez-Gonzalo, M., Losi, G., Chiavegato, A., Zonta, M., Cammarota, M., Brondi, M., … Carmignoto, G. (2010). An excitatory loop with astrocytes contributes to drive neurons to seizure threshold. *PLoS Biology, 8*(4), e1000352.

Grimaldi, G., Argyropoulos, G. P., Bastian, A., Cortes, M., Davis, N. J., Edwards, D. J., … Celnik, P. (2016). Cerebellar Transcranial direct current stimulation (ctDCS): A novel approach to understanding cerebellar function in health and disease. *The Neuroscientist, 22*(1), 83–97.

Hallett, M. (2007). Transcranial magnetic stimulation: a primer. *Neuron, 55*(2), 187–199.

Hammerer, D., Bonaiuto, J., Klein-Flugge, M., Bikson, M., & Bestmann, S. (2016). Selective alteration of human value decisions with medial frontal tDCS is predicted by changes in attractor dynamics. *Scientific Reports, 6*, 25160.

Hause, L. (1975). A mathematical model for transmembrane potentials secondary to extracellular fields. In *Electroanaesthesia: Biomedical and biophysical studies* (pp. 176–200). New York: Academic.

Haydon, P. G., & Carmignoto, G. (2006). Astrocyte control of synaptic transmission and neurovascular coupling. *Physiological Reviews, 86*(3), 1009–1031.

Herrmann, C. S., Rach, S., Neuling, T., & Struber, D. (2013). Transcranial alternating current stimulation: A review of the underlying mechanisms and modulation of cognitive processes. *Frontiers in Human Neuroscience, 7*, 279.

Hodgkin, A. L., & Huxley, A. F. (1952). A quantitative description of membrane current and its application to conduction and excitation in nerve. *The Journal of Physiology, 117*(4), 500–544.

Huisman, T. A. (2010). Diffusion-weighted and diffusion tensor imaging of the brain, made easy. *Cancer Imag, 10 Spec no A*, S163–S171.

Izhikevich, E. M. (2003). Simple model of spiking neurons. *IEEE Transactions on Neural Networks/a Publication of the IEEE Neural Networks Council, 14*(6), 1569–1572.

Izhikevich, E. M. (2007). *Dynamical systems in neuroscience*. MIT Press.

Jackson, M. P., Rahman, A., Lafon, B., Kronberg, G., Ling, D., Parra, L. C., & Bikson, M. (2016). Animal models of transcranial direct current stimulation: Methods and mechanisms. *Clinical Neurophysiology, 127*(11), 3425–3454.

Jayaram, G., Tang, B., Pallegadda, R., Vasudevan, E. V. L., Celnik, P., & Bastian, A. (2012). Modulating locomotor adaptation with cerebellar stimulation. *Journal of Neurophysiology, 107*(11), 2950–2957.

Jefferys, J. G. (1981). Influence of electric fields on the excitability of granule cells in Guinea-pig hippocampal slices. *The Journal of Physiology, 319*, 143–152.

Joucla, S., & Yvert, B. (2009). The "mirror" estimate: An intuitive predictor of membrane polarization during extracellular stimulation. *Biophysical Journal, 96*(9), 3495–3508.

Kabakov, A. Y., Muller, P. A., Pascual-Leone, A., Jensen, F. E., & Rotenberg, A. (2012). Contribution of axonal orientation to pathway-dependent modulation of excitatory transmission by direct current stimulation in isolated rat hippocampus. *Journal of Neurophysiology, 107*(7), 1881–1889.

Kanai, R., Chaieb, L., Antal, A., Walsh, V., & Paulus, W. (2008). Frequency-dependent electrical stimulation of the visual cortex. *Current Biology, 18*(23), 1839–1843.

Koessler, L., Colnat-Coulbois, S., Cecchin, T., Hofmanis, J., Dmochowski, J. P., Norcia, A. M., & Maillard, L. G. (2016). In-vivo measurements of human brain tissue conductivity using focal electrical current injection through intracerebral multicontact electrodes. LID. (1097-0193 (Electronic)). *Human Brain Mapping, 38*, 974–986.

Krause, B., Marquez-Ruiz, J., & Cohen Kadosh, R. (2013). The effect of transcranial direct current stimulation: A role for cortical excitation/inhibition balance? *Frontiers in Human Neuroscience, 7*, 602.

Kronberg, G., Bridi, M., Abel, T., Bikson, M., & Parra, L. C. (2016). Direct current stimulation modulates LTP and LTD: Activity dependence and dendritic effects. *Brain Stimulation: Basic, Translational, and Clinical Research in Neuromodulation.*

Laakso, I., Tanaka, S., Koyama, S., De Santis, V., & Hirata, A. (2015). Inter-subject variability in electric fields of motor cortical tDCS. *Brain Stimulation, 8*(5), 8.

Lafon, B., Rahman, A., Bikson, M., & Parra, L. C. (2016). Direct current stimulation alters neuronal input/output function. *Brain Stimulation: Basic, Translational, and Clinical Research in Neuromodulation, 10*, 36–45.

Liebetanz, D., Fregni, F., Monte-Silva, K. K., Oliveira, M. B., Amancio-Dos-Santos, A., Nitsche, M. A., & Guedes, R. C. (2006a). After-effects of transcranial direct current stimulation (tDCS) on cortical spreading depression. *Neuroscience Letters, 398*(1–2), 85–90.

Liebetanz, D., Klinker, F., Hering, D., Koch, R., Nitsche, M. A., Potschka, H., … Tergau, F. (2006b). Anticonvulsant effects of transcranial direct-current stimulation (tDCS) in the rat cortical ramp model of focal epilepsy. *Epilepsia, 47*(7), 1216–1224.

Logothetis, N. K., Kayser, C., & Oeltermann, A. (2007). In vivo measurement of cortical impedance spectrum in monkeys: Implications for signal propagation. *Neuron, 55*(5), 809–823.

Marquez-Ruiz, J., Leal-Campanario, R., Sanchez-Campusano, R., Molaee-Ardekani, B., Wendling, F., Miranda, P. C., … Delgado-Garcia, J. M. (2012). Transcranial direct-current stimulation modulates synaptic mechanisms involved in associative learning in behaving rabbits. *Proceedings of the National Academy of Sciences of the United States of America, 109*(17), 6710–6715.

Márquez-Ruiz, J., Leal-Campanario, R., Wendling, F., Ruffini, G., Gruart, A., & Delgado-García, J. M. (2014). Transcranial electrical stimulation in animals. In R. Cohen Kadosh (Ed.), *The stimulated brain* (pp. 117–144). Academic.

Mcintyre, C. C., & Grill, W. M. (1999). Excitation of central nervous system neurons by nonuniform electric fields. *Biophysical Journal, 76*(2), 878–888.

Minhas, P., Bansal, V., Patel, J., Ho, J. S., Diaz, J., Datta, A., & Bikson, M. (2010). Electrodes for high-definition transcutaneous DC stimulation for applications in drug delivery and electrotherapy, including tDCS. *Journal of Neuroscience Methods, 190*(2), 188–197.

Miranda, P. C., Correia, L., Salvador, R., & Basser, P. J. (2007). The role of tissue heterogeneity in neural stimulation by applied electric fields. *Conference Proceedings: Annual International Conference of the IEEE Engineering in Medicine and Biology Society IEEE Engineering in Medicine and Biology Society Annual Conference, 2007*, 1715–1718.

Miranda, P. C., Faria, P., & Hallett, M. (2009). What does the ratio of injected current to electrode area tell us about current density in the brain during tDCS? *Clinical Neurophysiology, 120*(6), 1183–1187.

Miranda, P. C., Hallett, M., & Basser, P. J. (2003). The electric field induced in the brain by magnetic stimulation: A 3-D finite-element analysis of the effect of tissue heterogeneity and anisotropy. *IEEE Transactions on Bio-medical Engineering, 50*(9), 1074–1085.

Miranda, P. C., Lomarev, M., & Hallett, M. (2006). Modeling the current distribution during transcranial direct current stimulation. *Clinical Neurophysiology, 117*(7), 1623–1629.

Miranda, P. C., Mekonnen, A., Salvador, R., & Ruffini, G. (2013). The electric field in the cortex during transcranial current stimulation. *NeuroImage, 70*, 48–58.

Moliadze, V., Antal, A., & Paulus, W. (2010). Electrode-distance dependent after-effects of transcranial direct and random noise stimulation with extracephalic reference electrodes. *Clinical Neurophysiology, 121*(12), 2165–2171.

Monai, H., Ohkura, M., Tanaka, M., Oe, Y., Konno, A., Hirai, H., … Hirase, H. (2016). Calcium imaging reveals glial involvement in transcranial direct current stimulation-induced plasticity in mouse brain. *Nature Communications, 7*, 11100.

Nitsche, M. A., Boggio, P. S., Fregni, F., & Pascual-Leone, A. (2009). Treatment of depression with transcranial direct current stimulation (tDCS): A review. *Experimental Neurology, 219*(1), 14–19.

Nitsche, M. A., Cohen, L. G., Wassermann, E. M., Priori, A., Lang, N., Antal, A., … Pascual-Leone, A. (2008). Transcranial direct current stimulation: State of the art 2008. *Brain Stimulation, 1*(3), 206–223.

Nitsche, M. A., & Paulus, W. (2000). Excitability changes induced in the human motor cortex by weak transcranial direct current stimulation. *The Journal of Physiology, 527*(Pt 3), 633–639.

Nitsche, M. A., & Paulus, W. (2001). Sustained excitability elevations induced by transcranial DC motor cortex stimulation in humans. (0028–3878 (Print)). *Neurology, 57*, 1899.

Nitsche, M. A., & Paulus, W. (2009). Noninvasive brain stimulation protocols in the treatment of epilepsy: Current state and perspectives. *Neurotherapeutics: The Journal of the American Society for Experimental NeuroTherapeutics, 6*(2), 244–250.

Oostendorp, T. F., Delbeke, J., & Stegeman, D. F. (2000). The conductivity of the human skull: Results of in vivo and in vitro measurements. *IEEE Transactions on Bio-medical Engineering, 47*(11), 1487–1492.

Opitz, A., Falchier, A., Yan, C. G., Yeagle, E. M., Linn, G. S., Megevand, P., … Schroeder, C. E. (2016). Spatiotemporal structure of intracranial electric fields induced by transcranial electric stimulation in humans and nonhuman primates. (2045-2322 (electronic)). *Scientific Reports, 6*, 31236. PST – epublish.

Opitz, A., Paulus, W., Will, S., Antunes, A., & Thielscher, A. (2015). Determinants of the electric field during transcranial direct current stimulation. (1095–9572 (Electronic)). *Neuroimage, 109*, 140.

Opitz, A., Windhoff, M., Heidemann, R. M., Turner, R., & Thielscher, A. (2011). How the brain tissue shapes the electric field induced by transcranial magnetic stimulation. *NeuroImage, 58*(3), 849–859.

Ozen, S., Sirota, A., Belluscio, M. A., Anastassiou, C. A., Stark, E., Koch, C., & Buzsaki, G. (2010). Transcranial electric stimulation entrains cortical neuronal populations in rats. *The Journal of neuroscience : the official journal of the Society for Neuroscience, 30*(34), 11476–11485.

Panatier, A., Vallee, J., Haber, M., Murai, K. K., Lacaille, J. C., & Robitaille, R. (2011). Astrocytes are endogenous regulators of basal transmission at central synapses. *Cell, 146*(5), 785–798.

Park, E.-H., Barreto, E., Gluckman, B. J., Schiff, S. J., & So, P. (2005). A model of the effects of applied electric fields on neuronal synchronization. *Journal of Computational Neuroscience, 19*(1), 53–70.

Parra, L. C., & Bikson, M. (2004). Model of the effect of extracellular fields on spike time coherence. *Conference Proceedings: Annual International Conference of the IEEE Engineering in Medicine and Biology Society IEEE Engineering in Medicine and Biology Society Annual Conference, 6*, 4584–4587.

Paulus, W., & Rothwell, J. C. (2016). Membrane resistance and shunting inhibition: Where biophysics meets state-dependent human neurophysiology. *The Journal of Physiology, 594*, 2719–2728.

Pelletier, S. J., & Cicchetti, F. (2015). Cellular and molecular mechanisms of action of transcranial direct current stimulation: Evidence from in vitro and in vivo models. *The International Journal of Neuropsychopharmacology/Official Scientific Journal of the Collegium Internationale Neuropsychopharmacologicum, 18*(2).

Peterchev, A. V., Jalinous, R., & Lisanby, S. H. (2008). A transcranial magnetic stimulator inducing near-rectangular pulses with controllable pulse width (cTMS). *IEEE Transactions on Biomedical Engineering, 55*(1), 257–266.

Peterchev, A. V., Wagner, T. A., Miranda, P. C., Nitsche, M. A., Paulus, W., Lisanby, S. H., … Bikson, M. (2012). Fundamentals of transcranial electric and magnetic stimulation dose: Definition, selection, and reporting practices. *Brain Stimulation, 5*(4), 435–453.

Pethig, R., & Kell, D. B. (1987). The passive electrical properties of biological systems: Their significance in physiology, biophysics and biotechnology. *Physics in Medicine and Biology, 32*(8), 933–970.

Plonsey, R., & Barr, R. C. (1998). Electric field stimulation of excitable tissue. *IEEE Engineering in Medicine and Biology Magazine: The Quarterly Magazine of the Engineering in Medicine & Biology Society, 17*(5), 130–137.

Plonsey, R., & Heppner, D. B. (1967). Considerations of quasi-Stationarity in electrophysiological systems. *B Math Biophys, 29*(4), 657–664.

Podda, M. V., Cocco, S., Mastrodonato, A., Fusco, S., Leone, L., Barbati, S. A., … Grassi, C. (2016). Anodal transcranial direct current stimulation boosts synaptic plasticity and memory in mice via epigenetic regulation of Bdnf expression. *Scientific Reports, 6*, 22180.

Prescott, S. A., De Koninck, Y., & Sejnowski, T. J. (2008). Biophysical basis for three distinct dynamical mechanisms of action potential initiation. *PLoS Computational Biology, 4*(10), e1000198.

Priori, A., Berardelli, A., Rona, S., Accornero, N., & Manfredi, M. (1998). Polarization of the human motor cortex through the scalp. *Neuroreport, 9*(10), 2257–2260.

Purpura, D. P., & Mcmurtry, J. G. (1965). Intracellular activities and evoked potential changes during polarization of motor cortex. *Journal of Neurophysiology, 28*, 166–185.

Radman, T., Ramos, R. L., Brumberg, J. C., & Bikson, M. (2009). Role of cortical cell type and morphology in subthreshold and suprathreshold uniform electric field stimulation in vitro. *Brain Stimulation, 2*(4), 215–228.

Radman, T., Su, Y., An, J. H., Parra, L. C., & Bikson, M. (2007). Spike timing amplifies the effect of electric fields on neurons: Implications for endogenous field effects. *The Journal of neuroscience : the official journal of the Society for Neuroscience, 27*(11), 3030–3036.

Rahman, A., Lafon, B., & Bikson, M. (2015). Multilevel computational models for predicting the cellular effects of noninvasive brain stimulation. *Progress in Brain Research, 222*, 25–40.

Rahman, A., Lafon, B., Parra, L. C., & Bikson, M. (2017). Direct current stimulation boosts synaptic gain and cooperativity in vitro. *The Journal of Physiology, 595*, 3535–3547.

Rahman, A., Reato, D., Arlotti, M., Gasca, F., Datta, A., Parra, L. C., & Bikson, M. (2013). Cellular effects of acute direct current stimulation: Somatic and synaptic terminal effects. *The Journal of Physiology, 591*(10), 2563–2578.

Rahman, A., Lafon, B., Parra, L. C., & Bikson, M. (2017). Direct current stimulation boosts synaptic gain and cooperativity in vitro. *The Journal of Physiology, 595*, 3535–3547.

Rampersad, S., Fau, S. D., Oostendorp, T., & Oostendorp, T. (2011). On handling the layered structure of the skull in transcranial direct current stimulation models. (1557-170X (Print)). *Conference Proceedings IEEE Engineering in Medicine and Biology Society, 2011*, 1989.

Ranck, J. B., Jr. (1975). Which elements are excited in electrical stimulation of mammalian central nervous system: A review. *Brain Research, 98*(3), 417–440.

Ranieri, F., Podda, M. V., Riccardi, E., Frisullo, G., Dileone, M., Profice, P., … Grassi, C. (2012). Modulation of LTP at rat hippocampal CA3-CA1 synapses by direct current stimulation. *Journal of Neurophysiology, 107*(7), 1868–1880.

Reato, D., Bikson, M., & Parra, L. C. (2015). Lasting modulation of in vitro oscillatory activity with weak direct current stimulation. *Journal of Neurophysiology, 113*(5), 1334–1341.

Reato, D., Cammarota, M., Parra, L. C., & Carmignoto, G. (2012). Computational model of neuron-astrocyte interactions during focal seizure generation. *Frontiers in Computational Neuroscience, 6*, 81.

Reato, D., Gasca, F., Datta, A., Bikson, M., Marshall, L., & Parra, L. C. (2013a). Transcranial electrical stimulation accelerates human sleep homeostasis. *PLoS Computational Biology, 9*(2), e1002898.

Reato, D., Rahman, A., Bikson, M., & Parra, L. C. (2010). Low-intensity electrical stimulation affects network dynamics by modulating population rate and spike timing. *The Journal of neuroscience : the official journal of the Society for Neuroscience, 30*(45), 15067–15079.

Reato, D., Rahman, A., Bikson, M., & Parra, L. C. (2013b). Effects of weak transcranial alternating current stimulation on brain activity-a review of known mechanisms from animal studies. *Frontiers in Human Neuroscience, 7*, 687.

Renart, A., de la Rocha, J., Bartho, P., Hollender, L., Parga, N., Reyes, A., & Harris, K. D. (2010). The asynchronous state in cortical circuits. *Science, 327*(5965), 587–590.

Rohan, J. G., Carhuatanta, K. A., Mcinturf, S. M., Miklasevich, M. K., & Jankord, R. (2015). Modulating hippocampal plasticity with in vivo brain stimulation. *The Journal of Neuroscience: The Official Journal of the Society for Neuroscience, 35*(37), 12824–12832.

Roth, B. J., Cohen, L. G., & Hallett, M. (1991). The electric field induced during magnetic stimulation. *Electroencephalography and Clinical Neurophysiology, 43*, 268–278.

Ruffini, G., Fox, M. D., Ripolles, O., Miranda, P. C., & Pascual-Leone, A. (2014). Optimization of multifocal transcranial current stimulation for weighted cortical pattern targeting from realistic modeling of electric fields. *NeuroImage, 89*, 216–225.

Ruffini, G., Wendling, F., Merlet, I., Molaee-Ardekani, B., Mekkonen, A., Salvador, R., … Miranda, P. (2013). Transcranial current brain stimulation (tCS):Models and technologies. *IEEE Transactions on Neural Systems and Rehabilitation Engineering, 21*(3), 333–345.

Rush, S., & Driscoll, D. A. (1968). Current distribution in the brain from surface electrodes. *Anesthesia and Analgesia, 47*(6), 717-723.

Rush, S., & Driscoll, D. A. (1969). Eeg electrode sensitivity – an application of reciprocity. *IEEE Transactions on Bio-medical Engineering, 16*(1), 15.

Sadleir, R. J., Vannorsdall, T. D., Schretlen, D. J., & Gordon, B. (2010). Transcranial direct current stimulation (tDCS) in a realistic head model. *NeuroImage, 51*(4), 1310–1318.

Salvador, R., Ramirez, F., V'Yacheslavovna, M., & Miranda, P. C. (2012). Effects of tissue dielectric properties on the electric field induced in tDCS: A sensitivity analysis. *34th Annual International Conference of the IEEE Engineering in Medicine and Biology Society (EMBC), San Diego*, 787–790.

Salvador, R., Wenger, C., & Miranda, P. C. (2015). Investigating the cortical regions involved in MEP modulation in tDCS. *Frontiers in Cellular Neuroscience, 9.*

Saturnino, G. B., Antunes, A., & Thielscher, A. (2015). On the importance of electrode parameters for shaping electric field patterns generated by tDCS. (1095–9572 (Electronic)). *Neuroimage, 120*, 25.

Schlaug, G., Renga, V., & Nair, D. (2008). Transcranial direct current stimulation in stroke recovery. *Archives of Neurology, 65*(12), 1571–1576.

Schwan, H. P. (1966). Alternating current electrode polarization. *Biophysik, 3*(2), 181–201.

Sehm, B., Hoff, M., Gundlach, C., Taubert, M., Conde, V., Villringer, A., & Ragert, P. (2013). A novel ring electrode setup for the recording of somatosensory evoked potentials during transcranial direct current stimulation (tDCS). *Journal of Neuroscience Methods, 212*(2), 234–236.

Stagg, C. J., & Nitsche, M. A. (2011). Physiological basis of transcranial direct current stimulation. *The Neuroscientist: A Review Journal Bringing Neurobiology, Neurology and Psychiatry, 17*(1), 37–53.

Svirskis, G., Baginskas, A., Hounsgaard, J., & Gutman, A. (1997). Electrotonic measurements by electric field-induced polarization in neurons: Theory and experimental estimation. *Biophysical Journal, 73*(6), 3004–3015.

Terney, D., Chaieb, L., Moliadze, V., Antal, A., & Paulus, W. (2008). Increasing human brain excitability by transcranial high-frequency random noise stimulation. *The Journal of Neuroscience, 28*(52), 14147–14155.

Terzuolo, C. A., & Bullock, T. H. (1956). Measurement of imposed voltage gradient adequate to modulate neuronal firing. *Proceedings of the National Academy of Sciences of the United States of America, 42*(9), 687–694.

Tofts, P. S. (1990). The distribution of induced currents in magnetic stimulation of the nervoussystem. *Physics in Medicine and Biology, 35*(8), 1119–1128.

Tranchina, D., & Nicholson, C. (1986). A model for the polarization of neurons by extrinsically applied electric fields. *Biophysical Journal, 50*(6), 1139–1156.

Tuch, D. S., Wedeen, V. J., Dale, A. M., George, J. S., & Belliveau, J. W. (2001). Conductivity tensor mapping of the human brain using diffusion tensor MRI. *Proceedings of the National Academy of Sciences of the United States of America, 98*(20), 11697–11701.

Vogels, T. P., Rajan, K., & Abbott, L. F. (2005). Neural network dynamics. *Annual Review of Neuroscience, 28*, 357–376.

Wagner, S., Fau, R. S., Aydin, U., Fau, A. U., Vorwerk, J., Fau, V. J., … Wolters, C. H. (2014a). Investigation of tDCS volume conduction effects in a highly realistic head model. (1741–2552 (Electronic)). *Journal of Neural Engineering, 11*, 016002.

Wagner, T., Eden, U., Rushmore, J., Russo, C. J., Dipietro, L., Fregni, F., … Valero-Cabre, A. (2014b). Impact of brain tissue filtering on neurostimulation fields: A modeling study. *NeuroImage, 85*(Pt 3), 1048–1057.

Woods, A. J., Antal, A., Bikson, M., Boggio, P. S., Brunoni, A. R., Celnik, P., … Nitsche, M. A. (2016). A technical guide to tDCS, and related non-invasive brain stimulation tools. *Clinical Neurophysiology: Official Journal of the International Federation of Clinical Neurophysiology, 127*(2), 1031–1048.

Xu, W., Wolff, B. S., & Wu, J. Y. (2014). Low-intensity electric fields induce two distinct response components in neocortical neuronal populations. *Journal of Neurophysiology, 112*(10), 2446–2456.

Yi, G.-S., Wang, J., Wei, X.-L., Tsang, K.-M., Chan, W.-L., Deng, B., & Han, C.-X. (2014). Exploring how extracellular electric field modulates neuron activity through dynamical analysis of a two-compartment neuron model. *Journal of Computational Neuroscience, 36*(3), 383–399.

Zaehle, T., Rach, S., & Herrmann, C. S. (2010). Transcranial alternating current stimulation enhances individual alpha activity in human EEG. *PLoS One, 5*(11), e13766.

Chapter 3
Mechanisms of Acute and After Effects of Transcranial Direct Current Stimulation

Marom Bikson, Walter Paulus, Zeinab Esmaeilpour, Greg Kronberg, and Michael A. Nitsche

Introduction

Understanding the mechanisms of action of central nervous system modulation with direct current stimulation (DCS) is an important endeavor, given the increasing usage of tDCS as a research tool in basic and applied studies, including trials exploring clinical potential. The scale and breadth of tDCS research requires careful consideration of tDCS mechanisms, namely tDCS-induced alterations of physiology and morphology to understand trial results and develop a consensus of its application as a research or treatment tool. In the absence of such understanding, retrospective or meta-analysis can be misguided, for example grouping studies that use different tDCS protocols, which are known from mechanistic studies to produce different and sometimes even opposite functional changes. Leveraging insights on mechanism will support the design of stimulation protocols resulting in optimized functional outcome, especially for clinical application. The parameter space for tDCS protocols (spanning

M. Bikson (✉)
Department of Biomedical Engineering, The City College of New York, New York, NY, USA
e-mail: bikson@ccny.cuny.edu

W. Paulus
Department of Clinical Neurophysiology, University Medical Center Göttingen, Göttingen, Germany

Z. Esmaeilpour · G. Kronberg
Department of Biomedical Engineering, The City College of the City University of New York, New York, NY, USA

M. A. Nitsche
Department of Psychology and Neurosciences, Leibniz Research Centre for Working Environment and Human Factors, Dortmund, Germany

University Medical Hospital Bergmannsheil, Bochum, Germany

H. Knotkova et al. (eds.), *Practical Guide to Transcranial Direct Current Stimulation*, https://doi.org/10.1007/978-3-319-95948-1_3

not just variation in dose but also when/how tDCS is combined with training) makes discovery of best practices (by trial-and-error) in human trials impractical. Indeed, many ongoing trials are encouraging, as modern insights on mechanism are integrated into trial design and significant increases in efficacy can be expected. Similarly, real population level effects of tDCS are reduced in effect-size by inter-subject variability – understanding tDCS mechanisms helps to explain this variability and point the way forward to individualize tDCS (including use of biomarkers) (Strube et al. 2016).

There is a broad base of knowledge regarding the mechanisms of action of tDCS, which spans decades but has rapidly increased during the last years. The first critical description of physiological and functional effects of DCS dates back to the 50s and 60s of the twentieth century in animal models and humans (for an overview see Nitsche et al. (2003a)). This work helped to define basic mechanisms including established polarity specific effects on both acute and lasting activity. The early stimulation approaches were then nearly forgotten until the turn of the century. Interest in tDCS was then increasing again, mainly based on experiments in humans showing neuroplastic effects of tDCS. Based on established neurophysiological effects in man predominantly derived from motor evoked potential studies – including polarity specific lasting changes – additional trials demonstrated effects on behavior and cognitive processes, as well as clinical symptoms in patients suffering from neurological and psychiatric symptoms. The demonstration that tDCS could influence a wide range of behaviors and disorders, spurred further research regarding identification of the mechanistic foundations and thus modeling as well as animal studies and experiments in humans were conducted to this aim. This work reinforced the basic findings on polarity specific changes in acute function (e.g. synaptic efficacy) as well as the modulation of plasticity; but modern mechanistic studies have focused on developing a deeper and more subtle understanding of mechanism including identification of new cellular targets, molecular cascades, forms of plasticity (e.g. long-term potentiation [LTP] vs. long-term depression [LTD]) dose response (at time non-linear), and a more subtle understanding on how tDCS can be specific to various indications (e.g. “functional targeting”; (Bikson and Rahman 2013)).

Studying the mechanisms of tDCS can be approached from various scales and is relevant for understanding the effects of DCS; these can be discerned into studies exploring the effects of tDCS at the microscopic (molecular, cellular), mesoscopic (small neuronal networks, defined cortical areas), and macroscopic (whole brain effects including functional connectivity) level (Rahman et al. 2013). For comprehension of the effects of tDCS, combining all these levels ranging from single cells in animal brain slices to large-scale brain networks in human and ultimately cognition and behavior is relevant, and different experimental approaches are suited to explore tDCS effects at these different levels of complexity (Fig. 3.1). In addition to considerations of scale, in regards to time the mechanisms of tDCS can be discerned in acute or primary effects, which emerge directly during stimulation, and after or secondary effects, which develop during stimulation, but outlast the intervention. We will follow this structure, starting with acute effects of the different levels of complexity, and then going on with tDCS after-effects. We then consider tDCS effects at the network level. Furthermore, we will describe morphological effects of tDCS and effects of tDCS on non-neuronal tissue, which have been comparatively less studied.

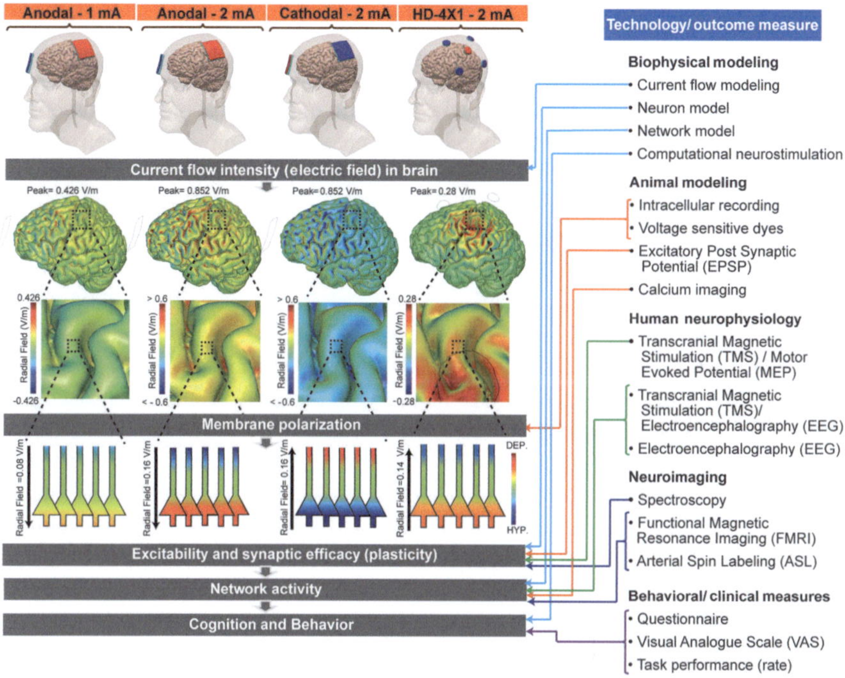

Fig. 3.1 Multi-scale effects and outcome measures of transcranial direct current stimulation. MRI-derived FEM models of current flow illustrate EF in cortex as a function of stimulation polarity, current intensity and electrode configuration. From macroscopic to microscopic level, a uniform EF along pyramidal neurons polarize membrane proportional to induced EF magnitude and direction. Neuronal excitability and plasticity is modulated by external electric field that in larger scale modulate network connectivity and ultimately cognition and behavior. tDCS effects can be probed using different techniques and experimental procedures regarding different scales

Regional Neuronal Effects of tDCS

Primary or Acute Effects

As with other forms of electrical stimulation (Mcintyre et al. 2004; Merrill et al. 2005; Rattay and Wenger 2010), the physiological effects of tDCS can be understood to derive from membrane polarization produced during stimulation. Weak DCS initiates the polarization of cell membranes; specifically the flow of electrical current produced by DCS results in sustained polarization of cell membranes exposed to this current flow (Bikson et al. 2004). Therefore, for the duration that DCS is applied the polarization is sustained. For example, if stimulation is applied for 20 min, then during that entire time the membranes of neurons would be slightly polarized. If tDCS is applied with a training task, then the polarization will be ongoing during the neuronal activity generated by the task. This in turn, would have the effect of changing how neurons process information related to the task (Lafon et al. 2017; Rahman et al. 2017) and their propensity for plasticity (Fritsch et al. 2010; Jackson et al. 2016; Kronberg et al. 2017).

Characterizing which cells (principal cells, interneurons, glia, endothelial cells…) are polarized, and more specifically which compartments within these cells (soma, dendrite, axon) is thus central for understanding the effects of DCS. As discussed below, the consequences of membrane polarization are multi-faceted and complex, spanning changes in action potential threshold and timing following neuronal soma polarization (Radman et al. 2007b) to changes in network coherence (Polania et al. 2011a; Reato et al. 2010) to changes in synaptic efficacy (Bikson et al. 2004; Dudel 1971) and plasticity (Fritsch et al. 2010; Kronberg et al. 2017) to morphological and molecular changes (Pelletier and Cicchetti 2014). Early studies referred to tDCS/DCS as 'polarizing current' (Bindman et al. 1964), reinforcing the idea that transduction is by membrane polarization. Contrasting to other brain stimulation techniques, DCS has the inherent feature that the polarization is sustained (does not recover or reverse as consequence of change in stimulation waveform). The well-recognized time dependence of tDCS/DCS plastic changes (Nitsche and Paulus 2000, 2001) presumably results from the need for sustained polarization, and so in some aspects may be unique to DCS.

A range of alternate transduction mechanisms have been historically ventured as alternative to membrane polarization such as ionic concentration changes somehow generated directly by DCS (e.g. iontophoresis of charged molecules/ions; (Gardner-Medwin 1983)), but to our knowledge no quantitative analysis, much less experimental evidence, exists for tDCS. Rather, as detailed throughout the remainder of this chapter, our mechanistic considerations typically start with the well-established principle of membrane polarization induced by extracellular direct current flow, and all other changes are presumed secondary to this membrane polarization.

The Polarization Effect and Acute DCS Polarity-Specific Excitability Changes

DC stimulation with electrodes on the scalp leads to current flow across the brain (Datta et al. 2009; Huang et al. 2017; Miranda et al. 2006; Opitz et al. 2016), with current from the anode flowing into the brain and current exiting the brain to the cathode. The flow of current around neurons results in polarization of cell membranes when some of this current crosses the membrane. Flow into a specific membrane compartment (from outside the neuron into it) will result in local membrane hyperpolarization, and flow out of another membrane compartment (from inside to out) will result in local membrane depolarization (Andreasen and Nedergaard 1996; Bikson et al. 2004). An often overlooked concept is that the physics of electrical stimulation dictate that any neuron exposed to extracellular DC stimulation will have some compartments that are depolarized while others are hyperpolarized (Bikson et al. 2004; Chan et al. 1988). Which compartments are polarized in which direction depends on the neuronal morphology relative to the DC electric field. Simplistically, for a typical cortical pyramidal cell, with a large apical dendrite pointed toward the cortical surface, a surface anode (positive electrode, generating a cortical inward current flow) will result in somatic (and basal dendrite) depolarization and apical dendrite hyperpolarization (Radman et al. 2009). For this same neuron, a surface cathode (negative electrode, generating cortical outward current flow) will result in opposite polarization effects (Fig. 3.2).

The importance of the somatic compartment in eliciting action potentials, and thereby determining cortical output, suggests somatic polarization plays a critical role in determining cortical excitability changes by DCS (Bikson et al. 2004; Bindman

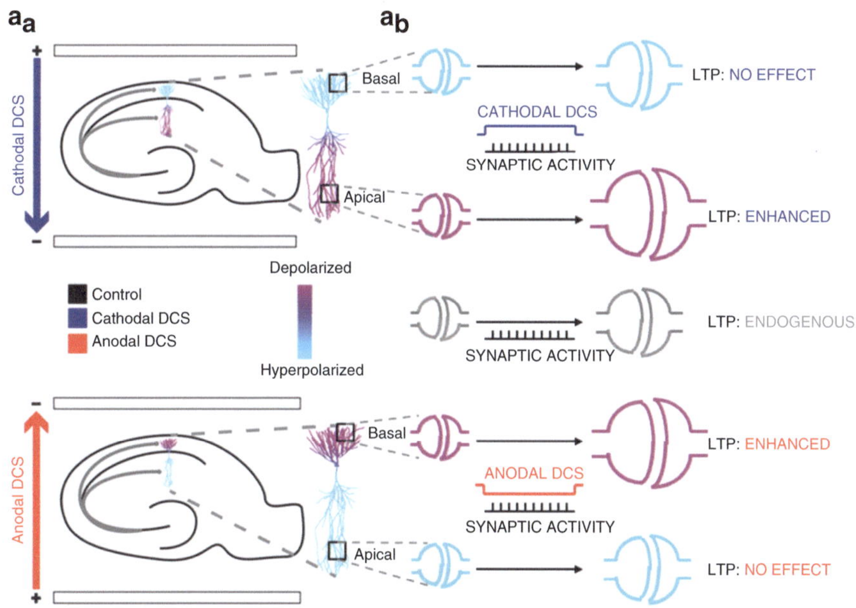

Fig. 3.2 DCS modulation of LTP and LTD depends on dendritic location and endogenous synaptic activity. DCS was applied during synaptic plasticity induction in hippocampal brain slices. The frequency of synaptic activity and dendritic location of plasticity induction were varied to study their role in determining DCS effects. (**a**$_a$) Schematic of hippocampal brain slice preparation, highlighting the membrane polarization of CA1 pyramidal neurons during each polarity of DCS. (**a**$_b$) Changes in synaptic strength in each dendritic compartment when DCS is applied during LTP induction. Both anodal and cathodal DCS can enhance LTP, but in different dendritic compartments, consistent with a pivotal role for DCS induced dendritic membrane depolarization. (**b**) In apical dendrites, cathodal DCS modulates both LTD and LTP induced by trains of synaptic activity at varying frequencies. Note that when synaptic activity is very weak (0.0167 Hz), DCS has no effect on synaptic strength. (**c**) DCS effects depend on the synaptic activity that stimulation is concurrent with (20 or 1 Hz) and the dendritic compartment (apical or basal). Plasticity modulation here is the ratio of the change in synaptic strength for each stimulation condition to the change in synaptic strength for corresponding control condition. Figure adapted from (Kronberg et al. 2017; with permission)

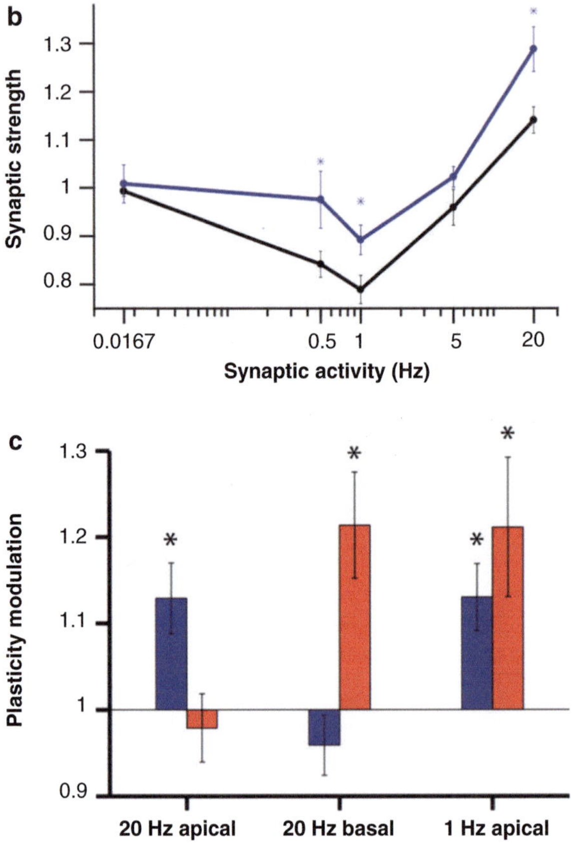

Fig. 3.2 (continued)

et al. 1964; Purpura and Mcmurtry 1965; Radman et al. 2007b), an idea we term the 'somatic doctrine.' Some of the earliest DCS findings in animals were changes in neuronal firing rate under electrodes consistent with surface-anode producing soma depolarization and surface-cathode producing soma hyper-polarization (Bindman et al. 1964; Purpura and Mcmurtry 1965). Ultimately, whether a neuron fires or not is not only determined by the soma, but by the integration of activity in all neuronal compartments including dendrites, axon, presynaptic terminal, axon hillock (see below). DC fields can modulate the functionality of these compartments, increasing the complexity of a purely 'somatic doctrine' (Kabakov et al. 2012; Kronberg et al. 2017; Rahman et al. 2013). None-the-less, the somatic doctrine has implicitly informed the rationale for most tDCS human trials – namely presumed excitation by the anode and inhibition by the cathode.

In accordance with a primary polarizing effect of DC stimulation, studies in humans have shown that tDCS for a few seconds, which does not induce after-effects, already induces stimulation polarity-dependent cortical excitability alterations as probed by transcranial magnetic stimulation (TMS) (Nitsche et al. 2007a; Nitsche and Paulus 2000). These seem not to relevantly depend on synaptic effects, since block of glutamatergic NMDA receptors and enhancement of GABAergic activity – the main synaptic drivers of cortical excitability – do not affect acute DC-induced excitability alterations. Furthermore, intracortical inhibition and facilitation, which are driven by GABAergic and glutamatergic synapses, are not relevantly affected by stimulation protocols which do not induce after effects (Nitsche et al. 2005). In contrast, block of voltage-gated ion channels, which should affect the impact of depolarizing stimulation on cortical excitability, abolishes excitability-enhancing effects of tDCS (Nitsche et al. 2003a). Excitability-enhancing effects of anodal tDCS and –reducing effects with cathodal tDCS in the human motor cortex (Nitsche and Paulus 2000) are in accordance with respective de- and hyperpolarization of the soma of pyramidal cells. However, the respective experiments cannot rule out an effect of tDCS on other structures, since the primary measure of motor cortex excitability – single pulse transcranial magnetic stimulation-generated motor evoked potentials – is an unspecific measure of cortico-spinal excitability.

In analogy to findings that tDCS acutely changes response to TMS in man, studies in animal models have demonstrated that responses to afferent micro-stimulation are acutely changed in the target neurons by direct current (Bikson et al. 2004; Kabakov et al. 2012; Lafon et al. 2017; Rahman et al. 2013). The modulation is polarity specific and for short duration DCS, the effects on evoked responses do not outlast the DCS.

Quantification of Polarization Effects with Coupling Constant

Precisely understanding tDCS requires a quantitative model, beginning with quantification of somatic, as well axon and dendrite, polarization during tDCS. Here, the coupling constant (also termed polarization length) is an important concept. Assumed that for weak electric fields (well below the threshold for action potential generation) the membrane polarization at any given compartment, including the soma, produced by DCS is linear with electric field intensity, for uniform electric fields, the membrane potential polarization can thus be expressed as: $V_{tm} = G*E$ where V_{tm} is the polarization of the compartment of interest (in: Volts), G is the coupling constant (in: V per V/m, or simply: m) and E is the electric field (in: V/m). For rat hippocampus and cortical neurons, the somatic coupling constant is in the range of 0.1–0.3 mm (Bikson et al. 2004; Deans et al. 2007; Radman et al. 2009). In ferret cortical neurons the coupling constant is similarly approximately 0.25 mm (Fröhlich and Mccormick 2010). Note that for humans, assuming scaling of sensitivity with total neuronal length (Joucla and Yvert 2009) somatic depolarization per V/m may be higher. The finding that higher stimulation intensities result in stronger effects of stimulation, within specific limits, in case of motor cortex tDCS in humans is in principle accordance with this coupling constant, although respective intensity-dependent effects have been only explored for after-effects of tDCS so far (Nitsche and Paulus 2000) and higher dose and altered brain state complicates dose response in humans (Giordano et al. 2017; Jamil et al. 2017).

An important consequence of the concept of the coupling constant (polarization length) is that a presumed linear polarization with DCS intensity means that there is no "threshold" for polarization; any field intensity will produce some level of polarization (Bikson et al. 2004). The central question is not if tDCS will polarize neurons at all but rather what is the consequence of that polarization, and specifically as tDCS is expected to produce only a small membrane potential change (e.g. less than a mV) what active brain processes "amplify" the effects of this polarization. Vice versa it has been argued that activation of neurons may via opening of ion channels shorten the time constant of the membrane and reduce the efficacy of tDCS (Paulus and Rothwell 2016). Characterizing the mechanisms of tDCS has thus focused on explaining how weak membrane polarization of specific cellular compartments leads to functional changes of ongoing activity.

Geometry of Stimulation Effects and Sensitivity of Soma, Dendrite, and Axon Compartments

Determining the coupling constant of the soma and other membrane compartments in humans to tDCS remains an important research question. The maximal depolarization of pyramidal neurons somas occurs when the electric field is parallel with the somato-dendritic axis which typically corresponds to an electric field radial (normal) to the cortical surface, while electric fields orthogonal to the somato-dendritic axis (along the cortical surface) do not produce significant somatic polarization (Bikson et al. 2004; Chan et al. 1988). The somatic coupling strength is generally related to the size of the cell and the dendritic asymmetry around the soma (Radman et al. 2009; Svirskis et al. 1997) making layer II/IV and layer 5 pyramidal neurons relatively sensitive to DCS polarization. For cortical pyramidal neurons, the typical polarity of somatic polarization is consistent with the 'somatic doctrine' (e.g., positive somatic depolarization for positive electric field). The polarity of the coupling constant is inverted (using our field direction convention) for CA1 pyramidal neurons due to their inverted morphology of the apical-dendrite branches relative to the field direction.

Experiments in humans support the direction-dependency of tDCS effects not only for antagonistic stimulation polarities, but also for the relation of cortical current flow angle in relation to neuronal orientation. It was shown that the position of the return electrode, and thus electrical field orientation, critically determines the efficacy of tDCS (Nitsche and Paulus 2000). Furthermore, with the same target electrode position, antagonistically placed return electrodes, which convert the direction of electrical field orientation, result in roughly converted effects of visual cortex stimulation on visual evoked potentials (Accornero et al. 2007; Antal et al. 2004a). Finally, studies showing that stimulation of distant, but connected areas affect primary motor cortex excitability are compatible with the concept that tDCS might affect primarily pyramidal output neurons (Boros et al. 2008; Rivera-Urbina et al. 2015).

A presumption of the somatic doctrine is that at the cortex under the anode electrode currents are radial and inward producing somatic depolarization, while at the cortex under the cathode current is radial and outward, producing somatic hyperpolarization. However, high-resolution modeling suggests that in convoluted human cortex, current is neither unidirectional nor dominantly radial (Rahman et al. 2013). Though the 'somatic doctrine' is based only on radially directed electrical current flow (normal to the cortical surface), during tDCS significant tangential current flow is also generated (along the cortical surface) (Rahman et al. 2013). Indeed, recent work suggests tangential currents may be more prevalent between and even under electrodes. Tangential currents cannot be ignored in considering the effects of tDCS. Moreover, due to cortical folding the direction of radial current flow under tDCS electrodes is not consistent, meaning there are clusters of both inward (depolarizing) and outward (hyperpolarizing) cortical current flow under either the anode or the cathode (Rahman et al. 2013). Due to the cortical convolutions, current is not unidirectional under electrodes, thus, under the cathode there may be isolated regions of inward cortical flow, and in those regions neuronal excitability may increase (Creutzfeldt et al. 1962).

For dendritic effects of DCS, the basal dendrite of pyramidal neurons will be polarized similarly as the soma, however the apical dendrite will be polarized in the opposite direction (Fig. 3.2) (Andreasen and Nedergaard 1996; Bikson et al. 2004). The dendrites are also electrically excitable. Animal studies with high intensity applied DC fields (~100 V/m) have shown that with sufficiently strong stimulation, active processes (spikes) can be triggered in the dendrites (Andreasen and Nedergaard 1996; Chan et al. 1988; Delgado-Lezama et al. 1999; Wong and Stewart 1992). Even if the electric fields induced during tDCS are not sufficient in themselves to trigger dendritic spikes, they are likely to alter ongoing voltage-dependent mechanisms and synaptic integration in dendrites (Cavarretta et al. 2014). Indeed, recent work suggests that DCS modulates synaptic plasticity in a manner consistent with dendritic polarization (Fig. 3.3; (Kronberg et al. 2017)). The role of dendritic polarization during tDCS remains an open question especially when considering processing of synaptic input.

It is also well established that axons are sensitive to applied electric fields (see below); the magnitude and direction of polarization is a function of neuronal and axonal morphology (Bullock and Hagiwara 1957; Salvador et al. 2011; Takeuchi and Takeuchi 1962). While the axon initial segment would likely be polarized in the same direction as the soma (Chan et al. 1988), for distal regions of long axons, this is not necessarily the case. Hence, it is useful to separately consider the axon initial segments (within a membrane space constant of the soma) and more distal axonal processes, which can be further divided into 'axons-of-passage' and afferent axons with terminations. Notably, for long straight axons-of-passage (e.g., Peripheral Nervous System, PNS) cathodal stimulation will be more effective than anodal stimulation in inducing depolarization (opposite to the somatic doctrine; (Bishop and Erlanger 1926)). It has been shown that weak DC fields can produce acute changes in CNS axon excitability (pre-synaptic/antidromic volley; (Bikson et al. 2004; Jefferys 1981; Kabakov et al. 2012)). The relevance of alteration of dendritic and axonal excitability by DC stimulation is underscored further by suggestions that not only radial, on which the somatic doctrine is based, but also tangential current flow might be relevant for DCS effects.

The involvement of non-pyramidal neurons in the effects of DC stimulation remains an open question. Because of their relatively symmetric dendritic morphology, interneuron somas are expected to polarize less than pyramidal neurons (Radman et al. 2009). Based on the 'somatic doctrine' their importance might then be assumed diminished. However, one cannot exclude polarizing effects of fields on dendrites and axons of interneurons. Moreover, interneurons represent a wide range of morphologies and size, including more asymmetric morphologies (Freund and Buzsaki 1996). An impact of DC fields on interneuron excitability has been shown in animal experimentation (Purpura and Mcmurtry 1965). Interneurons exert a powerful regional effect, including a role in plasticity and oscillations. An effect of paired-pulse facilitation in hippocampal slices may also suggest modulation of the activity of interneurons (Kabakov et al. 2012). Similarly at least for after-effects of tDCS, alteration of GABAergic-driven processes seems to be relevant, as shown in experiments in humans (Nitsche et al. 2005; Stagg et al. 2009a), although these experiments do not allow to conclude if these are direct or secondary effects of DC stimulation. Thus, the specific role of interneurons in the direct effect of tDCS remains an open question.

In summary, while it is convenient to assume a consistent direction of current flow under electrodes, such that brain regions under anode/cathode have uniform inward/outward direct current across the cortex, the situation in humans is more complex. The convoluted cortical surface in fact produces mixed directed currents even directly under each electrode (Lafon et al. 2017; Rahman et al. 2013). This in turn means that neurons will experience a mixed polarity of polarization. The morphology of neuronal processes is itself heterogeneous, and the role of dendrite and axon polarization independent of soma, should be considered.

Amplification: Enhancing Neuronal Sensitivity to DCS

Work quantifying how much current reaches the brain during tDCS (Datta et al. 2009; Huang et al. 2017; Miranda et al. 2006; Opitz et al. 2016) and the sensitivity of neurons to weak DCS has raised questions about how such minimal polarization (<1 mV) could result in functional/clinical changes especially considering that endogenous 'background' synaptic noise can exceed these levels (Magee and Cook 2000). In recent years, motivated by increased evidence that transcranial stimulation with weak currents has functional effects (Floel 2014), as well as ongoing questions about the role of endogenous electric fields that can have comparable electric fields (Fröhlich and Mccormick 2010), the mechanisms of amplification have been explored in animal studies.

At the level of a single neuron, the most evident non-linear response that could serve as a substrate for acute amplification is the threshold-based all-or-none action potential. Importantly, as the electric fields generated in the brain during tDCS are too weak to trigger action potentials in neurons at rest (e.g. ~20 mV membrane depolarization from rest to action potential threshold) we should consider instead modulation of ongoing action potential activity. At the single cell level, amplification could affect either: (1) the rate of action potential generation (rate effects); and/or (2) amplification through change in the timing of action potentials (timing effects). As discussed above, classic animal studies on weak direct current stimulation showed a change in ongoing action potential discharge rate that is roughly linear with electric field intensity and so membrane polarization by DCS (Bindman et al. 1964; Creutzfeldt et al. 1962; Purpura and Mcmurtry 1965; Terzuolo and Bullock 1956). In this sense, the amplification (gain) would relate to the sensitivity of discharge rate to DCS-induced membrane polarization. Interestingly, Terzuolo and Bullock (Terzuolo and Bullock 1956) reported a detectable change in neuronal firing rate at electric fields as small as 0.8 V/m, and postulated that this detection threshold would likely decrease with longer and more sophisticated experiments. Assuming that a 2 mA tDCS protocol generated a peak electric field in the brain of 0.5 V/m (Huang et al. 2017) leading to ~0.15 mV somatic polarization (Radman et al. 2009), and that across animal studies changes in firing rates of 7 Hz per mV membrane polarization have been reported (Carandini and Ferster 2000), a change in firing rate of approximately 1 Hz during conventional tDCS is plausible. Remarkably, recent work has shown that sub-mV depolarization of pyramidal neuron somas was sufficient to convert silent cells into place cells in the hippocampus (Lee et al. 2012).

Changes in AP timing (rather than discharge rate) could also serve to amplify the effects of weak membrane polarization produced by weak direct current stimulation (Radman et al. 2007b). In acute brain slice recordings and in a simple neuron model it was demonstrated that the resulting change in timing could be quantified simply by the induced membrane polarization times the inverse of the ramp slope. Thus, the inverse of the ramp-slope is a "gain/amplification" term because the shallower a ramp, the larger the timing change for any given small polarization by direct current stimulation. For example, based on an approximate 0.2 mV somatic polarization during 2 mA tDCS, then in response to a 1 mV/ms ramp slope, timing would change by 0.3 ms. Therefore, the amplification in this case can be understood as a larger change in action potential timing for a small DCS membrane polarization. This coupling sensitivity and the resulting timing changes were further confirmed by Anastassiou and colleagues (Anastassiou et al. 2010) using a more complex model. Though the basic principle of timing amplification is expected to generalize to other neuron types responding to an increasing synaptic input (Bikson et al. 2004), the most simple amplification equation makes specific assumptions about membrane properties and dynamics (Radman et al. 2007a) that may not extend to all neurons types (Radman et al. 2009). For acute effects of DC stimulation, amplification has not been studied in the human brain, but amplification seems to play a role in network after effects of tDCS (see below). For reasons not entirely clear, the maintenance of tDCS for minutes appears to play a key role in the generation of after-effects and thus increasing sensitivity, as discussed next.

DCS Modulation of Synaptic Efficacy and Polarization of Axon Terminals

A compelling topic of investigation about probable mechanisms of excitability changes induced by tDCS, is which types of neurons, and which neuronal compartments are involved. Regarding changes in synaptic efficacy a key question is: as invariably during tDCS half the dendrite will be polarized in the same direction as the soma and half of the dendrite will be polarized in the opposite direction (see above), how do polarity-specific changes arise? This question has been addressed in detail in animal models examining acute changes in evoked synaptic efficacy (excitability) during DCS.

Early work probing evoked responses in animal models indicated modulation in excitability, with the direction of evoked response change consistent with the somatic doctrine (Bindman et al. 1964; Creutzfeldt et al. 1962), though Bishop and O'Leary (1950) already noted deviations. Recent studies aimed at developing and validating animal models of transcranial electrical stimulation have shown modulation of TMS evoked potentials and visual evoked potentials consistent with the somatic doctrine (Cambiaghi et al. 2010, 2011). In a pioneering work using uniform electric fields in brain slices, Jefferys showed acute modulation of excitability (synaptically driven population spikes) in the dentate gyrus of hippocampal slices when electric fields were parallel to the primary target cell dendritic axis. The detected polarity-specific changes were consistent with somatic polarization, and no modulation occurred when the electric field was applied orthogonal to the primary dendritic axis (Jefferys 1981). The precise control of electric field angle is possible in brain slices and was leveraged in subsequent work.

For the hippocampal slice preparation, several deviations from the somatic doctrine were found (Bikson et al. 2004). Optical imaging with voltage sensitive dyes provided direct evidence that DC electric fields always produce bimodal polarization across target neurons such that somatic depolarization is associated with apical dendrite hyperpolarization, and vice-versa – yet weak interactions across compartments were observed. In addition, for synaptic inputs to the apical dendritic tuft, we reported modulation inconsistent with the somatic doctrine. Also in hippocampal slices, Kabakov et al. (2012) reported modulation of synaptic efficacy in a direction opposite to that expected from the somatic doctrine (noting inversion of dendrite morphology in CA1 pyramids relative to cortex). In this case, one may speculate that apical dendrite depolarization determines the direction of modulation despite somatic hyperpolarization (Bikson et al. 2004); though Kabakov et al. (2012) provides evidence suggesting dendritic polarization affects the magnitude but not direction of modulation. As noted, in cortical slices by Fritsch et al. (2010), modulation of evoked responses is indeed consistent with the somatic doctrine – a finding we have confirmed for four distinct afferent cortical synaptic pathways (Rahman et al. 2013). Variations across animal studies could be simply ascribed to differences in region/preparation, timescale (acute, long-term), and different forms of plasticity (BDNF dependent/independent), but this is speculative and provides little insight into tDCS. Rather, in attempt to reconcile these findings in a single framework, we cite evidence for and define the 'terminal-doctrine' to compliment the 'somatic-doctrine'.

The effects of tangential fields on synaptic efficacy were also explored (Bikson et al. 2004). Tangential fields are oriented perpendicular to the primary somato-dendritic axis, so they are expected to produce little somatic polarization, which was directly confirmed with intracellular recording. Surprisingly, electric fields applied tangentially were as effective at modulating synaptic efficacy as radially directed fields. The afferent axons run tangentially, so we speculated they might be the targets of stimulation. Exploring different pathways, we found that axon pathways with terminals pointed toward the anode were potentiated, while axon pathways with terminals pointed toward the cathode were inhibited. Kabakov et al. (2012) reported similar pathway specific dependence summarizing "the fEPSP is maximally suppressed when the AP travels toward the cathode, and either facilitated or remains unchanged when the excitatory signal [AP] propagates toward the anode". In addition, Kabakov et al. (2012) observed changes in paired-pulse facilitation that are consistent with pre-synaptic vesicular glutamate release. In a variety of tDCS studies different tDCS polarity resulted in behavioral effects in one direction only. E.g. in an implicit motor learning paradigm anodal tDCS facilitated reaction times (Nitsche et al. 2003a) whereas cathodal tDCS also induced a trendwise facilitation. One explanation could be that in case of anodal tDCS the somatic doctrine dominated whereas with cathodal tDCS more superficial horizontal afferents were facilitated.

We recently confirmed a similar directional sensitivity in cortical slices across 4 distinct pathways where electric fields applied tangentially to the surface (and so producing minimal somatic polarization) (Radman et al. 2009), modulated synaptic efficacy (Rahman et al. 2013). An impact of premotor and posterior parietal tDCS on primary motor cortex plasticity was reported for the human brain, which is in accordance with an involvement of afferent terminals in the plasticity effects of tDCS (Boros et al. 2008; Rivera-Urbina et al. 2015). A role for pre-synaptic modulation during DC stimulation is indeed not surprising and has been also historically observed. Purpura and McMurtry (1965) noted "although the [somatic] membrane changes produced by transcortical polarization current satisfactorily explains alterations in spontaneous discharges and evoked synaptic activities in [pyramidal tract] cell, it must be emphasized that the effects of polarizing current on other elements constituting the 'pre-synaptic,' interneuronal pathway to [pyramidal tract] cells also appear to be determinants of the overt changes observed in [pyramidal tract] cells activities." Bishop and O'Leary (1950) not only quantified pre-synaptic effects during DC stimulation in animals, they noted that pre-synaptic effects would complicate the interpretation of post-synaptic changes as well as themselves induce long-lasting aftereffects.

Cellular process terminals including axon terminals are especially sensitive to electric fields as a result of their morphology, and terminal polarization can modulate synaptic efficacy (independent of target soma polarization) (Awatramani et al. 2005; Bullock and Hagiwara 1957; Del Castillo and Katz 1954; Hubbard and Willis 1962a, b; Takeuchi and Takeuchi 1962). Moreover, this modulation is cumulative in time and endures after stimulation (Hubbard and Willis 1962b), has a temporal profile noted in classic DC experiments (Bindman et al. 1964), and suggests the possibility for plasticity. The direction of modulation in brain slice studies consistently suggests that terminal hyperpolarization enhanced efficacy, while depolarization inhibited efficacy. Paired-pulse analysis in a rabbit model suggested tDCS influences pre-synaptic sites (Márquez-Ruiz et al. 2012). Since tDCS induces significant tangential fields, the role of terminal polarization (independent of the 'somatic doctrine') remains a compelling and open question especially when taken together with the need for amplification and the role of synapses in plasticity.

Secondary or After-Effects

Beyond the acute effects of DC stimulation on membrane polarity, sufficiently long stimulation (for some minutes) induces after-effects, which can last for over 1 h, and under specific conditions more than 24 h after stimulation (Monte-Silva et al. 2013; Nitsche et al. 2003a; Nitsche and Paulus 2001). Several animal and human studies have speculated that processes linked to the dendrites are involved in the long-term effects of tDCS (e.g., glutamatergic receptors like n-methyl-D-aspartic receptor, NMDAR) (Liebetanz et al. 2002; Nitsche et al. 2003a; Yoon et al. 2012). Animal studies, some decades old, have suggested lasting changes in brain excitability by DCS. Animal studies in the 1960's established that weak DC current can produce lasting physical changes in neural activity, which cannot be explained as persistent 'reverberating circuit' of activation (Gartside 1968a, b). Especially notable are animal studies by Bindman and colleagues (Bindman et al. 1962), who recognized the importance of prolonged DC stimulation to produce polarity-specific lasting cortical excitability changes (>5 h) which informed their early work in tDCS of psychiatric disorders (Costain et al. 1964; Redfearn et al. 1964). Multi-minute stimulation was later adopted in humans to demonstrate polarity-specific lasting changes in cortical excitability by TMS (Nitsche et al. 2003a; Nitsche and Paulus 2000, 2001). Though these multi-minute protocols are now universally adopted in tDCS research, the mechanisms by which specifically prolonged stimulation protocols trigger plasticity have not been completely clarified.

General Framework for Synaptic Plasticity Modulation by DCS

Synaptic plasticity is considered central in brain plasticity, so synapses are an evident focus to explain lasting tDCS effects. Both in humans and animal studies changes in synaptically mediated evoked responses are considered reliable hallmarks of long-term plastic changes. Thus, much of modern animal studies on tDCS plasticity considered lasting changes in synaptic efficacy.

Electric fields generated by tDCS are sub-threshold, in the sense that they are too weak to trigger action potential in quiescent neurons – in the brain where neurons are not quiescent the actions of tDCS are considered to modulate ongoing activity. Modulatory effects on firing rate, timing, and synaptic efficacy have been demonstrated. Lasting changes in synaptic efficacy could be mediated through different paradigms, which are not necessarily exclusive:

1. Membrane polarization may trigger plastic synaptic changes in a manner independent of any ongoing, future, or past synaptic input or action potential generation (i.e., simply holding the membrane at an offset polarization initiates changes). However, in a cortical brain slice model (with no background activity), weak polarization was not sufficient to induce plastic changes in synaptic efficacy (Fritsch et al. 2010) (c.f. Ranieri et al. 2012). The concept is mute in humans since the cortex is always active; it was shown that alteration of cortical activity levels modulates tDCS effects (Antal et al. 2007; Thirugnanasambandam et al. 2011).
2. Changes in action potential rate or timing, secondary to neuronal polarization, may affect synaptic plasticity. Bindman et al. (1964) already stated "There is some evidence that a determining factor in producing long-lasting after effects is the change in the firing rate of neurons rather than the current flow that produces the changes." Classic animal studies indicated weak DC stimulation is sufficient to induce plastic changes (Bindman et al. 1964; Gartside 1968a).
3. Incremental polarization of the membrane in combination with ongoing synaptic activity may induce synaptic plasticity. The specific hypothesis here is that the generation of plasticity requires synaptic co-activation during DC stimulation. Fritsch et al. (2010) shows synaptic potentiation in-vitro under anodal stimulation only during synaptic stimulation of specific frequencies. In a rabbit study, DCS was combined with repeated somatosensory stimulation in-vivo, leading to acute polarity-specific changes, and lasting changes for the cathodal case (Márquez-Ruiz et al. 2012). If dependent on combined polarization and synaptic input, then synapse specific changes are plausible. If one assumes DCS exerts a post-synaptic priming effect (polarization of soma/dendrite) then co-activation of afferent synaptic input could be conceived as Hebbian reinforcement. This plasticity paradigm is broadly analogous to combining tDCS with a cognitive task or specific behavior that co-activates a targeted network or combining tDCS with TMS. Indeed, work showing the importance of

co-activation in cortical slices (Hess and Donoghue 1999; Rioult-Pedotti et al. 1998), influenced Nitsche and Paulus (2000) in developing tDCS. Importantly, unlike in brain slice and anesthetized animal models, the human cortex is constantly active such that tDCS is always applied in conjunction with ongoing synaptic input even if it is not explicitly paired with another intervention. However, plasticity-increasing effects are seen when tDCS is combined with peripheral nerve stimulation in humans (Rizzo et al. 2014), which supports this concept.

4. Incremental polarization of the membrane may boost ongoing endogenous synaptic plasticity. Clinically this fourth paradigm is analogous to combing tDCS with learning/training (Bolognini et al. 2010). For example, in the aforementioned rabbit study, DCS modulated ongoing synaptic habituation, similar to a model of associative learning (Márquez-Ruiz et al. 2012). An important implication of this paradigm is that DCS effects will depend on the nature of the endogenous plasticity that is paired with. For example, recent work in brain slices showed that DCS can modulate endogenous synaptic plasticity, but the direction and magnitude of this modulation depends on the dendritic location and pattern of endogenous synaptic activity (Fig. 3.3; Kronberg et al. 2017). As a result, both anodal and cathodal stimulation can enhance and diminish LTP depending on these parameters. In human motor cortex, tDCS modulates simultaneous LTP induction via paired associative stimulation (PAS) (Nitsche et al. 2007b). Moreover, LTP-like plasticity-inducing tDCS has been shown to foster motor learning, which is thought to critically depend on LTP, if applied synchronously with task performance (Nitsche et al. 2003b; Reis et al. 2009).
5. Meta-plasticity is defined as sustained polarization before, or potentially after, the generation of endogenous LTP that "primes" the brain to respond differently to potentiation. Evidence from brain slices (Ranieri et al. 2012) and in vivo animal experiments (Podda et al. 2016; Rohan et al. 2015) shows priming with DCS modulates subsequent tetanus-induced LTP in a polarity specific manner. A similar effect has been shown for the human motor cortex in case of priming PAS-induced LTP-like plasticity via anodal and cathodal tDCS. However, whether priming stimulation reduces or enhances subsequently induced plasticity might also critically depend on the inter-intervention interval (Fricke et al. 2011; Monte-Silva et al. 2010).
6. Changes in network dynamics where the generation of LTD/LTP is explained through intervention with ongoing oscillations and may manifest as lasting changes in oscillation dynamics (Reato et al. 2013a, 2015). Such modulation may reflect interference with the finely tuned excitatory-inhibitory synaptic balance during oscillations (Reato et al. 2010). Indeed, tDCS in humans was shown to alter oscillatory brain activity during (Hanley et al. 2016), but also after stimulation (Ardolino et al. 2005; Zaehle et al. 2010), and might also affect phase-coupling of oscillatory activity (Carter et al. 2015).

Decades of Research Characterizing DCS Changes of Neuronal Plasticity

It is remarkable that a decade before the widely-credited "discovery" of Long-Term Potentiation by trains of suprathreshold pulses by Bliss and Lomo (1973), animal studies had shown lasting changes in excitability following DCS lasting up to hours (Bindman et al. 1962). Moreover, DCS researchers had begun to address the underlying molecular mechanisms (Gartside 1968a, b) and translating results to humans. LTP/LTD induced by tetanic stimulation and by DC current may share some common molecular substrates (Gartside 1968b; Islam et al. 1995b; Ranieri et al. 2012).

Common forms of LTP/LTD are mediated by the NMDA receptor (Malenka and Bear 2004), which has been implicated in both long-term tDCS effects in humans (Liebetanz et al. 2002; Nitsche et al. 2003a, 2004) and in-vitro DCS-induced plasticity (Fritsch et al. 2010). Moreover, GABAergic activity – which reduces glutamatergic plasticity in animal slice preparations (Castro-Alamancos et al. 1995) seems to be reduced by both, cathodal and anodal tDCS, as shown for the human motor cortex (Stagg et al. 2009a). This combined mechanism might enhance the propensity of tDCS to induce plasticity in the human brain in vivo. Given the relevant involvement of calcium in NMDA receptor-dependent glutamatergic plasticity, it is not surprising that intracellular calcium content is increased by LTP-like plasticity-inducing DC stimulation in animal models (Islam et al. 1995), and that calcium channel block abolishes tDCS-induced LTP-like plasticity in humans (Nitsche et al. 2003a). The dependency of LTP and LTD induction on the amount of calcium influx – low increase results in LTD, high increase in LTP (Lisman 2001), and even higher increase might again diminish plasticity due to compensatory mechanisms – explains furthermore the switch from LTP- to LTD-like plasticity if stimulation lasts too long (Monte-Silva et al. 2013), or is accompanied by pharmacological intervention increasing calcium influx (Lugon et al. 2015).

Beyond these potential drivers of DC stimulation-induced plasticity, experiments in humans have revealed an important impact of neuromodulators, such as dopamine, acetylcholine, and serotonin. Alteration of the activity of these systems prominently impact the plasticity-inducing effects of DC stimulation (Fresnoza et al. 2014a, b; Grundey et al. 2012; Nitsche et al. 2012). Similarly, the BDNF/TrKB pathway is known to be a potent modulator of these common forms of LTP/LTD (Lu 2003) and this pathway has also been implicated in long-term tDCS effects in both humans and animals (Fritsch et al. 2010; Podda et al. 2016; Ranieri et al. 2012). Earlier work looked at accumulation of potential molecular targets of stimulated brain tissue, and beyond the impact of calcium (Islam et al. 1995a) found effects of DC stimulation on adenosine-sensitive cAMP (Hattori et al. 1990), and protein kinase C (Islam et al. 1995b), each of which play a role in LTP/LTD. Building on this, more recent in vivo animal work has shown long-term tDCS effects to be dependent on the adenosine A1 receptor (Márquez-Ruiz et al. 2012). While evidence is accumulating that DCS-induced plasticity shares molecular mechanisms with classic LTP/LTD, the manner in which the primary, polarizing effect of tDCS interacts with this molecular machinery remains an important area of research. Here experiments in humans show that combination of anodal tDCS and voltage-gated ion channel block not only abolish acute, polarization-dependent effects of tDCS, but also after-effects, which suggests an important role of polarization for the development of neuroplasticity (Nitsche et al. 2003a).

Furthermore, regarding contributing neurons, motor cortex studies in humans deliver relevant information adding to the results of pharmacological studies. Here, tDCS polarity-dependently alters intracortical inhibition and facilitation, which are driven by glutamatergic and GABAergic neurons. However, tDCS polarity-independently enhances I-wave facilitation, which is suppressed by GABAergic activity (Nitsche et al. 2005). Modulation of afferent activity to the primary motor cortex might be involved, since modulation of premotor activity by DC stimulation modifies intracortical inhibition and facilitation in a similar manner as primary motor cortex stimulation (Boros et al. 2008).

Given the complexity of plasticity, and how it underpins learning, there are open questions about how tDCS modulates synaptic function. Importantly, valuable research in this direction should not be confused with the absence of decades of literature (summarized above). Similarly, exhaustive work over the past decade showing nuance in how DCS modulates synaptic efficacy (such as state dependent effects) should not be conflated with a deficiency in existing knowledge. Rather, ongoing research on tDCS modulation of plasticity is more advanced than most other neuromodulation tools and indeed many drugs. These studies reflect the detail of ongoing work. Many of these investigations relate to variation in the direction of modulation, if anodal and cathodal stimulation always exhibit and inhibit synaptic efficacy – consistent with the ‘somatic doctrine’ – or if there are dose and brain-state specific reversals in direction.

Synaptic Plasticity and Galvanotropism

The kind of plasticity induced by tDCS so far refers to functional or synaptic plasticity. Another plasticity mechanism includes morphological alterations, like axonal growth and guidance, which might also be affected by DCS. It is well established that electric fields play a role as signals in the development and regeneration of the nervous system (Mccaig et al. 2005). Several studies have shown endogenous electric fields within growing and recovering tissue. Whether similar mechanisms may be relevant during DCS may come down to the sensitivity of growth to DCS relevant electric fields. As we review, axonal growth in vivo and in vitro has been demonstrated with applied fields at significantly higher intensities and for longer durations than tDCS (Mccaig and Rajnicek 1991).

The study of electric fields and cellular galvanotropism (induced growth by an electrical stimulus) has been linked to cell proliferation, development, membrane protein redistribution, and recovery from injury (Mccaig et al. 2005). We will focus here on the role of galvanotropism for tDCS relevant field intensities and durations. The first quantitative study in vitro by Marsh and Beams in 1946, exposed medullary explants from chicken embryos to ~60 V/m electric fields and demonstrated that neural processes grow preferentially towards the cathode and their development is suppressed towards the anode (Marsh and Beams 1946). In 1979 Jaffe and Poo assessed that neurites grow about three times faster towards the cathode at 70 V/m (Jaffe and Poo 1979). The lowest reported field values to induce galvanotropis are: 3 V/m applied for 20 min for locally induced fields (Patel and Poo 1984) and for uniform fields from 7 V/m applied during 16–20 h (Hinkle et al. 1981) to 10–50 V/m applied for 24 h (Patel and Poo 1982). The mean growth induced by DC fields is 0.4 μm per V/m per minute for local fields and 0.12 nm per V/m per minute for uniform fields (Patel and Poo 1982).

The effects of extracellular fields on nerve migration have been extensively characterized in vivo. In 1984, Pomeranz et al. applied 1 μA of current for 3 weeks to a sprouting rat nerve (Pomeranz et al. 1984). Hindpaw sensitivity was assessed before and after applying the field, finding an increase in responsiveness only when the cathode was placed in the direction of growth of the sprouting nerve (anodal stimulation). Physiological correlates were measured through histological studies showing an elevated number of neural fibers for anodal stimulation. In 1987, McDevitt et al. were the first to describe re-growth in mammals. They did a cut-suture intervention of the sciatic nerve and applied currents that generated fields of approximately 10 V/m for 20 days, each session lasting 30 min. Electromyographic activity was present in 67% of the animals that received stimulation with growth directed toward the cathode, and only in 17% with the reversed polarity (Mcdevitt et al. 1987). Supporting evidence is shown for an increase in neurofilament growth towards the cathode in damaged sciatic nerves (Politis et al. 1988) and for morphological regeneration after nerve transection (Roman et al. 1987). In addition, functional recovery was assessed by measuring various parameters of the rat's gait (Beveridge and Politis 1988).

Even endogenous injury potentials, which are presumed to have a functional role, are over an order of magnitude above tDCS fields (~10 V/m compared to <0.5 V/m). Given that studies on galvanotropism use much higher magnitude and longer duration DCS (typically ~100 V/m; (Palmer et al. 2000)), at first glance, effects of tDCS-relevant dose might be dismissed. However, assuming a linear dose-response (e.g. 0.12 nm per V/m minute) and considering the scale of individual synapse/dendrite spines, it is possible that even small morphological modifications have an important role in plastic changes underlying long term effects induced by tDCS. Indeed, the need for long-duration tDCS to produce after-effects may reflect cumulative galvanotropism. For example, 2 mA tDCS would, in theory, result in local electric fields of ~ 0.5 V/m, which over 20 min, could displace a neuronal process by 1.2 nm. Thus, during tDCS morphological reorientation of axon terminals and dendritic spines at synapses (rather than growth of axons over long distance) may be significant. To distinguish this local synaptic-cleft phenomena from conventional long range axon guidance, we call this "nano-galvanotropis". This conjecture reinforces our overall methodological theme that the relevance of animal studies to tDCS relies on both dose response (e.g. change per V/m) and outcome measures (e.g. plasticity vs. migration).

Network Effects of tDCS: Amplification and Recruitment

The consideration of how tDCS interacts with active networks (e.g. oscillations) is a major area of ongoing research: just as networks of coupled active neurons exhibit "emergent" network activity not apparent in isolated neurons, the application of DCS to active networks can produce responses not expected by single neurons. These responses are specific to the network architecture and activity (Reato et al. 2013b; Schmidt et al. 2014). Networks also provide an important substrate for amplification beyond the cell/synapse level. Ongoing studies on tDCS in humans has addressed modulation of EEG oscillations, while reports that DCS can alter "spontaneous rhythm" in animals span decades (Antal et al. 2004b; Dubner 1939; Marshall et al. 2011). Finally, modulation of oscillations are a substrate for changes in plasticity (Reato et al. 2013a, 2015).

Beyond the single neuronal level, amplification of networks might play a role in DCS effects. As discussed above, the initial action of DC stimulation remains to polarize all neurons subjected to the electric field (current flow inside the head). Our emphasis here is that tDCS generates electric fields across large areas of cortex and that polarization acts on every neuron in these brain regions. In considering the effects of tDCS on networks, a key concept is that the entire population of coupled neurons is polarized- this *coherent* polarization of the population provides a substrate for signal detection and for amplification (Parra and Bikson 2004; Reato et al. 2013b; Schmidt et al. 2014). In an oscillating network, DCS polarization of even a sub-set of neurons effects the whole population – in this way cells that in isolation might be less sensitive (e.g. interneurons) might be recruited to respond to tDCS (Reato et al. 2010).

Interestingly, at the single neuron scale the effective coupling constant for a neuron immersed in an active network may be enhanced compared to that of neurons in isolation (Reato et al. 2010) – meaning that by virtue of being in a network, a given compartment (soma) may be polarized directly by the field and indirectly by field actions on a collection of afferent neurons. In addition, in a network if tDCS is effective on a (more sensitive) upstream neuron, this will change synaptic activity at downstream neurons (Boros et al. 2008).

As described above, the concept that the threshold for electric field sensitivity would be "lower for modulation of the frequency of an already active neuron than for excitation of a silent one" (Terzuolo and Bullock 1956) is well established, but network activity adds another dimension to this. During many network activities, notably oscillations, neurons are near threshold and thus primed for firing. If a neuron is near threshold by virtue of network drive, then a small polarization may be influential in modulating the likelihood of firing. For example, a relatively small depolarization may be sufficient to trigger an action potential. Moreover, because the network is interconnected, activated neurons could synaptically trigger action potentials in other neurons. The whole process can be feed-forward such that a small DC electric field can induce a robust action potential discharge in a population. This has been demonstrated in brain slices and explained with quantitative models (Reato et al. 2010). This concept is interesting because it blurs the distinction between "supra-threshold" stimulation, such as TMS, and "sub-threshold" stimulation, as tDCS is commonly considered.

Mechanisms of network amplification are difficult to explore in the human brain directly, but functional imaging data are in accordance with enhanced glutamatergic activity during stimulation (Alekseichuk et al. 2016; Hone-Blanchet et al. 2016). Moreover, electroencephalography shows that DC stimulation enhances individual alpha activity (Spitoni et al. 2013), which is in good accordance with network amplification mechanisms of tDCS (Polania et al. 2011a).

Network Effects of tDCS: Consequences for Spread of Neuromodulation

Apart from the regional network effects of tDCS under or near the stimulation electrodes, remote effects on topographically distant cortical and subcortical areas were described relatively early for the human brain (Lang et al. 2005). There is no *a priori* rationale to ignore these regions in interpreting the behavioral and cognitive consequences of tDCS. These brain-wide changes might also further support network-scale amplification.

However, it was unclear whether those effects are caused by physiological spreading of cortical activity (i.e. one region being activated by tDCS and subsequently driving another region) or by physical current spread (i.e. during tDCS current flow). Simulation studies, which have been recently validated, are in favor of at least a partial contribution of spread of current flow (Datta et al. 2009; Huang et al. 2017). In addition, clear physiological effects of tDCS on remote areas have been described. Premotor anodal tDCS enhances intracortical facilitation of M1, most probably due to the activation of premotor-primary motor cortex afferents (Boros et al. 2008). Similarly, combined dorsal premotor and supplementary motor area (SMA) stimulation alters motor and somatosensory evoked potentials (Kirimoto et al. 2011). For parietal cortex stimulation, anodal tDCS enhanced, but cathodal tDCS reduced MEP amplitudes elicited by motor cortex TMS. Moreover, anodal tDCS over the posterior parietal cortex increased ipsilateral M1 intracortical inhibition and facilitation, as well as parietal-motor cortical connectivity (Rivera-Urbina et al. 2015). Furthermore, anodal tDCS over posterior parietal cortex increased cortico-cortical potentials elicited by TMS in both local and surrounding or contralateral regions (Romero Lauro et al. 2014).

Recently, functional connectivity approaches have been applied to explore cortical network alterations induced by tDCS in humans. For motor cortex stimulation under resting conditions, a fMRI study revealed that nodal minimum path length increased after anodal tDCS over M1, which means that functional connectivity of this area with topographically distant regions of the whole brain significantly decreased. In contrast to this generally reduced whole brain connectivity of M1, functional connectivity was enhanced between the primary motor cortex on the one hand, and premotor and superior parietal areas on the other (Polania et al. 2011b). In another study, cathodal tDCS of the primary motor cortex increased functional connectivity between the stimulated M1, and the contralateral M1 and premotor cortices (Stagg et al. 2009b). A similar effect of tDCS was described for anodal stimulation combined with motor practice in an EEG study, where functional connectivity was enhanced between primary motor, premotor, and sensorimotor areas in the high gamma band (Polania et al. 2011a). Moreover, anodal tDCS of the primary motor cortex alters cortico-subcortical connectivity of the motor cortex at rest. Specifically, it was shown to enhance connectivity with the ipsilateral caudate nucleus, and thalamus (Polania et al. 2012a). Alterations of intrinsic motor cortex connectivity by tDCS have also been demonstrated: cathodal stimulation increased local connectivity, most likely due to cortical noise reduction accomplished by the respective excitability and activity diminution, while anodal tDCS enhanced long-distance connectivity within this area (Polania et al. 2012b). Therefore it can be concluded by the results of these studies that motor cortex tDCS alters the connectivity of large parts of the motor network, and thus regional stimulation has network effects.

Such effects are not restricted to motor cortex tDCS. Stimulation of the dorsolateral prefrontal cortex has been demonstrated to induce widespread alterations of functional connectivity, including the default mode network, and attention-related networks in healthy subjects (Keeser et al. 2011; Pena-Gomez et al. 2012). Thus it can be concluded that the effects of DC stimulation in vivo are not restricted to the primary target area, but involve a larger set of connected areas. Since these effects are assumed to be activity-related, the impact of tDCS on remote areas might nevertheless differ from those stimulated directly by the intervention, because the polarizing effect by external application of an electrical field is missing. If and in which way this leads to different functional and physiological effects in these secondary areas remains to be shown.

Non-neuronal Effects of tDCS

So far, most research on DC stimulation was focused on neurons. However, additional cell types – including glia and endothelial cells – are affected by DC fields and might contribute to the neuromodulation outcomes. Here, it can be distinguished between (1) direct stimulation effects, reflecting direct polarization and modulation of these cell types by direct current fields; (2) indirect stimulation effects, reflecting changes in function secondary to direct excitatory neuronal activation that then influences these other cell types; and (3) modulatory effects, where the sensitivity of neurons to direct effects (e.g., their excitability) is influenced by these other cell types.

Glia cells represent the majority of cells in the CNS – the concept that they are just 'passive' support cells is outdated (Haydon and Carmignoto 2006) and their essential role in neuronal functions such as plasticity are being elucidated (Di Castro et al. 2011; Panatier et al. 2011). Astrocytes are particularly crucial in regulating synaptic transmission and plasticity, leading to the recent idea of a 'tripartite synapse' (Perea et al. 2009). While astrocytes are sensitive to small changes in membrane potential (Amzica et al. 2002) and their elongated processes are susceptible to polarization by DCS (Ruohonen and Karhu 2012), the effects of weak DCS on these cells remain relatively neglected in the literature (Gellner et al. 2016). However, a recent in vivo study in mice showed that tDCS induced astrocytic calcium waves in visual cortex, which appeared to drive plasticity of visually evoked potentials (Monai et al. 2016). It was unclear whether this effect was due to direct or indirect action on astrocytes, but this motivates more work in understanding the role of astrocytes in tDCS induced plasticity. In addition to effects in individual glia cells, a glial syncytium (an electrically coupled population of glial cells) might act to amplify field polarization. Just as a single cell (glia) experiences a biphasic polarization in response to DCS, the glial syncytium may experience a net biphasic polarization across the network axis. Another possible mechanism for DC modulation through glia cells relates to the concept of potassium 'spatial buffering'. Glia cells are thought to regulate extracellular potassium concentration through a polarization imbalance across their membrane, and the biphasic polarization induced by DC fields would be expected to drive the collection and release of potassium across the glia or glial syncytium ends. Indeed, Gardner-Medwin induced extracellular potassium transport by passing DC current and noted concentration changes in saline near the electrodes, which is mechanistically distinct from tissue changes (Gardner-Medwin 1983). Studies in brain slices however show no changes in extracellular potassium concentration with DC fields (Lian et al. 2003), though the brain slice preparation has distorted extracellular concentration control mechanisms (An et al. 2008).

Endothelial cells form the blood-brain barrier (BBB) that tightly regulates transport between the brain extracellular space and blood. Any direct action of DC stimulation on endothelial cells would thus have important consequence for brain function. Endothelial cells do not have processes and their spherical shape indicates peak polarization will be related to cell diameter (Kotnik et al. 2010). However, a compelling hypothesis is that the blood vessel network formed by the BBB might channel current flow in a manner that concentrates electric field across the BBB. The direct effects of tDCS current on vascular response remain an open and compelling question. There is abundant evidence that DC current affects vascular function in skin (Berliner 1997; Ledger 1992; Malty and Petrofsky 2007; Prausnitz 1996) and skin redness is inevitable under tDCS electrodes (Minhas et al. 2010) – with a component that is pressure related but a component that is in response to current flow (Ezquerro et al. 2016).

Vascular and neuronal functions in the brain are closely interrelated, as evidenced by functional Magnetic Resonance Imaging (fMRI). The relation is also complex, and it can be difficult to disentangle direct neuronal and potential direct vascular effects (Takano et al. 2011), including during tDCS. Wachter and colleagues (2011) reported a polarity specific change in blood perfusion during tDCS in the rat, in a direction consistent with the somatic doctrine, and speculated the direction specificity was consistent with a primary neuronal action. Furthermore, it was shown that high-intensity electrical stimulation could increase transport across the blood-brain barrier. This phenomenon was termed "electro-permeation" between cells, to distinguish it from electroporation of single cells (Lopez-Quintero et al. 2010). Taken together, there are reasons to assume that application of DC fields affect also non-neuronal cells of the CNS, but the paucity of experimental evidence requires further investigation on the ultimate impact on tDCS outcomes.

Concluding Remarks: Building on an Extensive Foundation of Mechanistic Studies

This chapter gave an overview about the current state of knowledge of the physiological effects of brain stimulation with weak DC fields. As can be derived from the available studies and concepts, knowledge is extensive but far from being complete. Whereas basic general mechanisms of action have been identified, especially at the microscopic cellular level and clinical neurophysiology, important identified questions await yet to be answered. The effects of tDCS may be complex in the sense that they are brain-state and dose (montage, current intensity, duration) dependent, such that different mechanisms are operant depending on the application. None-theless, certain basic principles, as highlighted in this review, are likely universal. Especially integration of knowledge across animal and human experiments at different levels of organization, is important to address this complexity.

What seems to be clear even at different physiological scales (from cellular to human neurophysiology), is that the general assumption that anodal DC stimulation enhances excitability and cathodal stimulation diminishes excitability is an over-simplification. Rather, the outcome of stimulation is to be qualified by protocol specifics. At the same time it's important to recognize that such over-simplifications are not germane to tDCS and exist across neuromodulation technologies (e.g. DBS) and pharmacology. tDCS research, more than other domains, has (1) over decades established a scientific foundation; (2) in this process addressed head-on limitations in existing understanding. It is a mistake to confuse ongoing discovery of nuance in DCS effects with a crisis in the fundamentals.

For example, ongoing experiments in animal models of direct current stimulation are beginning to provide insight into how neuromodulation by tDCS cannot be explained as a monolithic "sliding-scale" of excitability (where regions under the anode are "excited" while regions under the cathode are "de-excited"). Brain function and disease are complex and so their influence by DC stimulation is similarly complex. Moving beyond the "somatic doctrine", polarization of dendrites, axon terminals, and astrocytes can no longer be ignored. The effects of polarization in each of these compartments are likely to vary with their activity state (e.g. membrane potential, neurotransmitter tone, ion channel state), with effects being amplified by increased ongoing activity. Importantly, this may support modulation of plasticity specifically in the most active synapses. This also implies that tDCS may have vastly different effects depending on the form of endogenous plasticity (e.g. driven by dendritic or somatic spikes).

Which neuronal processes are modulated and how, will depend on the tDCS montage used and the state of the underlying network. The rational advancement of tDCS thus requires progressing from the sliding-scale approach (applied indiscriminately across cognitive applications and indications) and addressing these mechanistic and targeting issues. With increased recognition of complexity, the need for translational animal studies, that are properly designed, becomes increasingly clear. Following the organization in this chapter, this includes considering the effects of DCS at three scales: membrane compartment polarization, synaptic efficacy, and network effects. While brain function is evidently understood to span across these levels, this among other structures introduced here, provide a path forward toward framing of new hypotheses. Combining animal experimentation with human experimental work, and new approaches like computational neurostimulation (Bestmann 2015) will help to comprehend the mechanisms of action of DC stimulation further, which will be the essential pre-condition to develop stimulation protocols which allow clearly defined and targeted interventions in basic and applied neuroscience.

Literature

Accornero, N., Voti, P. L., La Riccia, M., & Gregori, B. (2007). Visual evoked potentials modulation during direct current cortical polarization. *Experimental Brain Research, 178*(2), 261–266.

Alekseichuk, I., Diers, K., Paulus, W., & Antal, A. (2016). Transcranial electrical stimulation of the occipital cortex during visual perception modifies the magnitude of BOLD activity: A combined tES-fMRI approach. *NeuroImage, 140*, 110–117.

Amzica, F., Massimini, M., & Manfridi, A. (2002). Spatial buffering during slow and paroxysmal sleep oscillations in cortical networks of glial cells in vivo. *The Journal of Neuroscience, 22*(3), 1042–1053.

An, J. H., Su, Y., Radman, T., & Bikson, M. (2008). Effects of glucose and glutamine concentration in the formulation of the artificial cerebrospinal fluid (ACSF). *Brain Research, 1218*, 77–86.

Anastassiou, C. A., Montgomery, S. M., Barahona, M., Buzsáki, G., & Koch, C. (2010). The effect of spatially inhomogeneous extracellular electric fields on neurons. *Journal of Neuroscience, 30*(5), 1925–1936.

Andreasen, M., & Nedergaard, S. (1996). Dendritic electrogenesis in rat hippocampal CA1 pyramidal neurons: Functional aspects of Na+ and Ca2+ currents in apical dendrites. *Hippocampus, 6*(1), 79–95.

Antal, A., Nitsche, M. A., Kruse, W., Kincses, T. Z., Hoffmann, K.-P., & Paulus, W. (2004a). Direct current stimulation over V5 enhances visuomotor coordination by improving motion perception in humans. *Journal of Cognitive Neuroscience, 16*(4), 521–527.

Antal, A., Terney, D., Poreisz, C., & Paulus, W. (2007). Towards unravelling task-related modulations of neuroplastic changes induced in the human motor cortex. *European Journal of Neuroscience, 26*(9), 2687–2691.

Antal, A., Varga, E. T., Kincses, T. Z., Nitsche, M. A., & Paulus, W. (2004b). Oscillatory brain activity and transcranial direct current stimulation in humans. *Neuroreport, 15*(8), 1307–1310.

Ardolino, G., Bossi, B., Barbieri, S., & Priori, A. (2005). Non-synaptic mechanisms underlie the after-effects of cathodal transcutaneous direct current stimulation of the human brain. *The Journal of Physiology, 568*(Pt 2), 653–663.

Awatramani, G. B., Price, G. D., & Trussell, L. O. (2005). Modulation of transmitter release by presynaptic resting potential and background calcium levels. *Neuron, 48*(1), 109–121.

Berliner, M. N. (1997). Skin microcirculation during tapwater iontophoresis in humans: Cathode stimulates more than anode. *Microvascular Research, 54*(1), 74–80.

Bestmann, S. (2015). Computational neurostimulation: Models for bridging physiology and behavior. Brain stimulation: Basic, translational, and clinical research in. *Neuromodulation, 8*(2), 435.

Beveridge, J. A., & Politis, M. J. (1988). Use of exogenous electric current in the treatment of delayed lesions in peripheral nerves. *Plastic and Reconstructive Surgery, 82*(4), 573–579.

Bikson, M., Inoue, M., Akiyama, H., Deans, J. K., Fox, J. E., Miyakawa, H., & Jefferys, J. G. (2004). Effects of uniform extracellular DC electric fields on excitability in rat hippocampal slices in vitro. *The Journal of Physiology, 557*(1), 175–190.

Bikson, M., & Rahman, A. (2013). Origins of specificity during tDCS: Anatomical, activity-selective, and input-bias mechanisms. *Frontiers in Human Neuroscience, 7*, 688.

Bindman, L. J., Lippold, O., & Redfearn, J. (1962). Long-lasting changes in the level of the electrical activity of the cerebral cortex produced by polarizing currents. *Nature, 196*(4854), 584–585.

Bindman, L. J., Lippold, O., & Redfearn, J. (1964). The action of brief polarizing currents on the cerebral cortex of the rat (1) during current flow and (2) in the production of long-lasting after-effects. *The Journal of Physiology, 172*(3), 369–382.

Bishop, G., & Erlanger, J. (1926). The effects of polarization upon the activity of vertebrate nerve. *American Journal of Physiology--Legacy Content, 78*(3), 630–657.

Bishop, G., & O'Leary, J. (1950). The effects of polarizing currents on cell potentials and their significance in the interpretation of central nervous system activity. *Electroencephalography and Clinical Neurophysiology, 2*(1), 401–416.

Bliss, T. V., & Lomo, T. (1973). Long-lasting potentiation of synaptic transmission in the dentate area of the anaesthetized rabbit following stimulation of the perforant path. *The Journal of Physiology, 232*(2), 331–356.

Bolognini, N., Fregni, F., Casati, C., Olgiati, E., & Vallar, G. (2010). Brain polarization of parietal cortex augments training-induced improvement of visual exploratory and attentional skills. *Brain Research, 1349*, 76–89.

Boros, K., Poreisz, C., Munchau, A., Paulus, W., & Nitsche, M. A. (2008). Premotor transcranial direct current stimulation (tDCS) affects primary motor excitability in humans. *The European Journal of Neuroscience, 27*(5), 1292–1300.

Bullock, T. H., & Hagiwara, S. (1957). Intracellular recording from the giant synapse of the squid. *The Journal of General Physiology, 40*(4), 565–577.

Cambiaghi, M., Teneud, L., Velikova, S., Gonzalez-Rosa, J., Cursi, M., Comi, G., & Leocani, L. (2011). Flash visual evoked potentials in mice can be modulated by transcranial direct current stimulation. *Neuroscience, 185*, 161–165.

Cambiaghi, M., Velikova, S., Gonzalez-Rosa, J. J., Cursi, M., Comi, G., & Leocani, L. (2010). Brain transcranial direct current stimulation modulates motor excitability in mice. *European Journal of Neuroscience, 31*(4), 704–709.

Carandini, M., & Ferster, D. (2000). Membrane potential and firing rate in cat primary visual cortex. *Journal of Neuroscience, 20*(1), 470–484.

Carter, M. J., Maslovat, D., & Carlsen, A. N. (2015). Anodal transcranial direct current stimulation applied over the supplementary motor area delays spontaneous antiphase-to-in-phase transitions. *Journal of Neurophysiology, 113*(3), 780–785.

Castro-Alamancos, M. A., Donoghue, J. P., & Connors, B. W. (1995). Different forms of synaptic plasticity in somatosensory and motor areas of the neocortex. *The Journal of Neuroscience, 15*(7 Pt 2), 5324–5333.

Cavarretta, F., Carnevale, N. T., Tegolo, D., & Migliore, M. (2014). Effects of low frequency electric fields on synaptic integration in hippocampal CA1 pyramidal neurons: Implications for power line emissions. *Frontiers in Cellular Neuroscience, 8*, 310.

Chan, C., Hounsgaard, J., & Nicholson, C. (1988). Effects of electric fields on transmembrane potential and excitability of turtle cerebellar Purkinje cells in vitro. *The Journal of Physiology, 402*, 751–771.

Costain, R., Redfearn, J., & Lippold, O. (1964). A controlled trial of the therapeutic effects of polarization of the brain in depressive illness. *The British Journal of Psychiatry, 110* (469),786–799.

Creutzfeldt, O. D., Fromm, G. H., & Kapp, H. (1962). Influence of transcortical dc currents on cortical neuronal activity. *Experimental Neurology, 5*(6), 436–452.

Datta, A., Bansal, V., Diaz, J., Patel, J., Reato, D., & Bikson, M. (2009). Gyri-precise head model of transcranial direct current stimulation: Improved spatial focality using a ring electrode versus conventional rectangular pad. *Brain Stimulation, 2*(4), 201–207. e201.

Deans, J. K., Powell, A. D., & Jefferys, J. G. (2007). Sensitivity of coherent oscillations in rat hippocampus to AC electric fields. *The Journal of Physiology, 583*(2), 555–565.

Del Castillo, J., & Katz, B. (1954). Changes in end-plate activity produced by pre-synaptic polarization. *The Journal of Physiology, 124*(3), 586–604.

Delgado-Lezama, R., Perrier, J. F., & Hounsgaard, J. (1999). Local facilitation of plateau potentials in dendrites of turtle motoneurones by synaptic activation of metabotropic receptors. *The Journal of Physiology, 515*(Pt 1), 203–207.

Di Castro, M. A., Chuquet, J., Liaudet, N., Bhaukaurally, K., Santello, M., Bouvier, D., ... Volterra, A. (2011). Local Ca2+ detection and modulation of synaptic release by astrocytes. *Nature Neuroscience, 14*(10), 1276–1284.

Dubner, H. H. (1939). Factors controlling brain potentials in the cat. Ph D, University of Chicago, Springfield, IL.

Dudel, J. (1971). The effect of polarizing current on action potential and transmitter release in crayfish motor nerve terminals. *Pflügers Archiv, 324*(3), 227–248.

Ezquerro, F., Moffa, A. H., Bikson, M., Khadka, N., Aparicio, L. V., Bd, S.-J., ... Pereira, A. C. (2016). *The influence of skin redness on blinding in transcranial direct current stimulation studies: A crossover trial.* Neuromodulation: Technology at the Neural Interface.

Floel, A. (2014). tDCS-enhanced motor and cognitive function in neurological diseases. *NeuroImage, 85*(Pt 3), 934–947.

Fresnoza, S., Paulus, W., Nitsche, M. A., & Kuo, M. F. (2014a). Nonlinear dose-dependent impact of D1 receptor activation on motor cortex plasticity in humans. *The Journal of Neuroscience, 34*(7), 2744–2753.

Fresnoza, S., Stiksrud, E., Klinker, F., Liebetanz, D., Paulus, W., Kuo, M. F., & Nitsche, M. A. (2014b). Dosage-dependent effect of dopamine D2 receptor activation on motor cortex plasticity in humans. *The Journal of Neuroscience, 34*(32), 10701–10709.

Freund, T. F., & Buzsaki, G. (1996). Interneurons of the hippocampus. *Hippocampus, 6*(4), 347–470.

Fricke, K., Seeber, A. A., Thirugnanasambandam, N., Paulus, W., Nitsche, M. A., & Rothwell, J. C. (2011). Time course of the induction of homeostatic plasticity generated by repeated transcranial direct current stimulation of the human motor cortex. *Journal of Neurophysiology, 105*(3), 1141–1149.

Fritsch, B., Reis, J., Martinowich, K., Schambra, H. M., Ji, Y., Cohen, L. G., & Lu, B. (2010). Direct current stimulation promotes BDNF-dependent synaptic plasticity: Potential implications for motor learning. *Neuron, 66*(2), 198–204.

Fröhlich, F., & Mccormick, D. A. (2010). Endogenous electric fields may guide neocortical network activity. *Neuron, 67*(1), 129–143.

Gardner-Medwin, A. (1983). Analysis of potassium dynamics in mammalian brain tissue. *The Journal of Physiology, 335*, 393–426.

Gartside, I. B. (1968a). Mechanisms of sustained increases of firing rate of neurones in the rat cerebral cortex after polarization: Reverberating circuits or modification of synaptic conductance? *Nature, 220*(5165), 382–383.

Gartside, I. B. (1968b). Mechanisms of sustained increases of firing rate of neurones in the rat cerebral cortex after polarization: Role of protein synthesis. *Nature, 220*(5165), 383–384.

Gellner, A. K., Reis, J., & Fritsch, B. (2016). Glia: A neglected player in non-invasive direct current brain stimulation. *Frontiers in Cellular Neuroscience, 10*, 188.
Giordano, J., Bikson, M., Kappenman, E. S., Clark, V. P., Coslett, H. B., Hamblin, M. R., … Mckinley, R. A. (2017). Mechanisms and effects of transcranial direct current stimulation. *Dose-Response, 15*(1), 1559325816685467.
Grundey, J., Thirugnanasambandam, N., Kaminsky, K., Drees, A., Skwirba, A. C., Lang, N., … Nitsche, M. A. (2012). Rapid effect of nicotine intake on neuroplasticity in non-smoking humans. *Frontiers in Pharmacology, 3*, 186.
Hanley, C. J., Singh, K. D., & Mcgonigle, D. J. (2016). Transcranial modulation of brain oscillatory responses: A concurrent tDCS-MEG investigation. *NeuroImage, 140*, 20–32.
Hattori, Y., Moriwaki, A., & Hori, Y. (1990). Biphasic effects of polarizing current on adenosine-sensitive generation of cyclic AMP in rat cerebral cortex. *Neuroscience Letters, 116*(3), 320–324.
Haydon, P. G., & Carmignoto, G. (2006). Astrocyte control of synaptic transmission and neurovascular coupling. *Physiological Reviews, 86*(3), 1009–1031.
Hess, G., & Donoghue, J. P. (1999). Facilitation of long-term potentiation in layer II/III horizontal connections of rat motor cortex following layer I stimulation: Route of effect and cholinergic contributions. *Experimental Brain Research, 127*(3), 279–290.
Hinkle, L., Mccaig, C. D., & Robinson, K. R. (1981). The direction of growth of differentiating neurones and myoblasts from frog embryos in an applied electric field. *The Journal of Physiology, 314*, 121–135.
Hone-Blanchet, A., Edden, R. A., & Fecteau, S. (2016). Online effects of transcranial direct current stimulation in real time on human prefrontal and striatal metabolites. *Biological Psychiatry, 80*(6), 432–438.
Huang, Y., Liu, A. A., Lafon, B., Friedman, D., Dayan, M., Wang, X., … Parra, L. C. (2017). Measurements and models of electric fields in the in vivo human brain during transcranial electric stimulation. *eLife, 6*, e18834.
Hubbard, J., & Willis, W. (1962a). Hyperpolarization of mammalian motor nerve terminals. *The Journal of Physiology, 163*(1), 115–137.
Hubbard, J. I., & Willis, W. D. (1962b). Mobilization of transmitter by hyperpolarization. *Nature, 193*(4811), 174–175.
Islam, N., Aftabuddin, M., Moriwaki, A., Hattori, Y., & Hori, Y. (1995a). Increase in the calcium level following anodal polarization in the rat brain. *Brain Research, 684*(2), 206–208.
Islam, N., Moriwaki, A., & Hori, Y. (1995b). Co-localization of c-fos protein and protein kinase C gamma in the rat brain following anodal polarization. *Indian Journal of Physiology and Pharmacology, 39*(3), 209–215.
Jackson, M. P., Rahman, A., Lafon, B., Kronberg, G., Ling, D., Parra, L. C., & Bikson, M. (2016). Animal models of transcranial direct current stimulation: Methods and mechanisms. *Clinical Neurophysiology, 127*(11), 3425–3454.
Jaffe, L. F., & Poo, M. M. (1979). Neurites grow faster towards the cathode than the anode in a steady field. *The Journal of Experimental Zoology, 209*(1), 115–128.
Jamil, A., Batsikadze, G., Kuo, H. I., Labruna, L., Hasan, A., Paulus, W., & Nitsche, M. A. (2017). Systematic evaluation of the impact of stimulation intensity on neuroplastic after-effects induced by transcranial direct current stimulation. *The Journal of Physiology, 595*(4), 1273–1288.
Jefferys, J. (1981). Influence of electric fields on the excitability of granule cells in Guinea-pig hippocampal slices. *The Journal of Physiology, 319*, 143–152.
Joucla, S., & Yvert, B. (2009). The "mirror" estimate: An intuitive predictor of membrane polarization during extracellular stimulation. *Biophysical Journal, 96*(9), 3495–3508.
Kabakov, A. Y., Muller, P. A., Pascual-Leone, A., Jensen, F. E., & Rotenberg, A. (2012). Contribution of axonal orientation to pathway-dependent modulation of excitatory transmission by direct current stimulation in isolated rat hippocampus. *Journal of Neurophysiology, 107*(7), 1881–1889.

Keeser, D., Meindl, T., Bor, J., Palm, U., Pogarell, O., Mulert, C., … Padberg, F. (2011). Prefrontal transcranial direct current stimulation changes connectivity of resting-state networks during fMRI. *The Journal of Neuroscience, 31*(43), 15284–15293.

Kirimoto, H., Ogata, K., Onishi, H., Oyama, M., Goto, Y., & Tobimatsu, S. (2011). Transcranial direct current stimulation over the motor association cortex induces plastic changes in ipsilateral primary motor and somatosensory cortices. *Clinical Neurophysiology, 122*(4), 777–783.

Kotnik, T., Pucihar, G., & Miklavcic, D. (2010). Induced transmembrane voltage and its correlation with electroporation-mediated molecular transport. *The Journal of Membrane Biology, 236*(1), 3–13.

Kronberg, G., Bridi, M., Abel, T., Bikson, M., & Parra, L. C. (2017). Direct current stimulation modulates LTP and LTD: Activity dependence and dendritic effects. *Brain Stimulation, 10*(1), 51–58.

Lafon, B., Rahman, A., Bikson, M., & Parra, L. C. (2017). Direct current stimulation alters neuronal input/output function. *Brain Stimulation, 10*(1), 36–45.

Lang, N., Siebner, H. R., Ward, N. S., Lee, L., Nitsche, M. A., Paulus, W., … Frackowiak, R. S. (2005). How does transcranial DC stimulation of the primary motor cortex alter regional neuronal activity in the human brain? *The European Journal of Neuroscience, 22*(2), 495–504.

Ledger, P. W. (1992). Skin biological issues in electrically enhanced transdermal delivery. *Advanced Drug Delivery Reviews, 9*(2–3), 289–307.

Lee, D., Lin, B. J., & Lee, A. K. (2012). Hippocampal place fields emerge upon single-cell manipulation of excitability during behavior. *Science, 337*(6096), 849–853.

Lian, J., Bikson, M., Sciortino, C., Stacey, W. C., & Durand, D. M. (2003). Local suppression of epileptiform activity by electrical stimulation in rat hippocampus in vitro. *The Journal of Physiology, 547*(Pt 2), 427–434.

Liebetanz, D., Nitsche, M. A., Tergau, F., & Paulus, W. (2002). Pharmacological approach to the mechanisms of transcranial DC-stimulation-induced after-effects of human motor cortex excitability. *Brain, 125*(10), 2238–2247.

Lisman, J. E. (2001). Three Ca2+ levels affect plasticity differently: The LTP zone, the LTD zone and no man's land. *The Journal of Physiology, 532*(Pt 2), 285.

Lopez-Quintero, S. V., Datta, A., Amaya, R., Elwassif, M., Bikson, M., & Tarbell, J. M. (2010). DBS-relevant electric fields increase hydraulic conductivity of in vitro endothelial monolayers. *Journal of Neural Engineering, 7*(1), 16005.

Lu, B. (2003). BDNF and activity-dependent synaptic modulation. *Learning & Memory, 10*(2), 86–98.

Lugon, M. D. M. V., Batsikadze, G., Fresnoza, S., Grundey, J., Kuo, M.-F., Paulus, W., … Nitsche, M. A. (2015). Mechanisms of nicotinic modulation of glutamatergic neuroplasticity in humans. *Cerebral Cortex*, bhv252.

Magee, J. C., & Cook, E. P. (2000). Somatic EPSP amplitude is independent of synapse location in hippocampal pyramidal neurons. *Nature Neuroscience, 3*(9), 895–903.

Malenka, R. C., & Bear, M. F. (2004). LTP and LTD: An embarrassment of riches. *Neuron, 44*(1), 5–21.

Malty, A. M., & Petrofsky, J. (2007). The effect of electrical stimulation on a normal skin blood flow in active young and older adults. *Medical Science Monitor, 13*(4), CR147–CR155.

Márquez-Ruiz, J., Leal-Campanario, R., Sánchez-Campusano, R., Molaee-Ardekani, B., Wendling, F., Miranda, P. C., … Delgado-García, J. M. (2012). Transcranial direct-current stimulation modulates synaptic mechanisms involved in associative learning in behaving rabbits. *Proceedings of the National Academy of Sciences, 109*(17), 6710–6715.

Marsh, G., & Beams, H. W. (1946). In vitro control of growing chick nerve fibers by applied electric currents. *Journal of Cellular and Comparative Physiology, 27*, 139–157.

Marshall, L., Kirov, R., Brade, J., Molle, M., & Born, J. (2011). Transcranial electrical currents to probe EEG brain rhythms and memory consolidation during sleep in humans. *PLoS One, 6*(2), e16905.

Mccaig, C. D., & Rajnicek, A. M. (1991). Electrical fields, nerve growth and nerve regeneration. *Experimental Physiology, 76*(4), 473–494.
Mccaig, C. D., Rajnicek, A. M., Song, B., & Zhao, M. (2005). Controlling cell behavior electrically: Current views and future potential. *Physiological Reviews, 85*(3), 943–978.
Mcdevitt, L., Fortner, P., & Pomeranz, B. (1987). Application of weak electric field to the hindpaw enhances sciatic motor nerve regeneration in the adult rat. *Brain Research, 416*(2), 308–314.
Mcintyre, C. C., Grill, W. M., Sherman, D. L., & Thakor, N. V. (2004). Cellular effects of deep brain stimulation: Model-based analysis of activation and inhibition. *Journal of Neurophysiology, 91*(4), 1457–1469.
Merrill, D. R., Bikson, M., & Jefferys, J. G. (2005). Electrical stimulation of excitable tissue: Design of efficacious and safe protocols. *Journal of Neuroscience Methods, 141*(2), 171–198.
Minhas, P., Bansal, V., Patel, J., Ho, J. S., Diaz, J., Datta, A., & Bikson, M. (2010). Electrodes for high-definition transcutaneous DC stimulation for applications in drug delivery and electrotherapy, including tDCS. *Journal of Neuroscience Methods, 190*(2), 188–197.
Miranda, P. C., Lomarev, M., & Hallett, M. (2006). Modeling the current distribution during transcranial direct current stimulation. *Clinical Neurophysiology, 117*(7), 1623–1629.
Monai, H., Ohkura, M., Tanaka, M., Oe, Y., Konno, A., Hirai, H., … Hirase, H. (2016). Calcium imaging reveals glial involvement in transcranial direct current stimulation-induced plasticity in mouse brain. *Nature Communications, 7*, 11100.
Monte-Silva, K., Kuo, M.-F., Hessenthaler, S., Fresnoza, S., Liebetanz, D., Paulus, W., & Nitsche, M. A. (2013). Induction of late LTP-like plasticity in the human motor cortex by repeated non-invasive brain stimulation. *Brain Stimulation, 6*(3), 424–432.
Monte-Silva, K., Kuo, M. F., Liebetanz, D., Paulus, W., & Nitsche, M. A. (2010). Shaping the optimal repetition interval for cathodal transcranial direct current stimulation (tDCS). *Journal of Neurophysiology, 103*(4), 1735–1740.
Nitsche, M., Fricke, K., Henschke, U., Schlitterlau, A., Liebetanz, D., Lang, N., … Paulus, W. (2003a). Pharmacological modulation of cortical excitability shifts induced by transcranial direct current stimulation in humans. *The Journal of Physiology, 553*(1), 293–301.
Nitsche, M. A., Doemkes, S., Karakoese, T., Antal, A., Liebetanz, D., Lang, N., … Paulus, W. (2007a). Shaping the effects of transcranial direct current stimulation of the human motor cortex. *Journal of Neurophysiology, 97*(4), 3109–3117.
Nitsche, M. A., Jaussi, W., Liebetanz, D., Lang, N., Tergau, F., & Paulus, W. (2004). Consolidation of human motor cortical neuroplasticity by D-cycloserine. *Neuropsychopharmacology, 29*(8), 1573–1578.
Nitsche, M. A., Muller-Dahlhaus, F., Paulus, W., & Ziemann, U. (2012). The pharmacology of neuroplasticity induced by non-invasive brain stimulation: Building models for the clinical use of CNS active drugs. *The Journal of Physiology, 590*(19), 4641–4662.
Nitsche, M. A., & Paulus, W. (2000). Excitability changes induced in the human motor cortex by weak transcranial direct current stimulation. *The Journal of Physiology, 527*(3), 633–639.
Nitsche, M. A., & Paulus, W. (2001). Sustained excitability elevations induced by transcranial DC motor cortex stimulation in humans. *Neurology, 57*(10), 1899–1901.
Nitsche, M. A., Roth, A., Kuo, M. F., Fischer, A. K., Liebetanz, D., Lang, N., … Paulus, W. (2007b). Timing-dependent modulation of associative plasticity by general network excitability in the human motor cortex. *The Journal of Neuroscience, 27*(14), 3807–3812.
Nitsche, M. A., Schauenburg, A., Lang, N., Liebetanz, D., Exner, C., Paulus, W., & Tergau, F. (2003b). Facilitation of implicit motor learning by weak transcranial direct current stimulation of the primary motor cortex in the human. *Journal of Cognitive Neuroscience, 15*(4), 619–626.
Nitsche, M. A., Seeber, A., Frommann, K., Klein, C. C., Rochford, C., Nitsche, M. S., … Antal, A. (2005). Modulating parameters of excitability during and after transcranial direct current stimulation of the human motor cortex. *The Journal of Physiology, 568*(1), 291–303.

Opitz, A., Falchier, A., Yan, C.-G., Yeagle, E. M., Linn, G. S., Megevand, P., & Thielscher, A. (2016). Spatiotemporal structure of intracranial electric fields induced by transcranial electric stimulation in humans and nonhuman primates. *Scientific Reports, 6,* 31236.

Palmer, A. M., Messerli, M. A., & Robinson, K. R. (2000). Neuronal galvanotropism is independent of external ca(2+) entry or internal ca(2+) gradients. *Journal of Neurobiology, 45*(1), 30–38.

Panatier, A., Vallee, J., Haber, M., Murai, K. K., Lacaille, J. C., & Robitaille, R. (2011). Astrocytes are endogenous regulators of basal transmission at central synapses. *Cell, 146*(5), 785–798.

Parra, L. C., & Bikson, M. (2004). Model of the effect of extracellular fields on spike time coherence. In *Engineering in Medicine and Biology Society. IEMBS'04. 26th Annual International Conference of the IEEE, 2004. IEEE* (pp. 4584–4587).

Patel, N., & Poo, M. M. (1982). Orientation of neurite growth by extracellular electric fields. *The Journal of Neuroscience, 2*(4), 483–496.

Patel, N. B., & Poo, M. M. (1984). Perturbation of the direction of neurite growth by pulsed and focal electric fields. *The Journal of Neuroscience, 4*(12), 2939–2947.

Paulus, W., & Rothwell, J. C. (2016). Membrane resistance and shunting inhibition: where biophysics meets state–dependent human neurophysiology. *The Journal of Physiology, 594*(10), 2719–2728.

Pelletier, S. J., & Cicchetti, F. (2014). Cellular and molecular mechanisms of action of transcranial direct current stimulation: Evidence from in vitro and in vivo models. *The International Journal of Neuropsychopharmacology, 18*(2), pyu047.

Pena-Gomez, C., Sala-Lonch, R., Junque, C., Clemente, I. C., Vidal, D., Bargallo, N., … Bartres-Faz, D. (2012). Modulation of large-scale brain networks by transcranial direct current stimulation evidenced by resting-state functional MRI. *Brain Stimulation, 5*(3), 252–263.

Perea, G., Navarrete, M., & Araque, A. (2009). Tripartite synapses: Astrocytes process and control synaptic information. *Trends in Neurosciences, 32*(8), 421–431.

Podda, M. V., Cocco, S., Mastrodonato, A., Fusco, S., Leone, L., Barbati, S. A., … Grassi, C. (2016). Anodal transcranial direct current stimulation boosts synaptic plasticity and memory in mice via epigenetic regulation of Bdnf expression. *Scientific Reports, 6*, 22180.

Polania, R., Nitsche, M. A., & Paulus, W. (2011a). Modulating functional connectivity patterns and topological functional organization of the human brain with transcranial direct current stimulation. *Human Brain Mapping, 32*(8), 1236–1249.

Polania, R., Paulus, W., Antal, A., & Nitsche, M. A. (2011b). Introducing graph theory to track for neuroplastic alterations in the resting human brain: A transcranial direct current stimulation study. *NeuroImage, 54*(3), 2287–2296.

Polania, R., Paulus, W., & Nitsche, M. A. (2012a). Modulating cortico-striatal and thalamo-cortical functional connectivity with transcranial direct current stimulation. *Human Brain Mapping, 33*(10), 2499–2508.

Polania, R., Paulus, W., & Nitsche, M. A. (2012b). Reorganizing the intrinsic functional architecture of the human primary motor cortex during rest with non-invasive cortical stimulation. *PLoS One, 7*(1), e30971.

Politis, M. J., Zanakis, M. F., & Albala, B. J. (1988). Facilitated regeneration in the rat peripheral nervous system using applied electric fields. *The Journal of Trauma, 28*(9), 1375–1381.

Pomeranz, B., Mullen, M., & Markus, H. (1984). Effect of applied electrical fields on sprouting of intact saphenous nerve in adult rat. *Brain Research, 303*(2), 331–336.

Prausnitz, M. R. (1996). Do high-voltage pulses cause changes in skin structure? *Journal of Controlled Release, 40*(3), 321–326.

Purpura, D. P., & Mcmurtry, J. G. (1965). Intracellular activities and evoked potential changes during polarization of motor cortex. *Journal of Neurophysiology, 28*(1), 166–185.

Radman, T., Datta, A., & Peterchev, A. V. (2007a). In vitro modulation of endogenous rhythms by AC electric fields: Syncing with clinical brain stimulation. *The Journal of Physiology, 584*(2), 369–370.

Radman, T., Ramos, R. L., Brumberg, J. C., & Bikson, M. (2009). Role of cortical cell type and morphology in subthreshold and suprathreshold uniform electric field stimulation in vitro. *Brain Stimulation, 2*(4), 215–228.e3.

Radman, T., Su, Y., An, J. H., Parra, L. C., & Bikson, M. (2007b). Spike timing amplifies the effect of electric fields on neurons: Implications for endogenous field effects. *Journal of Neuroscience, 27*(11), 3030–3036.

Rahman, A., Lafon, B., Parra, L. C., & Bikson, M. (2017). Direct current stimulation boosts synaptic gain and cooperativity in vitro. *The Journal of Physiology, 595*, 3535–3547.

Rahman, A., Reato, D., Arlotti, M., Gasca, F., Datta, A., Parra, L. C., & Bikson, M. (2013). Cellular effects of acute direct current stimulation: Somatic and synaptic terminal effects. *The Journal of Physiology, 591*(10), 2563–2578.

Ranieri, F., Podda, M. V., Riccardi, E., Frisullo, G., Dileone, M., Profice, P., … Grassi, C. (2012). Modulation of LTP at rat hippocampal CA3-CA1 synapses by direct current stimulation. *Journal of Neurophysiology, 107*(7), 1868–1880.

Rattay, F., & Wenger, C. (2010). Which elements of the mammalian central nervous system are excited by low current stimulation with microelectrodes? *Neuroscience, 170*(2), 399–407.

Reato, D., Bikson, M., & Parra, L. C. (2015). Lasting modulation of in vitro oscillatory activity with weak direct current stimulation. *Journal of Neurophysiology, 113*(5), 1334–1341.

Reato, D., Gasca, F., Datta, A., Bikson, M., Marshall, L., & Parra, L. C. (2013a). Transcranial electrical stimulation accelerates human sleep homeostasis. *PLoS Computational Biology, 9*(2), e1002898.

Reato, D., Rahman, A., Bikson, M., & Parra, L. C. (2010). Low-intensity electrical stimulation affects network dynamics by modulating population rate and spike timing. *Journal of Neuroscience, 30*(45), 15067–15079.

Reato, D., Rahman, A., Bikson, M., & Parra, L. C. (2013b). Effects of weak transcranial alternating current stimulation on brain activity—A review of known mechanisms from animal studies. *Frontiers in Human Neuroscience, 7*, 687.

Redfearn, J., Lippold, O., & Costain, R. (1964). Preliminary account of the clinical effects of polarizing the brain in certain psychiatric disorders. *The British Journal of Psychiatry, 110*(469), 773–785.

Reis, J., Schambra, H. M., Cohen, L. G., Buch, E. R., Fritsch, B., Zarahn, E., … Krakauer, J. W. (2009). Noninvasive cortical stimulation enhances motor skill acquisition over multiple days through an effect on consolidation. *Proceedings of the National Academy of Sciences of the United States of America, 106*(5), 1590–1595.

Rioult-Pedotti, M.-S., Friedman, D., Hess, G., & Donoghue, J. P. (1998). Strengthening of horizontal cortical connections following skill learning. *Nature Neuroscience, 1*(3), 230–234.

Rivera-Urbina, G. N., Batsikadze, G., Molero-Chamizo, A., Paulus, W., Kuo, M. F., & Nitsche, M. A. (2015). Parietal transcranial direct current stimulation modulates primary motor cortex excitability. *The European Journal of Neuroscience, 41*(6), 845–855.

Rizzo, V., Terranova, C., Crupi, D., Sant'angelo, A., Girlanda, P., & Quartarone, A. (2014). Increased transcranial direct current stimulation after effects during concurrent peripheral electrical nerve stimulation. *Brain stimulation, 7*(1), 113–121.

Rohan, J. G., Carhuatanta, K. A., Mcinturf, S. M., Miklasevich, M. K., & Jankord, R. (2015). Modulating hippocampal plasticity with in vivo brain stimulation. *The Journal of Neuroscience, 35*(37), 12824–12832.

Roman, G. C., Strahlendorf, H. K., Coates, P. W., & Rowley, B. A. (1987). Stimulation of sciatic nerve regeneration in the adult rat by low-intensity electric current. *Experimental Neurology, 98*(2), 222–232.

Romero Lauro, L. J., Rosanova, M., Mattavelli, G., Convento, S., Pisoni, A., Opitz, A., … Vallar, G. (2014). TDCS increases cortical excitability: Direct evidence from TMS-EEG. *Cortex, 58*, 99–111.

Ruohonen, J., & Karhu, J. (2012). tDCS possibly stimulates glial cells. *Clinical Neurophysiology, 123*(10), 2006–2009.

Salvador, R., Silva, S., Basser, P. J., & Miranda, P. C. (2011). Determining which mechanisms lead to activation in the motor cortex: A modeling study of transcranial magnetic stimulation using realistic stimulus waveforms and sulcal geometry. *Clinical Neurophysiology, 122*(4), 748–758.

Schmidt, S. L., Iyengar, A. K., Foulser, A. A., Boyle, M. R., & Fröhlich, F. (2014). Endogenous cortical oscillations constrain neuromodulation by weak electric fields. *Brain Stimulation, 7*(6), 878–889.

Spitoni, G. F., Cimmino, R. L., Bozzacchi, C., Pizzamiglio, L., & Di Russo, F. (2013). Modulation of spontaneous alpha brain rhythms using low-intensity transcranial direct-current stimulation. *Frontiers in Human Neuroscience, 7*, 529.

Stagg, C. J., Best, J. G., Stephenson, M. C., O'Shea, J., Wylezinska, M., Kincses, Z. T., … Johansen-Berg, H. (2009a). Polarity-sensitive modulation of cortical neurotransmitters by transcranial stimulation. *Journal of Neuroscience, 29*(16), 5202–5206.

Stagg, C. J., O'Shea, J., Kincses, Z. T., Woolrich, M., Matthews, P. M., & Johansen-Berg, H. (2009b). Modulation of movement-associated cortical activation by transcranial direct current stimulation. *The European Journal of Neuroscience, 30*(7), 1412–1423.

Strube, W., Bunse, T., Nitsche, M. A., Nikolaeva, A., Palm, U., Padberg, F., … Hasan, A. (2016). Bidirectional variability in motor cortex excitability modulation following 1 mA transcranial direct current stimulation in healthy participants. *Physiology Reports, 4*(15), e12884.

Svirskis, G., Gutman, A., & Hounsgaard, J. (1997). Detection of a membrane shunt by DC field polarization during intracellular and whole cell recording. *Journal of Neurophysiology, 77*(2), 579–586.

Takano, Y., Yokawa, T., Masuda, A., Niimi, J., Tanaka, S., & Hironaka, N. (2011). A rat model for measuring the effectiveness of transcranial direct current stimulation using fMRI. *Neuroscience Letters, 491*(1), 40–43.

Takeuchi, A., & Takeuchi, N. (1962). Electrical changes in pre-and postsynaptic axons of the giant synapse of Loligo. *The Journal of General Physiology, 45*(6), 1181–1193.

Terzuolo, C., & Bullock, T. (1956). Measurement of imposed voltage gradient adequate to modulate neuronal firing. *Proceedings of the National Academy of Sciences, 42*(9), 687–694.

Thirugnanasambandam, N., Grundey, J., Adam, K., Drees, A., Skwirba, A. C., Lang, N., … Nitsche, M. A. (2011). Nicotinergic impact on focal and non-focal neuroplasticity induced by non-invasive brain stimulation in non-smoking humans. *Neuropsychopharmacology, 36*(4), 879–886.

Wachter, D., Wrede, A., Schulz-Schaeffer, W., Taghizadeh-Waghefi, A., Nitsche, M. A., Kutschenko, A., … Liebetanz, D. (2011). Transcranial direct current stimulation induces polarity-specific changes of cortical blood perfusion in the rat. *Experimental Neurology, 227*(2), 322–327.

Wong, R. K., & Stewart, M. (1992). Different firing patterns generated in dendrites and somata of CA1 pyramidal neurones in Guinea-pig hippocampus. *The Journal of Physiology, 457*, 675–687.

Yoon, K. J., Oh, B.-M., & Kim, D.-Y. (2012). Functional improvement and neuroplastic effects of anodal transcranial direct current stimulation (tDCS) delivered 1day vs. 1week after cerebral ischemia in rats. *Brain Research, 1452*, 61–72.

Zaehle, T., Rach, S., & Herrmann, C. S. (2010). Transcranial alternating current stimulation enhances individual alpha activity in human EEG. *PLoS One, 5*(11), e13766.

Chapter 4
Current Methods and Approaches of Noninvasive Direct Current–Based Neuromodulation Techniques

Walter Paulus and Alberto Priori

Introduction

In the last 20 years several techniques for inducing excitability changes based upon the delivery of direct current (DC) over the skin overlying different structures of the central nervous system became available to experimental and clinical neuroscientists. Transcranial direct current stimulation (tDCS) refers to DC delivery on the scalp over the cerebral cortex (Nitsche and Paulus 2000; Priori et al. 1998), cerebellar DC stimulation refers to delivering DC current over the cerebellum (Ferrucci et al. 2015), and transcutaneous spinal DC stimulation (tsDCS) refers to the delivery of DC currents over the spinal cord (Cogiamanian et al. 2012).

Electrodes

Any transcranial electric stimulation technique needs to transfer the electric current by at least two electrodes, a target electrode and a return electrode. Multiple electrodes may be used as well both for the target and for the return electrode in order to shape the current flow. The types of electrode used for tDCS encompass metal electrodes usually covered by sponges, conductive rubber electrodes or plastic electrodes providing some mm of space for being filled with a contact medium such as conductive cream or any combination of it. Electrode fixation is usually achieved

W. Paulus (✉)
Department of Clinical Neurophysiology, University Medical Center Göttingen, Göttingen, Germany
e-mail: wpaulus@med.uni-goettingen.de

A. Priori
"Aldo Ravelli" Research Center for Neurotechnology and Experimental Brain Therapeutics, University of Milan Medical School, Milan, Italy

H. Knotkova et al. (eds.), *Practical Guide to Transcranial Direct Current Stimulation*, https://doi.org/10.1007/978-3-319-95948-1_4

by the aid of elastic straps, or head gears attached in various ways to the subject head. No ideal fixation system so far exists. The straps may still allow some movement over time during a tDCS session. Over-tightening the straps may lead to evacuation of saline from the electrode sponges. At the conductive electrode electrochemical reactions take place. Therefore the electrode should contact the skin by intermediate gel or saline solution in a sponge as a buffer between electrode and skin – with sufficient electrolyte volume preventing chemicals formed at the electrode from reaching the skin (Palm et al. 2014). In order to confine the electrode surface to the size of the electrode neither too much gel nor too much saline solution should be applied. In general, precise location of electrodes needs to be documented and kept constant to minimize variability (Saturnino et al. 2015). For example, even the position of the connecting electrode wire should be documented to provide maximum potential for replication (e.g., wire oriented to back of head, behind the ear, etc.).

The shape and the size of electrodes and/or sponges significantly alters the distribution of current delivered to the scalp and the brain (Saturnino et al. 2015). Small electrodes enable a more focused stimulation of smaller brain areas ending up e.g. in selective modulation of muscles targeting thenar or hypothenar (Nitsche et al. 2007). Large electrodes such as those conventionally used (Nitsche and Paulus 2000) with an area of 35 cm^2 provide the advantage that at first glance a not so precise allocation of the electrode position is needed. However in the light of the calculations made by Saturnino (Saturnino et al. 2015) and others small deviations from a standard electrode allocation may result in a substantial variability. Variability may be further enhanced and complicated by local thinnings of the skull which as a current running pathway may guide current through areas of locally reduced resistance somewhat independent of the location of larger electrodes (Opitz et al. 2015) (Fig. 4.1).

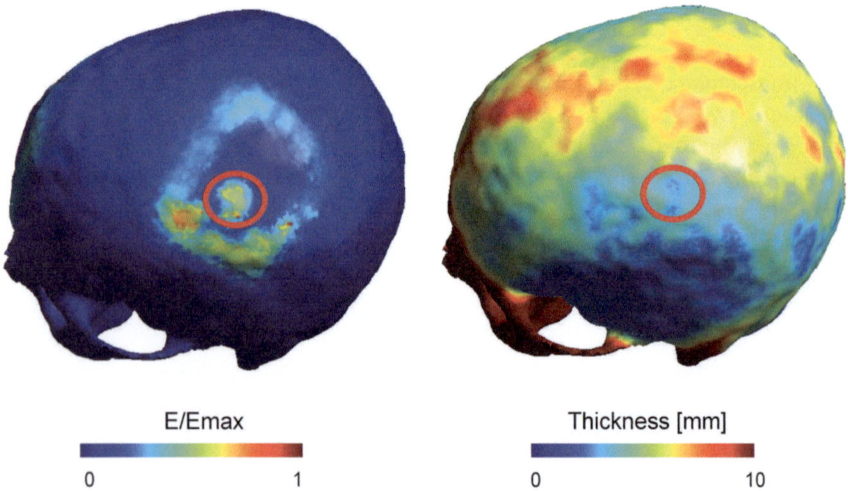

Fig. 4.1 Skull thickness (right). Red areas mark thick skull, blue areas thin skull ("temporal window" also used in ultrasound investigation). Red circle marks local thinning. On the left side electrical flow induced by a 7*5 cm electrode is calculated. Current drawn to the electrode edges is seen as well as a current pathway caused by the local thinning (red circle)

This problem can be circumvented by smaller electrodes which however need higher allocation precision (Woods et al. 2015) (*see also* Chap. 7, "Methodological Considerations for Selection of tDCS Approach, Protocols and Devices").

At the motor cortex this can be comparatively easy achieved by transcranial magnetic stimulation, other methods incorporate the International 10-20 (or 10-5) Electrode Placement System or commercially available neuronavigation systems.

With larger electrodes one should keep in mind that the conducting gel in larger electrodes guides electric current towards the edges of the electrodes, in fact a kind of ring stimulation may be taking place – although this scenario might particularly apply for the skin, but not the brain level. While other electrodes have been designed for defibrillation purposes with decreasing conductivities towards the electrode edges to enforce a more homogeneous current distribution, these electrode types have so far not been employed in transcranial stimulation techniques (Saturnino et al. 2015).

Usually the target electrode is placed above the target area. The return electrode(s) play a decisive role for guiding electric current through the intended brain or spinal cord areas. The early study by Nitsche and Paulus (2000) already showed that out of a number of different return electrodes only the one placed at the contralateral forehead provided effects during stimulation (Nitsche and Paulus 2000). In the spinal cord, the position of the return electrode influences the level of distribution of the maximum current density (Parazzini et al. 2014a) (Figs. 4.2 and 4.3).

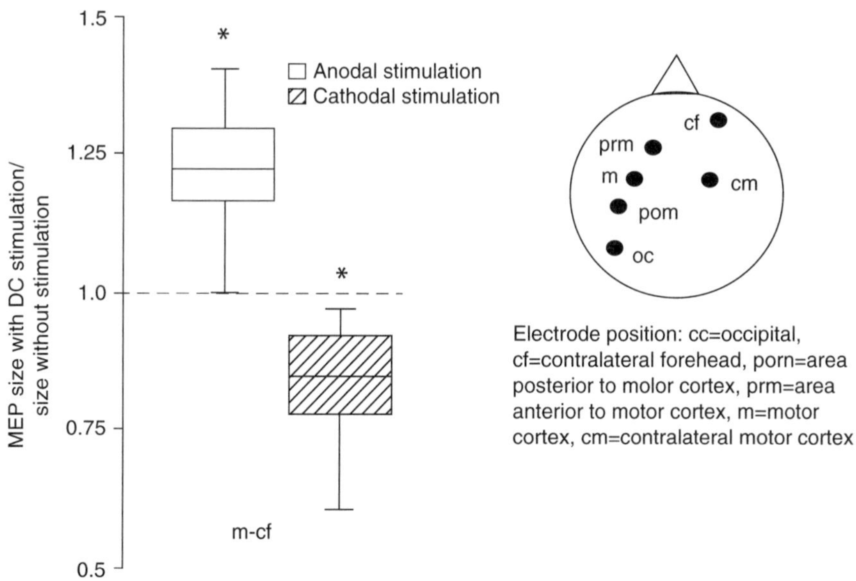

Fig. 4.2 Cortical excitability change during current flow showing rapidly induced effects of weak DC stimulation on the size of the motor evoked potential (MEP) in the right abductor digiti minimi (ADM) muscle, revealed by transcranial magnetic stimulation (TMS), using the motor cortex—contralateral forehead arrangement. MEP amplitudes during stimulation are normalized by division by MEP amplitudes without stimulation. During DC stimulation, the MEP amplitude increased with anodal and decreased with cathodal current stimulation. An effect was only seen with the m-cf montage. (Taken from Nitsche and Paulus 2000; with permission)

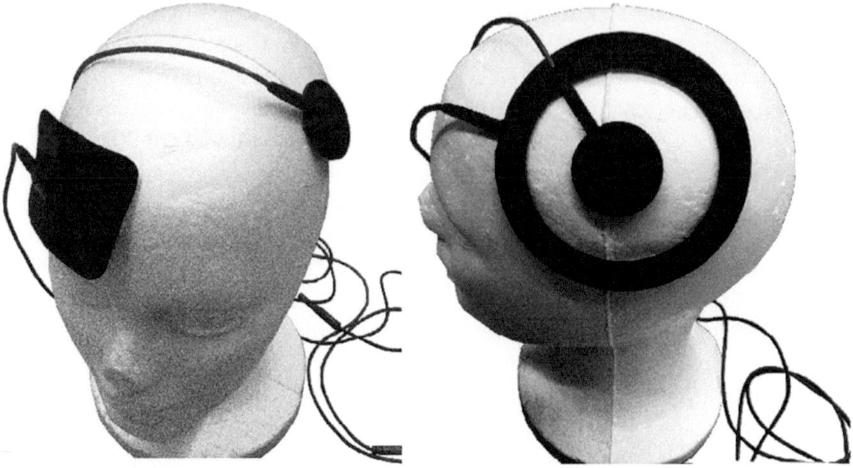

Fig. 4.3 Electrode montages can be realized in a conventional "bipolar" (top) or "center-surround" mode (bottom). (From Heise et al. 2016). The outer ring has the disadvantage that current flow cannot be controlled for compensation at thinner or thicker skull areas

Large return electrodes with an area of about 100 cm^2 have been suggested as a tool to dilute current intensity below threshold for excitation of brain tissue (Nitsche et al. 2007). Extracephalic electrodes have been discussed as another means to circumvent stimulation of the brain areas beneath cephalic return electrodes. In order to achieve comparable after effects sizes however stimulation intensity has to be doubled, at least with a return electrode at the arm (Moliadze et al. 2010b). Many modelling studies have suggested optimized current flows by the use of multichannel electrode arrays e.g. (Minhas et al. 2010; Ruffini et al. 2014). These arrays need individual calculations of electrode positions, commercial programs as well as shareware programs (e.g. www.simnibs.de) are available. It should be noted that these models have not been physiologically validated in most cases (Fig. 4.4).

Stimulation Protocols

In contrast to tACS with its capability for on-line entrainment of brain function, tDCS is essentially a method for induction of plastic after effects, although it was shown very early that 4 s of anodal tDCS increases and cathodal tDCS decreases excitability (Nitsche and Paulus 2000). Most of the available literature has dose-titrated systematically required physical parameters by single pulse TMS at the motor cortex. At least 0.6 mA intensity with a stimulation duration of at least 3 min was necessary to induce after effects (Nitsche & Paulus, 2000). In order to achieve an anodal excitatory after effects of 1 h a stimulation duration

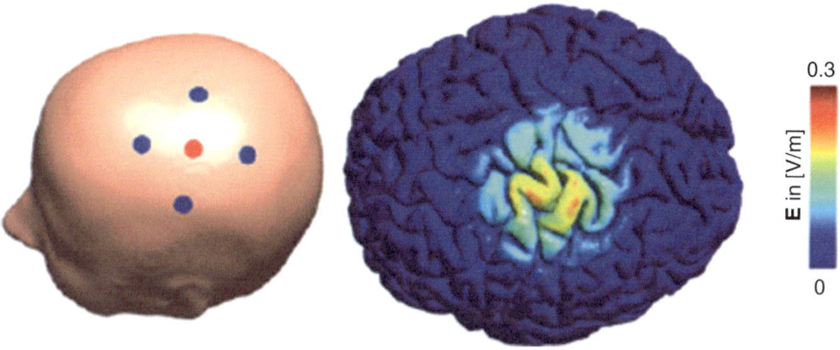

Fig. 4.4 A specific form of center-surround stimulation encompasses 4 surrounding electrodes called high-definition tDCS by (Minhas et al. 2010). Any other combination of (more) electrodes in the centre or both more or less electrodes in the surround is possible. If a constant current flow of 25% in each of the surround electrodes is to be guaranteed then a split channel connecting 4 electrodes must be used summing up to 100% in the center, with consistent impedance for the 4 electrodes. (Taken from Saturnino et al. 2015)

of 13 min is required (Nitsche and Paulus 2001), for cathodal inhibition 9 min are sufficient (Nitsche et al. 2003b). The original expectation that longer stimulation durations inevitably lead to longer plastic after effects is not true. After 26 min of continuous anodal stimulation the excitatory after effects switch into inhibition (Monte-Silva et al. 2013). Excitatory after effects can be achieved if the 26 min stimulation duration is interrupted by an either 3 min or 20 min interval, in these cases extending into the 24 h range (Monte-Silva et al. 2013). Also variation of stimulation intensity may induce a reversal of the sign of the after effects. While 1 mA cathodal stimulation intensity leads to inhibition a switch to 2 mA amplitude causes cathodally induced excitation (Batsikadze et al. 2013). All these data were derived from and are confined to resting relaxed subjects. In case of attentional challenge the after effects collapse and tend to reverse; anodal tDCS under finger tapping leads to reduction of MEP after effects sizes below baseline (Antal et al. 2007). A possible explanation for this behaviour might be that in activated neurons channels may open leaving a smaller range of membrane potential alteration induced by transcranial electrical stimulation methods (Paulus and Rothwell 2016). In line with these MEP results, also behavioural data show deviations from the simple rule – anodal tDCS~ excitation, cathodal tDCS ~inhibition. Furthermore, excitation and inhibition from tDCS may not be synonymous with functional changes in task performance (e.g., excitation may not equal faster reaction time in all cases and may be dependent on the inherent systems engaged in a given behavioural task). For example, in an implicit motor learning paradigm involving motor reaction times anodal tDCS improved reaction times, at odds with the MEP inhibition by anodal tDCS during finger tapping. Furthermore, cathodal tDCS also improved reaction times, albeit non-significantly (Nitsche et al. 2003c). Hence, the application of anodal current does not mean necessarily facilitation of a given function and vice versa for cathodal polarity. Some effects may be related to much more complex neurochemical, metabolic and plastic changes occurring in the central nervous system often uncoupled from excitability changes at least as assessed by TMS. Thus, operating on the simple assumption that anode equals excitation and cathode equals inhibition may be ill advised.

As a corollary, the stimulation parameters obtained effectively at the motor cortex provided a gross impression which intensities and stimulation durations might be best suited for stimulation of other areas. However, in the case of patients every item has to be reconsidered. Stroke patients having had loss of brain tissue being replaced by CSF will probably need very different tDCS in terms of electrode placement and stimulation parameters. Thinner CSF will lead to higher electric fields in the underlying brain (Opitz et al. 2015), hence in older patients with brain atrophy (i.e, more CSF) it may be the case that current levels reaching the brain are less than would be achieved in younger adults. This however awaits experimental verification. As a consequence each new specific experimental protocol should incorporate a titration of stimulation parameters. Furthermore individual efficacy varies considerably even with the standard TMS protocol at the motor cortex. A substantial number of subjects behave in an opposite direction when compared to the overall group level, both in tDCS and other neurostimulation applications. Individual adjustment of stimulation protocols by current flow calculations may end up at a theoretical limit when cortical folding is taken into account. Suppose a target area incorporates a cortical gyrus including the crown and both opposing walls, anodal stimulation at one side will by opposed by cathodal stimulation at the opposite wall. Thus, current flow direction in relation to neuronal orientation will be in opposite directions. Switching to tACS or tRNS, which may end up with after effects similar to tDCS might provide an improvement in the present context (Moliadze et al. 2010a, 2012; Terney et al. 2008). Another way to guide tDCS after effects in a wanted direction will be the combination with neuropharmacology. If the sodium channel blocker carbamazepine is combined with tDCS only inhibitory effects survive (Nitsche et al. 2003a). L-Dopa in a medium dosage of 100 mg switched anodal excitation into inhibition, and stabilized excitability-diminishing effects of cathodal tDCS (Kuo et al. 2008), vice versa serotonin reuptake inhibition guides inhibitory cathodal after effects into excitation, and enhances excitatory effects of anodal tDCS (Nitsche et al. 2009). Boosting tDCS after effects by co-application of citalopram in the treatment of depression has been confirmed in a large multi-center study (Brunoni et al. 2013). Many more effects of these and other drugs have been published beyond the scope of this contribution (Nitsche et al. 2012). Nonetheless, drugs may substantially affect the effects induced by DC-based transcutaneous techniques and pharmacological influences should be carefully considered in designing and interpreting the results of clinical studies in patients. Different results obtained with tDCS by different groups, can be explained by differences in ongoing pharmacological treatments.

Sham Stimulation

In a large study on depression encompassing 120 patients the placebo response with 2 mA anodal tDCS amounted to – 18.2% on the Montgomery Asberg Rating Scale as compared with the tDCS response of – 39.5% (Brunoni et al. 2013). As in any drug or other interventional study proper control for sham stimulation effects is a big issue. Usually a fade in fade out protocol is used to imitate some initial skin sensation in order to assure a subject's or patient's feeling real stimulation. In any case the subject should be questioned after the stimulation about his own rating if sham or real tDCS has been applied. A few issues have to be considered. Up to about 1 mA amplitude it is difficult for unexperienced subjects to differentiate between sham and real tDCS (Ambrus et al. 2012). With 2 mA current strength tDCS stimulation comfort is lower at stimulation onset in young and older adults and, overall, lower for young participants (Wallace et al. 2016).

With conventional 35 cm^2 electrodes active stimulation at 2 mA can be identified at above chance levels with an accuracy never exceeding 65% (Wallace et al. 2016). Stimulators will have to be modified in order provide some itching during the whole stimulation procedure at higher intensities for proper blinding. With 3 mA tDCS intensity stimulation starts to become painful. Smaller electrodes per se do not increase skin sensations (Turi et al. 2014). Other issues of importance for blinding (parallel design, skin erythema, double blinding, repeated measures conditions and others) have been discussed recently (Woods et al. 2016).

The usual approach of blinding participants for plasticity-inducing protocols is to apply a "sham" stimulation protocol, which encompasses ramping stimulation up and down like in the real stimulation condition, but to stimulate with the target intensity only for a few seconds. Participants will feel the initial itching/tingling sensation, but the stimulation duration is too short to induce after effects. For 1 mA tDCS with an electrode size of 25 cm^2, this method has been shown to reliably blind participants (Gandiga et al. 2006). Stronger stimulation will induce larger sensations, and thus compromise blinding, especially under repeated measures conditions (Nitsche et al. 2003b; Opitz et al. 2015). In crossover studies, this might however not be a relevant problem (Palm et al. 2014). Alternative approaches are application of topical anaesthetics to abolish skin sensations (Parazzini et al. 2014a) or an active control condition (i.e. stimulation over an area irrelevant for the task under study). Since the occurrence of skin damage seems to be not reliably associated with cutaneous sensation (Parazzini et al. 2013), local anaesthetics should not put participants specifically at risk. Blinding of the experimenter with regard to the specific stimulation protocol is accomplished by use of stimulators that include a sham stimulation function, thus keeping the experimenter unaware of the specific stimulation condition. Even here, however, the presence of skin erythema, which is due to tDCS-induced vasodilation (Parazzini et al. 2014b), can compromise blinding. Skin erythema is reliably reduced by acetylsalicylate, or topical application of ketoprofen (Parazzini et al. 2014b; Paulus and Rothwell 2016). Thus, for reliable double-blinding, a couple of approaches are available, which should be chosen carefully due to the specific experimental design. Other approaches for testing the specificity of the effects are assessing the effects of opposite stimulation polarities, or testing the effect on different central nervous system areas.

Cerebellar Direct Current Stimulation

In the last 10 years several pieces of evidence demonstrated that delivering DC over the cerebellum can modulate its functions. Ferrucci et al. (2008) firstly reported that delivering DC with one electrode over the cerebellum and the other over the right shoulder (Fig. 4.5) for few minutes at 2 mA, specifically decreased the rate of improvement of a working memory task. Interestingly, stimulation over the dorsolateral prefrontal cortex induced the opposite effect, whereas sham stimulation failed to induce any change. Additionally, cerebellar stimulation did not influence the visual evoked potential, therefore ruling out any possible effect through influence over the visual system. Though indirect, this was the first report about the behavioural and cognitive effects of DC stimulation of the cerebellum. A further step forward were the physiological experiments reported by Galea et al. (2009) who observed that cathodal cerebellar DC stimulation (2 mA) can modulate cerebellar-brain inhibition assessed by transcranial magnetic

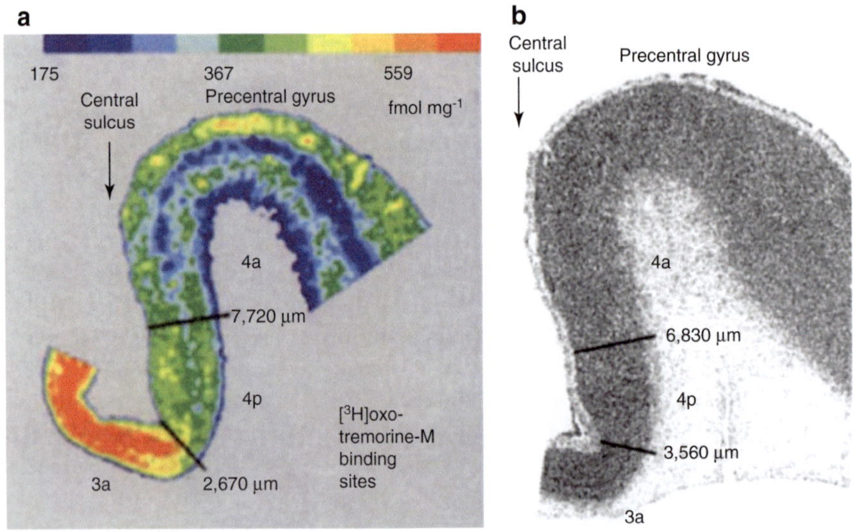

Fig. 4.5 **(a, b)** Allocation of the motor cortex area 4a and 4p in the anterior wall of the human motor cortex. (Taken from Geyer et al. 1996). Current flow may be more perpendicular in the sulcus than at the crown, favouring tDCS effects in a sulcal as compared to a crown located area. However, this is currently a hotly debated notion. In contrast, it is accepted that the same electric field will result in different current flow directions regarding neuron positions at the crown or the skull. The human motor cortex, area 4a and 4p, a mostly allocated in the anterior wall of the precentral gyrus and not at the crown

stimulation. Again, sham stimulation failed to induce any physiological change. These two seminal papers prompted several groups to test the effects of cerebellar DC stimulation on different behavioural and neurophysiological variables (for recent reviews see Ferrucci and Priori 2014; Grimaldi et al. 2014, 2016). The hypothesis is that in spite of the highly folded pattern DC stimulation can influence the excitability of cerebellar cortex, ultimately modulating its inhibition over the cerebellar nuclei, and therefore their efferent output projections to the brain. Modelling studies showed that the electric field generated by cerebellar DC stimulation variably goes deep into the posterior cranial fossa in relation with gender and age: the field apparently is deeper in children and woman (Parazzini et al. 2013, 2014b) (Fig. 4.6).

Besides the observations of the effects induced by cerebellar DC stimulation in normal subjects, there are also interesting studies in patients with ataxia and Parkinson's disease. Benussi et al. (Benussi et al. 2015) reported that in 19 patients with ataxia of different etiologies, a single session anodal cerebellar DC stimulation (20 min, 2 mA) –but not sham stimulation— transiently improves symptoms and motor coordination in patients with ataxia. The cerebellum is also involved in the pathophysiology of movement disorders other than cerebellar ataxia as for instance Parkinson's disease (Mirdamadi 2016; Wu and Hallett 2013). With the hypothesis of modulating the motor cortical excitability during levodopa induced dyskinesias, Ferrucci et al. (2016) tested a group of 9 patients with Parkinson's disease with anodal and sham DC stimulation (20 min, 2 mA) either over the cerebellum or over the motor cortical areas for 5 days: anodal –but not sham-- DC stimulation over both sites failed to change the UPDRS III but significantly improved the UPDRS IV related to involuntary movements. Minichino et al. (2014) assessed sleep quality of a group of 25 euthymic patients with bipolar disorder and found that sleep distrurbance-dependent daytime dysfunction significantly decreased after 3 consecutive weeks of treatment (20 min, 2 mA). In 14 patients with depression cerebellar DC stimulation with the other electrode over the prefrontal cortex was also found effective (Ho et al. 2014). Ten-session anodal cerebellar tDCS (twice a day, 20 min 2 mA) with the other electrode over the prefrontal cortex in treatment resistant obsessive compulsive disorder improved obsessive symptoms but not depression by some 26% for 3 months, thus making DC stimulation an attractive possibility in the management of obsessive compulsive disorder (Bation et al. 2016).

Transcutaneous Spinal Direct Current Stimulation

The third target for DC based non invasive neuromodulation techniques is the spinal cord. Eccles et al. in the sixties observed that polarizing DC currents delivered over the exposed cat spinal cord elicited consistent and remarkable changes in motoneuronal function in the ventral horn (Eccles et al. 1962).

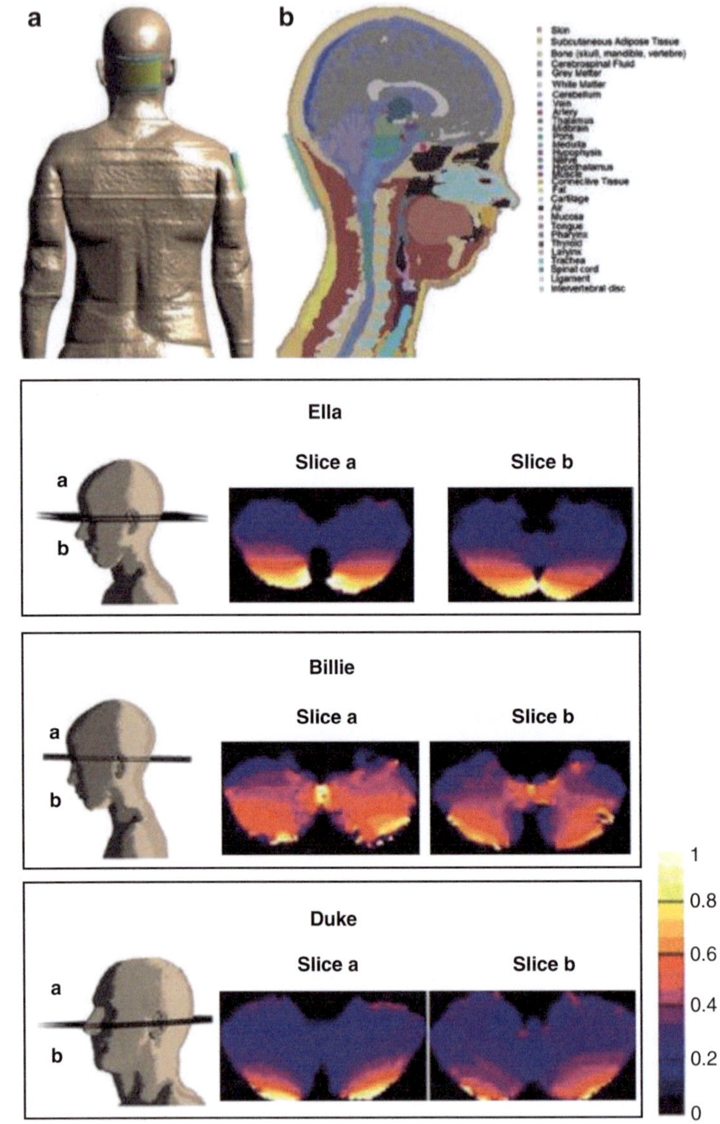

Fig. 4.6 Position of electrodes for transcutaneous cerebellar DC stimulation shown on a model used for current estimation. (From Parazzini et al. 2014a, b. with permission). Top, (**a**) electrode (green and light blue) position viewed from the back; the active electrode is over the cerebellum and the return electrode over the left shoulder. The active electrode can also be smaller and placed over a single cerebellar hemisphere, the return electrode can also be placed in other position over the head or face (not shown). Top, (**b**) a sagittal MRI reconstruction showing the tissues below the electrode; different tissues are identified by different colours shown on the right. Bottom: current density amplitude distributions below the electrode for cerebellar DC stimulation in three different subjects (Ella, Billie, Duke) modelled on a transversal MRI slice passing through the electrode; current density is plotted according to the colour scale on the right. Note that the current density distribution varies in different subjects and tends to spread anteriorly in the adolescent Billie (middle), whereas remains localized to cerebellar hemispheres in the adult male subject Duke (bottom) and has an intermediate distribution in the adult female Ella (top)

Starting from the observation by Eccles and coworkers, the Milano group assessed the effects of delivering DC over the thoracic human spinal cord (Cogiamanian et al. 2008) by transcutaneous thoracic spinal DC stimulation (Fig. 4.6). The conduction along the lemniscal system was assessed by somatosensory evoked potentials (SEP) elicited by stimulation of the tibial nerve in healthy subjects. The SEP amplitude decreased after anodal DC stimulation and increased (not significantly) after cathodal DC stimulation. Interestingly thoracic DC stimulation failed to change the SEP evoked by median nerve stimulation, thus demonstrating that the effect of DC was spatially restricted to the sensory fibres travelling in the spinal cord below the stimulating electrode but not in other places. Further studies found that a similar effect appeared for the spinothalamic system (Truini et al. 2011) and corticospinal fibers (Bocci et al. 2015). Nierat et al. (2014) found that cathodal tsDCS at cervical level increased significantly the volume of air inhaled or exhaled in a single breath (Tidal Volume) in a group of healthy subjects, possibly modulating the descending input over phrenic motoneurones. Several other studies tested the effects of tsDCS on segmental reflexes. For instance, Winkler et al. (2010) found that tsDCS modulated the H-reflex post-activation depression in a polarity dependent manner, Cogiamanian et al. (2011) found that tsDCS modulated the nociceptive flexion reflex in humans. Bocci et al. (2014) tested the effects of tsDCS on spinal motorneuron excitability: they found that cathodal-tsDCS dramatically increases motor unit number estimation (MUNE) values following cervical polarization, while sham and anodal polarization had no significant effect. At the same time, cathodal-tsDCS dampened the peripheral silent period in respect to sham and anodal conditions. The authors concluded that tsDCS, possibly also through supraspinal effects, could provide a novel therapeutic tool in managing several pathological conditions characterized by reduced motor unit recruitment (Fig. 4.7).

Anodal tsDCS in restless leg syndrome decreased for a short time symptoms on the VAS, whereas application of sham stimulation had no effects (Heide et al. 2014) supporting the pathophysiological concept of spinal cord hyperexcitability in RLS. Hubli et al. (2013) assessed the effects of tsDCS on spinal reflexes in patients with complete spinal cord injury reporting that reflexes improved after anodal tsDCS concluding that anodal tsDCS can modulate spinal neuronal circuitries after SCI.

Direct Current–Based Noninvasive Neuromodulation Techniques at Home

Among various advantages of tDCS over rTMS, there is the possibility of delivering stimulation at home. Yet, DC-based techniques are relatively cheap, safe, and the devices are small, easily portable, and wearable. The patients and their caregivers

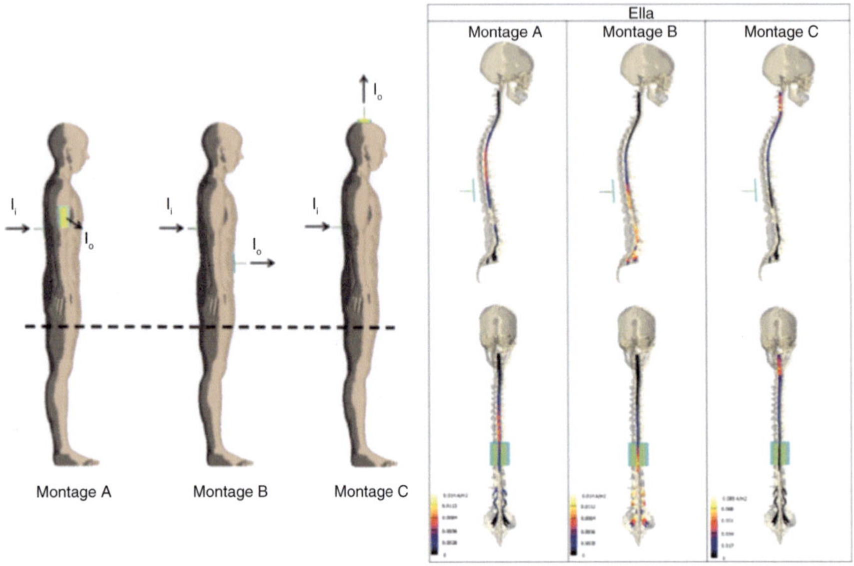

Fig. 4.7 Position of electrodes for transcutaneous spinal DC stimulation shown on a model used for current distribution estimation. (From Parazzini et al. 2014a). Left: with the active electrode over the lower thoracic spinal cord, three different positions of the return electrode (I0) are shown from the left to the right: left shoulder, abdominal wall, and vertex. Right: current density distribution (top: lateral view, bottom: viewed from the back) within the spinal cord keeping the green active electrode over the lower thoracic spinal cord, with three different positions of the return electrode shown from the left to the right: left shoulder, abdominal wall, and vertex. Current density is graphically expressed according to the colour scale. Note that when the return electrode is placed over the right shoulder the maximum current density is in the thoracic spinal cord above the level of the electrode, when the return electrode is on the abdominal wall the maximum current density is below the lower half of the stimulating electrode, and when the return electrode is on the vertex the maximum current density is in the cervical spinal cord. Hence, different positions of the return electrode can focus the current distribution at different spinal cord levels

can easily learn how to place the electrodes for different types of brain, cerebellar and spinal cord DC stimulation. At difference from TMS related techniques, though the great feasibility and accessibility of DC-based techniques can be dangerous because it makes it easy using tDCS as a "toy", without medical supervision, the simplicity of the technique and of the devices allows the treatment of large populations of patients at home (Priori et al. 2009). Andrade (2013) effectively and safely used tDCS at home in a patient with clozapine refractory auditory hallucinations. Mortensen et al. (2016) found that tDCS at home is well-tolerated by patients with upper limb impairment following intracerebral hemorrage and the authors found that anodal tDCS increased the grip strength thus representing a feasible add-on treatment for home rehabilitation. Kasschau et al. (2016) reported the use of a telemedicine platform to monitor the use of tDCS at home in a group of patients with multiple sclerosis concluding that remotely supervised tDCS can be safe and reliable in multiple sclerosis, further expanding the patient access to the technique. Hyvarinen et al. (2016) found domiciliary tDCS safe and feasible for tinnitus. In conclusion, the possibility of home delivery of tDCS opens the avenue to a treatment that will be feasible in large population of patients without entering a hospital. This has also obvious implications for developing countries or countries where there are great distances to be covered before finding a hospital.

Conclusions

Available evidence shows that non-invasive DC-based neuromodulation techniques can influence the function of different structures in the human brain, cerebellum, and spinal cord. Although the effects can vary from subject to subject in relation with different factors (age, gender, concomitant drug consumption), the excitability changes induced have potential clinical relevance for therapeutic purposes. In addition, the techniques discussed above share feasibility for use at home and the safety that warrant their possible use in large population of patients. Much remains to be done, especially for the development of standardized protocols of DC stimulation in different neuropsychiatric disorders.

References

Ambrus, G. G., Al-Moyed, H., Chaieb, L., Sarp, L., Antal, A., & Paulus, W. (2012). The fade-in – short stimulation – fade out approach to sham tDCS – reliable at 1 mA for naive and experienced subjects, but not investigators. *Brain Stimulation, 5*(4), 499–504.

Andrade, C. (2013). Once- to twice-daily, 3-year domiciliary maintenance transcranial direct current stimulation for severe, disabling, clozapine-refractory continuous auditory hallucinations in schizophrenia. *The Journal of ECT, 29*(3), 239–242.

Antal, A., Terney, D., Poreisz, C., & Paulus, W. (2007). Towards unravelling task-related modulations of neuroplastic changes induced in the human motor cortex. *The European Journal of Neuroscience, 26*(9), 2687–2691.

Bation, R., Poulet, E., Haesebaert, F., Saoud, M., & Brunelin, J. (2016). Transcranial direct current stimulation in treatment-resistant obsessive-compulsive disorder: An open-label pilot study. *Progress in Neuro-Psychopharmacology & Biological Psychiatry, 65*, 153–157.

Batsikadze, G., Moliadze, V., Paulus, W., Kuo, M. F., & Nitsche, M. A. (2013). Partially non-linear stimulation intensity-dependent effects of direct current stimulation on motor cortex excitability in humans. *The Journal of Physiology, 591*(7), 1987–2000.

Benussi, A., Koch, G., Cotelli, M., Padovani, A., & Borroni, B. (2015). Cerebellar transcranial direct current stimulation in patients with ataxia: A double-blind, randomized, sham-controlled study. *Movement Disorders, 30*(12), 1701–1705.

Bocci, T., Santarcangelo, E., Vannini, B., Torzini, A., Carli, G., Ferrucci, R., et al. (2015). Cerebellar direct current stimulation modulates pain perception in humans. *Restorative Neurology and Neuroscience, 33*(5), 597–609.

Bocci, T., Vannini, B., Torzini, A., Mazzatenta, A., Vergari, M., Cogiamanian, F., et al. (2014). Cathodal transcutaneous spinal direct current stimulation (tsDCS) improves motor unit recruitment in healthy subjects. *Neuroscience Letters, 578*, 75–79.

Brunoni, A. R., Valiengo, L., Baccaro, A., Zanao, T. A., de Oliveira, J. F., Goulart, A., et al. (2013). The sertraline vs. electrical current therapy for treating depression clinical study: Results from a factorial, randomized, controlled trial. *JAMA Psychiatry, 70*(4), 383–391.

Cogiamanian, F., Ardolino, G., Vergari, M., Ferrucci, R., Ciocca, M., Scelzo, E., et al. (2012). Transcutaneous spinal direct current stimulation. *Frontiers in Psychiatry, 3*, 63.

Cogiamanian, F., Vergari, M., Pulecchi, F., Marceglia, S., & Priori, A. (2008). Effect of spinal transcutaneous direct current stimulation on somatosensory evoked potentials in humans. *Clinical Neurophysiology, 119*(11), 2636–2640. S1388-2457(08)00879-1 [pii].

Cogiamanian, F., Vergari, M., Schiaffi, E., Marceglia, S., Ardolino, G., Barbieri, S., et al. (2011). Transcutaneous spinal cord direct current stimulation inhibits the lower limb nociceptive flexion reflex in human beings. *Pain, 152*(2), 370–375. S0304-3959(10)00675-5 [pii].

Eccles, J. C., Kostyuk, P. G., & Schmidt, R. F. (1962). The effect of electric polarization of the spinal cord on central afferent fibres and on their excitatory synaptic action. *The Journal of Physiology, 162*, 138–150.

Ferrucci, R., Cortese, F., Bianchi, M., Pittera, D., Turrone, R., Bocci, T., et al. (2016). Cerebellar and motor cortical transcranial stimulation decrease levodopa-induced dyskinesias in Parkinson's disease. *Cerebellum, 15*(1), 43–47.

Ferrucci, R., Cortese, F., & Priori, A. (2015). Cerebellar tDCS: How to do it. *Cerebellum, 14*(1), 27–30.

Ferrucci, R., Marceglia, S., Vergari, M., Cogiamanian, F., Mrakic-Sposta, S., Mameli, F., et al. (2008). Cerebellar transcranial direct current stimulation impairs the practice-dependent proficiency increase in working memory. *Journal of Cognitive Neuroscience, 20*(9), 1687–1697.

Ferrucci, R., & Priori, A. (2014). Transcranial cerebellar direct current stimulation (tcDCS): Motor control, cognition, learning and emotions. *NeuroImage, 85*(Pt 3), 918–923.

Galea, J. M., Jayaram, G., Ajagbe, L., & Celnik, P. (2009). Modulation of cerebellar excitability by polarity-specific noninvasive direct current stimulation. *The Journal of Neuroscience, 29*(28), 9115–9122. 29/28/9115 [pii].

Gandiga, P. C., Hummel, F. C., & Cohen, L. G. (2006). Transcranial DC stimulation (tDCS): A tool for double-blind sham-controlled clinical studies in brain stimulation. *Clinical Neurophysiology, 117*, 845–850.

Geyer, S., Ledberg, A., Schleicher, A., Kinomura, S., Schormann, T., Burgel, U., et al. (1996). Two different areas within the primary motor cortex of man. *Nature, 382*(6594), 805–807.

Grimaldi, G., Argyropoulos, G. P., Bastian, A., Cortes, M., Davis, N. J., Edwards, D. J., et al. (2016). Cerebellar transcranial direct current stimulation (ctDCS): A novel approach to understanding cerebellar function in health and disease. *The Neuroscientist, 22*(1), 83–97.

Grimaldi, G., Argyropoulos, G. P., Boehringer, A., Celnik, P., Edwards, M. J., Ferrucci, R., et al. (2014). Non-invasive cerebellar stimulation--a consensus paper. *Cerebellum, 13*(1), 121–138.

Heide, A. C., Winkler, T., Helms, H. J., Nitsche, M. A., Trenkwalder, C., Paulus, W., et al. (2014). Effects of transcutaneous spinal direct current stimulation in idiopathic restless legs patients. *Brain Stimulation, 7*(5), 636–642.

Heise, K. F., Kortzorg, N., Saturnino, G. B., Fujiyama, H., Cuypers, K., Thielscher, A., et al. (2016). Evaluation of a modified high-definition electrode montage for transcranial alternating current stimulation (tACS) of pre-central areas. *Brain Stimulation.*

Ho, K. A., Bai, S., Martin, D., Alonzo, A., Dokos, S., Puras, P., et al. (2014). A pilot study of alternative transcranial direct current stimulation electrode montages for the treatment of major depression. *Journal of Affective Disorders, 167*, 251–258.

Hubli, M., Dietz, V., Schrafl-Altermatt, M., & Bolliger, M. (2013). Modulation of spinal neuronal excitability by spinal direct currents and locomotion after spinal cord injury. *Clinical Neurophysiology, 124*(6), 1187–1195.

Hyvarinen, P., Mendonca, C., Santala, O., Pulkki, V., & Aarnisalo, A. A. (2016). Auditory localization by subjects with unilateral tinnitus. *The Journal of the Acoustical Society of America, 139*(5), 2280–2289.

Kasschau, M., Reisner, J., Sherman, K., Bikson, M., Datta, A., & Charvet, L. E. (2016). Transcranial direct current stimulation is feasible for remotely supervised home delivery in multiple sclerosis. *Neuromodulation, 19*(8), 824–831.

Kuo, M.-F., Paulus, W., & Nitsche, M. A. (2008). Boosting focally-induced brain plasticity by dopamine. *Cerebral Cortex, 18*(3), 648–651.

Minhas, P., Bansal, V., Patel, J., Ho, J. S., Diaz, J., Datta, A., et al. (2010). Electrodes for high-definition transcutaneous DC stimulation for applications in drug delivery and electrotherapy, including tDCS. *Journal of Neuroscience Methods, 190*(2), 188–197. S0165-0270(10)00266-9 [pii].

Minichino, A., Bersani, F. S., Spagnoli, F., Corrado, A., De Michele, F., Calo, W. K., et al. (2014). Prefronto-cerebellar transcranial direct current stimulation improves sleep quality in euthymic bipolar patients: a brief report. *Behavioural Neurology, 2014*, 876521.

Mirdamadi, J. L. (2016). Cerebellar role in Parkinson's disease. *Journal of Neurophysiology, 01132*, 02015.

Moliadze, V., Antal, A., & Paulus, W. (2010a). Boosting brain excitability by transcranial high frequency stimulation in the ripple range. *The Journal of Physiology, 588*(Pt 24), 4891–4904.

Moliadze, V., Antal, A., & Paulus, W. (2010b). Electrode-distance dependent after-effects of transcranial direct and random noise stimulation with extracephalic reference electrodes. *Clinical Neurophysiology, 121*(12), 2165–2171.

Moliadze, V., Atalay, D., Antal, A., & Paulus, W. (2012). Close to threshold transcranial electrical stimulation preferentially activates inhibitory networks before switching to excitation with higher intensities. *Brain Stimulation, 5*(4), 505–511.

Monte-Silva, K., Kuo, M.-F., Hessenthaler, S., Fresnoza, S., Liebetanz, D., Paulus, W., et al. (2013). Induction of late LTP-like plasticity in the human motor cortex by repeated non-invasive brain stimulation. *Brain Stimulation, 6*(3), 424–432.

Mortensen, J., Figlewski, K., & Andersen, H. (2016). Combined transcranial direct current stimulation and home-based occupational therapy for upper limb motor impairment following intracerebral hemorrhage: A double-blind randomized controlled trial. *Disability and Rehabilitation, 38*(7), 637–643.

Nierat, M. C., Similowski, T., & Lamy, J. C. (2014). Does trans-spinal direct current stimulation alter phrenic motoneurons and respiratory neuromechanical outputs in humans? A double-blind, sham-controlled, randomized, crossover study. *Journal of Neuroscience, 34*(43), 14420–14429.

Nitsche, M. A., Doemkes, S., Karakose, T., Antal, A., Liebetanz, D., Lang, N., et al. (2007). Shaping the effects of transcranial direct current stimulation of the human motor cortex. *Journal of Neurophysiology, 97*(4), 3109–3117.

Nitsche, M. A., Fricke, K., Henschke, U., Schlitterlau, A., Liebetanz, D., Lang, N., et al. (2003a). Pharmacological modulation of cortical excitability shifts induced by transcranial direct current stimulation in humans. *The Journal of Physiology, 553*(Pt 1), 293–301.

Nitsche, M. A., Kuo, M. F., Karrasch, R., Wachter, B., Liebetanz, D., & Paulus, W. (2009). Serotonin affects transcranial direct current-induced neuroplasticity in humans. *Biological Psychiatry, 66*(5), 503–508. S0006-3223(09)00422-3 [pii].

Nitsche, M. A., Müller-Dahlhaus, F., Paulus, W., & Ziemann, U. (2012). The pharmacology of neuroplasticity induced by non-invasive brain stimulation: Building models for the clinical use of CNS active drugs. *The Journal of Physiology, 590*, 4641–4662.

Nitsche, M. A., Nitsche, M. S., Klein, C. C., Tergau, F., Rothwell, J. C., & Paulus, W. (2003b). Level of action of cathodal DC polarisation induced inhibition of the human motor cortex. *Clinical Neurophysiology, 114*(4), 600–604.

Nitsche, M. A., & Paulus, W. (2000). Excitability changes induced in the human motor cortex by weak transcranial direct current stimulation. *The Journal of Physiology, 527*(Pt 3), 633–639.

Nitsche, M. A., & Paulus, W. (2001). Sustained excitability elevations induced by transcranial DC motor cortex stimulation in humans. *Neurology, 57*(10), 1899–1901.

Nitsche, M. A., Schauenburg, A., Lang, N., Liebetanz, D., Exner, C., Paulus, W., et al. (2003c). Facilitation of implicit motor learning by weak transcranial direct current stimulation of the primary motor cortex in the human. *Journal of Cognitive Neuroscience, 15*(4), 619–626.

Opitz, A., Paulus, W., Will, S., Antunes, A., & Thielscher, A. (2015). Determinants of the electric field during transcranial direct current stimulation. *NeuroImage, 109*, 140–150.

Palm, U., Feichtner, K. B., Hasan, A., Gauglitz, G., Langguth, B., Nitsche, M. A., et al. (2014). The role of contact media at the skin-electrode interface during transcranial direct current stimulation (tDCS). *Brain Stimulation, 7*(5), 762–764.

Parazzini, M., Fiocchi, S., Liorni, I., Rossi, E., Cogiamanian, F., Vergari, M., et al. (2014a). Modeling the current density generated by transcutaneous spinal direct current stimulation (tsDCS). *Clinical Neurophysiology, 125*(11), 2260–2270. S1388-2457(14)00173-4 [pii].

Parazzini, M., Rossi, E., Ferrucci, R., Fiocchi, S., Liorni, I., Priori, A., et al. (2013). Computational model of cerebellar transcranial direct current stimulation. *Conference Proceedings: Annual International Conference of the IEEE Engineering in Medicine and Biology Society, 2013*, 237–240.

Parazzini, M., Rossi, E., Ferrucci, R., Liorni, I., Priori, A., & Ravazzani, P. (2014b). Modelling the electric field and the current density generated by cerebellar transcranial DC stimulation in humans. *Clinical Neurophysiology, 125*(3), 577–584.

Paulus, W., & Rothwell, J. C. (2016). Membrane resistance and shunting inhibition: Where biophysics meets state-dependent human neurophysiology. *The Journal of Physiology, 594*(10), 2719–2728.

Priori, A., Berardelli, A., Inghilleri, M., Pedace, F., Giovannelli, M., & Manfredi, M. (1998). Electrical stimulation over muscle tendons in humans. Evidence favouring presynaptic inhibition of Ia fibres due to the activation of group III tendon afferents. *Brain, 121*(Pt 2), 373–380.

Priori, A., Hallett, M., & Rothwell, J. C. (2009). Repetitive transcranial magnetic stimulation or transcranial direct current stimulation? *Brain Stimulation, 2*(4), 241–245. S1935-861X(09)00012-6 [pii].

Ruffini, G., Fox, M. D., Ripolles, O., Miranda, P. C., & Pascual-Leone, A. (2014). Optimization of multifocal transcranial current stimulation for weighted cortical pattern targeting from realistic modeling of electric fields. *NeuroImage, 89*, 216–225.

Saturnino, G. B., Antunes, A., & Thielscher, A. (2015). On the importance of electrode parameters for shaping electric field patterns generated by tDCS. *NeuroImage, 120*, 25–35.

Terney, D., Chaieb, L., Moliadze, V., Antal, A., & Paulus, W. (2008). Increasing human brain excitability by transcranial high-frequency random noise stimulation. *The Journal of Neuroscience, 28*(52), 14147–14155.

Truini, A., Vergari, M., Biasiotta, A., La Cesa, S., Gabriele, M., Di Stefano, G., et al. (2011). Transcutaneous spinal direct current stimulation inhibits nociceptive spinal pathway conduction and increases pain tolerance in humans. *European Journal of Pain, 15*(10), 1023–1027.

Turi, Z., Ambrus, G. G., Ho, K. A., Sengupta, T., Paulus, W., & Antal, A. (2014). When size matters: Large electrodes induce greater stimulation-related cutaneous discomfort than smaller electrodes at equivalent current density. *Brain Stimulation, 7*(3), 460–467.

Wallace, D., Cooper, N. R., Paulmann, S., Fitzgerald, P. B., & Russo, R. (2016). Perceived comfort and blinding efficacy in randomised sham-controlled transcranial direct current stimulation (tDCS) trials at 2 mA in young and older healthy adults. *PLoS One, 11*(2), e0149703.

Winkler, T., Hering, P., & Straube, A. (2010). Spinal DC stimulation in humans modulates post-activation depression of the H-reflex depending on current polarity. *Clinical Neurophysiology, 121*(6), 957–961. S1388-2457(10)00054-4 [pii].

Woods, A. J., Antal, A., Bikson, M., Boggio, P. S., Brunoni, A. R., Celnik, P., et al. (2016). A technical guide to tDCS, and related non-invasive brain stimulation tools. *Clinical Neurophysiology, 127*(2), 1031–1048.

Woods, A. J., Bryant, V., Sacchetti, D., Gervits, F., & Hamilton, R. (2015). Effects of electrode drift in transcranial direct current stimulation. *Brain Stimulation, 8*(3), 515–519.

Wu, T., & Hallett, M. (2013). The cerebellum in Parkinson's disease. *Brain, 136*(Pt 3), 696–709.

Chapter 5
Transcranial Direct Current Stimulation Modulation of Neurophysiological Functional Outcomes: Neurophysiological Principles and Rationale

Helena Knotkova, Michael A. Nitsche, and Rafael Polania

Introduction

Exploring the physiological effects of tDCS is of utmost importance for the field due to numerous reasons. First, physiological measures allow the quantification of basic effects of tDCS, and thus help to develop and tailor stimulation protocols based on parameters like magnitude, duration, and focality of effects. Second, combination of tDCS with physiological measures can help to improve mechanistic understanding of neuroplasticity of the human brain. Third, physiologically defined tDCS protocols are relevant to develop targeted and rationally based stimulation procedures for modification of psychological and behavioral processes, both in basic, but also in applied clinical studies. Nowadays, numerous neurophysiological and functional imaging tools are available which allow to monitor physiological alterations induced by tDCS in the human brain. For monitoring regional effects of tDCS of a specific target region, these include evoked potential measures, which enable monitoring of tDCS effects over sensory and motor cortices, event-related potentials, EEG, combination of transcranial magnetic stimulation (TMS) and EEG, and neuroimaging tools such as magnetic

H. Knotkova
MJHS Institute for Innovation in Palliative Care, New York, NY, USA

Department of Family and Social Medicine, Albert Einstein College of Medicine, Bronx, NY, USA

M. A. Nitsche
Department of Psychology and Neurosciences, Leibniz Research Centre for Working Environment and Human Factors, Dortmund, Germany

University Medical Hospital Bergmannsheil, Bochum, Germany

R. Polania (✉)
ETH Zurich, Decision Neuroscience Lab, Department of Health Sciences and Technology, Zurich, Switzerland
e-mail: rafael.polania@hest.ethz.ch

H. Knotkova et al. (eds.), *Practical Guide to Transcranial Direct Current Stimulation*, https://doi.org/10.1007/978-3-319-95948-1_5

resonance tomography, and positron emission tomography for exploration of physiological effects also over association cortices. Some of these techniques do also allow to disentangle the effects of tDCS to afferent structures of the target area, and thus to monitor the impact of tDCS on specific neuronal populations. Adding pharmacological interventions enable to explore the impact of tDCS on spefific neurotransmitters, ion channels, and receptors, or allow to disentangle the sometimes complex impact of the activity state of transmitters on tDCS effects. Depending on the specific technique, these allow monitoring of cortical excitability or activity. On the other hand, tools like functional magnetic resonance tomography and EEG allow monitoring of network effect of stimulation, by correlating activity indices of remote cerebral areas. EEG allows monitoring of associated cortical activity with high temporal, but less spatial precision, whereas fMRI enables also identification of cortico-subcortical connectivity with high spatial sensitivity. Respective studies have shown during the last years that tDCS are not restricted to a specific targeted area, but induce alterations of connectivity of distributed cerebral networks. Beyond pure physiological results at the regional and network level, combination of tDCS and cognitive or behavioral interventions with physiological monitoring might furthermore be suited to obtain information about the physiological background of task-related effects of tDCS, which is of specific relevance due to the state-dependent neuromodulatory effects of this intervention.

In this chapter, an overview about neurophysiological effects of tDCS on the human brain is given. It will cover the main fields which have been explored so far with regard to regional and network effects of tDCS, but also include emerging techniques which hold promise to reveal substantial information about tDCS-induced neuromodulation.

Regional Effects of tDCS

tDCS accomplishes its effects via electrodes positioned to affect one or more target areas. For these target areas, electrical fields are induced which are sufficiently strong to induce physiological effects at the sites of neuronal tissue, i.e. primary effects like membrane polarization, and secondary neuroplastic effects, which go along with excitability alterations and modulation of spontaneous neuronal activity. These effects under the target areas should be discerned from remote effects of tDCS on functionally connected neuronal population, which are thought to be elicited via activity alterations of the target area, but do not include respective physical polarization effects. For exploring regional physiological effects of the stimulation technique, the primary motor cortex is the most frequently used model, because it is relatively easy to access by non-invasive brain stimulation because of its surface-near position, and a couple of tools are available to explore stimulation-induced physiological effects. Physiological effects of tDCS on other cortical areas, however, have been also explored, which is relevant, because due to differences of cortical architecture, receptor distribution, and anatomical factors, it cannot be taken for granted that motor cortex tDCS effects translate one-to-one to other areas.

Motor Cortex

The majority of studies exploring physiological effects of tDCS has been conducted for the primary motor cortex. Beyond monitoring of tDCS-induced excitability alterations via transcranial magnetic stimulation (TMS) (Fig. 5.1), a couple of studies explored tDCS effects on cortical activity via functional imaging approaches such as EEG, fMRI, and PET.

Primary effects of tDCS are thought to depend on membrane polarization of the targeted neurons, causing an alteration of cortical excitability which depends on the direction of current flow in relation to neuronal orientation. Early TMS experiments support this view by showing that stimulation for a few seconds alters motor cortex excitability, as demonstrated by modulation of single pulse TMS-elicited motor evoked potentials (MEPs), a relatively unspecific parameter of cortico-spinal excitability. MEPs were enhanced by the anode positioned over the motor cortex, while cathodal tDCS resulted in an excitability diminution. In accordance with the proposed electrical field direction sensitivity of tDCS effects, in these experiments only motor cortex vs contralateral supraorbital electrode positions induced respective effects (Nitsche and Paulus 2000). In accordance with the polarization hypothesis, voltage-gated ion channel block prevented acute effects of tDCS, while pharmacological alteration of the glutamatergic system by NMDA receptor block or of the GABA-ergic system via benzodiazepines, which would affect synaptic tDCS effects, did not alter respective excitability changes (Liebetanz et al. 2002, Nitsche et al. 2003c, Nitsche et al. 2004b). Likewise, TMS double pulse stimulation protocols, which monitor synaptically driven excitability alterations were not affected by these tDCS protocols (Nitsche et al. 2005).

Secondary physiological effects of motor cortex tDCS emerge with stimulation durations for a few minutes. Similar to the acute effects, anodal stimulation enhances and cathodal tDCS reduces motor cortex excitability, as explored for single pulse TMS-elicited MEP amplitudes (Nitsche and Paulus 2000, 2001; Nitsche et al. 2003b). These effects were accomplished with specific stimulation protocols (1 mA current intensity, 35 cm^2 electrode size, stimulation duration for up to 20 min in healthy young adults). Hereby, stimulation for 5 and 7 min induce relatively short lasting after-effects, while 9 min or longer tDCS prolong after-effect duration for 30–90 min. The duration of these MEP alterations is in the range of early phase long term potentiation- and depression-like plasticity (Malenka and Bear 2004). Combination of TMS with pharmacological interventions have shown that the respective excitability alterations depend on the glutamatergic system, because block of NMDA receptors with dextromethorphan abolished any after-effects of tDCS (Liebetanz et al. 2002; Nitsche et al. 2003c), whereas the NMDA receptor agonist d-cycloserine prolonged the after-effects of anodal tDCS (Nitsche et al. 2004a). Supporting evidence comes from TMS studies with double pulse stimulation TMS protocols, which show reduced intracortical inhibition, but enhanced facilitation, after anodal tDCS, but reversed effects after cathodal tDCS (Nitsche et al. 2005). For both measures, NMDA receptors are involved. Furthermore, and in accordance with the relevance of NMDA receptors for

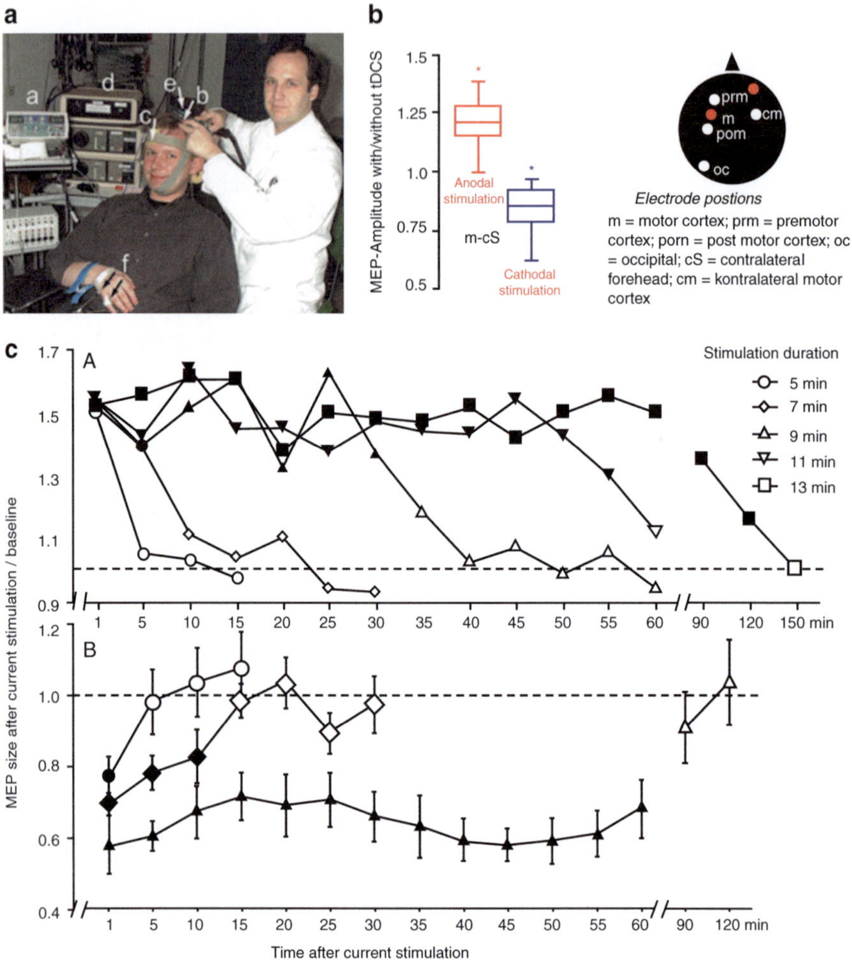

Fig. 5.1 Motor cortex TMS for monitoring tDCS-induced excitability changes. (**a**) shows the experimental setup. Current source is a constant current stimulator (a). The stimulator is connected with a stimulation electrode over the motor cortex (b), and a reference electrode positioned over the contralateral orbit (c). The impact of tDCS on cortical excitability is monitored by transcranial magnetic stimulation (TMS, d – stimulator, e – coil) of the representation area of the abductor digiti minimi muscle. Motor evoked potentials are recorded from this muscle via surface electromyography electrodes (f). (**b**) shows motor evoked potential (MEP) alterations induced by short tDCS (4 s), which induces no after-effects. (**c**) depicts after-effects of anodal (A) and cathodal (B) motor cortex tDCS, as monitored by baseline-standardized TMS-generated MEP amplitudes. (With permission of Klinische Neurophysiologie, J Physiol, Neurology, and Clin Neurophysiol; Nitsche et al. Klin Neurophys 2002, Clin Neurophysiol 2003, Nitsche & Paulus J Physiol 2000, Neurology 2001)

the after-effects of tDCS, which have calcium channel properties, the calcium dependence of the after-effects of tDCS is substantiated by the fact that block of voltage-gated calcium channels via flunarizin prevented the formation of excitability enhancement by anodal tDCS (Nitsche et al. 2003c). Studies combining pharmacology with TMS to explore the physiology of tDCS after effects furthermore show that dopaminergic as well as nicotinergic receptor activity is required for the after effects of tDCS, since block of respective receptors or receptor hypoactivity due to nicotine withdrawal in smokers abolished after effects of tDCS (Nitsche et al. 2006; Grundey et al. 2012). With regard to the contribution of GABAergic effects, combination of tDCS with the benzodiazepine lorazepam, which enhances already active GABA receptors, did not lead to major effect differences on stimulation-induced MEP alterations (Nitsche et al. 2004b). TMS-evoked I-waves however, which are reduced by GABA activity, were enhanced by anodal and cathodal tDCS (Nitsche et al. 2005). This at first sight puzzling result is explained by a magnetic resonance spectroscopy (MRS) study, which revealed that independent from stimulation polarity tDCS reduces GABA activity (Stagg et al. 2009). Beyond the above-mentioned transmitter systems, serotonin activation has a relevant impact on tDCS-induced excitability alterations, as it enhances amplitude and duration of MEP alterations induced by anodal tDCS, whereas it converts the inhibitory effects of cathodal tDCS into inhibition (Nitsche et al. 2009; Kuo et al. 2016). Electrophysiological studies furthermore helped to define the level of action of tDCS. Comparison of tDCS-driven MEP alterations obtained via TMS, which activates corticospinal tract neurons indirectly via its impact on intracortical neurons, and high voltage transcranial electrical stimulation (TES), which directly activates corticospinal tract neurons, shows that only TMS-evoked MEPs were affected in accordance with a primary intracortical effect (Nitsche and Paulus 2000, 2001; Nitsche et al. 2003b). This assumption is supported by a study in which spinal tract recordings were performed after tDCS, which showed a primary effect of tDCS on the amplitude of cortically evoked I-waves, and by results of two studies which demonstrated that intracortical motor cortex inhibition and facilitation were modulated by tDCS-induced excitability alterations of the premotor and posterior parietal cortex, which are both relevantly connected with the primary motor cortex (Boros et al. 2008; Rivera-Urbina et al. 2015).

All above-mentioned physiological effects were obtained with the "classic" stimulation protocols, as outlined above. For adjustment of stimulation protocols to obtain optimal physiological effects, within these limits stronger and longer stimulation increase the alteration and duration of TMS-induced MEP amplitude changes (Nitsche and Paulus 2000, 2001; Nitsche et al. 2003b). It could however been shown that too strong and long stimulation convert the direction of MEP alterations. 20 min tDCS with 2 mA resulted in an excitability enhancement after cathodal tDCS, whereas 26 min anodal tDCS with 1 mA reduced MEP amplitudes (Batsikadze et al. 2013; Monte-Silva et al. 2013). Given that tDCS effects are calcium-dependent, and that in animal experimentation low calcium increase result in LTD, and high calcium increase in LTP (Lisman 2001), it can be speculated that this shift of MEP alterations is caused by enhancing calcium concentration in case of cathodal tDCS to the LTP-inducing range, whereas in case of prolonged anodal tDCS, calcium overflow causes counter-regulatory neuronal activities. Indeed the respective conversion of plasticity in case of anodal tDCS is abolished by calcium channel block (Monte-Silva et al. 2013). In contrast, tDCS-dependent MEP alterations can be relevantly prolonged if LTP- and LTD-like plasticity-inducing protocols are repeated within a time window critical for late phase plasticity induction in animal models, i.e. application of the second intervention within a time window of 30 min (Monte-Silva et al. 2010, 2013). Here anodal tDCS induces after effects lasting for more than 24 h after plasticity induction, and these effects are NMDA receptor dependent, because block of these receptors abolishes respective MEP alterations. Interestingly, for stimulation protocols falling short of inducing prolonged neuroplastic effects, the impact of repeated stimulation within relatively short intervals seems to be more mixed and heterogeneous (Fricke et al. 2011).

Physiological effects of tDCS are object to intra- and interindividual variability, which is not surprising given that the primary physiological effect is a slight modulation of resting membrane potentials. Wiethoff et al. (2014) found excitability enhancements following anodal tDCS in about 75% of all participants, while below 50% had lower MEP amplitudes after cathodal tDCS. Intra-individual variability seems to be lower, with about 70% of participants showing similar MEP results for an inter-session tDCS interval for up to a year (López-Alonso et al. 2015). Sources for this variability of effects might be handedness, brain state according to task performance or muscle contraction, genetic polymorphisms, or differences in availability of neurotransmitters or receptor activity, head size, and presence of neurological or psychiatric dieases, amongst others (Nitsche et al. 2006; Antal et al. 2007, 2010; Kuo et al. 2008; Hasan et al. 2011; Thirugnanasambandam et al. 2011; Grundey et al. 2012; Schade et al. 2012; Kessler et al. 2013). The relative contribution of these factors to variability of physiological tDCS effects is unknown so far. Sensitivity to TMS might have predictive value for the magnitude of MEP alterations induced at least by anodal tDCS, as shown in a retrospective analysis, where subjects displaying higher TMS sensitivity reacted stronger to tDCS (Labruna et al. 2016). If this is caused by anatomical or physiological factors, and if this means that individual intensity adjustment of tDCS based on TMS sensitivity will reduce variability is unclear at present.

Beyond tDCS-induced cortical excitability alterations, tDCS effects on human motor cortex activity were explored in a couple of studies. For oscillatory brain activity, in resting EEG motor cortex cathodal stimulation increased delta and theta activity in one study (Ardolino et al. 2005). In another study, increased power of the theta and alpha frequency bands was described after both, anodal and cathodal tDCS (Pellicciari et al. 2013). Enhanced theta and alpha power were also described in another study during anodal tDCS, while cathodal stimulation reduced delta power (Roy et al. 2014). tDCS was furthermore shown to modulate event related desynchronisation of mu rhythm polarity dependently (Matsumoto et al. 2010; Kasashima et al. 2012; Lapenta et al. 2013; Kasuga et al. 2015). For motor cortex-related blood flow alterations, which are indexing cortical activity, induced by tDCS, a PET study showed increase after anodal, and decrease after cathodal tDCS under resting conditions (Lang et al. 2005). Similar effects during stimulation were obtained in a PET study measuring blood flow alterations during tDCS combined with motor task performance. For fMRI, BOLD measures under resting conditions showed enhancement of blood flow in the primary motor cortex after anodal tDCS in resting conditions in one study, but not in another with similar relatively short stimulation conditions (repeated stimulation for some seconds, Antal et al. 2011; Kwon et al. 2008). Zheng et al. (2011) describe blood flow enhancements during and after anodal tDCS, but reductions after cathodal tDCS for the arterial spin labelling (ASL) method, which might have superior sensitivity for detection of blood flow changes (Fig. 5.2). Task-related BOLD signal changes seem also to be somewhat heterogeneous, and might depend on stimulation parameters. Whereas Baudewig et al. (2001) did not identify tDCS-induced BOLD activity changes after 5 min tDCS in the primary motor cortex, such effects were seen in later studies, in which more extended stimulation protocols were applied (Jang et al. 2009; Stagg

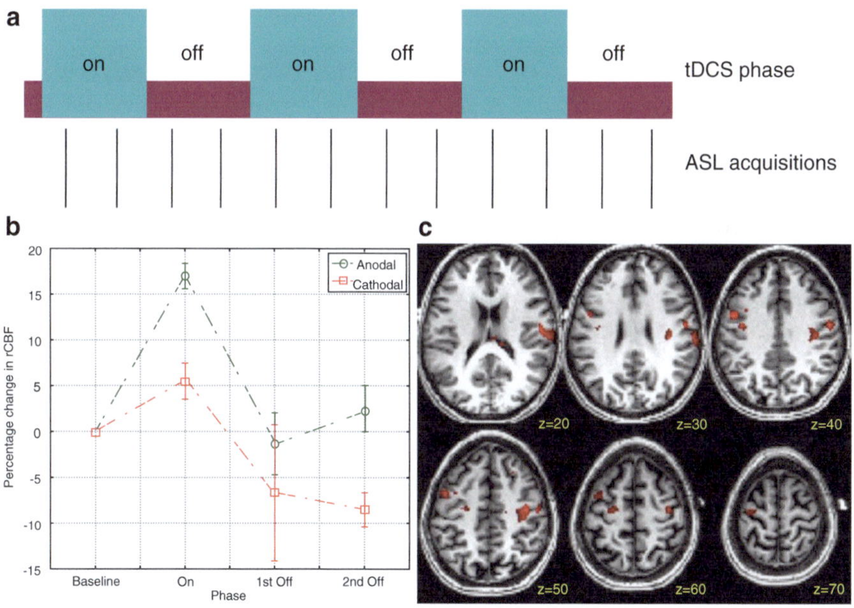

Fig. 5.2 Blood flow alterations induced by motor cortex tDCS. In this study, arterial spin labeling (ASL) was used to explore cerebral blood flow changes induced by anodal and cathodal tDCS. (**a**) shows interleaved tDCS-off and tDCS-on design while acquiring ASL images, where two ASL images were acquired at each on phase and two ASL images were acquired at each off phase, beginning with a baseline consisting of three ASL acquisitions. (**b**) shows the average changes in rCBF (normalized to zero) for the first OFF-ON-OFF of anodal and cathodal stimulation across all subjects. The description *1st off* and *2nd OFF* refers to the two acquisitions after the end of the stimulation and reflects the trend in rCBF after the stimulation has been turned off. (**c**) displays the averaged distribution of CBF response across the entire brain space correlated with the timecourse obtained from the VOI under the electrode for the anodal condition. Significant correlations ($p < 0.001$, uncorrected at the group level) were overlaid onto a single spatially standardized brain (Zheng et al. 2011, with permission by the authors, and Neuroimage)

et al. 2009; Kwon and Jang 2011). Thus taken together, beyond polarity-dependent cortical excitability changes, tDCS results in similar effects on cortical activity, as shown by EEG, PET, and fMRI studies.

The study results described so far were conducted with the "classic" electrode arrangement with relatively large target electrodes positioned over the hand area of the primary motor cortex. This stimulation procedure elicits relatively diffuse effects, affecting different movement representations relatively unspecifically (Nitsche et al. 2007), and might tackle also adjacent areas, such as the premotor cortex (Boros et al. 2008), although at least under task performance conditions, physiological specificity of tDCS effects might be determined also by synergistic effects on task-related activations (Polanía et al. 2011b). The focality of stimulation can be enhanced by reducing the size of the target electrode, and adjusting stimulation intensity accordingly to keep current density constant (Nitsche et al. 2007). Reduction of the motor cortex electrode size in this study limited MEP alterations during and after tDCS to a hand muscle representation covered by the small electrode, but left an adjacent hand muscle representation not covered by the electrode unaffected. Another electrode arrangement which was developed for more focal stimulation is so-called high-definition (HD) tDCS. Here, a central relatively small target electrode is surrounded by 4 return electrodes (Edwards et al. 2013). The efficacy of this electrode arrangement to induce MEP alterations is similar to the classic electrode arrangement (Kuo et al. 2013). Enhanced focality of this electrode arrangement is suggested by modelling approaches, but physiological evidence for respective higher focality of stimulation effects is limited (Edwards et al. 2013).

The majority of motor cortex physiological tDCS studies was so far conducted for small hand muscles. The respective motor cortical sub-field has the advantage that it is situated relatively superficially, and thus easy to be influenced by non-invasive brain stimulation. Moreover, sophisticated TMS protocols do exist for this area which allow monitoring of specific cortical subsystems, such as intracortical inhibition, facilitation, I-wave facilitation, amongst others, which are not in each case similarly well established for other motor cortex regions. However, tDCS exerts physiological effects also on other sub-compartments of the primary motor cortex. Only a limited amount of studies is available for physiological effects of stimulation of proximal muscles of the upper limb is available. It was however shown that anodal tDCS of the motor cortex representation enhances the activation of the contralateral biceps brachii muscle significantly, as shown by surface electromyography (Krishnan et al. 2014). For TMS-elicited MEP alterations in this muscle at rest, however, no significant effects of anodal tDCS were described (Mccambridge et al. 2015). Similarly, cathodal tDCS of the biceps brachii representation has not been shown to alter MEP amplitudes so far, however, it was suggested to suppress ipsilateral projections to propriospinal neurons of the proximal upper limb (Bradnam et al. 2011). Interestingly, in the same study cathodal tDCS suppressed MEP in a contralateral distal hand muscle. This pattern of results argues against missing efficacy of this specific stimulation protocol. The relatively minor plasticity effects of tDCS on proximal upper limb muscles might be caused by relatively low proneness of these muscles to undergo neuroplastic changes. Alternatively, differences in orientation or position of these neurons might require adjusted stimulation protocols. For the pharyngeal motor cortex, initial evidence is available that anodal tDCS enhances, whereas cathodal tDCS reduces respective MEP amplitudes (Jefferson et al. 2009). For physiological effects of tDCS on lower extremity muscles, an MEP enhancement was described in the resting and pre-contracted anterior tibial muscle after anodal tDCS, while cathodal stimulation over the primary motor cortex had no effect (Jeffery et al. 2007). In accordance, anodal, but not cathodal tDCS improved maximal pinch force (Tanaka et al. 2009). BOLD fMRI results were showing no direct effects on the stimulated primary motor cortex in another study, but indicative for increased activity of the ipsilateral sma and decreased activity of contralateral primary motor cortex, as compared to sham stimulation (Kim et al. 2012). Thus so far no protocols are available which reduce leg motor cortex excitability, whereas the physiological impact of anodal tDCS on lower extremities movement representations seem to be similar to those of hand muscle representation stimulation. Similar to proximal muscles of the upper extremity, limited effects might be caused by a minor propensity for plasticity in lower extremities, different neuronal orientations, or also caused by the larger electrode to brain distance, as compared to the motor cortex hand area.

Taken together, for motor cortex tDCS numerous studies are available which favour a polarity-dependent effect on cortical excitability and activity. Whereas the primary effect of tDCS seems to depend on subthreshold membrane polarization, after effects involve modification of the strength of glutamatergic synapses, and reduced GABAergic activity. The neuromodulatory effects of tDCS imply that beyond speficic limits of stimulation intensity and duration, the impact of tDCS on cortical excitability converts its direction. Less studies are available which explore the effect of tDCS on cortical activity via functional imaging tools, and respective results are less clear-cut. Physiological mechanisms of action have been best clarified for hand muscle representations, but effects are also obtained for other motor cortex areas. Especially for these protocols, studies which systematically explore protocol parameters suited to induce optimal effects are missing.

Sensory Cortices

Somatosensory Cortex

Effects of tDCS on neurophysiological function of the somatosensory cortex can be evaluated by means of changes in the somatosensory evoked potentials (SEPs) or somatosensory evoked magnetic fields (SEFs), changes in brain's hemodynamic response, or at the behavioral level by effects on measures of somatosensory perception (Dieckhöfer et al. 2006; Sugawara et al. 2015; Kojima et al. 2015; Wang et al. 2015; Grundmann et al. 2011; Rehmann et al. 2016; Song et al. 2011; and others).

SEPs represent electrical potentials generated in sensory pathways at peripheral, spinal, subcortical and cortical levels, elicited by electrical stimulation of a peripheral nerve (usually the median or posterior tibial nerves). A comprehensive overview of SEP components, normal waveforms and clinical interpretations can be found in Mauguiere (1999). SEP evaluations often include low-frequency SEP components, such as N20, P20, P22, N30, P35, or P60; neuroanatomical studies suggest that generator sources for these components are located cortically, including area 1,2 (component P60) or 3b (N20) of the primary sensory cortex (S1) or in the motor cortex (e.g. component P35). Further, SEP evaluations may also include high-frequency oscillations (HFOs; ~600 Hz) which are believed to be at least partially generated by postsynaptic activities in S1 as well as by subcortical generators, such as presynaptic terminals of thalamo-cortical pathways to S1 (Curio et al. 1994, 1997; Curio 2000; Dieckhöfer et al. 2006). Some SEP evaluations employ a paired-pulse paradigm, which typically involves evaluation of the N20 (N20-P25) component after stimulation of the median nerve with two stimuli delivered in a short interval (~30 ms), and is based on the premise that the resulting second N20 response shows a reduction in its amplitude when compared to the first pulse (Ragert et al. 2004a). The strength of the paired-pulse suppression depends on the interstimulus interval, but – contrary to the single-pulse SEP response -- shows only weak dependence on stimulus intensity; only the N20-P25 component shows some intensity effects. Here higher intensities result in stronger paired-pulse suppression (Ragert et al. 2004b). The paired-pulse suppression is believed to arise from inhibition generated by intracortical networks and it has been used as a marker of cortical excitability.

Evidence up to date indicates that tDCS delivered over the somatosensory cortex exerts different effects on low- and high-frequency SEPs, and the effects depend on tDCS modality. Nine minutes of cathodal tDCS at 1 mA applied to the somatosensory cortex in healthy subjects (Dieckhöfer et al. 2006) resulted in a long-lasting reduction of the low-frequency N20 SEP component after contralateral median nerve stimulation (Fig. 5.3). This finding corroborates evidence for an inhibitory effect of cathodal tDCS on the excitability of the human cortex (Nitsche and Paulus 2000). Accordingly, application of cathodal tDCS to the somatosensory cortex has been shown to have similar effect on paired-pulse suppression of SEPs (Rehmann et al. 2016), reduces tactile acuity (Rogalewski et al. 2004), and also resulted in decreased amplitudes of laser-evoked potentials (LEPs) and decreased pain perception in experimentally induced pain (Antal et al. 2008).

Application of anodal tDCS over S1 in Dieckhofer's study (Dieckhöfer et al. 2006) had no significant effects on low-frequency SEPs. Notably, when applied over the *sensorimotor* cortex, anodal tDCS resulted in increased amplitudes of P25/N33, N33/P40 and P22/N30 in another study (Matsunaga 2004). Anodal tDCS over S1 had no effects on LEPs, or pain perception (Antal et al. 2008). As for tactile acuity, anodal tDCS over S1 had no effect if applied for 10 min (Rogalewski et al. 2004), but an increase in tactile acuity was observed after an extended (20 min) stimulation (Ragert et al. 2008a, b), and anodal tDCS delivered over S1 also had an

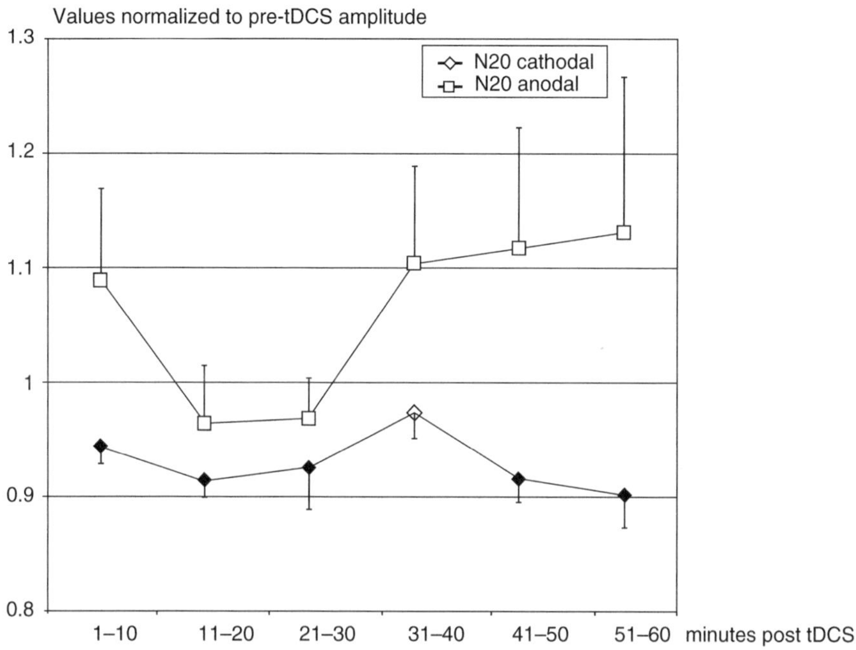

Fig. 5.3 After-effects of anodal and cathodal tDCS on somatosensory-evoked potentials. Time course changes in N20 amplitude evoked by stimulation of the contralateral median nerve following 9 min polarization with 1 mA DC current. Filled symbols indicate significant differences between SEP amplitudes after polarization and baseline. Error bars indicate standard error of means (From Dieckhöfer et al. 2006, Fig. 3, with permission)

excitatory effect on paired-pulse suppression of SEPs in a paired-pulse paradigm study (Rehmann et al. 2016).

For the high frequency SEP component (600 Hz oscilations, HFOs), no effects from anodal or cathodal tDCS over S1 were observed (Dieckhöfer et al. 2006). This finding is in accordance with evidence that the generators of HFOs are localized subcortically and therefore distant from the local effects of tDCS.

Some evidence of tDCS effects on the somatosensory cortex originates from studies employing evaluation of somatosensory evoked magnetic fields (SEFs). Evaluations of SEFs following median nerve stimulation focused on three main components: N20, P35 and P60 (Huttunen et al. 2006; Sugawara et al. 2015). In a study by Suguwara et al. (2015), anodal tDCS (15 min at 1 mA; electrodes 35 cm^2) over the somatosensory cortex had a significant effect on somatosensory evoked magnetic fields, increasing the source strength of P60. As noted above, it is believed that the generator for this component is located within areas 1 and 2 (Huttunen et al. 2006; and others). The component P35, which is believed origin from the motor cortex (Kawamura et al. 1996), was unchanged. Notably, the source strength of both components increased, if tDCS was delivered over the motor cortex.

Accordingly, tDCS delivered over the motor association cortex has been shown to induce plastic changes in the ipsilateral primary motor as well as somatosensory cortices (Kirimoto et al. 2011).

In summary, existing studies indicate that tDCS effects on neurophysiological activity of the somatosensory cortex depend on multiple factors including tDCS modality, such as anodal or cathodal tDCS, tDCS-targeted area, including its location (cortical or subcortical) of the neural generators of the response.

Visual Cortex

In the visual system, polarity-specific tDCS effects were demonstrated, too.

Anodal tDCS enhances excitabilty of the visual cortex. In a study by Sczesny-Kaiser et al. (2016), real or sham tDCS were applied in healthy subjects over V1 in a randomized, double-blinded design over four consecutive days. Excitability parameters were measured by analyzing paired stimulation-elicited visual-evoked potentials (ps-VEP) and by measuring phosphene thresholds before and after a stimulation period of 4 days. Compared with sham-tDCS, anodal tDCS resulted in increased ps-VEP ratios (Fig. 5.4) and reduced phosphene thresholds (Sczesny-Kaiser et al. 2016). Decreased phosphene thresholds after anodal tDCS over the occipital cortex have been also observed by Antal et al. (2003a, b). However, anodal tDCS over the visual cortex did not result in significant changes of contrast perception thresholds (Antal et al. 2001), possibly due to a ceiling effect.

Cathodal tDCS has been shown to increase thresholds for moving as well as stationary phosphenes in studies by Antal et al. (2003a, b), but had no effects on phosphene thresholds or VEPs in a study by Sczesny-Kaiser et al. (2016). Further, Accornero et al. (2007) evaluated changes in amplitudes and latencies of VEP component P100 (VEP-P100) in healthy subjects after anodal and cathodal tDCS applied for 3 and 10 min at 1 mA, with an extracephalic position of the return electrode (Accornero et al. 2007). In this study, anodal tDCS resulted in reduced VEP-P100 amplitude, whereas cathodal polarization significantly increased the amplitude, and no significant changes were observed in the VEP-P100 latencies.

Auditory Cortex

Very few tDCS studies have focused on tDCS modulation of sensory processing in the auditory cortex (Vines et al. 2006; Mathys et al. 2010; Chen et al. 2014a, b; Impey and Knott, 2015; Impey et al. 2016). The available studies mostly employed event-related potentials (ERPs) as an objective neural measure of information processing pertaining to early pre-attentive auditory processes such as sensory gating indexed by the ERP component P50, sensory discrimination indexed by the mismatch negativity (MMN) component, or novelty detection indexed by P3a; as well

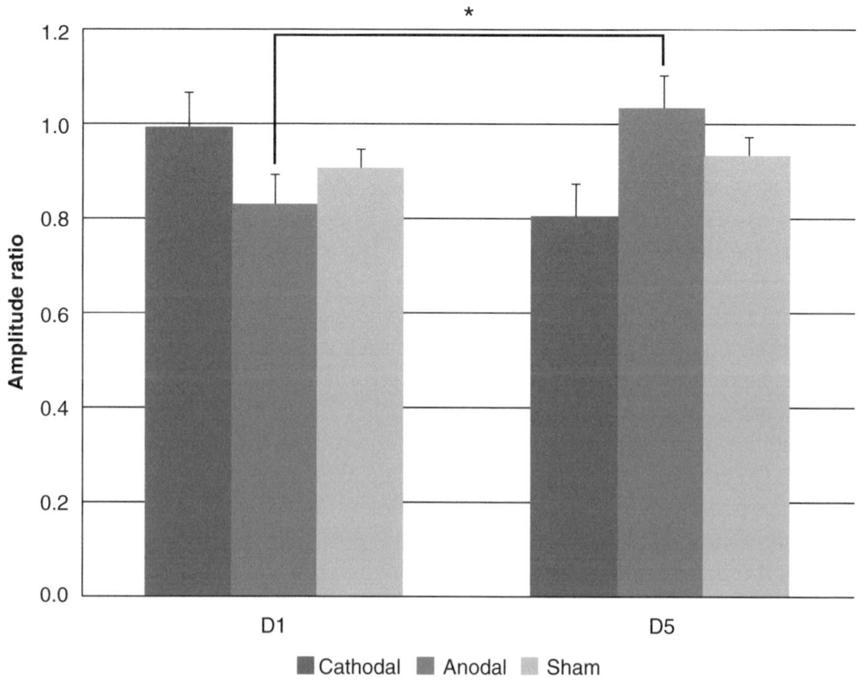

Fig. 5.4 Effects oft DCS on paired-stimulation VEP (psVEP). Mean amplitude ratios of all three groups on day 1 (D1) and day 5 (D5) are plotted. *significance level, $p < 0.017$. Error bars indicate standard error of the mean (From Sczesny-Kaiser et al. 2016, Fig. 5, with permission)

as to assess higher order auditory processes, such as attentional allocation ad processing speed indexed by P3b (Impey et al. 2016).

Early findings by Zaehle and colleagues (Zaehle et al. 2011) indicate that anodal tDCS over the auditory cortex increases amplitudes of the auditory P50, whereas cathodal tDCS over the primary and secondary auditory cortex (Vines et al. 2006; Mathys et al. 2010) resulted in decreased pitch discrimination and pitch memory performance. Further, pilot findings by Impey and Knott (2015) and a subsequent study by Impey et al. (2016) have suggested that an application of anodal tDCS over the temporal lobe in healthy subjects can increase auditory discrimination indexed by MMN, and that this modulation is baseline-dependent: anodal tDCS over the temporal cortex improved MMN-indexed auditory discrimination, compared to sham stimulation, particularly in individuals with relatively low sensory discrimination performance. In contrast, reduced MMN amplitudes with cathodal tDCS, compared to baseline assessment were obtained particularly in individuals with relatively high level task performance. These studies point toward the importance of the use of neurophysiological markers stratified by the baseline response when examining tDCS modulatory impact on cerebral functions.

Association Areas

Assocation areas are defined as cortical regions which receive projections from specific primary sensory or motor cortices. In addition, multimodal association areas receive sensory imput from different sensory modalities and various specific association areas and play a crucial role in multisensory integration. The posterior multimodal association area relates to bodily spatial awareness, as well as to reading, naming, and emotional components of speech. The anterior association area together with the limbic association area is involved in multimodal integration of past experience and processes of conditioning. Previous research employing rTMS indicates that modulation of multisensory integration, such as an integration of the proprioceptive, somatosensory and visual input, is possible (Tsakiris et al. 2008; Azanon and Haggard 2009). Accordingly, at the behavioral level tDCS has been shown to alter multisensory input, such as visuomotor coordination (Antal et al. 2004; Kwon et al. 2015) or visuomotor learning (Antal et al. 2004b; Shah et al. 2013), as well as processes pertaining to various cognitive domains, including risk taking behavior, planning ability, or behavioral inhibition. Further, in a study by Lapenta et al. (2014), tDCS has been shown to modulate inhibitory control as indexed by ERPs, and at the behavioral level reduced food consumption. In this study, active tDCS over the dorsolateral prefrontal cortex (anode right/cathode left) reduced the frontal N2 component and increased the P3 component of responses to No-go stimuli, as compared to sham, and these physiological effects were paralleled by reduced food craving and caloric intake. Increased No-go P3d amplitudes are in general interpreted as indicators that increased cognitive resources are recruited to achieve inhibition (Albert et al. 2010; Yang et al. 2009; Pfefferbaum et al. 1985; and others). In the study by Campanella et al. (2017) tDCS over the right inferior frontal cortex (rIFC, a neural substrate crucial for inhibitory control), but not sham stimulation, resulted in reduced P3d amplitudes in a Go/No-go task, indicating that boosting rIFC may specifically enhance inhibitory skills by decreasing the neural activity needed to correctly inhibit the response. Modulatory effects of tDCS on P3 ERP components have also been observed in other studies. A study by Conti et al. (2014) examined the effects of DLPFC modulation by single and repetitive tDCS on prefrontal visual P3 ERP components under neutral and drug cue exposition in crack-cocaine addicted subjects. Significant differences were found in P3-related parameters when comparing group of stimulation (active vs. sham tDCS) and number of sessions (single vs. repetitive tDCS). Specifically, P3 amplitudes in the left DLPFC after a single active tDCS application increased during neutral cues and decreased during crack-related cues, while opposite effects were observed in the sham group. Furthermore, significant increases of P3 DLPFC activity under both, neutral and crack-related cues (Fig. 5.5) were obtained bilaterally after five tDCS applications on five alternated days as compared to activity measured before the first tDCS application. When compared to the effects of a single dose, the multiple tDCS application increased P3 amplitudes not only in the DLPFC, but also in a wider array of prefrontal areas, including presumably the frontopolar cortex,

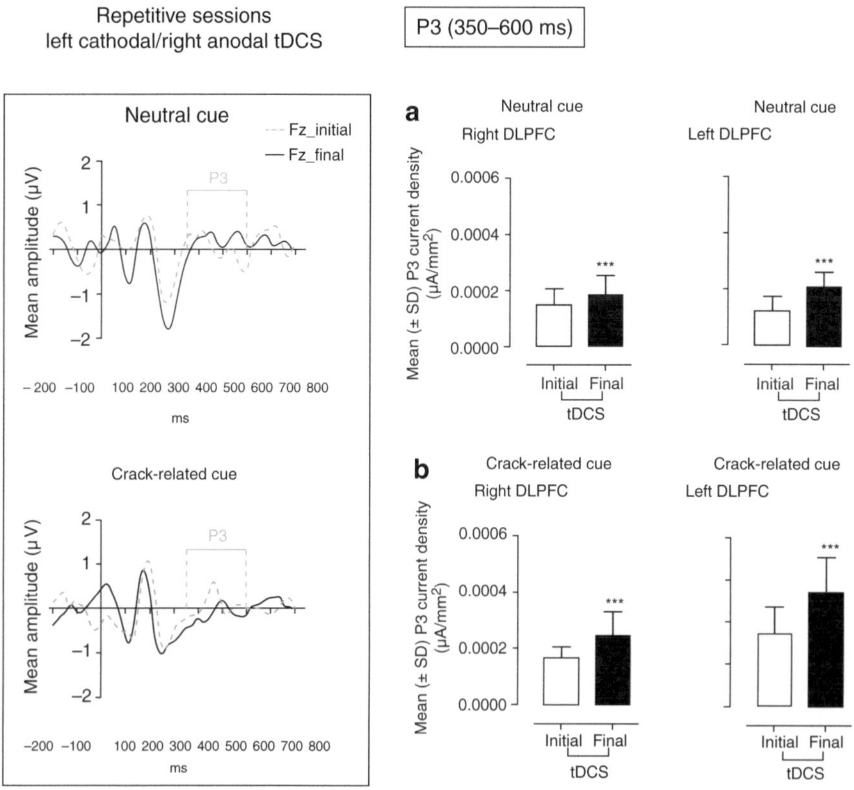

Fig. 5.5 Event Related Potentials (ERPs) evoked by neutral or crack-related visual stimuli at baseline (initial) and after five (final) applications of bilateral (left cathodal/right anodal) transcranial Direct Current Stimulation (tDCS, 2 mA, 35 cm², for 20 min) in crack-cocaine addicts at frontal site (Fz) Fz (according to 10–20 EEG international system). Current density in the P3 segment (350–600 ms) elicited by neutral (**a**) or crack-related (**b**) cue presentation in the right and left Dorsolateral Prefrontal Cortex (DLPFC) at the baseline (initial) and at the end of five sessions (final) of bilateral tDCS (n = 6) over the DLPFC ***p < 0.0001 (Wilcoxon signed rank test when comparing initial vs. final). (From Conti et al. 2014, Fig. 4, with permission)

orbitofrontal cortex and anterior cingulate cortex, when subjects were visualizing crack-related cues. These effects may reflect rescuing of prefrontal cognitive control that might have clinical potential for addiction management (Conti et al. 2014). Another study (Faehling and Plewnia 2016) focused on tDCS modulation of cognitive control upon negative emotional distraction. In this study, healthy subjects performed working memory tasks with neutral or emotionally loaded distraction during sham or real tDCS at intensities of 0.5–1.5 mA, with the anode placed over the left DLPFC, and the cathode over the right deltoid muscle. The late positive potential (LLP) – an ERP that indexes attention allocation, was recorded during tDCS/sham. The results show that in the sham group a valence-specific increase of the early portion of the LPP (eLPP, 250–500 ms) was associated with less emotional distraction, and tDCS had an intensity-related effect on this correlation. The later part of LLP (lLLP, 500–1000 ms) correlated with reaction time regardless of valence, while a general effect of tDCS on LLPs was not detected. These findings support the notion that the changes of eLPP reflect effective compensation for behavioral distraction by negative stimuli and thus points toward a neuronal mechanism for effective control of the emotional bias.

Overall, the findings up to date indicate that tDCS can impact on activity of neuronal networks of brain association areas and can modulate outcomes at both neurophysiological and behavioral levels.

Network Effects: Functional Imaging

A large body of research suggests that goal-directed behavior depends on an efficient integration of neural activity where several connected but widely distributed areas linking whole brain regions, cell populations, and individual cortical neurons, closely interact to generate an action or choice. In a typical goal-directed choice scenario, we must first process incoming sensory signals, then recognize the alternatives for choice, compute their values and the difference between them, followed by a mapping of these computations to locations in space and finally execute the appropriate action (Rangel et al. 2008; Rangel and Hare 2010; Polanía et al. 2014, 2015; Grueschow et al. 2015). But the question is: How can the brain achieve such a fast an efficient integration of information in a quickly changing environment? Synchronized neural activity in the brain appears to be a fundamental mechanism for such cognitive processes requiring an efficient large-scale integration of distributed neural activity, supporting both neural communication and plasticity (Polanía et al. 2012a, b; Siegel et al. 2012).

Based on the physiological effects observed in primary motor and other cortices described in the previous sections of this chapter, it can be speculated that tDCS could be used as tool to modulate more complex cognitive functions involving the type of goal-directed choice described above that are predominant in our everyday life. This also suggests that tDCS could potentially be used to resolve whether certain brain regions are indeed causally involved in specific behaviors based on, for instance, neuroimaging studies which are limited by their correlative nature. For example, based on prior neuroimaging work implicating the frontopolar cortex (FPC) in exploratory reward learning behavior (Daw et al. 2006), it was investigated whether upregulating and downregulating neuronal excitability with anodal or cathodal tDCS it is possible to show that the FPC is indeed causally involved for this type of complex behavior (Raja et al. 2015). The investigators found that that applying different types of tDCS (anodal or cathodal) over FPC indeed causes participants to explore more or less in uncertain environments, thus establishing a causal role for the FPC in regulating both exploration and exploitation behavior in humans.

Beyond behavior at the level of individual decisions, many of the proposed links between social decision making (and social learning) also come from neuroimaging studies in healthy participants and thus rely on correlations between task parameters and brain activity, thus once more raising the question of whether the observed neural responses are merely correlated with the observed behavior in social settings or whether they play a causal part. Based on a prior neuroimaging study implicating activity in the lateral prefrontal cortex (LPFC) in compliance with social norms (Spitzer et al. 2007), it was investigated in a subsequent tDCS study whereas this brain region is indeed implicated in this type of complex social behavior (Ruff et al. 2013). The investigators showed that LPFC is indeed involved in both voluntary and sanction-induced norm compliance (Fig. 5.6). Interestingly, both types of compliance could be changed by varying the neural excitability of this brain region with anodal or cathodal tDCS, but they were affected in opposite ways. Thus, once more using tDCS as a tool to test the link between activity and in this case complex social behaviors, the results of this study revealed that LPFC is a key biological prerequisite for social norm compliance, a socially important aspect of human behavior.

Despite the fact that in the above-mentioned examples tDCS was used to resolve whether certain brain regions are indeed causally involved in specific behaviors, the effects underlying these tDCS-induced modulations in the human brain, which are afterwards reflected in modulations of behavior, remain incompletely understood. For instance, from these studies (Ruff et al. 2013; Raja et al. 2015) it is unknown whether the observed effects on behavior are due to tDCS-induced alterations of activity underneath the electrode, and if it is the case, it is unknown what type of alterations are induced by the stimulation. On the other hand it could be hypothesized that one important aspect of the tDCS-induced functional effects could be attributed to learning- or task-related synaptic connections. Hereby, tDCS-induced effects might modulate functional connectivity between segregated cortical areas in the task under study.

Electrophysiological and neuroimaging methods such as electroencephalography (EEG) and functional magnetic resonance imaging (fMRI) have been used as tools to noninvasively acquire information regarding the neural activity of the brain with their respective spatial–temporal advantages and dis-advantages. In the last decade, these methods have been used as powerful tools to study the architecture of human brain functional networks at the large scale level both during rest (Keeser et al. 2011; Polanía et al. 2011b; Peña-Gómez et al. 2012), and also during the planning and execution of goal-directed actions (Antal et al. 2011; Saiote et al. 2013). Hence, the use of methods such as EEG and fMRI combined with noninvasive brain stimulation might be an appropriate starting point to elucidate the impact of tDCS-induced neuroplasticity on human brain functional networks on how these are linked to the observed changes in behavior.

In the following sections we provide insights on how different imaging and statistical methods can be used to track for tDCS-induced brain network effects in humans. We start by using the primary motor cortex as an example region, where

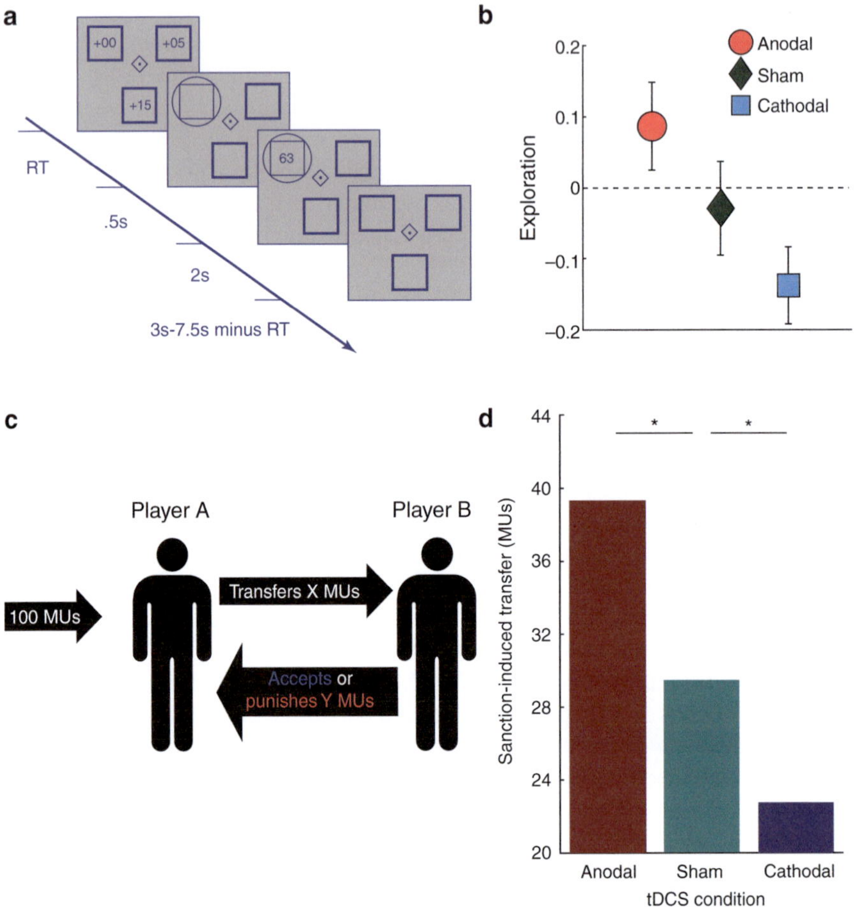

Fig. 5.6 (**a**) Brief description of the Bandit (Explore/Exploit) Task: Participants selected among three virtual slot machines (squares) whose payout values drifted independently and randomly across trials. The randomly-varying monetary rewards required participants to continuously learn about the slot machines payout values to maximize their monetary payoffs. At the start of each trial, participants saw three bonuses (numbers in first screen) that had to be added to the slot machine's underlying payout value to determine the total reward. After participants made their choice (circle), the total reward was displayed (last screen). The Degree of exploration on each trial was defined as the amount of monetary reward the participant was willing to give up by not selecting the highest-paying option and instead explore. (**b**) Effects of tDCS on Explore/Exploit behavior: Anodal stimulation over the FPC led to an increase in exploration, whereas cathodal stimulation decreased exploration, relative to inactive sham stimulation that left exploration unaffected. (**c**) Brief description of the norm compliance task: Both players (**a** and **b**) receive 25 initial monetary units (MUs). Player **a** is given an additional 100 MUs that she can share with player B by sending a transfer X (in multiples of 10 MUs). In a subsequent decision stage, Player B can either accept X or invest Y MUs from her initial endowment to punish player A and therefore reducing A's payoff by 5 × Y MUs. Player A is aware of this possible sanction; any increase in transfers for punishment relative to baseline rounds therefore measures sanction-induced norm compliance. (**d**) Effects of tDCS on norm compliance: Higher values indicate that the punishment threat led to a larger adjustment of transfers toward the fairness norm of an equal split, thus, suggesting that anodal tDCS over the rLPFC enhances fairness in the presence of sanction-induced norms, whereas cathodal tDCS induces the opposite effect

the tDCS-induced effects on brain networks have been more systematically studied relative to other brain areas and cognitive tasks, and then we complement this knowledge with more recent studies attempting to investigate tDCS-induced effects on higher cognitive functions and their associated brain networks.

tDCS-induced Global Network Effects

Characterization of complex human brain networks has been of increasing interest in the recent years using graph theory as a mathematical approach (Bullmore and Sporns 2009). This approach allows examining the functional connectivity architecture of the brain, which provides information regarding its organization linked to the capability of integration and transfer of information within and between different regions. Using this computational methodology in combination with EEG, it was investigated whether tDCS-induced excitability changes are expressed in modifications of the functional cortical architecture in humans when anodal tDCS was applied over the primary motor cortex (M1) during the execution of a simple motor task (Polanía et al. 2011a). The authors found a prominent increase in synchronization of regions involved in motor task performance in the gamma band (between 60 and 90 Hz) but also enhanced synchronization between the primary motor area, premotor and sensorimotor areas. Based on these results, it is tempting to speculate that tDCS-related increases of functional synchronization when applied over M1 is relevant for the beneficial effects of anodal tDCS on motor learning observed in a large number of reports in the past decade (Nitsche et al. 2003a; Reis et al. 2009). Based on this evidence, it is well possible to hypothesize that an important aspect of the beneficial effect of excitatory anodal tDCS might be that it enhances strengthening of dynamical task-related synaptic connections.

In a second study, the same authors aimed to explore whether tDCS-induced functional connectivity changes can be identified by a voxel-based graph theoretical approach in BOLD fMRI (Polanía et al. 2011b), thus exploiting the high spatial resolution offered by this non-invasive imaging technique (however, this time during resting state fMRI measurements). The graph theoretical analysis revealed once more a reconfiguration of the functional brain networks: Anodal stimulation over M1 combined with cathodal stimulation over the contralateral fronto-polar cortex during rest induces a global decrease in the long distance topological functional coupling of the left M1 with the rest of the brain. In other words, the number of direct functional connections from the left M1 to topologically distant brain areas significantly decreased. Interestingly, this result was accompanied by an increase of the functional coupling between M1 and neighbored topological regions such as the left premotor, and left parietal cortex, which is in line with the results found in the initial EEG study (Polanía et al. 2011a). Extending the previously postulated hypothesis (that anodal stimulation over M1 enhances strengthening of dynamical task-related synaptic connections (Polanía et al. 2011a)), the results of the resting state fMRI study suggest that excitatory anodal stimulation over M1 preconditions the task-related cortical motor areas by enhancing functional coupling within these cortical regions.

Beyond the effects on M1, tDCS in combination with fMRI has been recently used to understand the brain mechanisms underlying more complex behaviors. One such behavior crucial in many aspects of interactions with the environment is inhibitory control, which reflects the ability to suppress proponent responses. Neuroimaging studies have implicated a network of regions that together form the "stopping network" that supports the processes involved in inhibitory control. This network includes the pre-supplementary motor area (preSMA) as a key player in the implementation of inhibitory control of motor actions, which actively interacts with other brain regions such as the dorsolateral prefrontal cortex (DLPFC), medial prefrontal cortex (mPFC), and posterior parietal cortex (PPC) (Ray Li et al. 2006). Based on this evidence, researchers used tDCS in combination with fMRI to investigate the potential causal role of preSMA on inhibitory control (Yu, Tseng et al. 2015). In line with their hypothesis, investigators found that applying anodal tDCS over the preSMA leads to a significant improvement of inhibitory control in healthy participants. Interestingly, these behavioral improvements where accompanied by an increased activation in the preSMA following anodal DCS as opposed to the sham condition when stopping processes occurred. Additionally, a subsequent connectivity analysis revealed increased coupling with the ventro-medial prefrontal cortex (vmPFC), a region relatively remote with respect to the preSMA, but the only region whose activation difference was predictive of the individual improvement in behavioral performance. Hence, the results of this study further support the notion that the neural mechanisms behind the short and rapid behavioral improvement brought forth by tDCS may be quite different from, yet functionally connected to, the region/network targeted by the stimulation also in more complex cognitive functions.

tDCS-induced Local Network Effects

Coming back to tDCS-induced effects on M1 connectivity, it is also well possible that induced network effects also take place at the level of local circuits. Following this idea, researchers investigated the hypothesis that the relatively long-lasting synaptic modification induced by tDCS over M1 results in the alteration of associations among populations within M1 neurons which may be reflected in a change of its intrinsic functional architecture (Polanía et al. 2012c). This hypothesis is based on the fact that the intrinsic horizontal neuronal connections within M1 have been found to exhibit short-term and long-term plasticity, which is a strong substrate for learning-related map reorganization (Iezzi et al. 2011; Sanes 2000). Such a tDCS-generated alteration of intrinsic connectivity might help to explain the previously reported impact of tDCS on motor learning (Nitsche et al. 2003c; Reis et al. 2009). Thus, in this study the authors based their graph theory analysis focused on resting-state BOLD fMRI measurements within the M1. For anodal tDCS, the authors did not find any region where the connectivity degree significantly increased or decreased, however they found that nodes belonging to a cluster around the arm/hand region of M1 (located at approximately the center of the tDCS electrode) communicate more efficiently with the rest of the M1 network. This pattern of results suggests that the increase in efficient connections does not depend on an increase in the total number of functional connections, but is rather due to an efficient reorganization of the functional network. These results therefore provide important evidence indicating that the promotion of LTP-like plasticity induced by anodal tDCS (Fritsch et al. 2010) might be related to an efficient reorganization of the functional architecture of M1.

In a different study, researchers used a type of brain scan called magnetic resonance spectroscopy (MRS) to gain insights into the neuro-chemical mechanisms by which tDCS induces its effects at the level of local circuits (Stagg et al. 2009). The levels of a chemical called GABA (a neurotransmitter molecule that inhibits the activity of nerve cells) were measured in the primary motor cortex before and after healthy participants received tDCS over M1. The results revealed that anodal stimulation leads to a significant decrease in the GABA concentration in the cortex. In contrast, inhibitory, cathodal stimulation leads to a significant decrease in glutamate, with a correlated decrease in GABA. Crucially, this finding is in line with the hypothesis that LTP-like plasticity within the neocortex is critically dependent on GABA modulation (Trepel and Racine 2000), thus further supporting the notion of tDCS being capable of inducing LTP-like plasticity alterations in local neural circuits.

Using this knowledge, in a recent study investigators used tDCS as a mean to test the theoretical proposal that cognitive function is tightly related to the maintenance of detailed cortical balance, where synaptic inputs received by cortical neurons is balanced such that excitatory and inhibitory currents are precisely matched and stable firing preserved (Okun and Lampl 2008; Haider and Mccormick 2009). This hypothesis was tested using an associative learning task in humans where the prediction is that when stimuli are paired together, their neuronal activity patterns should exhibit representational overlap at the local circuit level, a consequence of the increase in strength of mediating excitatory connections (Barron et al. 2016). To assess the consequences of cortical rebalancing, the investigators used fMRI to track changes in representational overlap of the learned associations over time, before combining this approach with anodal tDCS in order to induce a local reduction in cortical GABA. In an extremely fascinating finding, the investigators showed that cortical memories can be re-exposed by reduction in local GABA concentrations, induced via tDCS. Interestingly, the extent to which the memory is re-expressed occurs in proportion to the tDCS-induced GABA reduction. Thus, this finding provides a clear example into how tDCS in combination with different neuroimaging modalities (MRS and fMRI) can be used to reveal the neural mechanisms of rather complex cognitive processes at the level of local neural circuits in healthy humans.

tDCS-induced Cortico-Subcortical Network Effects

Many of the tDCS-induced effects when the stimulation is applied over M1 can be readily explained by the effect of tDCS within the primary motor cortex (Nitsche and Paulus 2000; Stagg et al. 2009; Polanía et al. 2012c) and also due to alterations of task-related cortical connectivity of motor areas by enhancing functional coupling within these cortical regions (Polanía et al. 2011a; Stagg et al. 2014). However, some other functional effects of tDCS are more compatible with an additional alteration of subcortical areas. For instance, it has been shown that tDCS over M1 induces changes in thermal and mechanical sensory percepts and produces long lasting pain relief in chronic pain patients (Fenton et al. 2009). These effects have been attributed to suppression of thalamic sensory pathways following motor cortex stimulation. Additionally, motor cortex tDCS improves gait and bradykinesia in patients suffering from Parkinson's disease (PD) (Benninger et al. 2010), which might be caused by tDCS-induced alterations of basal ganglia function. The results of these studies suggest that cortico-striato-thalamo-cortical circuits might be modulated by transcranial cortical stimulation. Thus based on this evidence, it could be hypothesized that anodal tDCS over M1 would increase the functional connectivity between striatal and thalamic regions and cortical regions associated with motor function. Once more based on resting-state fMRI measurements, it was found that anodal tDCS over left M1 enhanced functional connectivity between the left primary motor cortex and the ipsilateral thalamus (Polanía et al. 2012d). Additionally, functional connectivity of the caudate nucleus, which receives afferents from the cortex and the thalamus, with associative areas such as the superior parietal cortex was enhanced. In line with these findings, in another work it was shown that tDCS over the primary sensori-motor cortex in anaesthetized animals not only affects cortical neurons, but also facilitates activation of neurons in subcortical motor systems (Bolzoni et al. 2013). In addition, it was shown that this subcortical facilitation greatly outlasts (by more than 1 h) the period of transcranial polarization. These studies carried out both in humans and animals provide new evidence of plasticity at subcortical levels, the mechanisms for which remain to be investigated. These findings are of great interest for clinical translational applications considering that anodal stimulation over the motor cortex has been shown to improve gait and bradykinesia in patients suffering from PD (Benninger et al. 2010), where it was speculated whether thalamic activity could be theoretically modulated by cortical stimulation. The results of the above mentioned studies are indeed in favor for connectivity-driven indirect effects of tDCS on thalamic function.

Beyond the effects on M1, tDCS in combination with fMRI has been recently used to understand the brain mechanisms underlying more complex behaviors involving higher cognitive functions, which most likely also actively involve the action of subcortical brain circuits. One such behavior which has received considerable attention in the last few years, is value-based decision-making, sometimes also known as economic decision-making (Krajbich and Dean 2015). Compelling evidence has shown that making decisions based on subjective values involve a large network of regions including cortical areas such as the ventromedial prefrontal cortex (vmPFC) and dopaminergic subcortical structures such as the ventral striatum (VS), substantia nigra (SN) and ventral tegmental area (VTA) that in turn project to numerous cortical areas in the brain including the vmPFC (Williams and Goldman-Rakic 1991; Clithero and Rangel 2013). Using tDCS applied over the frontopolar cortex combined with fMRI, a group of researchers investigated whereas vmPFC causally supports choices based on subjective preferences in a task where healthy participants had to make attractiveness ratings of a series of faces while being scanned with fMRI before and after receiving tDCS over the FPC (Chib et al. 2013). In line with their hypotheses, following anodal stimulation of vmPFC, participants found the presented faces significantly more attractive. The fMRI analyses revealed that activity in the vmPFC was correlated with attractiveness ratings for all participants both before and after stimulation, however, with no specific effects induced by the stimulation. However, in a subsequent interaction analysis in order to test for the specific effects of tDCS, the investigators found that, following stimulation, activity in the ventral midbrain was more positively correlated with attractiveness ratings. In a subsequent connectivity analysis, the investigators examined the network effects of VMPFC stimulation on other brain regions with special interest in regions encompassing the ventral midbrain dopaminergic areas. Strikingly, they found that the same ventral midbrain region found in the interaction analysis was more functionally coupled with activity in the vmPFC following stimulation. Thus, providing crucial evidence that functional connectivity between vmPFC and ventral midbrain is enhanced by anodal tDCS applied over the vmPFC. The results of this work have once more implications for clinical applications. Given that midbrain regions such as SN/VTA neurons lie deep within the brain, the primary means of influencing them in neuro-pathologies affecting midbrain dopaminergic structures have been with systematic pharmacological interventions, however, it precludes from region-specific interventions (Miyamoto et al. 2012). Alternatives, when the pharmacological interventions fail to deliver the desired effects, include the implantation of deep brain stimulators (Mayberg et al. 2005), however, at the expense of invasive and high risk chirurgical procedures. As shown by the above-mentioned example study (Chib et al. 2013), networks of interconnected brain areas can be stimulated with tDCS to influence deep brain regions, thus making tDCS a promising tool to noninvasively modulate subcortical activity and functions that may be disrupted in neuropsychiatric disorders.

Conclusions

The studies presented in this section provide important evidence that long-lasting synaptic modifications induced by tDCS, which result in behavioral improvements, might include an alteration of associations among populations of neurons involved in the respective task-relevant functional networks. These series of studies have important clinical implications given that functional connectivity loss and alterations have been observed in many neurological diseases such as stroke (Wang et al. 2010), Alzheimer's disease (AD) (Stam et al. 2007), Schizophrenia (Zhou et al. 2007), among many others (Van Den Heuvel and Pol 2010). Thus the combination of tDCS, non-invasive brain imaging techniques and computational methods provide a new and promising platform to track for functional recovery and to correlate these changes with behavioral improvements in both health and disease.

Concluding Remarks

Insight into neurophysiological effects of tDCS on targeted neuronal populations as well as on complex cerebral networks provides the crucial foundation for advancing both research and clinical applications of tDCS. Quantification of tDCS effects using advanced neurophysiological and functional imaging tools represent an important stepping stone towards the development of parameter-tailored stimulation protocols in order to improve mechanistic understanding of neuroplasticity of the human brain, to elucidate the link between changes in cerebral activity and modification of functional and behavioral outcomes, as well as to facilitate the development of physiologically justified tDCS treatment protocols for clinical applications in neurorehabilitation, psychiatry or pain management. Despite enormous progress in mapping and understanding tDCS effects in recent years, many questions remain unanswered or only poorly understood. Among them stands out the gap in understanding the sources of inter-individual and intra-individual variability in tDCS effects at the molecular, cellular, systemic and functional/behavioral level. Regardless, tDCS bears great potential for modulation of neurophysiological outcomes in health and disease.

References

Accornero, N., Voti, P. L., La Riccia, M., & Gregori, B. (2007). Visual evoked potentials modulation during direct current cortical polarization. *Experimental Brain Research, 178*(2), 261–266.

Albert, J., López-Martín, S., & Carretié, L. (2010). Emotional context modulates response inhibition: Neural and behavioral data. *NeuroImage, 49*(1), 914–921.

Antal, A., Brepohl, N., Poreisz, C., Boros, K., Csifcsak, G., & Paulus, W. (2008). Transcranial direct current stimulation over somatosensory cortex decreases experimentally induced acute pain perception. *The Clinical Journal of Pain, 24*(1), 56–63.

Antal, A., Chaieb, L., Moliadze, V., Monte-Silva, K., Poreisz, C., Thirugnanasambandam, N., & Paulus, W. (2010). Brain-derived neurotrophic factor (BDNF) gene polymorphisms shape cortical plasticity in humans. *Brain Stimulation, 3*(4), 230–237.

Antal, A., Kincses, T. Z., Nitsche, M. A., & Paulus, W. (2003a). Manipulation of phosphene thresholds by transcranial direct current stimulation in man. *Experimental Brain Research, 150*(3), 375–378.

Antal, A., Kincses, T. Z., Nitsche, M. A., & Paulus, W. (2003b). Modulation of moving phosphene thresholds by transcranial direct current stimulation of V1 in human. *Neuropsychologia, 41*(13), 1802–1807.

Antal, A., Nitsche, M. A., Kincses, T. Z., Kruse, W., Hoffmann, K. P., & Paulus, W. (2004a). Facilitation of visuo-motor learning by transcranial direct current stimulation of the motor and extrastriate visual areas in humans. *European Journal of Neuroscience, 19*(10), 2888–2892.

Antal, A., Nitsche, M. A., Kruse, W., Kincses, T. Z., Hoffmann, K. P., & Paulus, W. (2004b). Direct current stimulation over V5 enhances visuomotor coordination by improving motion perception in humans. *Journal of Cognitive Neuroscience, 16*(4), 521–527.

Antal, A., Nitsche, M. A., & Paulus, W. (2001). External modulation of visual perception in humans. *Neuroreport, 12*(16), 3553–3555.

Antal, A., Polania, R., Schmidt-Samoa, C., Dechent, P., & Paulus, W. (2011). Transcranial direct current stimulation over the primary motor cortex during fMRI. *NeuroImage, 55*(2), 590–596.

Antal, A., Terney, D., Poreisz, C., & Paulus, W. (2007). Towards unravelling task-related modulations of neuroplastic changes induced in the human motor cortex. *European Journal of Neuroscience, 26*(9), 2687–2691.

Ardolino, G., Bossi, B., Barbieri, S., & Priori, A. (2005). Non-synaptic mechanisms underlie the after-effects of cathodal transcutaneous direct current stimulation of the human brain. *The Journal of Physiology, 568*(2), 653–663.

Azanon, E., & Haggard, P. (2009). Somatosensory processing and the body representation. *Cortex, 45*(9), 1078–1084.

Barron, H. C., Vogels, T. P., Emir, U. E., Makin, T. R., O'Shea, J., Clare, S., … Behrens, T. E. J. (2016). Unmasking latent inhibitory connections in human cortex to reveal dormant cortical memories. *Neuron, 90*, 191–203.

Batsikadze, G., Moliadze, V., Paulus, W., Kuo, M. F., & Nitsche, M. A. (2013). Partially non-linear stimulation intensity-dependent effects of direct current stimulation on motor cortex excitability in humans. *The Journal of Physiology, 591*(7), 1987–2000.

Baudewig, J., Nitsche, M. A., Paulus, W., & Frahm, J. (2001). Regional modulation of BOLD MRI responses to human sensorimotor activation by transcranial direct current stimulation. *Magnetic Resonance in Medicine, 45*(2), 196–201.

Benninger, D. H., Lomarev, M., Lopez, G., Wassermann, E. M., Li, X., Considine, E., & Hallett, M. (2010). Transcranial direct current stimulation for the treatment of Parkinson's disease. *Journal of Neurology, Neurosurgery & Psychiatry, 81*(10), 1105–1111.

Bolzoni, F., Pettersson, L. G., & Jankowska, E. (2013). Evidence for long-lasting subcortical facilitation by transcranial direct current stimulation in the cat. *The Journal of Physiology, 591*(13), 3381–3399.

Boros, K., Poreisz, C., Münchau, A., Paulus, W., & Nitsche, M. A. (2008). Premotor transcranial direct current stimulation (tDCS) affects primary motor excitability in humans. *European Journal of Neuroscience, 27*(5), 1292–1300.

Bradnam, L. V., Stinear, C. M., & Byblow, W. D. (2011). Cathodal transcranial direct current stimulation suppresses ipsilateral projections to presumed propriospinal neurons of the proximal upper limb. *Journal of Neurophysiology, 105*(5), 2582–2589.

Bullmore, E., & Sporns, O. (2009). Complex brain networks: Graph theoretical analysis of structural and functional systems. *Nature Reviews Neuroscience, 10*(3), 186–198.

Campanella, S., Schroder, E., Monnart, A., Vanderhasselt, M. A., Duprat, R., Rabijns, M., … Baeken, C. (2017). Transcranial direct current stimulation over the right frontal inferior cortex decreases neural activity needed to achieve inhibition: A double-blind ERP study in a male population. *Clinical EEG and Neuroscience, 48*(3), 176–188.

Chen, J. C., Hämmerer, D., D'Ostilio, K., Casula, E. P., Marshall, L., Tsai, C. H., … Edwards, M. J. (2014a). Bi-directional modulation of somatosensory mismatch negativity with transcranial direct current stimulation: An event related potential study. *The Journal of Physiology, 592*(4), 745–757.

Chen, J. C., Hämmerer, D., Strigaro, G., Liou, L. M., Tsai, C. H., Rothwell, J. C., & Edwards, M. J. (2014b). Domain-specific suppression of auditory mismatch negativity with transcranial direct current stimulation. *Clinical Neurophysiology, 125*(3), 585–592.

Chib, V. S., Yun, K., Takahashi, H., & Shimojo, S. (2013). Noninvasive remote activation of the ventral midbrain by transcranial direct current stimulation of prefrontal cortex. *Translational Psychiatry, 3*, e268.

Clithero, J. A., & Rangel, A. (2013). Informatic parcellation of the network involved in the computation of subjective value. *Social Cognitive and Affective Neuroscience, 9*(9), 1289–1302.

Conti, C. L., Moscon, J. A., Fregni, F., Nitsche, M. A., & Nakamura-Palacios, E. M. (2014). Cognitive related electrophysiological changes induced by non-invasive cortical electrical stimulation in crack-cocaine addiction. *The International Journal of Neuropsychopharmacology, 17*(9), 1465–1475.

Curio, G. (2000). Linking 600-Hz "spikelike" EEG/MEG wavelets ("sigma-bursts") to cellular substrates: concepts and caveats. *Journal of Clinical Neurophysiology, 17*(4), 377–396. 11012041.

Curio, G., Mackert, B. M., Burghoff, M., Koetitz, R., Abraham-Fuchs, K., & Härer, W. (1994). Localization of evoked neuromagnetic 600 Hz activity in the cerebral somatosensory system. *Electroencephalography and Clinical Neurophysiology, 91*(6), 483–487.

Curio, G., Mackert, B. M., Burghoff, M., Neumann, J., Nolte, G., Scherg, M., & Marx, P. (1997). Somatotopic source arrangement of 600 Hz oscillatory magnetic fields at the human primary somatosensory hand cortex. *Neuroscience Letters, 234*(2), 131–134.

Daw, N. D., O'Doherty, J. P., Dayan, P., Seymour, B., & Dolan, R. J. (2006). Cortical substrates for exploratory decisions in humans. *Nature, 441*, 876–879.

Dieckhöfer, A., Waberski, T. D., Nitsche, M., Paulus, W., Buchner, H., & Gobbelé, R. (2006). Transcranial direct current stimulation applied over the somatosensory cortex–differential effect on low and high frequency SEPs. *Clinical Neurophysiology, 117*(10), 2221–2227.

Edwards, D., Cortes, M., Datta, A., Minhas, P., Wassermann, E. M., & Bikson, M. (2013). Physiological and modeling evidence for focal transcranial electrical brain stimulation in humans: A basis for high-definition tDCS. *NeuroImage, 74*, 266–275.

Faehling, F., & Plewnia, C. (2016). Controlling the emotional bias: Performance, late positive potentials, and the effect of anodal transcranial direct current stimulation (tDCS). *Frontiers in Cellular Neuroscience, 10*, 159. PubMed PMID: 27378856.

Fenton, B. W., Palmieri, P. A., Boggio, P., Fanning, J., & Fregni, F. (2009). A preliminary study of transcranial direct current stimulation for the treatment of refractory chronic pelvic pain. *Brain Stimulation, 2*(2), 103–107.

Fricke, K., Seeber, A. A., Thirugnanasambandam, N., Paulus, W., Nitsche, M. A., & Rothwell, J. C. (2011). Time course of the induction of homeostatic plasticity generated by repeated transcranial direct current stimulation of the human motor cortex. *Journal of Neurophysiology, 105*(3), 1141–1149.

Fritsch, B., Reis, J., Martinowich, K., Schambra, H. M., Ji, Y., Cohen, L. G., & Lu, B. (2010). Direct current stimulation promotes BDNF-dependent synaptic plasticity: Potential implications for motor learning. *Neuron, 66*(2), 198–204.

Grueschow, M., Polania, R., Hare, T. A., & Ruff, C. C. (2015). Automatic versus choice-dependent value representations in the human brain. *Neuron, 85*(4), 874–885.

Grundey, J., Thirugnanasambandam, N., Kaminsky, K., Drees, A., Skwirba, A. C., Lang, N., … Nitsche, M. A. (2012). Neuroplasticity in cigarette smokers is altered under withdrawal and partially restituted by nicotine exposition. *The Journal of Neuroscience, 32*(12), 4156–4162.

Grundmann, L., Rolke, R., Nitsche, M. A., Pavlakovic, G., Happe, S., Treede, R. D., … Bachmann, C. G. (2011). Effects of transcranial direct current stimulation of the primary sensory cortex on somatosensory perception. *Brain Stimulation, 4*(4), 253–260.

Haider, B., & Mccormick, D. A. (2009). Rapid neocortical dynamics: Cellular and network mechanisms. *Neuron, 62*, 171–189.

Hasan, A., Nitsche, M. A., Rein, B., Schneider-Axmann, T., Guse, B., Gruber, O., … Wobrock, T. (2011). Dysfunctional long-term potentiation-like plasticity in schizophrenia revealed by transcranial direct current stimulation. *Behavioural Brain Research, 224*(1), 15–22.

Huttunen, J., Komssi, S., & Lauronen, L. (2006). Spatial dynamics of population activities at S1 after median and ulnar nerve stimulation revisited: An MEG study. *NeuroImage, 32*(3), 1024–1031.

Iezzi, E., Suppa, A., Conte, A., Li Voti, P., Bologna, M., & Berardelli, A. (2011). Short-term and long-term plasticity interaction in human primary motor cortex. *European Journal of Neuroscience, 33*(10), 1908–1915.

Impey, D., de la Salle, S., & Knott, V. (2016). Assessment of anodal and cathodal transcranial direct current stimulation (tDCS) on MMN-indexed auditory sensory processing. *Brain and Cognition, 105*, 46–54. PMID: 27054908.

Impey, D., & Knott, V. (2015). Effect of transcranial direct current stimulation (tDCS) on MMN-indexed auditory discrimination: A pilot study. *Journal of Neural Transmission, 122*(8), 1175–1185.

Jang, S. H., Ahn, S. H., Byun, W. M., Kim, C. S., Lee, M. Y., & Kwon, Y. H. (2009). The effect of transcranial direct current stimulation on the cortical activation by motor task in the human brain: An fMRI study. *Neuroscience Letters, 460*(2), 117–120.

Jefferson, S., Mistry, S., Singh, S., Rothwell, J., & Hamdy, S. (2009). Characterizing the application of transcranial direct current stimulation in human pharyngeal motor cortex. *American Journal of Physiology. Gastrointestinal and Liver Physiology, 297*(6), G1035–G1040.

Jeffery, D. T., Norton, J. A., Roy, F. D., & Gorassini, M. A. (2007). Effects of transcranial direct current stimulation on the excitability of the leg motor cortex. *Experimental Brain Research, 182*(2), 281–287.

Kasashima, Y., Fujiwara, T., Matsushika, Y., Tsuji, T., Hase, K., Ushiyama, J., … Liu, M. (2012). Modulation of event-related desynchronization during motor imagery with transcranial direct current stimulation (tDCS) in patients with chronic hemiparetic stroke. *Experimental Brain Research, 221*(3), 263–268.

Kasuga, S., Matsushika, Y., Kasashima-Shindo, Y., Kamatani, D., Fujiwara, T., Liu, M., & Ushiba, J. (2015). Transcranial direct current stimulation enhances mu rhythm desynchronization during motor imagery that depends on handedness. *Laterality: Asymmetries of Body, Brain and Cognition, 20*(4), 453–468.

Kawamura, T., Nakasato, N., Seki, K., Kanno, A., Fujita, S., Fujiwara, S., & Yoshimoto, T. (1996). Neuromagnetic evidence of pre-and post-central cortical sources of somatosensory evoked responses. *Electroencephalography and Clinical Neurophysiology/Evoked Potentials Section, 100*(1), 44–50.

Keeser, D., Meindl, T., Bor, J., Palm, U., Pogarell, O., Mulert, C., … Padberg, F. (2011). Prefrontal transcranial direct current stimulation changes connectivity of resting-state networks during fMRI. *The Journal of Neuroscience, 31*, 15284–15293.

Kessler, S. K., Minhas, P., Woods, A. J., Rosen, A., Gorman, C., & Bikson, M. (2013). Dosage considerations for transcranial direct current stimulation in children: A computational modeling study. *PLoS One, 8*(9), e76112.

Kim, C. R., Kim, D. Y., Kim, L. S., Chun, M. H., Kim, S. J., & Park, C. H. (2012). Modulation of cortical activity after anodal transcranial direct current stimulation of the lower limb motor cortex: A functional MRI study. *Brain Stimulation, 5*(4), 462–467.

Kirimoto, H., Ogata, K., Onishi, H., Oyama, M., Goto, Y., & Tobimatsu, S. (2011). Transcranial direct current stimulation over the motor association cortex induces plastic changes in ipsilateral primary motor and somatosensory cortices. *Clinical Neurophysiology, 122*(4), 777–783.

Kojima, S., Onishi, H., Miyaguchi, S., Kotan, S., Sugawara, K., Kirimoto, H., & Tamaki, H. (2015). Effects of cathodal transcranial direct current stimulation to primary somatosensory cortex on short-latency afferent inhibition. *Neuroreport, 26*(11), 634–637.

Krajbich, I., & Dean, M. (2015). How can neuroscience inform economics? *Current Opinion Behavioral Science, 5*, 51–57.

Krishnan, C., Ranganathan, R., Kantak, S. S., Dhaher, Y. Y., & Rymer, W. Z. (2014). Anodal transcranial direct current stimulation alters elbow flexor muscle recruitment strategies. *Brain Stimulation, 7*(3), 443–450.

Kuo, H. I., Bikson, M., Datta, A., Minhas, P., Paulus, W., Kuo, M. F., & Nitsche, M. A. (2013). Comparing cortical plasticity induced by conventional and high-definition 4× 1 ring tDCS: A neurophysiological study. *Brain Stimulation, 6*(4), 644–648.

Kuo, H. I., Paulus, W., Batsikadze, G., Jamil, A., Kuo, M. F., & Nitsche, M. A. (2016). Chronic enhancement of serotonin facilitates excitatory transcranial direct current stimulation-induced neuroplasticity. *Neuropsychopharmacology, 41*(5), 1223.

Kuo, M. F., Paulus, W., & Nitsche, M. A. (2008). Boosting focally-induced brain plasticity by dopamine. *Cerebral Cortex, 18*(3), 648–651.

Kwon, Y. H., & Jang, S. H. (2011). The enhanced cortical activation induced by transcranial direct current stimulation during hand movements. *Neuroscience Letters, 492*(2), 105–108.

Kwon, Y. H., Kang, K. W., Son, S. M., & Lee, N. K. (2015). Is effect of transcranial direct current stimulation on visuomotor coordination dependent on task difficulty? *Neural Regeneration Research, 10*(3), 463–466.

Kwon, Y. H., Ko, M. H., Ahn, S. H., Kim, Y. H., Song, J. C., Lee, C. H., … Jang, S. H. (2008). Primary motor cortex activation by transcranial direct current stimulation in the human brain. *Neuroscience Letters, 435*(1), 56–59.

Labruna, L., Jamil, A., Fresnoza, S., Batsikadze, G., Kuo, M. F., Vanderschelden, B., … Nitsche, M. A. (2016). Efficacy of anodal transcranial direct current stimulation is related to sensitivity to transcranial magnetic stimulation. *Brain Stimulation, 9*(1), 8–15.

Lang, N., Siebner, H. R., Ward, N. S., Lee, L., Nitsche, M. A., Paulus, W., … Frackowiak, R. S. (2005). How does transcranial DC stimulation of the primary motor cortex alter regional neuronal activity in the human brain? *European Journal of Neuroscience, 22*(2), 495–504.

Lapenta, O. M., Di Sierve, K., de Macedo, E. C., Fregni, F., & Boggio, P. S. (2014). Transcranial direct current stimulation modulates ERP-indexed inhibitory control and reduces food consumption. *Appetite, 83*, 42–48.

Lapenta, O. M., Minati, L., Fregni, F., & Boggio, P. S. (2013). Je pense donc je fais: transcranial direct current stimulation modulates brain oscillations associated with motor imagery and movement observation. *Frontiers in human neuroscience, 7*, 256.

Liebetanz, D., Nitsche, M. A., Tergau, F., & Paulus, W. (2002). Pharmacological approach to the mechanisms of transcranial DC-stimulation-induced after-effects of human motor cortex excitability. *Brain, 125*(10), 2238–2247.

Lisman, J. E. (2001). Three Ca2+ levels affect plasticity differently: The LTP zone, the LTD zone and no man's land. *The Journal of Physiology, 532*(2), 285–285.

López-Alonso, V., Fernández-Del-Olmo, M., Costantini, A., Gonzalez-Henriquez, J. J., & Cheeran, B. (2015). Intra-individual variability in the response to anodal transcranial direct current stimulation. *Clinical Neurophysiology, 126*(12), 2342–2347.

Malenka, R. C., & Bear, M. F. (2004). LTP and LTD: An embarrassment of riches. *Neuron, 44*(1), 5–21.

Mathys, C., Loui, P., Zheng, X., & Schlaug, G. (2010). Non-invasive brain stimulation applied to Heschl's gyrus modulates pitch discrimination. *Frontiers in Psychology, 1*, 193.

Matsumoto, J., Fujiwara, T., Takahashi, O., Liu, M., Kimura, A., & Ushiba, J. (2010). Modulation of mu rhythm desynchronization during motor imagery by transcranial direct current stimulation. *Journal of Neuroengineering and Rehabilitation, 7*(1), 1.

Matsunaga, K., Nitsche, M. A., Tsuji, S., & Rothwell, J. C. (2004). Effect of transcranial DC sensorimotor cortex stimulation on somatosensory evoked potentials in humans. *Clinical Neurophysiology, 115*(2), 456–460.

Mauguiere, F. (1999). Somatosensory evoked potentials: Normal responses, abnormal waveforms and clinical applications in neurological diseases. In E. Niedermeyer & F. Lopes Da Silva (Eds.), *Electrocephalography: Basic principles,clinical applications and related fields* (pp. 1014–1058). Baltimore: Williams and Wilkins.

Mayberg, H. S., Lozano, A. M., Voon, V., Mcneely, H. E., Seminowicz, D., Hamani, C., … Kennedy, S. H. (2005). Deep brain stimulation for treatment-resistant depression. *Neuron, 45*, 651–660.

Merritt, K., McGuire, P., & Egerton, A. (2013). Relationship between glutamate dysfunction and symptoms and cognitive function in psychosis. *Frontiers in Psychiatry, 4*, 151.

Mccambridge, A. B., Stinear, J. W., & Byblow, W. D. (2015). 'I-wave' recruitment determines response to tDCS in the upper limb, but only so far. *Brain Stimulation, 8*(6), 1124–1129.

Miyamoto, S., Miyake, N., Jarskog, L. F., Fleischhacker, W. W., & Lieberman, J. A. (2012). Pharmacological treatment of schizophrenia: A critical review of the pharmacology and clinical effects of current and future therapeutic agents. *Molecular Psychiatry, 17*, 1206–1227.

Monte-Silva, K., Kuo, M. F., Hessenthaler, S., Fresnoza, S., Liebetanz, D., Paulus, W., & Nitsche, M. A. (2013). Induction of late LTP-like plasticity in the human motor cortex by repeated non-invasive brain stimulation. *Brain Stimulation, 6*(3), 424–432.

Monte-Silva, K., Kuo, M. F., Liebetanz, D., Paulus, W., & Nitsche, M. A. (2010). Shaping the optimal repetition interval for cathodal transcranial direct current stimulation (tDCS). *Journal of Neurophysiology, 103*(4), 1735–1740.

Nitsche, M. A., Doemkes, S., Karakoese, T., Antal, A., Liebetanz, D., Lang, N., … Paulus, W. (2007). Shaping the effects of transcranial direct current stimulation of the human motor cortex. *Journal of Neurophysiology, 97*(4), 3109–3117.

Nitsche, M. A., Fricke, K., Henschke, U., Schlitterlau, A., Liebetanz, D., Lang, N., … Paulus, W. (2003a). Pharmacological modulation of cortical excitability shifts induced by transcranial direct current stimulation in humans. *The Journal of Physiology, 553*(1), 293–301.

Nitsche, M. A., Jaussi, W., Liebetanz, D., Lang, N., Tergau, F., & Paulus, W. (2004a). Consolidation of human motor cortical neuroplasticity by D-cycloserine. *Neuropsychopharmacology, 29*(8), 1573–1578.

Nitsche, M. A., Kuo, M. F., Karrasch, R., Wächter, B., Liebetanz, D., & Paulus, W. (2009). Serotonin affects transcranial direct current–induced neuroplasticity in humans. *Biological Psychiatry, 66*(5), 503–508.

Nitsche, M. A., Lampe, C., Antal, A., Liebetanz, D., Lang, N., Tergau, F., & Paulus, W. (2006). Dopaminergic modulation of long-lasting direct current-induced cortical excitability changes in the human motor cortex. *European Journal of Neuroscience, 23*(6), 1651–1657.

Nitsche, M. A., Liebetanz, D., Schlitterlau, A., Henschke, U., Fricke, K., Frommann, K., … Tergau, F. (2004b). GABAergic modulation of DC stimulation-induced motor cortex excitability shifts in humans. *European Journal of Neuroscience, 19*(10), 2720–2726.

Nitsche, M. A., Nitsche, M. S., Klein, C. C., Tergau, F., Rothwell, J. C., & Paulus, W. (2003b). Level of action of cathodal DC polarisation induced inhibition of the human motor cortex. *Clinical Neurophysiology, 114*(4), 600–604.

Nitsche, M. A., & Paulus, W. (2000). Excitability changes induced in the human motor cortex by weak transcranial direct current stimulation. *The Journal of Physiology, 527*(3), 633–639.

Nitsche, M. A., & Paulus, W. (2001). Sustained excitability elevations induced by transcranial DC motor cortex stimulation in humans. *Neurology, 57*(10), 1899–1901.

Nitsche, M. A., Schauenburg, A., Lang, N., Liebetanz, D., Exner, C., Paulus, W., & Tergau, F. (2003c). Facilitation of implicit motor learning by weak transcranial direct current stimulation of the primary motor cortex in the human. *Journal of Cognitive Neuroscience, 15*(4), 619–626.

Nitsche, M. A., Seeber, A., Frommann, K., Klein, C. C., Rochford, C., Nitsche, M. S., … Paulus, W. (2005). Modulating parameters of excitability during and after transcranial direct current stimulation of the human motor cortex. *The Journal of Physiology, 568*(1), 291–303.

Okun, M., & Lampl, I. (2008). Instantaneous correlation of excitation and inhibition during ongoing and sensory-evoked activities. *Nature Neuroscience, 11*, 535–537.

Pellicciari, M. C., Brignani, D., & Miniussi, C. (2013). Excitability modulation of the motor system induced by transcranial direct current stimulation: A multimodal approach. *NeuroImage, 83*, 569–580.

Peña-Gómez, C., Sala-Lonch, R., Junqué, C., Clemente, I. C., Vidal, D., Bargalló, N., … Bartrés-Faz, D. (2012). Modulation of large-scale brain networks by transcranial direct current stimulation evidenced by resting-state functional MRI. *Brain Stimulation, 5*, 252–263.

Pfefferbaum, A., Ford, J. M., Weller, B. J., & Kopell, B. S. (1985). ERPs to response production and inhibition. *Electroencephalography and Clinical Neurophysiology, 60*(5), 423–434.

Polanía, R., Krajbich, I., Grueschow, M., & Ruff, C. C. (2014). Neural oscillations and synchronization differentially support evidence accumulation in perceptual and value-based decision making. *Neuron, 82*(3), 709–720.

Polanía, R., Moisa, M., Opitz, A., Grueschow, M., & Ruff, C. C. (2015). The precision of value-based choices depends causally on fronto-parietal phase coupling. *Nature Communications, 6, 8090.*

Polanía, R., Nitsche, M. A., Korman, C., Batsikadze, G., & Paulus, W. (2012a). The importance of timing in segregated theta phase-coupling for cognitive performance. *Current Biology, 22*(14), 1314–1318.

Polanía, R., Nitsche, M. A., & Paulus, W. (2011a). Modulating functional connectivity patterns and topological functional organization of the human brain with transcranial direct current stimulation. *Human Brain Mapping, 32*(8), 1236–1249.

Polanía, R., Paulus, W., Antal, A., & Nitsche, M. A. (2011b). Introducing graph theory to track for neuroplastic alterations in the resting human brain: A transcranial direct current stimulation study. *NeuroImage, 54*(3), 2287–2296.

Polanía, R., Paulus, W., & Nitsche, M. A. (2012b). Noninvasively decoding the contents of visual working memory in the human prefrontal cortex within high-gamma oscillatory patterns. *Journal of Cognitive Neuroscience, 24*(2), 304–314.

Polanía, R., Paulus, W., & Nitsche, M. A. (2012c). Reorganizing the intrinsic functional architecture of the human primary motor cortex during rest with non-invasive cortical stimulation. *PLoS One, 7*(1), e30971.

Polanía, R., Paulus, W., & Nitsche, M. A. (2012d). Modulating cortico-striatal and thalamo-cortical functional connectivity with transcranial direct current stimulation. *Human Brain Mapping, 33*(10), 2499–2508.

Ragert, P., Becker, M., Tegenthoff, M., Pleger, B., & Dinse, H. R. (2004a). Sustained increase of somatosensory cortex excitability by 5 Hz repetitive transcranial magnetic stimulation studied by paired median nerve stimulation in humans. *Neuroscience Letters, 356*(2), 91–94.

Ragert, P., Franzkowiak, S., Schwenkreis, P., Tegenthoff, M., & Dinse, H. R. (2008a). Improvement of tactile perception and enhancement of cortical excitability through intermittent theta burst rTMS over human primary somatosensory cortex. *Experimental Brain Research, 184*(1), 1–11.

Ragert, P., Schmidt, A., Altenmüeller, E., & Dinse, H. R. (2004b). Superior tactile performance and learning in professional pianists: Evidence for meta-plasticity in musicians. *European Journal of Neuroscience, 19*(2), 473–478.

Ragert, P., Vandermeeren, Y., Camus, M., & Cohen, L. G. (2008b). Improvement of spatial tactile acuity by transcranial direct current stimulation. *Clinical Neurophysiology, 119*(4), 805–811.

Raja, B. A., Polanía, R., Hare, T. A., & Ruff, C. C. (2015). Transcranial stimulation over Frontopolar cortex elucidates the choice attributes and neural mechanisms used to resolve exploration–exploitation trade-offs. *The Journal of Neuroscience, 35*(43), 14544–14556.

Rangel, A., Camerer, C., & Montague, P. R. (2008). A framework for studying the neurobiology of value-based decision making. *Nature Reviews Neuroscience, 9*(7), 545–556.

Rangel, A., & Hare, T. (2010). Neural computations associated with goal-directed choice. *Current Opinion in Neurobiology, 20*(2), 262–270.

Ray Li, C.-S., Huang, C., Constable, R. T., & Sinha, R. (2006). Imaging response inhibition in a stop-signal task: Neural correlates independent of signal monitoring and post-response processing. *The Journal of Neuroscience, 26*, 186–192.

Rehmann, R., Sczesny-Kaiser, M., Lenz, M., Gucia, T., Schliesing, A., Schwenkreis, P., … Höffken, O. (2016). Polarity-specific cortical effects of transcranial direct current stimulation in primary somatosensory cortex of healthy humans. *Frontiers in Human Neuroscience, 10*, 208.

Reis, J., Schambra, H. M., Cohen, L. G., Buch, E. R., Fritsch, B., Zarahn, E., … Krakauer, J. W. (2009). Noninvasive cortical stimulation enhances motor skill acquisition over multiple days through an effect on consolidation. *Proceedings of the National Academy of Sciences, 106*(5), 1590–1595.

Rivera-Urbina, G. N., Batsikadze, G., Molero-Chamizo, A., Paulus, W., Kuo, M. F., & Nitsche, M. A. (2015). Parietal transcranial direct current stimulation modulates primary motor cortex excitability. *European Journal of Neuroscience, 41*(6), 845–855.

Rogalewski, A., Breitenstein, C., Nitsche, M. A., Paulus, W., & Knecht, S. (2004). Transcranial direct current stimulation disrupts tactile perception. *European Journal of Neuroscience, 20*(1), 313–316.

Roy, A., Baxter, B., & He, B. (2014). High-definition transcranial direct current stimulation induces both acute and persistent changes in broadband cortical synchronization: A simultaneous tDCS–EEG study. *IEEE Transactions on Biomedical Engineering, 61*(7), 1967–1978.

Ruff, C. C., Ugazio, G., & Fehr, E. (2013). Changing social norm compliance with noninvasive brain stimulation. *Science, 342*, 482–484.

Saiote, C., Polanía, R., Rosenberger, K., Paulus, W., & Antal, A. (2013). High-frequency TRNS reduces BOLD activity during visuomotor learning. *PLoS One, 8*(3), e59669.

Sanes, J. N. (2000). Motor cortex rules for learning and memory. *Current Biology, 10*, R495–R497.

Schade, S., Moliadze, V., Paulus, W., & Antal, A. (2012). Modulating neuronal excitability in the motor cortex with tDCS shows moderate hemispheric asymmetry due to subjects' handedness: A pilot study. *Restorative Neurology and Neuroscience, 30*(3), 191–198.

Sczesny-Kaiser, M., Beckhaus, K., Dinse, H. R., Schwenkreis, P., Tegenthoff, M., & Höffken, O. (2016). Repetitive transcranial direct current stimulation induced excitability changes of primary visual cortex and visual learning effects—A pilot study. *Frontiers in Behavioral Neuroscience, 10*, 116.

Shah, B., Nguyen, T. T., & Madhavan, S. (2013). Polarity independent effects of cerebellar tDCS on short term ankle visuomotor learning. *Brain Stimulation, 6*(6), 966–968.
Siegel, M., Donner, T. H., & Engel, A. K. (2012). Spectral fingerprints of large-scale neuronal interactions. *Nature Reviews Neuroscience, 13*(2), 121–134.
Song, S., Sandrini, M., & Cohen, L. G. (2011). Modifying somatosensory processing with non-invasive brain stimulation. *Restorative Neurology and Neuroscience, 29*(6), 427–437.
Spitzer, M., Fischbacher, U., Herrnberger, B., Grön, G., & Fehr, E. (2007). The neural signature of social norm compliance. *Neuron, 56*, 185–196.
Stagg, C. J., Bachtiar, V., Amadi, U., Gudberg, C. A., Ilie, A. S., Sampaio-Baptista, C., … Near, J. (2014). Local GABA concentration is related to network-level resting functional connectivity. *eLife, 3*, e01465.
Stagg, C. J., Best, J. G., Stephenson, M. C., O'Shea, J., Wylezinska, M., Kincses, Z. T., … Johansen-Berg, H. (2009). Polarity-sensitive modulation of cortical neurotransmitters by transcranial stimulation. *The Journal of Neuroscience, 29*(16), 5202–5206.
Stam, C. J., Jones, B. F., Nolte, G., Breakspear, M., & Scheltens, P. (2007). Small-world networks and functional connectivity in Alzheimer's disease. *Cerebral Cortex, 17*(1), 92–99.
Sugawara, K., Onishi, H., Yamashiro, K., Kojima, S., Miyaguchi, S., Kirimoto, H., … Kameyama, S. (2015). The effect of anodal transcranial direct current stimulation over the primary motor or somatosensory cortices on somatosensory evoked magnetic fields. *Clinical Neurophysiology, 126*(1), 60–67.
Tanaka, S., Hanakawa, T., Honda, M., & Watanabe, K. (2009). Enhancement of pinch force in the lower leg by anodal transcranial direct current stimulation. *Experimental Brain Research, 196*(3), 459–465.
Thirugnanasambandam, N., Grundey, J., Adam, K., Drees, A., Skwirba, A. C., Lang, N., … Nitsche, M. A. (2011). Nicotinergic impact on focal and non-focal neuroplasticity induced by non-invasive brain stimulation in non-smoking humans. *Neuropsychopharmacology, 36*(4), 879–886.
Trepel, C., & Racine, R. J. (2000). GABAergic modulation of neocortical long-term potentiation in the freely moving rat. *Synapse, 35*(2), 120–128.
Tsakiris, M., Costantini, M., & Haggard, P. (2008). The role of the right temporo-parietal junction in maintaining a coherent sense of one's body. *Neuropsychologia, 46*(12), 3014–3018.
Van Den Heuvel, M. P., & Pol, H. E. H. (2010). Exploring the brain network: A review on resting-state fMRI functional connectivity. *European Neuropsychopharmacology, 20*(8), 519–534.
Vines, B. W., Schnider, N. M., & Schlaug, G. (2006). Testing for causality with transcranial direct current stimulation: Pitch memory and the left supramarginal gyrus. *Neuroreport, 17*(10), 1047–1050.
Wang, L., Yu, C., Chen, H., Qin, W., He, Y., Fan, F., … Woodward, T. S. (2010). Dynamic functional reorganization of the motor execution network after stroke. *Brain, 133*(4), 1224–1238.
Wang, Y., Hao, Y., Zhou, J., Fried, P. J., Wang, X., Zhang, J., … Manor, B. (2015). Direct current stimulation over the human sensorimotor cortex modulates the brain's hemodynamic response to tactile stimulation. *European Journal of Neuroscience, 42*(3), 1933–1940.
Wiethoff, S., Hamada, M., & Rothwell, J. C. (2014). Variability in response to transcranial direct current stimulation of the motor cortex. *Brain Stimulation, 7*(3), 468–475.
Williams, S. M., & Goldman-Rakic, P. S. (1991). Characterization of the dopaminergic innervation of the primate frontal cortex using a dopamine-specific antibody. *Cerebral Cortex, 3*, 199–222.
Yang, B., Yang, S., Zhao, L., Yin, L., Liu, X., & An, S. (2009). Event-related potentials in a go/Nogo task of abnormal response inhibition in heroin addicts. *Science in China Series C: Life Sciences, 52*(8), 780–788.
Yu, J., Tseng, P., Hung, D. L., Wu, S.-W., & Juan, C.-H. (2015). Brain stimulation improves cognitive control by modulating medial-frontal activity and preSMA-vmPFC functional connectivity. *Human Brain Mapping, 36*, 4004–4015.

Zaehle, T., Beretta, M., Jäncke, L., Herrmann, C. S., & Sandmann, P. (2011). Excitability changes induced in the human auditory cortex by transcranial direct current stimulation: Direct electrophysiological evidence. *Experimental Brain Research, 215*(2), 135–140.

Zheng, X., Alsop, D. C., & Schlaug, G. (2011). Effects of transcranial direct current stimulation (tDCS) on human regional cerebral blood flow. *NeuroImage, 58*(1), 26–33.

Zhou, Y., Liang, M., Jiang, T., Tian, L., Liu, Y., Liu, Z., … Kuang, F. (2007). Functional dysconnectivity of the dorsolateral prefrontal cortex in first-episode schizophrenia using resting-state fMRI. *Neuroscience Letters, 417*(3), 297–302.

Chapter 6
Safety of Transcranial Direct Current Stimulation

Pnina Grossman, Adam J. Woods, Helena Knotkova, and Marom Bikson

Introduction

The goal of this chapter is to review the safety of transcranial Direct Current Stimulation (tDCS), focusing only on reported Serious Adverse Effects in human trials and irreversible brain damage as reported in animal models. As such, this chapter is based on and expands upon the 2016 safety consensus published in *Brain Stimulation* (Bikson et al. 2016). For the purposes of this chapter, and following the approach set in the 2016 consensus, the analysis relies on (1) outcomes from human trials, including reports of serious adverse events and imaging changes; (2) results from animal models, including histologically observable tissue; and (3) predictions from computational modeling to the limited extent they inform the interpretation of experimental data. In accordance with WHO-delineated definitions (www.who.int/medicines/areas/quality_safety/safety_efficacy/.../definitions.pdf), we distinguish

P. Grossman
Department of Biomedical Engineering, The City College of the City University of New York, Grove School of Engineering, New York, NY, USA

A. J. Woods
Center for Cognitive Aging and Memory (CAM), McKnight Brain Institute, Department of Clinical and Health Psychology, College of Public Health and Health Professions, University of Florida, Gainesville, FL, USA

H. Knotkova
MJHS Institute for Innovation in Palliative Care, New York, NY, USA

Department of Family and Social Medicine, Albert Einstein College of Medicine, Bronx, NY, USA

M. Bikson (✉)
Department of Biomedical Engineering, The City College of New York, New York, NY, USA
e-mail: bikson@ccny.cuny.edu

H. Knotkova et al. (eds.), *Practical Guide to Transcranial Direct Current Stimulation*, https://doi.org/10.1007/978-3-319-95948-1_6

between adverse *events* (which are potentially coincidental and so not necessarily causal to application of tDCS) and adverse *effects* (for which there is a rational basis to establish causally related to application of tDCS). Tolerability or transient adverse cognitive and behavioral changes that are not associated with Serious Adverse Effects are not taken into account for the purposes of this chapter since they fall outside the stated operational definition of safety.

Electrical stimulation in animals, including epicranial stimulation, is referred to as Direct Current Stimulation (DCS), as opposed to tDCS, to distinguish it from human electrical stimulation. Human data in this chapter relies on reports of serious adverse events in published trials in which subjects are not typically exhaustively tested for injury per se or followed for an extensive period, providing an inherent limitation to any conclusions but not evidence for risk. There are limited prospective studies on tDCS safety in humans (Nitsche et al. 2004; Sawyer et al. 1989). In considering data from animal studies, we focus on understanding the translation of findings (e.g. dose scaling) to humans. Data from translational animal studies support establishing tDCS safety limits only in the context of detectable irreversible brain damage. Importantly, we avoid speculation regarding *theoretical* risks of tDCS including any that based on extrapolation from reports in which no specific link to tDCS has been established (e.g. inferring the potential risks of low intensity direct current based on the known risks of high intensity current). It is easy to confuse theoretical concern in the absence of evidence as a rationale to "call for caution" or suggest an inherent risk. While it is certainly valuable to identify factors that may change susceptibility to stimulation safety risks (e.g. children have smaller heads), this cannot justify claiming such susceptibilities incur a known safety risk without rational analysis. This is especially important when such unjustified claims can distract from evidence-based considerations, unduly restrict a trial or even prevent access to treatment. All this is not to suggest a cavalier approach to tDCS safety, rather, it is to encourage careful distinction between inferences based on evidence (even if incomplete) and speculation based on philosophy (e.g. children are different so tDCS is risky) or conclusions drawn from absence of evidence (e.g. tDCS has not been tested for over 20 years so long-term use is risky).

It is important to clarify that exclusion of subjects from participation in clinical trials because of preexisting co-morbidities (e.g. exclusion of subject with epilepsy from studies on efficacy for depression, and exclusion of subjects with depression from epilepsy studies) reduces the number of complicated (atypical presentation) cases tested with tDCS. Notably, when such exclusion is not explicitly justified for safety reasons then it likely reflects experimental design (e.g. depression post stroke is considered a different illness to depression of another etiology) rather than real concern regarding risk. Nonetheless, such "conservative" exclusions, as well as subject-specific safety monitoring protocols applied in the absence of evidence for risk, can be a source of confusion with regards to safety norms and are therefore noted in this chapter where relevant.

Operator intentions when applying tDCS (e.g. the stated goal of a trial), the efficacy of tDCS in eliciting desired outcomes (Brunoni et al. 2012), and the presumed mechanisms of tDCS (Medeiros et al. 2012) are not within the scope of this chapter as they do not necessarily influence safety (though they might influence separate risk/benefit consideration). Similarly, potential neuroprotective effects are not within our scope (Kim et al. 2010), except for cases in which they inform safety. Data from animal experiments are limited to non-invasive or epicranial electrode techniques, since the safety profile for implanted electrodes that directly contact the brain is markedly different (e.g. implanted electrodes produce electrochemical byproducts not relevant for non-invasive techniques such as tDCS). The conclusions derived from this chapter regarding safety, which mirror those of prior review and consensus statements, may inform ongoing ethical and regulatory decisions while not directly commenting on them (Fregni et al. 2015).

Definitions and Considerations of Dose Metrics for tDCS Safety

The terms "anodal" and "cathodal" can be misleading in tDCS, including in the context of safety, as both polarity electrodes are always present (there is always an anode electrode and a cathode electrode) and all current that enters the brain must exit, passing through brain regions between the electrodes (Bikson et al. 2010). Indeed, the folding of the cortex (sulci and gyri) results in cortical current flow polarity inversions with respect to the cortical surface even under a single electrode (Datta et al. 2009). Therefore, we do not attempt here to develop separate safety criterion in humans for "anodal" or "cathodal" tDCS. For the purposes of aggregating number of stimulation sessions, so-called "anodal" and "cathodal" tDCS are naturally collapsed, and tDCS safety data across polarities are grouped except where there are specific hypotheses to consider polarity specific effects. For animal DCS studies we not distinguish between polarity specific results, rather we collapse across polarities to obtain a conservative injury estimate. While differences in the two polarities with regard to injury thresholds and mechanisms are expected (depending on the mechanism of injury) here we are concerned with the minimum threshold regardless of polarity. An exception to collapsing across polarities will be made in our discussion of testing on seizures, where, for reasons explained in that section, the positions of the cathode and anode are noted.

We review data from human trials of tDCS by dose (Fig. 6.1). To obtain a coherent meta-analysis of tDCS, inevitably some testing conditions are collapsed (Nitsche et al. 2015) (e.g. electrode size, age and medical condition in a comparison of 1 mA intensity in adults with epilepsy using 25 cm^2 electrodes vs. 1 mA intensity in healthy children using 35 cm^2 electrodes). It is conventional to assume that risk increases monotonically with current intensity or duration (e.g. all else being equal, decreasing current from 2 mA to 1 mA maintains or reduces theoretical risk). In some sections, we aggregate data by current and/or duration (e.g. total number of sessions at 1 mA and 10 min), and we assume a monotonic dose-response relationship (e.g. the safety of 1 mA is supported by the total number of sessions at 1 mA or more). However, this collapsing of data is inherently problematic precisely

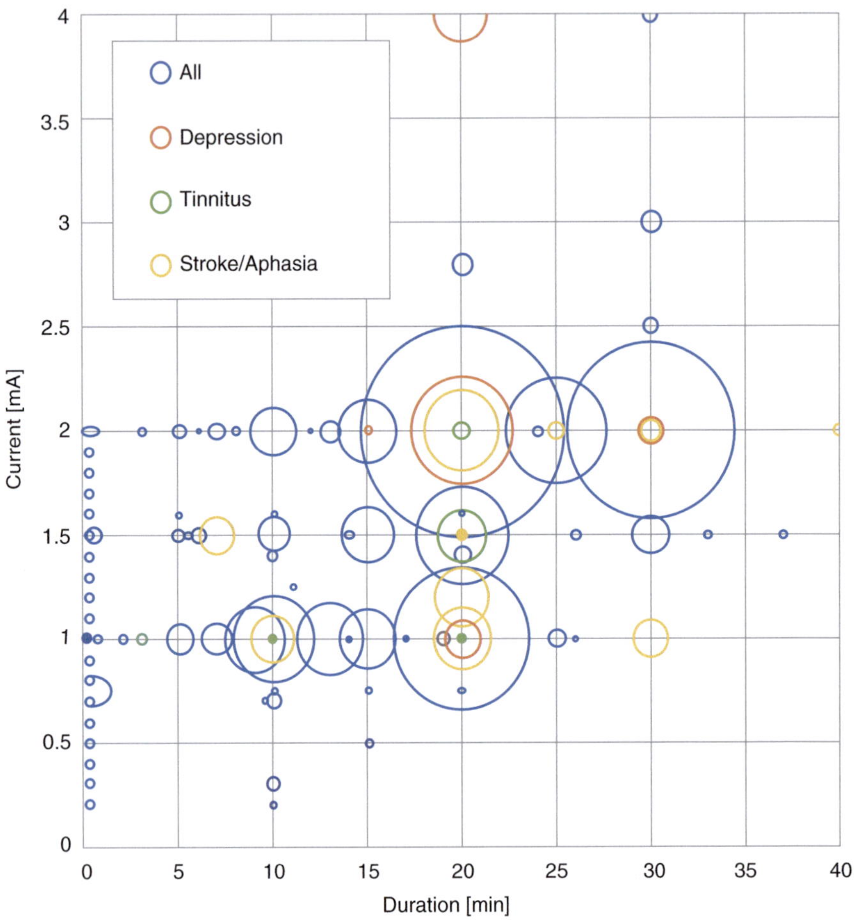

Fig. 6.1 tDCS sessions applied to date to all subjects, or those with depression, tinnitus or stroke/aphasia, by current and duration. Area of bubble corresponds to number of sessions applied at experimental conditions

because it ignores all other factors such as pre-existing morbidity. Evaluating risk factors by considering theoretically vulnerable (susceptible) populations have been addressed in the 2016 consensus (Bikson et al. 2016).

Prior efforts to assess tDCS safety proposed safety standards based on summary metrics (Liebetanz et al. 2009; Sundaram et al. 2009) such as charge (which combines stimulation intensity and time), current density (which combines intensity and electrode size), or charge density (which combines intensity, time, duration, and electrode size). On the one hand, summary metrics are appealing because they simplify analysis (e.g. 1 mA for 10 min, 2 mA for 5 min, and 10 mA for 1 min are equivalent from the perspective of charge). But, basing safety standards on summary metrics presupposes that critical details are not lost in combining terms such as current and duration. Moreover, it assumes no important interaction between dose terms and other factors such as inclusion criteria or brain state. Summary metrics are based on simple math (e.g. electrode charge density is charge divides by electrode area) rather than any detail model of the tissue or current flow patterns. For this last reason, there is a mismatch between summary metrics based on dose (what is applied outside the body) and complex or subject-specific current flow in the brain. Any reliance on a summary metric is further limited by the absence of established mechanisms for injury; this makes it difficult to know which stimulation properties are most relevant to safety and, hence, how to select relevant summary metrics. Thus, while useful in other contexts, safety discussion based on summary metrics is limited in this chapter.

There are additional "distributed" metrics of stimulation that can be predicted based on the underlying tissue properties and are not single values, but rather distributed values specific to locations within the brain. These include **current density** (in mA/m^2) that reflects the current flow distribution and intensity through the body. **Electric field** (in V/m) is current density multiplied by local tissue resistivity. The peak current density or electric field represents the maximum value at any point in space, which can be further restricted by head region such as peak current density in the brain or skin. **Power density** (in mW/m^3) is electric field multiplied by current density. The electric field predicts neuronal activation threshold more meaningfully than current density, but it is very sensitive to assumptions on local tissue resistivity. It is also not established whether injury is linked to neuronal activation (e.g. excitotoxic) or other factors. The above tissue properties are not time dependent, but can be combined with time in new metrics.

To control for unsafe tDCS practice, studies in which electrodes were not prepared following established methods are excluded. For included studies, stimulation is applied over skin that is not compromised by a pre-existing burn or injury (e.g. open wound) and is thus largely homogenous. Acne, however, is typically not an exclusion for electrode locations. Skin preparation does not typically include significant abrasion (intended to remove epidermis; (Shiozawa et al. 2013)), though cleaning of the skin/hair with saline or alcohol is sometimes used (Dasilva et al. 2011). Standard tDCS electrodes (pads) are typically square 5 × 5 cm or 5 × 7 cm, though both smaller and larger electrode assemblies have been explored (Nitsche et al. 2007). There is relatively limited data on circular pads. Standard tDCS electrode assemblies use either metal or conductive rubber electrodes (Kronberg and Bikson 2012). Electrolytes are most commonly isotonic saline (saturated in a sponge that wraps around the electrode), but conductive gels and/or creams have also been used. The details of electrode assembly design are considered important for tolerability and skin safety. For example, it is important to maintain a minimal distance between the electrode and skin, as well as the area of the electrode compared to the electrolyte-skin area (Kronberg and Bikson 2012). Pad electrodes, by virtue of size and materials, are typically limited in number to a maximum of 3–4. High-Definition (HD) electrodes are circular ~1 cm diameter with a sintered Ag/AgCl electrode and conductive gel or paste (Minhas et al. 2010). Because of this smaller size, a higher number and density of HD electrodes may be applied on the scalp (Dmochowski et al. 2012, 2013). When one or more HD electrodes are used, tDCS is called High-Definition tDCS (HD-tDCS) regardless of the number of electrodes or if stimulation is optimized for focality or intensity (Dmochowski et al. 2011). Except when indicated, our analysis is not specific to electrode design (e.g. HD-tDCS is "conventional" as long as meeting current, duration, and charge limits).

Definition and Considerations of Serious Adverse Effects for tDCS Safety

Following the evidence-based approach established in the 2016 consensus (Bikson et al. 2016), this chapter considers tDCS safety to indicate the absence of a Serious Adverse Effect, including brain tissue injury, related to tDCS application. It is necessary to precisely define this threshold for safety for clinical trials and separately for experiments in translational animal models.

Based on a prior consensus (Bikson et al. 2016), which in turn adapted prior standards including International and US guidelines on serious adverse events from medical devices (including the Office of Human Research and Protection (OHRP) of the U.S. Department of Health And Human Services (HSS); FDA regulations at 21 CFR 312.32[a]; 1996 International Conference on Harmonization E-6 Guidelines for Good Clinical Practice; ISO/DIS 14155 – Clinical investigations of medical devices in humans, good clinical practices, 2008), this chapter classifies a Serious Adverse Effect related to tDCS as a documented event that:

1. Is reported in a published clinical trial AND
2. Based upon scientific judgment is determined to be caused or aggravated by the application of direct current to the head, such that serious adverse *events* not linked to stimulation are excluded, even if they are subject to reporting requirements AND
3. EITHER Results in irreversible damage of brain tissue OR
4. Results in lasting disability or incapacity with a substantial disruption of a person's ability to conduct normal life functions, i.e., the adverse effect resulted in an unwanted significant, persistent or permanent change, impairment, damage or disruption in the patient's body function/structure, physical activities and/or quality of life OR
5. Results in otherwise unexpected inpatient hospitalization or prolongation of existing hospitalization, where emergency room visits that do not result in admission to the hospital should be evaluated for one of the other serious outcomes (e.g., life-threatening; required intervention to prevent permanent impairment or damage; other serious medically important event) OR
6. Results in death or is life-threatening where the patient was at substantial risk of dying as a result of the adverse event, or use was discontinued based on evidence tDCS might have resulted in death OR
7. Medical or surgical intervention was considered necessary to mitigate risk of permanent imminent impairment of a body function due to tDCS, or to prevent or minimize permanent damage to a body due to tDCS

Per criteria 1, our analysis is restricted to events reported in the scientific literature from human trials. A report meeting any of criteria 3 through 6, but not 2, would be a serious adverse *event*. As explicitly defined above, for the purpose of this chapter a Serious Adverse Effect requires a causal link with tDCS application. For example, serious adverse events potentially related only to a pre-existing condition or other activity in the trial (e.g. a fall unrelated to stimulation) would not meet the above criteria. Similarly, study dropouts are not necessarily Serious Adverse Effects. Reversible skin irritation not requiring medical intervention to prevent permanent injury would not meet the above criteria. Sensation and transient pain (tingling, itching) are similarly not relevant for safety though they impact tolerability and compliance. Changes in clinical symptoms are not considered a Serious Adverse Effect, unless proven to meet the above criteria; nor are transient decrements in cognition or behavior (Pirulli et al. 2014). As defined for this chapter, absence of a reported serious adverse event indicates lack of evidence for a Serious Adverse Effect.

Theoretical long-lasting changes in neuronal morphology (e.g. spine density, synaptic plasticity) or EEG activity (e.g. alpha oscillation power, ERP magnitude) are not considered a Serious Adverse Effect unless proven to meet the above criteria. Clinical and animal studies exploring long-lasting changes remain an important but challenging area of research.

Because establishing causality (and thus meeting criteria for a Serious Adverse Effect) can be difficult, human subject protection protocols often adopt predetermined and measurable stopping criteria to manage adverse events. Specific rules for subject withdrawal and/or trial cessation are designed to minimize risk in a real-time manner, which is distinct from a trial designed to establish safety. For example, in a trial of tDCS for epilepsy, stop criteria may include: (1) discontinuation of the session if the frequency of interictal discharges or seizures increases by 60% above baseline in the 2 h after stimulation or (2) cessation of the study if over 40% of subjects in a stimulation study have a 60% increase of seizure frequency in the first 36 h after tDCS. Such rules provide an objective standard for an investigator deciding whether a given event was serious enough to *potentially cause harm* to the patient regardless of causality. Then, in later analysis and discussion, a determination of *probable causality* can be decided. This methodology errs on the side of safety for ongoing trials. However as defined here, subject withdrawal or session/trial stop for a serious event is not necessarily a Serious Adverse Effect until causality is established.

As the case across medical research, in some tDCS trials insufficient data are collected, or details reported, to confirm causality of adverse events or whether a dropout might relate to a Serious Adverse Effect. Methods for subject monitoring and potential standardization in tolerability/safety outcomes is not in the scope of this chapter but has been considered elsewhere. Cases where causality with tDCS application is ambiguous do not meet this chapter's standard for a Serious Adverse Effect, but such examples show the desirability for more detailed reporting on adverse events.

If tDCS is applied with the intention to produce an abnormal brain state, for example to interrupt normal brain processing, then the abnormal brain state would be expected and appropriate safety measures would be in place if needed (e.g. hospitalization). Therefore, this is not considered a Serious Adverse Effect. In this sense (extrapolating from related fields and standards), the intentional generation of a seizure by electroconvulsive therapy (ECT) or magnetic seizure therapy (MST) is not a Serious Adverse Effect, while the unintentional generation of seizures in rTMS is a Serious Adverse Effect.

One potential limitation of using "evidence-based" causality to establish the criterion of Severe Adverse Effect is that it may not be possible to empirically determine whether causal relationships exist between very rare events and tDCS due to lack of data. In the absence of sufficient data to establish these links, the causality criterion of severe adverse effects may theoretically obscure very uncommon but causally related events, creating a bias toward judging tDCS to be safe. Nonetheless, sham-controlled trials are the best way to empirically assess adverse effects, including serious ones, and this chapter addresses the scale of data collected to date.

Assumptions Regarding Dose-Response Curves for Safety Data from Animal Studies

In summarizing animal safety data, the approach adopted here was to use the lowest current intensity documented to produce a measurable destructive brain tissue response in an animal model at any stimulation duration. This approach has its own limitations and assumptions. In any given experimental series, the limitations on both the precision of current increments tested and the number of animals tested will limit validation of a single lowest damage threshold. Alternatively, the entire data set may consolidate a curve-fit to extrapolate a minimum damage threshold. Though the quality of curve fit may support this approach, assumptions on the type of dose-response curve for damage will profoundly influence the resulting extrapolation, notably to low doses not actually tested. For example, dose-response projections based on injury at moderate intensity would ignore if lower intensities might in fact provide protection from injury (e.g.. also called "hormetic" dose response; (Calabrese, 2016; Calabrese et al. 2015)). Especially in the absence of a mechanistic explanation for damage supporting a particular dose-response curve, accumulation of data from different model systems and varying lesion measures we avoided extrapolation beyond tested stimulation intensities. For the same reason, we avoided putative summary-metrics of damage, such as charge or charge-density; but as the animal trials cited used stimulation durations equal to or greater than clinical tDCS, limits based simply on current can be considered conservative with regards to summary metrics influenced by time – assuming a monotonic relationship between stimulation duration and injury at any given intensity.

Additional assumptions about dose-response relationships are made. Experimental studies are often limited in time points for measurement (since the collection of tissue for analysis often requires terminal procedures), so we assume that damage is irreversible and that delayed damage responses cannot be excluded. Again, without an established mechanism for damage, we limit ourselves here to reported data.

The sensitivity of damage detection is evidently limited by the experimental measures. In addition, the relative sensitivity of animal tissue to DCS versus human tissue to tDCS is unclear. While arbitrary safety factors are sometimes applied in developing guidance, our goal here is to summarize injury evidence. In developing human safety guidelines, it is prudent not to approach injury thresholds, especially with montage and inter-individual differences. Consolidated animal DCS safety data, when scaled to the human case using computational models, indicates that at least with regards to manifest tissue damage, current conventional tDCS protocols are orders of magnitude below injury threshold.

DCS Safety Data from Animal Lesion Studies and Translational Models

Data on DCS lesion threshold in animals have been used to support the safety of existing tDCS protocols, with evidence demonstrating the wide gap between current tDCS protocols and DCS lesion thresholds, provides some reassurance (Bikson et al. 2009; Liebetanz et al. 2009). However, with increasing adoption of tDCS, these data warrant updating.

The issues when basing human safety standards on animal histology thresholds were previous outlined (Sawyer et al. 1989) and include: (1) potential differences in susceptibility of animal and human tissue to damage; (2) experimental limits on detecting various modes of damage including assumptions about dose-response relationships; (3) difference in scale from rodent (or other nonhuman) to human gross anatomy; (4) difference in method of stimulation (e.g. transdermal vs. epicranial). The use of animal models provides the distinct advantage of being able to histologically assess the impact of current on brain tissue. The results from animal models can thereby inform current threshold limits and, in addition, be used to validate and improve the computational models used for determining predictive safety thresholds in humans.

Tissue damage from animal studies using electrodes in direct contact with the brain or using other waveforms (e.g. AC) are largely inappropriate (and potentially misleading) for establishing tDCS safety guidelines (Bikson et al. 2009). Here, results from three groups of testing safety thresholds for epicranial DCS are consolidated, acknowledging the limitations of the different methods of lesion detection (e.g. hematoxylin-eosin (H&E) staining is potentially less sensitive than the direct staining of neurodegeneration by Fluoro-Jade C): (i) Liebetanz and colleagues

(Liebetanz et al. 2009), (ii) Fritsch and colleagues (unpublished data), (iii) Jankord and colleagues (unpublished data). In all cases DCS was applied to the surface of a rat skull using a relatively small electrode-contact (defined as the electrolyte-skull interface) compared to the return electrode on the body. The lowest DCS intensity at which histological damage was detected in the three studies were as follows: (i) Liebetanz, 500 μA applied through 2.1 mm diameter circular electrode-contact for 10 min (return electrode on the chest), assessed by H&E stain (used for histological assessment of tissue following current exposure); (ii) Fritsch, 600 μA applied through 4 mm diameter circular electrode-contact for 20 min (return electrode on the chest), assessed by FluoroJade C stain; (iii) Jankord, 500 μA applied through 5 × 5 mm square electrode-contact for 60 min (return electrode behind the neck), assessed by H&E stain.

To scale these results to humans, we developed a high-resolution rat model and predicted brain current flow produced for each montage used. The predicted minimum induced current density for detected damage was 12, 17, and 6.3 A/m^2 for Liebetanz et al. Fritsch et al. and Jankord et al. respectively. By comparing resulting peak current density (or electric field) per applied mA in the rat brain to the peak electric field produced per mA in the human brain, we are able to propose a scaling factor from DCS to tDCS. Specifically, the scaling factor allows us to predict how much current should be applied in the human using a representative montage (M1-SO adult) to approximate the brain electric field produced in a rat for a given current. Note the M1-SO montage is among the most commonly used in tDCS but does not produce the theoretically maximum brain electric field. Applying this scaling factor to the current intensity damage threshold observed in rat allows us to predict a current intensity damage threshold in humans. The scaling factor determined was 288 for Fritsch et al. 240 for Liebetanz et al. and 134 for the Jankord et al. studies. Combining the reported current-thresholds for damage in animal models with the respective rat-to-human scaling factors results in a predicted human damage threshold of 173 mA based on Fritsch, 120 mA based on Liebetanz, and 67 mA based on Jankord. These scaled values are over an order of magnitude above maximum currents levels used during tDCS. Differences across animal models are expected and arise from additional dose metrics (e.g. time, which model based scaling does not account for), and which are neglected for the purpose of the chapter. If separate scaling factors are used (e.g. average electrode current density as opposed to model based scaling) or additional dose metrics considered, then different animal-to-human scaling factors would be predicted for each study. *This analysis does not in any way constitute an endorsement for the use of such high current in humans but serves only to illustrate the vast difference between current producing observable tissue damage in animal models and current used in conventional tDCS.*

Kim et al. (2010) assessed whether anodal DCS increases pre-existing infarct volume in a rat stroke model 2 days post-injury. Their results showed no increase in volume at the doses tested (0.785 cm^2 epicranial electrode, 0.1 mA for 20 min), and a potential neuro-protective effect. Cathodal DCS at 0.2 mA has also been shown to have a protective effect for ischemic stroke in rats (Baba et al. 2009). These results suggest that the safety threshold predicted above extends to post-injury models. Results in the mouse model differ from those in the rat. Peruzzotti-Jametti and colleagues (2013) suggest anodal stimulation induced an increase in the post-ischemic lesion volume and augmented blood brain barrier derangement in a mouse model with 1.2 mm diameter epicranial stimulation at 0.25 mA for 40 min total, while cathodal stimulation had a protective effect. Importantly, decreased mouse head volume compared to the rat suggests a further scaling factor – which if ≥2 brings this result in line with those in healthy rats. However, it is important to note that several studies in the acute and subacute phase of recovery have been successfully conducted in humans (see above) without reported serious adverse events (Cho and Cha 2015; Fusco et al. 2014b; Kim et al. 2014; Sattler et al. 2015; Tahtis et al. 2014).

tDCS Safety Data from Human Trials and Models

There is direct support for the safety of tDCS as applied thus far in controlled human trials (previously reviewed in (Brunoni et al. 2011, 2012)). Though mild skin erythema is common during tDCS, it is not inherently hazardous (Guarienti et al. 2015) and resolves after stimulation. tDCS was not found to produce edema or injurious alterations of the blood-brain barrier or cerebral tissue detectable by MRI (Nitsche et al. 2004), though non-injurious reversible changes in brain perfusion are plausible (Mielke et al. 2013; Wachter et al. 2011) as a result of direct action on endothelial cells or indirectly via modulation of neuronal (metabolic) activity.

During tDCS the ratio of current density in the skin to the brain is predicted to exceed 10:1 (Minhas et al. 2011). If one assumes comparable sensitivity to injury of skin and brain, then the tolerability to tDCS evidenced by lack of skin lesions provides indirect support for safety with respect to the brain. For example, tDCS produces negligible temperature changes in the skin (Minhas et al. 2010), making direct injury from brain heating improbable. Poor electrode skin contact (dry sponges) will lead to skin irritation (e.g. by dramatically reducing the stimulation area, which increases current density). In rare cases, poorly designed or prepared electrodes produced skin lesions (Frank et al. 2010; Palm et al. 2014; Rodríguez et al. 2014; Wang et al. 2015). If these are attributed to electrochemical reactions produced locally at the electrode (Bikson et al. 2009; Minhas et al. 2010), it would not be relevant for brain injury since chemical products above the skin surface are not expected to diffuse into the brain. Important factors in electrode design and preparation have been reviewed (Woods et al. 2015).

The maximum current density generated in the brain will vary according to montage and head anatomy for a given applied current. The resulting current density can be quantified using computational models and demonstrated experimentally (Edwards et al. 2013). In susceptible populations, current flow to the head may be further altered by pathological changes in the cranium or brain tissue such as stroke. This may also be the case in patients with post-surgical or trauma-induced skull defects or post-stroke encephalomalacia (Datta et al. 2011, 2010). In children, further divergence from expected current flow may be attributable to an immature brain anatomy (Gillick et al. 2014; Kessler et al. 2013). Across heads and montages, the maximum predicted brain current density (0.23 A/m^2 for a small adult head and 0.32 A/m^2 for pediatric head) remains substantially below injury threshold levels found in animals (6.3–17 A/m^2, described in detail below). Peak current densities in the modeling literature (spanning head sizes, model parameterization and tDCS dose) range from 0.0828 to 0.211 A/m^2 (Laakso and Hirata 2013; Mekonnen et al. 2012; Rampersad et al. 2014; Sadleir et al. 2010). At these predicted current densities, we are not aware of any well-defined theoretical risk for brain injury by tDCS based on experiments or modeling.

Controlled human studies involving the general population, susceptible subjects (e.g. children), and potentially susceptible (e.g. subjects with altered neuroanatomy or neurophysiology) populations support safety in tDCS application (Grecco et al. 2014a, b; Mattai et al. 2011; Vestito et al. 2014). We are aware of no direct evidence from human trials involving tDCS that suggests tissue damage or behavioral changes indicative of irreversible brain injury. Though methodology and rigor for reporting adverse events in tDCS are inconsistent across studies (Brunoni et al. 2011a; Kessler et al. 2012; Mcintire et al. 2014; Morales-Quezada et al. 2015; Nitsche et al. 2003; Poreisz et al. 2007; Raimundo et al. 2012; Russo et al. 2013; Tadini et al. 2011) human trials (per IRB guidance) should have specifically designed safety monitoring and reporting. Especially given the severity of a serious adverse event as defined above and mandatory reporting requirements defined in CFR, the lack of Serious Adverse Effect report in any trial supports the absence of occurrence. A meta-analysis of the aggregate number of tDCS sessions failed to identify even a single record of Serious Adverse Effect related to tDCS across >33,200 sessions. Among these over 1000 subjects received tDCS repeatedly (multiple sessions across days) without Serious Adverse Effect (Fig. 6.2).

The acceleration in the number of publications is not associated with a general increase in trial size (number of subjects) or period of trial (number of sessions per trial). This is consistent with tDCS being adopted by increasingly more independent groups as well increased activity within groups, and so more investigators in general. Demographics suggest a majority of sessions were applied to healthy subjects. This is consistent with the use of tDCS to study normal brain function under the assumption tDCS is minimal risk. The treatment of a broad range of indications has been explored by tDCS. Distribution of sessions by medical indications often reflects the size of trials rather than number of publications (e.g. tinnitus) (Fig. 6.3). The distribution and diversity of clinical trials with tDCS support the generalization of overall safety findings.

There are also data on individual patients who have received over 100 treatment sessions of tDCS without any indication of adverse effects arising from cumulative exposure. These include a patient with schizophrenia who received maintenance

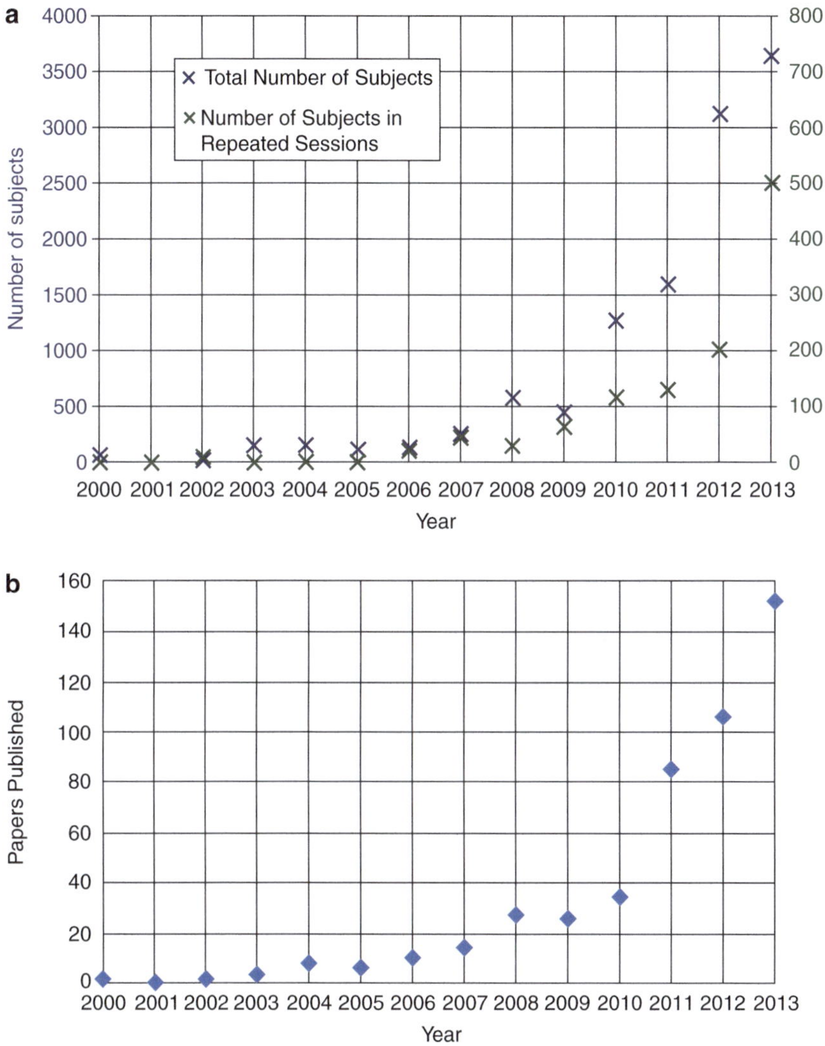

Fig. 6.2 (**a**) Total number of subjects who received tDCS and total number of subjects who received repeated sessions (more than 4 sessions per week) per year (**b**) Total number of tDCS papers published per year

tDCS once to twice daily on a domiciliary basis over a three-year period (i.e. > 1000 sessions) (Andrade 2013); and patients with depression who received multiple courses of tDCS (>100 sessions in total) safely, assessed with structured questionnaires of side effects and formal neuropsychological testing (Tadini et al. 2011). Further, 33 healthy volunteers received up to 30 sessions of tDCS over the course of 6 weeks (2 mA, 20 min, high-performance adhesive electrodes) without a serious adverse event (Paneri et al. 2015).

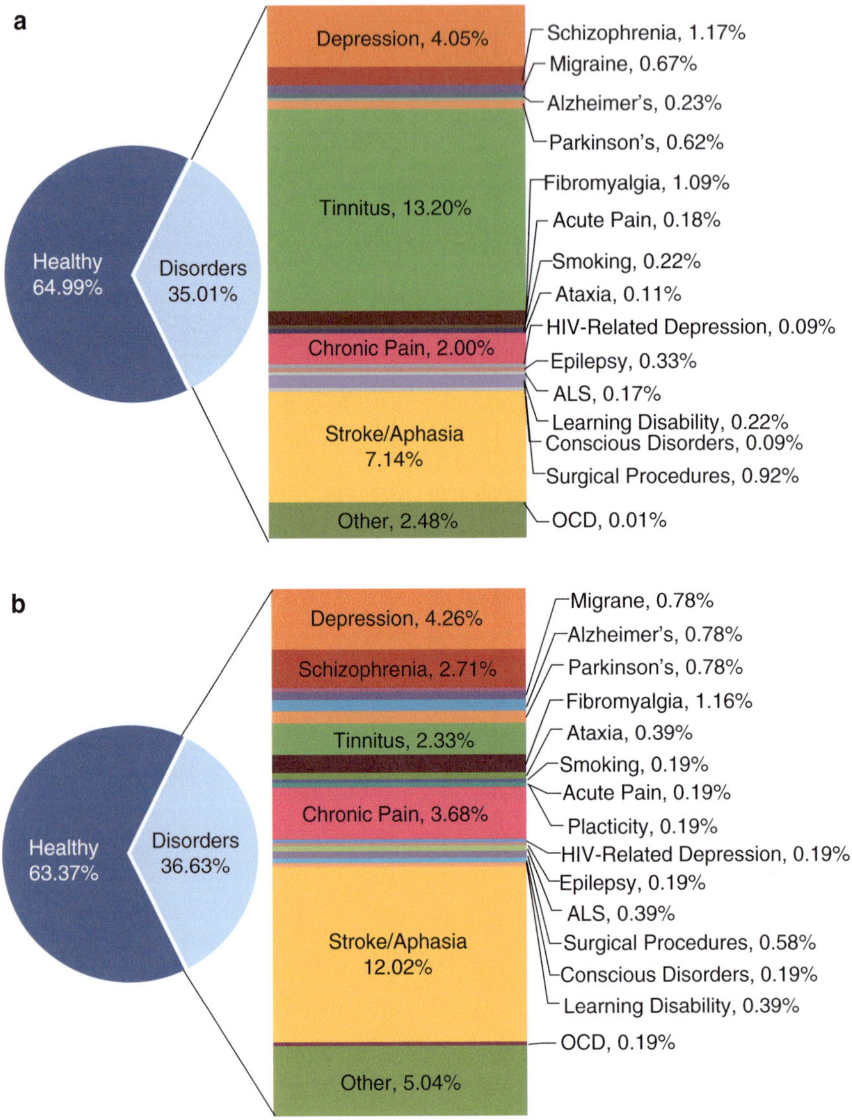

Fig. 6.3 Medical conditions of subjects treated with tDCS, as reported in the papers analyzed (**a**). Papers published by medical conditions of subjects (**b**)

To our knowledge, the US FDA considers trials of tDCS as non-significant-risk, which means tDCS is without reasonable expectation of any Serious Adverse Effect (as defined here). The FDA requires reporting of "unanticipated" adverse events. As of the publication of this chapter, the FDA "MedWatch" database search returns no reports for "tDCS" or "transcranial Direct Current Stimulation." A similar research status approval is in place from Health Canada and internationally (Fregni et al. 2015).

tDCS Special Consideration for Safety in Children

As is typical for most investigational techniques, experience with tDCS in children has been limited compared to adults, and applications in the developing brain require additional considerations. Fewer than 5% of published tDCS studies include pediatric populations. In children, considerations include potential modification of dosing for both safety and efficacy. Specific systems and techniques for recording, side-effects, potential adverse events and effects, and tolerability measures are required.

In trials involving children, at least 2800 sessions have been applied across nearly 500 subjects. No Serious Adverse Effects have been reported. tDCS has been investigated in children with a variety of diagnoses including cerebral palsy, stroke, encephalitis, epilepsy, schizophrenia, and attention-deficit hyperactivity disorder (Andrade 2013; Aree-uea et al. 2014; Auvichayapat et al. 2013; Cosmo et al. 2015; Duarte Nde et al. 2014; Gillick et al. 2015; Grecco et al. 2014a, b, c; Mattai et al. 2011; San-Juan et al. 2011a; Young et al. 2013). According to clinicaltrials.gov, current studies in pediatric applications of tDCS include perinatal stroke, cerebral palsy, dystonia, childhood-onset schizophrenia, attention deficit hyperactivity disorder, and autism. The relatively limited nature of this tDCS experience across pediatric populations as compared to that of adults is shown in Fig. 6.4. Combining this emerging pediatric evidence with the larger animal and

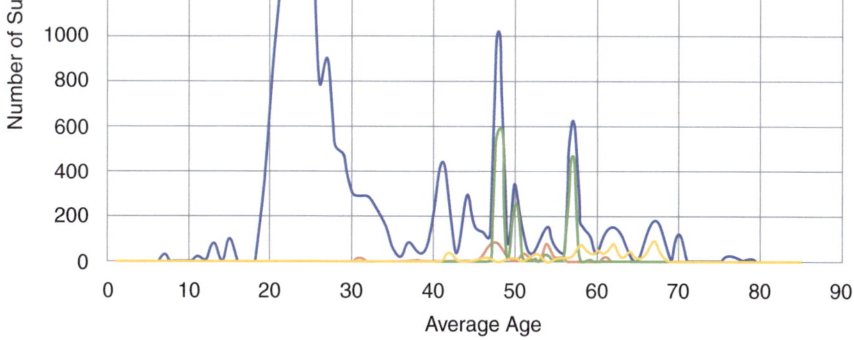

Fig. 6.4 Number of subjects to date who received tDCS sessions by average age. Articles that provided age data of subjects were included, and the average age, rounded down to the closest year, was applied to all subjects in paper. Number of subjects with depression, tinnitus and stroke/aphasia by age were also noted. These medical conditions were included because they had the largest number of subjects

adult experience suggests tDCS within the same ranges of dosing and duration can be considered minimal risk, based on current evidence, in school-aged children.

tDCS Special Considerations for Safety in Aging Populations

Given the increasingly older demographic of our national population, there is a growing interest in tDCS as a mechanism for stabilizing, or even enhancing, cognitive functioning in older adults (Anton et al. 2015). It is established that particular aspects of cognitive decline, even during "normal" aging (Salthouse 2010), are exacerbated by incipient neurodegenerative diseases. It is important to distinguish between increased risks arising from unrelated comorbidities in these subjects, such as increased risk of seizures and other comorbid medical conditions, including neurodegenerative disease (Stephen and Brodie 2000), from evidence that aging subjects are at increased risk for Serious Adverse Effects during tDCS. As in other situations, exclusion of subjects from tDCS human trials for pre-existing conditions is not necessarily evidence by itself for increased risk.

Building on the results of a recent review in this content area (Hsu et al. 2015), we identified a total of 19 tDCS studies that targeted a range of motor and cognitive abilities (Berryhill and Jones 2012; Boggio et al. 2010; Fertonani et al. 2014; Flöel et al. 2012; Goodwill et al. 2013; Hardwick and Celnik 2014; Harty et al. 2014; Holland et al. 2011; Jones et al. 2015; Liebetanz et al. 2009; Manenti et al. 2013; Meinzer et al. 2014; Meinzer et al. 2013; Parikh and Cole 2015; Park et al. 2014; Puri et al. 2015; Ross et al. 2011; Sandrini et al. 2014; Zhou et al. 2015). These 19 studies included over 500 participants whose mean ages were in the mid to late 60's. Across studies, participants received between 1 and 10 sessions of tDCS, with a duration of 5–30 min, at an intensity of 1 to 2 mA. Five studies failed to report any safety data (Berryhill and Jones 2012; Flöel et al. 2012; Jones et al. 2015; Puri et al. 2015; Ross et al. 2011) (which this chapter considers evidence for the absence of a serious adverse event), and one reportedly asked about side effects but failed to report any data (Hardwick and Celnik 2014). None of the remaining 13 studies reported any adverse events (serious or otherwise). Five studies made limited comments about all participants tolerating treatment well (Manenti et al. 2014; Parikh and Cole 2015; Park et al. 2014; Sandrini et al. 2014; Zhou et al. 2015), and the other eight reported expected sensory experiences (e.g., itching, tingling, burning) that were generally indistinguishable from those reported by participants receiving sham stimulation.

If effective, tDCS could be particularly beneficial for treating cognitive, motor, and psychiatric symptoms of neurodegenerative diseases, as well as decline in health associated with normal aging (see reviews by (Elder and Taylor 2014; Hsu et al. 2015)). We identified 15 studies that evaluated the effects of tDCS on patients with Alzheimer's disease (Boggio et al. 2009, 2012; Cotelli et al. 2014a; Ferrucci et al. 2008; Khedr et al. 2014; Suemoto et al. 2014), Parkinson's Disease (Benninger et al. 2010; Boggio et al. 2006; Doruk et al. 2014; Fregni et al. 2006a; Kaski et al. 2014; Manenti et al. 2014), Dementia with Lewy Bodies (Elder et al. 2015), Corticobasal degeneration (Manenti et al. 2015), and Frontotemporal dementia (Cotelli et al. 2014b). In all, there were over 275 subjects (some assigned to sham conditions) who received between 7 and 30 min of stimulation in each of 1 to 10 sessions with an intensity of between 1 and 2.8 mA. Ten studies comment on safety. One patient was removed from treatment after experiencing delirium caused by pneumonia, and another patient experienced a bout of diarrhea and could not attend some of the tDCS sessions (Suemoto et al. 2014). Neither of these events appear to be attributable to tDCS and thus are not considered Serious Adverse Effects for this chapter. Four studies reported typical side effects (e.g., itching, tingling, burning) (Doruk et al. 2014; Elder et al. 2015; Suemoto et al. 2014), as well as temporary headache and dizziness (Khedr et al. 2014). It is also worthwhile to note that a review of eight tDCS studies in the geriatric depression literature found no major side effects of stimulation (Gálvez et al. 2015).

Overall, there were no unexpected or serious adverse events in >40 studies with >600 older adults regardless of cognitive or disease status. There is thus no current evidence for increased risk of Serious Adverse Effects with aging subjects.

Risk of tDCS-Related Seizures and Use in Epilepsy

As defined for our purposes, a Serious Adverse Effect for tDCS would include the triggering of a seizure, either in healthy individuals, individuals with epilepsy or others predisposed to seizures, with evidence that tDCS was causally related to the ictal event. Encouragingly, no such instances have been reported in published human trials.

Clinical experience with tDCS in epilepsy patients indicates the procedure is well-tolerated and safe (Brunoni et al. 2012). When a cathode electrode is positioned over epileptogenic cortex, there may be a mild anti-epileptogenic effect, manifest as reduced interictal discharge frequency (San-Juan et al. 2015). There have been several studies investigating the effect of tDCS with the cathode positioned over the targeted cortex on reducing seizure frequency and focal hyperexcitability in partial onset seizures (six original studies published in English in a recently published meta-analysis, (San-Juan et al. 2015)). In a randomized, sham-controlled study applying a single session of tDCS (1 mA, 20 min) with the cathode over the epileptogenic zone and the anode placed over an area without epileptiform activity, there was a significant reduction in the frequency of interictal epileptiform discharges, with a trend towards decrease in seizure frequency (Fregni et al. 2006b). In another study involving 36 children with partial epilepsy, a single session of tDCS (1 mA, 20 min) with the cathode directed toward the target suppressed epileptiform activity for 48 h and demonstrated seizure reduction (Auvichayapat et al. 2013). Several case reports and small case series similarly suggest tDCS is well-tolerated with the cathode over epileptogenic cortex (San-Juan et al. 2011b; Yook et al. 2011), including transient reduction in spike frequency in continuous spike and waves during slow wave sleep (Faria et al. 2012). As with other indication, while ongoing research on efficacy and dose optimization to enhance effect size is warranted, in regards to safety (as defined for the purposes of this chapter) there is no evidence for increased risk for patients with epilepsy.

Special Considerations for Susceptible Populations and Subjects with Implants

In the 33 studies considered of tDCS in persons with stroke published since 2014, there are 2 studies reporting minor adverse events (Gillick et al. 2015; Kim et al. 2014) including mild headache, sleepiness, and various sensations. In addition, there are few reports of dropouts with 14 out of 507 total participants from 6 studies (Cho and Cha 2015; Fusco et al. 2014a; Gillick et al. 2015; Lee and Chun 2014; Smit et al. 2015; Wu et al. 2015) across 33 studies. Reporting criteria and reasons for dropouts vary and include personal reasons (e.g. unrelated medical problems, refusal to participate, etc.) that were not Serious Adverse Effects as defined in this chapter. To date, we identified no persistent decrements in behavioral performance or mood reported as a consequence of tDCS trials in stroke populations.

A theoretical concern is that the presence of skull defects may increase risk by creating a "funnel" of current through the skull, resulting in local concentrations of current density in the brain. Electrical field modeling suggests that typical tDCS protocols administered over a range of skull defects may result in local increase in current density compared to the intact-skull case, under worst-case theoretical conditions corresponding to a six-fold increase in brain current density (Datta et al. 2010; Opitz et al. 2015). This does not exceed the current density threshold for injury reported in animal models. Increases in brain current density can be prevented or minimized by adjusting electrode montage. The exclusion of subjects from some human trials because of pre-existing implants is not evidence for increased risk of a Serious Adverse Effect.

Treatment-emergent (hypo)mania (TEM) is a potential Serious Adverse Effect that can occur in depressed patients during pharmacologic antidepressant treatment, for instance, in up to 2.3% of patients with unipolar depression (Benvenuti et al. 2008). There are four stand-alone case reports in literature (Arul-Anandam et al. 2010; Baccaro et al. 2010; Brunoni et al. 2011b; Gálvez et al. 2011) and some reports in randomized clinical trials (Brunoni et al. 2013; Loo et al. 2012) of mania or hypomania induction after tDCS treatment. Most of these episodes resolved spontaneously when tDCS was withheld for a few days or with either small dose adjustments or introduction of a new pharmacotherapy. It is not possible to disentangle with confidence which intervention, or indeed if both interventions, was responsible for the symptoms and thus these were not Serious Adverse *Effects* as per the definition of this chapter. Thus, in trials for depression, more than 4160 sessions have been applied across more than 430 subjects without a documented Serious Adverse Effect.

For subjects with implants, *theoretical* concerns about increased susceptibility to tDCS include (1) injury to the brain related to changes in brain current flow pattern as a result of a conductive implant and/or associated skull defect, that can lead to a local current concentration, and (2) damage or disruption of device function, especially when the device includes an electrical sensing component (such as a pacemaker). Theoretical concern about interactions with pacemakers increases for extracephalic electrodes but remains hypothetical (Parazzini et al. 2013). Though exclusion of subjects with preexisting implants, especially head implants, is common in tDCS trials as a precautionary measure (Brunoni et al. 2012) – there is no evidence of injury to a subject with an implant and no theoretical risk of injury based on modeling. Limited ongoing experience with tDCS in subjects with both DBS and cortical electrode arrays (the latter for pre-epilepsy surgical monitoring) suggests that stimulation is tolerated (Esmaeilpour et al. 2017; Huang et al. 2017; Opitz et al. 2016). Thus, while pre-existing implants remain a theoretical concern, neither theory nor limited clinical experience establish evidence for increased risk of Serious Adverse Effects.

Extended Use and Home Use

With growing indications and data supporting extended (e.g. weeks of) treatment, home use, as opposed to in-clinic administration, is expected to become more common. Indeed, there is growing evidence that beneficial effects may be compounded with repeated sessions (Monte-Silva et al. 2013), including when paired with cognitive/behavioral programs (e.g. cognitive or physical exercises for recovery of function; see Chang et al. 2015; Mortensen et al. 2015; Tippett et al. 2015). Therefore, extended tDCS sessions over time may be essential to the effectiveness of many treatments. Home use may also be helpful to either sustain or continue an initial therapeutic benefit, possibly spanning months (e.g. 100+ sessions) (Andrade 2013; Ho et al. 2015). While testing remains limited (Hagenacker et al. 2014), in the context of human trials with approved equipment, there has been no established Serious Adverse Effects for home-use (including self-directed) tDCS. However, it is critical to distinguish between clinical trials of tDCS where home-use is carefully monitored and only specialized equipment is used, with any other approaches where the equipment and/or protocols are not medical grade. Only the former is within the scope of this chapter, and standards for medical grade home-use (e.g. Remote Supervised tDCS) are summarized next.

Importantly, the clinical study of tDCS with home use must be both safe and reliable. This means procedure must be reproducible and compliance measurable. Guidelines for home use in tDCS clinical trials have been developed, governed by remote-supervision through a telemedicine platform (Charvet et al. 2015). Critical to this "remote supervised tDCS" approach is specially-designed equipment that both carefully regulates and records use. Comprehensive training procedures and safety checks at each step can guide safe self-application or application by caregiver or other proxy (Kasschau et al. 2015).

Conclusions

This chapter examined safety of tDCS based on an explicit and limited definition of evidence of safety – which directly derives from the 2016 tDCS safety consensus. (Bikson et al. 2016). While recognizing the "absence of evidence is not evidence of absence," this approach is strictly data (evidence) limited, in the sense that we do not suggest injury where there is no proof. This chapter does not make specific recommendations or propose guidelines regarding new protocols (e.g. a new dose in a new population). Lack of evidence for risk should not be confused with suggesting that for any tDCS protocol safety monitoring is not important. As with any investigational technique, vigilance is warranted, and responsibility to manage risk rests with the trial sponsors and requires independent ethics review. But, at the same time, unscientific concerns (e.g. calls for "caution" ignoring existing evidence) can, in fact, impede research.

We show evidence supporting the fact that brain injury by DCS in animal models occurs at size-corrected intensities over an order of magnitude above the intensities used in conventional tDCS. To date, based on a total of over 33,000 sessions and over 1000 subjects who received repeated tDCS sessions, there is no evidence for irreversible injury produced by conventional tDCS protocols within a wide range of stimulation parameters ($\leq$40 min, $\leq$4 mA, $\leq$7.2 C). This analysis mirrors and updates the 2016 tDCS safety consensus (Bikson et al. 2016). These general conclusions are also in agreement with other analyses of safety (Antal et al. 2017; Moffa et al. 2017; Poreisz et al. 2007; Woods et al. 2015).

References

Andrade, C. (2013). Once- to twice-daily, 3-year domiciliary maintenance transcranial direct current stimulation for severe, disabling, clozapine-refractory continuous auditory hallucinations in schizophrenia. *The Journal of ECT, 29*, 239–242.

Antal, A., Alekseichuk, I., Bikson, M., Brockmöller, J., Brunoni, A. R., Chen, R., … Paulus, W. (2017). Low intensity transcranial electric stimulation: Safety, ethical, legal regulatory and application guidelines. *Clinical Neurophysiology, 128*, 1774–1809.

Anton, S. D., Woods, A. J., Ashizawa, T., Barb, D., Buford, T. W., Carter, C. S., … Pahor, M. (2015). Successful aging: Advancing the science of physical independence in older adults. *Ageing Research Reviews, 24*, 304–327.

Aree-uea, B., Auvichayapat, N., Janyacharoen, T., Siritaratiwat, W., Amatachaya, A., Prasertnoo, J., … Auvichayapat, P. (2014). Reduction of spasticity in cerebral palsy by anodal transcranial direct current stimulation. *Journal of the Medical Association of Thailand, 97*, 954–962.

Arul-Anandam, A. P., Loo, C., & Mitchell, P. (2010). Induction of hypomanic episode with transcranial direct current stimulation. *The Journal of ECT, 26*, 68–69.

Auvichayapat, N., Rotenberg, A., Gersner, R., Ngodklang, S., Tiamkao, S., Tassaneeyakul, W., & Auvichayapat, P. (2013). Transcranial direct current stimulation for treatment of refractory childhood focal epilepsy. *Brain Stimulation, 6*, 696–700.

Baba, T., Kameda, M., Yasuhara, T., Morimoto, T., Kondo, A., Shingo, T., … Date, I. (2009). Electrical stimulation of the cerebral cortex exerts antiapoptotic, angiogenic, and anti-inflammatory effects in ischemic stroke rats through phosphoinositide 3-kinase/Akt signaling pathway. *Stroke, 40*, e598–e605.

Baccaro, A., Brunoni, A. R., Bensenor, I. M., & Fregni, F. (2010). Hypomanic episode in unipolar depression during transcranial direct current stimulation. *Acta Neuropsychiatrica, 22*, 316–318.

Benninger, D. H., Lomarev, M., Lopez, G., Wassermann, E. M., Li, X., Considine, E., & Hallett, M. (2010). Transcranial direct current stimulation for the treatment of Parkinson's disease. *Journal of Neurology, Neurosurgery, and Psychiatry, 81*, 1105–1111.

Benvenuti, A., Rucci, P., Miniati, M., Papasogli, A., Fagiolini, A., Cassano, G. B., … Frank, E. (2008). Treatment-emergent mania/hypomania in unipolar patients. *Bipolar Disorders, 10*, 726–732.

Berryhill, M. E., & Jones, K. T. (2012). tDCS selectively improves working memory in older adults with more education. *Neuroscience Letters, 521*, 148–151.

Bikson, M., Datta, A., & Elwassif, M. (2009). Establishing safety limits for transcranial direct current stimulation. *Clinical Neurophysiology, 120*, 1033–1034.

Bikson, M., Datta, A., Rahman, A., & Scaturro, J. (2010). Electrode montages for tDCS and weak transcranial electrical stimulation: Role of "return" electrode's position and size. *Clinical Neurophysiology, 121*, 1976–1978.

Bikson, M., Grossman, P., Thomas, C., Zannou, A. L., Jiang, J., Adnan, T., … Woods, A. J. (2016). Safety of transcranial direct current stimulation: Evidence based update 2016. *Brain Stimulation, 9*, 641–661.

Boggio, P. S., Campanhã, C., Valasek, C. A., Fecteau, S., Pascual-Leone, A., & Fregni, F. (2010). Modulation of decision-making in a gambling task in older adults with transcranial direct current stimulation. *The European Journal of Neuroscience, 31*, 593–597.

Boggio, P. S., Ferrucci, R., Mameli, F., Martins, D., Martins, O., Vergari, M., … Priori, A. (2012). Prolonged visual memory enhancement after direct current stimulation in Alzheimer's disease. *Brain Stimulation, 5*, 223–230.

Boggio, P. S., Ferrucci, R., Rigonatti, S. P., Covre, P., Nitsche, M., Pascual-Leone, A., & Fregni, F. (2006). Effects of transcranial direct current stimulation on working memory in patients with Parkinson's disease. *Journal of the Neurological Sciences, 249*, 31–38.

Boggio, P. S., Khoury, L. P., Martins, D. C. S., Covre, P., Nitsche, M., Pascual-Leone, A., & Fregni, F. (2009). Temporal cortex direct current stimulation enhances performance on a visual recognition memory task in Alzheimer disease. *Journal of Neurology, Neurosurgery, and Psychiatry, 80*, 444–447.

Brunoni, A. R., Amadera, J., Berbel, B., Volz, M. S., Rizzerio, B. G., & Fregni, F. (2011a). A systematic review on reporting and assessment of adverse effects associated with transcranial direct current stimulation. *The International Journal of Neuropsychopharmacology, 14*, 1133–1145.

Brunoni, A. R., Nitsche, M. A., Bolognini, N., Bikson, M., Wagner, T., Merabet, L., … Fregni, F. (2012). Clinical research with transcranial direct current stimulation (tDCS): Challenges and future directions. *Brain Stimulation, 5*, 175–195.

Brunoni, A. R., Valiengo, L., Baccaro, A., Zanão, T. A., de Oliveira, J. F., Goulart, A., … Fregni, F. (2013). The sertraline vs. electrical current therapy for treating depression clinical study: Results from a factorial, randomized, controlled trial. *JAMA Psychiatry, 70*, 383–391.

Brunoni, A. R., Valiengo, L., Zanao, T., de Oliveira, J. F., Bensenor, I. M., & Fregni, F. (2011b). Manic psychosis after sertraline and transcranial direct-current stimulation. *The Journal of Neuropsychiatry and Clinical Neurosciences, 23*, E4–E5.

Calabrese, E. J. (2016). Preconditioning is hormesis part I: Documentation, dose-response features and mechanistic foundations. *Pharmacological Research, 110*, 242–264.

Calabrese, E. J., Dhawan, G., Kapoor, R., Iavicoli, I., & Calabrese, V. (2015). HORMESIS: A fundamental concept with widespread biological and biomedical applications. *Gerontology, 62*, 530–535.

Chang, W.-J., Bennell, K. L., Hodges, P. W., Hinman, R. S., Liston, M. B., & Schabrun, S. M. (2015). Combined exercise and transcranial direct current stimulation intervention for knee osteoarthritis: Protocol for a pilot randomised controlled trial. *BMJ Open, 5*, e008482.

Charvet, L. E., Kasschau, M., Datta, A., Knotkova, H., Stevens, M. C., Alonzo, A., … Bikson, M. (2015). Remotely-supervised transcranial direct current stimulation (tDCS) for clinical trials: Guidelines for technology and protocols. *Frontiers in Systems Neuroscience, 9*(26).

Cho, H.-S., & Cha, H.-G. (2015). Effect of mirror therapy with tDCS on functional recovery of the upper extremity of stroke patients. *Journal of Physical Therapy Science, 27*, 1045–1047.

Cosmo, C., Baptista, A. F., & de Sena, E. P. (2015). Contribution of transcranial direct current stimulation on inhibitory control to assess the neurobiological aspects of attention deficit hyperactivity disorder: Randomized controlled trial. *JMIR Research Protocols, 4*, e56.

Cotelli, M., Manenti, R., Brambilla, M., Petesi, M., Rosini, S., Ferrari, C., … Miniussi, C. (2014a). Anodal tDCS during face-name associations memory training in Alzheimer's patients. *Frontiers in Aging Neuroscience, 6*, 38.

Cotelli, M., Manenti, R., Petesi, M., Brambilla, M., Cosseddu, M., Zanetti, O., … Borroni, B. (2014b). Treatment of primary progressive aphasias by transcranial direct current stimulation combined with language training. *Journal of Alzheimer's Disease, 39*, 799–808.

Dasilva, A. F., Volz, M. S., Bikson, M., & Fregni, F. (2011). Electrode positioning and montage in transcranial direct current stimulation. *Journal of Visualized Experiments*.

Datta, A., Baker, J. M., Bikson, M., & Fridriksson, J. (2011). Individualized model predicts brain current flow during transcranial direct-current stimulation treatment in responsive stroke patient. *Brain Stimulation, 4*, 169–174.

Datta, A., Bansal, V., Diaz, J., Patel, J., Reato, D., & Bikson, M. (2009). Gyri-precise head model of transcranial direct current stimulation: Improved spatial focality using a ring electrode versus conventional rectangular pad. *Brain Stimulation, 2*, 201–207, 207.e1.

Datta, A., Bikson, M., & Fregni, F. (2010). Transcranial direct current stimulation in patients with skull defects and skull plates: High-resolution computational FEM study of factors altering cortical current flow. *NeuroImage, 52*, 1268–1278.

Dmochowski, J. P., Bikson, M., Datta, A., Richardson, J., Fridriksson, J., & Parra, L. C. (2012). On the role of electric field orientation in optimal design of transcranial current stimulation. *Conference Proceedings: Annual International Conference of the IEEE Engineering in Medicine and Biology Society, 2012*, 6426–6429.

Dmochowski, J. P., Datta, A., Bikson, M., Su, Y., & Parra, L. C. (2011). Optimized multi-electrode stimulation increases focality and intensity at target. *Journal of Neural Engineering, 8*, 046011.

Dmochowski, J. P., Datta, A., Huang, Y., Richardson, J. D., Bikson, M., Fridriksson, J., & Parra, L. C. (2013). Targeted transcranial direct current stimulation for rehabilitation after stroke. *NeuroImage, 75*, 12–19.

Doruk, D., Gray, Z., Bravo, G. L., Pascual-Leone, A., & Fregni, F. (2014). Effects of tDCS on executive function in Parkinson's disease. *Neuroscience Letters, 582*, 27–31.

Duarte Nde, A. C., Grecco, L. A. C., Galli, M., Fregni, F., & Oliveira, C. S. (2014). Effect of transcranial direct-current stimulation combined with treadmill training on balance and functional performance in children with cerebral palsy: A double-blind randomized controlled trial. *PLoS One, 9*, e105777.

Edwards, D., Cortes, M., Datta, A., Minhas, P., Wassermann, E. M., & Bikson, M. (2013). Physiological and modeling evidence for focal transcranial electrical brain stimulation in humans: A basis for high-definition tDCS. *NeuroImage, 74*, 266–275.

Elder, G. J., Firbank, M. J., Kumar, H., Chatterjee, P., Chakraborty, T., Dutt, A., & Taylor, J. P. (2015). Effects of transcranial direct current stimulation upon attention and visuoperceptual function in Lewy body dementia: A preliminary study. *International Psychogeriatrics, 28*, 1–7.

Elder, G. J., & Taylor, J.-P. (2014). Transcranial magnetic stimulation and transcranial direct current stimulation: Treatments for cognitive and neuropsychiatric symptoms in the neurodegenerative dementias? *Alzheimer's Research & Therapy, 6*, 74.

Esmaeilpour, Z., Milosevic, M., Azevedo, K., Khadka, N., Navarro, J., & Brunoni, A. (2017). Proceedings #21. Intracranial voltage recording during transcranial direct current stimulation (tDCS) in human subjects with validation of a standard model. *Brain Stimulation, 10*, e72–e75.

Faria, P., Fregni, F., Sebastião, F., Dias, A. I., & Leal, A. (2012). Feasibility of focal transcranial DC polarization with simultaneous EEG recording: Preliminary assessment in healthy subjects and human epilepsy. *Epilepsy & Behavior, 25*, 417–425.

Ferrucci, R., Mameli, F., Guidi, I., Mrakic-Sposta, S., Vergari, M., Marceglia, S., … Priori, A. (2008). Transcranial direct current stimulation improves recognition memory in Alzheimer disease. *Neurology, 71*, 493–498.

Fertonani, A., Brambilla, M., Cotelli, M., & Miniussi, C. (2014). The timing of cognitive plasticity in physiological aging: A tDCS study of naming. *Frontiers in Aging Neuroscience, 6*, 131.

Flöel, A., Suttorp, W., Kohl, O., Kürten, J., Lohmann, H., Breitenstein, C., & Knecht, S. (2012). Non-invasive brain stimulation improves object-location learning in the elderly. *Neurobiology of Aging, 33*, 1682–1689.

Frank, E., Wilfurth, S., Landgrebe, M., Eichhammer, P., Hajak, G., & Langguth, B. (2010). Anodal skin lesions after treatment with transcranial direct current stimulation. *Brain Stimulation, 3*, 58–59.

Fregni, F., Boggio, P. S., Santos, M. C., Lima, M., Vieira, A. L., Rigonatti, S. P., … Pascual-Leone, A. (2006a). Noninvasive cortical stimulation with transcranial direct current stimulation in Parkinson's disease. *Movement Disorders, 21*, 1693–1702.

Fregni, F., Nitsche, M. A., Loo, C. K., Brunoni, A. R., Marangolo, P., Leite, J., … Bikson, M. (2015). Regulatory considerations for the clinical and research use of transcranial direct current stimulation (tDCS): Review and recommendations from an expert panel. *Clinical Research and Regulatory Affairs, 32*, 22–35.

Fregni, F., Thome-Souza, S., Nitsche, M. A., Freedman, S. D., Valente, K. D., & Pascual-Leone, A. (2006b). A controlled clinical trial of cathodal DC polarization in patients with refractory epilepsy. *Epilepsia, 47*, 335–342.

Fusco, A., Assenza, F., Iosa, M., Izzo, S., Altavilla, R., Paolucci, S., & Vernieri, F. (2014a). The ineffective role of cathodal tDCS in enhancing the functional motor outcomes in early phase of stroke rehabilitation: An experimental trial. *BioMed Research International, 2014*, 547290.

Fusco, A., Iosa, M., Venturiero, V., De Angelis, D., Morone, G., Maglione, L., … Paolucci, S. (2014b). After vs. priming effects of anodal transcranial direct current stimulation on upper extremity motor recovery in patients with subacute stroke. *Restorative Neurology and Neuroscience, 32*, 301–312.

Gálvez, V., Alonzo, A., Martin, D., Mitchell, P. B., Sachdev, P., & Loo, C. K. (2011). Hypomania induction in a patient with bipolar II disorder by transcranial direct current stimulation (tDCS). *The Journal of ECT, 27*, 256–258.

Gálvez, V., Ho, K.-A., Alonzo, A., Martin, D., George, D., & Loo, C. K. (2015). Neuromodulation therapies for geriatric depression. *Current Psychiatry Reports, 17*, 59.

Gillick, B. T., Feyma, T., Menk, J., Usset, M., Vaith, A., Wood, T. J., … Krach, L. E. (2015). Safety and feasibility of transcranial direct current stimulation in pediatric hemiparesis: Randomized controlled preliminary study. *Physical Therapy, 95*, 337–349.

Gillick, B. T., Kirton, A., Carmel, J. B., Minhas, P., & Bikson, M. (2014). Pediatric stroke and transcranial direct current stimulation: Methods for rational individualized dose optimization. *Frontiers in Human Neuroscience, 8*, 739.

Goodwill, A. M., Reynolds, J., Daly, R. M., & Kidgell, D. J. (2013). Formation of cortical plasticity in older adults following tDCS and motor training. *Frontiers in Aging Neuroscience, 5*, 87.

Grecco, L. A. C., de Almeida Carvalho Duarte, N., Mendonça, M. E., Cimolin, V., Galli, M., Fregni, F., & Santos Oliveira, C. (2014a). Transcranial direct current stimulation during treadmill training in children with cerebral palsy: A randomized controlled double-blind clinical trial. *Research in Developmental Disabilities, 35*, 2840–2848.

Grecco, L. A. C., Duarte, N. A. C., Zanon, N., Galli, M., Fregni, F., & Oliveira, C. S. (2014b). Effect of a single session of transcranial direct-current stimulation on balance and spatiotemporal gait variables in children with cerebral palsy: A randomized sham-controlled study. *Brazilian Journal of Physical Therapy, 18*, 419–427.

Grecco, L. A. C., Mendonça, M. E., Duarte, N. A. C., Zanon, N., Fregni, F., & Oliveira, C. S. (2014c). Transcranial direct current stimulation combined with treadmill gait training in delayed neuro-psychomotor development. *Journal of Physical Therapy Science, 26*, 945–950.

Guarienti, F., Caumo, W., Shiozawa, P., Cordeiro, Q., Boggio, P. S., Benseñor, I. M., … Brunoni, A. R. (2015). Reducing transcranial direct current stimulation-induced erythema with skin pretreatment: Considerations for sham-controlled clinical trials. *Neuromodulation, 18*, 261–265.

Hagenacker, T., Bude, V., Naegel, S., Holle, D., Katsarava, Z., Diener, H. C., & Obermann, M. (2014). Patient-conducted anodal transcranial direct current stimulation of the motor cortex alleviates pain in trigeminal neuralgia. *The Journal of Headache and Pain, 15*, 78.

Hardwick, R. M., & Celnik, P. A. (2014). Cerebellar direct current stimulation enhances motor learning in older adults. *Neurobiology of Aging, 35*, 2217–2221.

Harty, S., Robertson, I. H., Miniussi, C., Sheehy, O. C., Devine, C. A., McCreery, S., & O'Connell, R. G. (2014). Transcranial direct current stimulation over right dorsolateral prefrontal cortex enhances error awareness in older age. *The Journal of Neuroscience, 34*, 3646–3652.

Ho, K.-A., Bai, S., Martin, D., Alonzo, A., Dokos, S., & Loo, C. K. (2015). Clinical pilot study and computational modeling of Bitemporal transcranial direct current stimulation, and safety of repeated courses of treatment, in major depression. *The Journal of ECT, 31*, 226–233.

Holland, R., Leff, A. P., Josephs, O., Galea, J. M., Desikan, M., Price, C. J., … Crinion, J. (2011). Speech facilitation by left inferior frontal cortex stimulation. *Current Biology, 21*, 1403–1407.

Hsu, W.-Y., Ku, Y., Zanto, T. P., & Gazzaley, A. (2015). Effects of noninvasive brain stimulation on cognitive function in healthy aging and Alzheimer's disease: A systematic review and meta-analysis. *Neurobiology of Aging, 36*, 2348–2359.

Huang, Y., Liu, A. A., Lafon, B., Friedman, D., Dayan, M., Wang, X., … Parra, L. C. (2017). Measurements and models of electric fields in the in vivo human brain during transcranial electric stimulation. *eLife, 6*, e18834.

Jones, K. T., Stephens, J. A., Alam, M., Bikson, M., & Berryhill, M. E. (2015). Longitudinal neurostimulation in older adults improves working memory. *PLoS One, 10*, e0121904.

Kaski, D., Dominguez, R. O., Allum, J. H., Islam, A. F., & Bronstein, A. M. (2014). Combining physical training with transcranial direct current stimulation to improve gait in Parkinson's disease: A pilot randomized controlled study. *Clinical Rehabilitation, 28*, 1115–1124.

Kasschau, M., Sherman, K., Haider, L., Frontario, A., Shaw, M., Datta, A., … Charvet, L. (2015). A protocol for the use of remotely-supervised transcranial direct current stimulation (tDCS) in multiple sclerosis (MS). *Journal of Visualized Experiments*.

Kessler, S. K., Minhas, P., Woods, A. J., Rosen, A., Gorman, C., & Bikson, M. (2013). Dosage considerations for transcranial direct current stimulation in children: A computational modeling study. *PLoS One, 8*, e76112.

Kessler, S. K., Turkeltaub, P. E., Benson, J. G., & Hamilton, R. H. (2012). Differences in the experience of active and sham transcranial direct current stimulation. *Brain Stimulation, 5*, 155–162.

Khedr, E. M., Gamal, N. F. E., El-Fetoh, N. A., Khalifa, H., Ahmed, E. M., Ali, A. M., … Karim, A. A. (2014). A double-blind randomized clinical trial on the efficacy of cortical direct current stimulation for the treatment of Alzheimer's disease. *Frontiers in Aging Neuroscience, 6*, 275.

Kim, S. J., Kim, B. K., Ko, Y. J., Bang, M. S., Kim, M. H., & Han, T. R. (2010). Functional and histologic changes after repeated transcranial direct current stimulation in rat stroke model. *Journal of Korean Medical Science, 25*, 1499–1505.

Kim, Y. J., Ku, J., Cho, S., Kim, H. J., Cho, Y. K., Lim, T., & Kang, Y. J. (2014). Facilitation of corticospinal excitability by virtual reality exercise following anodal transcranial direct current stimulation in healthy volunteers and subacute stroke subjects. *Journal of Neuroengineering and Rehabilitation, 11*, 124.

Kronberg, G., & Bikson, M. (2012). Electrode assembly design for transcranial direct current stimulation: A FEM modeling study. *Conference Proceedings: Annual International Conference of the IEEE Engineering in Medicine and Biology Society, 2012*, 891–895.

Laakso, I., & Hirata, A. (2013). Computational analysis shows why transcranial alternating current stimulation induces retinal phosphenes. *Journal of Neural Engineering, 10*, 046009.

Lee, S. J., & Chun, M. H. (2014). Combination transcranial direct current stimulation and virtual reality therapy for upper extremity training in patients with subacute stroke. *Archives of Physical Medicine and Rehabilitation, 95*, 431–438.

Liebetanz, D., Koch, R., Mayenfels, S., König, F., Paulus, W., & Nitsche, M. A. (2009). Safety limits of cathodal transcranial direct current stimulation in rats. *Clinical Neurophysiology, 120*, 1161–1167.

Loo, C. K., Alonzo, A., Martin, D., Mitchell, P. B., Galvez, V., & Sachdev, P. (2012). Transcranial direct current stimulation for depression: 3-week, randomised, sham-controlled trial. *The British Journal of Psychiatry, 200*, 52–59.

Manenti, R., Bianchi, M., Cosseddu, M., Brambilla, M., Rizzetti, C., Padovani, A., … Cotelli, M. (2015). Anodal transcranial direct current stimulation of parietal cortex enhances action naming in Corticobasal Syndrome. *Frontiers in Aging Neuroscience, 7*, 49.

Manenti, R., Brambilla, M., Petesi, M., Ferrari, C., & Cotelli, M. (2013). Enhancing verbal episodic memory in older and young subjects after non-invasive brain stimulation. *Frontiers in Aging Neuroscience, 5*, 49.

Manenti, R., Brambilla, M., Rosini, S., Orizio, I., Ferrari, C., Borroni, B., & Cotelli, M. (2014). Time up and go task performance improves after transcranial direct current stimulation in patient affected by Parkinson's disease. *Neuroscience Letters, 580*, 74–77.

Mattai, A., Miller, R., Weisinger, B., Greenstein, D., Bakalar, J., Tossell, J., … Gogtay, N. (2011). Tolerability of transcranial direct current stimulation in childhood-onset schizophrenia. *Brain Stimulation, 4*, 275–280.

Mcintire, L. K., Mckinley, R. A., Goodyear, C., & Nelson, J. (2014). A comparison of the effects of transcranial direct current stimulation and caffeine on vigilance and cognitive performance during extended wakefulness. *Brain Stimulation, 7*, 499–507.

Medeiros, L. F., de Souza, I. C. C., Vidor, L. P., de Souza, A., Deitos, A., Volz, M. S., … Torres, I. L. (2012). Neurobiological effects of transcranial direct current stimulation: A review. *Frontiers in Psychiatry, 3*, 110.

Meinzer, M., Lindenberg, R., Antonenko, D., Flaisch, T., & Flöel, A. (2013). Anodal transcranial direct current stimulation temporarily reverses age-associated cognitive decline and functional brain activity changes. *The Journal of Neuroscience, 33*, 12470–12478.

Meinzer, M., Lindenberg, R., Sieg, M. M., Nachtigall, L., Ulm, L., & Flöel, A. (2014). Transcranial direct current stimulation of the primary motor cortex improves word-retrieval in older adults. *Frontiers in Aging Neuroscience, 6*, 253.

Mekonnen, A., Salvador, R., Ruffini, G., & Miranda, P. C. (2012). The relationship between transcranial current stimulation electrode montages and the effect of the skull orbital openings. *Conference Proceedings: Annual International Conference of the IEEE Engineering in Medicine and Biology Society, 2012*, 831–834.

Mielke, D., Wrede, A., Schulz-Schaeffer, W., Taghizadeh-Waghefi, A., Nitsche, M. A., Rohde, V., & Liebetanz, D. (2013). Cathodal transcranial direct current stimulation induces regional, long-lasting reductions of cortical blood flow in rats. *Neurological Research, 35*, 1029–1037.

Minhas, P., Bansal, V., Patel, J., Ho, J. S., Diaz, J., Datta, A., & Bikson, M. (2010). Electrodes for high-definition transcutaneous DC stimulation for applications in drug delivery and electrotherapy, including tDCS. *Journal of Neuroscience Methods, 190*, 188–197.

Minhas, P., Datta, A., & Bikson, M. (2011). Cutaneous perception during tDCS: Role of electrode shape and sponge salinity. *Clinical Neurophysiology, 122*, 637–638.

Moffa, A. H., Brunoni, A. R., Fregni, F., Palm, U., Padberg, F., Blumberger, D. M., … Loo, C. K. (2017). Safety and acceptability of transcranial direct current stimulation for the acute treatment of major depressive episodes: Analysis of individual patient data. *Journal of Affective Disorders, 221*, 1–5.

Monte-Silva, K., Kuo, M.-F., Hessenthaler, S., Fresnoza, S., Liebetanz, D., Paulus, W., & Nitsche, M. A. (2013). Induction of late LTP-like plasticity in the human motor cortex by repeated non-invasive brain stimulation. *Brain Stimulation, 6*, 424–432.

Morales-Quezada, L., Cosmo, C., Carvalho, S., Leite, J., Castillo-Saavedra, L., Rozisky, J. R., & Fregni, F. (2015). Cognitive effects and autonomic responses to transcranial pulsed current stimulation. *Experimental Brain Research, 233*, 701–709.

Mortensen, J., Figlewski, K., & Andersen, H. (2015). Combined transcranial direct current stimulation and home-based occupational therapy for upper limb motor impairment following intracerebral hemorrhage: A double-blind randomized controlled trial. *Disability and Rehabilitation, 38*, 1–7.

Nitsche, M. A., Bikson, M., & Bestmann, S. (2015). On the use of meta-analysis in Neuromodulatory non-invasive brain stimulation. *Brain Stimulation, 8*, 666–667.

Nitsche, M. A., Doemkes, S., Karaköse, T., Antal, A., Liebetanz, D., Lang, N., … Paulus, W. (2007). Shaping the effects of transcranial direct current stimulation of the human motor cortex. *Journal of Neurophysiology, 97*, 3109–3117.

Nitsche, M. A., Liebetanz, D., Lang, N., Antal, A., Tergau, F., & Paulus, W. (2003). Safety criteria for transcranial direct current stimulation (tDCS) in humans. *Clinical Neurophysiology, 114*, 2220–2222; author reply 2222–2223.

Nitsche, M. A., Niehaus, L., Hoffmann, K. T., Hengst, S., Liebetanz, D., Paulus, W., & Meyer, B. U. (2004). MRI study of human brain exposed to weak direct current stimulation of the frontal cortex. *Clinical Neurophysiology, 115*, 2419–2423.

Opitz, A., Falchier, A., Yan, C.-G., Yeagle, E., Linn, G., Megevand, P., … Schroeder, C. (2016). Spatiotemporal structure of intracranial electric fields induced by transcranial electric stimulation in humans and nonhuman primates. *Scientific Reports, 6*, 31236.

Opitz, A., Paulus, W., Will, S., Antunes, A., & Thielscher, A. (2015). Determinants of the electric field during transcranial direct current stimulation. *NeuroImage, 109*, 140–150.

Palm, U., Feichtner, K. B., Hasan, A., Gauglitz, G., Langguth, B., Nitsche, M. A., … Padberg, F. (2014). The role of contact media at the skin-electrode interface during transcranial direct current stimulation (tDCS). *Brain Stimulation, 7*, 762–764.

Paneri, B., Khadka, N., Patel, V., Thomas, C., Tyler, W., Parra, L. C., & Bikson, M. (2015). The tolerability of transcranial electrical stimulation used across extended periods in a naturalistic context by healthy individuals. *PeerJ Prepr, 3*

Parazzini, M., Rossi, E., Rossi, L., Priori, A., & Ravazzani, P. (2013). Numerical estimation of the current density in the heart during transcranial direct current stimulation. *Brain Stimulation, 6*, 457–459.

Parikh, P. J., & Cole, K. J. (2015). Effects of transcranial direct current stimulation on the control of finger force during dexterous manipulation in healthy older adults. *PLoS One, 10*, e0124137.

Park, S.-H., Seo, J.-H., Kim, Y.-H., & Ko, M.-H. (2014). Long-term effects of transcranial direct current stimulation combined with computer-assisted cognitive training in healthy older adults. *Neuroreport, 25*, 122–126.

Peruzzotti-Jametti, L., Cambiaghi, M., Bacigaluppi, M., Gallizioli, M., Gaude, E., Mari, S., … Leocani, L. (2013). Safety and efficacy of transcranial direct current stimulation in acute experimental ischemic stroke. *Stroke, 44*, 3166–3174.

Pirulli, C., Fertonani, A., & Miniussi, C. (2014). Is neural hyperpolarization by cathodal stimulation always detrimental at the behavioral level? *Frontiers in Behavioral Neuroscience, 8*, 226.

Poreisz, C., Boros, K., Antal, A., & Paulus, W. (2007). Safety aspects of transcranial direct current stimulation concerning healthy subjects and patients. *Brain Research Bulletin, 72*, 208–214.

Puri, R., Hinder, M. R., Fujiyama, H., Gomez, R., Carson, R. G., & Summers, J. J. (2015). Duration-dependent effects of the BDNF Val66Met polymorphism on anodal tDCS induced motor cortex plasticity in older adults: A group and individual perspective. *Frontiers in Aging Neuroscience, 7*, 107.

Raimundo, R. J. S., Uribe, C. E., & Brasil-Neto, J. P. (2012). Lack of clinically detectable acute changes on autonomic or thermoregulatory functions in healthy subjects after transcranial direct current stimulation (tDCS). *Brain Stimulation, 5*, 196–200.

Rampersad, S. M., Janssen, A. M., Lucka, F., Aydin, Ü., Lanfer, B., Lew, S., … Oostendorp, T. F. (2014). Simulating transcranial direct current stimulation with a detailed anisotropic human head model. *IEEE Transactions on Neural Systems and Rehabilitation Engineering, 22*, 441–452.

Rodríguez, N., Opisso, E., Pascual-Leone, A., & Soler, M. D. (2014). Skin lesions induced by transcranial direct current stimulation (tDCS). *Brain Stimulation, 7*, 765–767.

Ross, L. A., McCoy, D., Coslett, H. B., Olson, I. R., & Wolk, D. A. (2011). Improved proper name recall in aging after electrical stimulation of the anterior temporal lobes. *Frontiers in Aging Neuroscience, 3*, 16.

Russo, R., Wallace, D., Fitzgerald, P. B., & Cooper, N. R. (2013). Perception of comfort during active and sham transcranial direct current stimulation: A double blind study. *Brain Stimulation, 6*, 946–951.

Sadleir, R. J., Vannorsdall, T. D., Schretlen, D. J., & Gordon, B. (2010). Transcranial direct current stimulation (tDCS) in a realistic head model. *NeuroImage, 51*, 1310–1318.

Salthouse, T. A. (2010). Selective review of cognitive aging. *Journal of the International Neuropsychological Society, 16*, 754–760.

Sandrini, M., Brambilla, M., Manenti, R., Rosini, S., Cohen, L. G., & Cotelli, M. (2014). Noninvasive stimulation of prefrontal cortex strengthens existing episodic memories and reduces forgetting in the elderly. *Frontiers in Aging Neuroscience, 6*, 289.

San-Juan, D., Calcáneo J de, D. D. C., González-Aragón, M. F., Bermúdez Maldonado, L., Avellán, A. M., Argumosa, E. V., & Fregni, F. (2011a). Transcranial direct current stimulation in adolescent and adult Rasmussen's encephalitis. *Epilepsy & Behavior, 20*, 126–131.

San-Juan, D., Mayorga, A. P. M., Anschel, D. J., Avellán, A. M., González-Aragón, M. F., & Cole, A. J. (2011b). The double generalization phenomenon in juvenile absence epilepsy. *Epilepsy & Behavior, 21*, 318–320.

San-Juan, D., Morales-Quezada, L., Orozco Garduño, A. J., Alonso-Vanegas, M., González-Aragón, M. F., Espinoza López, D. A., … Fregni, F. (2015). Transcranial direct current stimulation in epilepsy. *Brain Stimulation, 8*, 455–464.

Sattler, V., Acket, B., Raposo, N., Albucher, J. F., Thalamas, C., Loubinoux, I., … Simonetta-Moreau, M. (2015). Anodal tDCS combined with radial nerve stimulation promotes hand motor recovery in the acute phase after ischemic stroke. *Neurorehabilitation and Neural Repair, 29*, 743–754.

Sawyer, D. W., Donowitz, G. R., & Mandell, G. L. (1989). Polymorphonuclear neutrophils: An effective antimicrobial force. *Reviews of Infectious Diseases, 11*(Suppl 7), S1532–S1544.

Shiozawa, P., da Silva, M. E., Raza, R., Uchida, R. R., Cordeiro, Q., Fregni, F., & Brunoni, A. R. (2013). Safety of repeated transcranial direct current stimulation in impaired skin: A case report. *The Journal of ECT, 29*, 147–148.

Smit, M., Schutter, D. J. L. G., Nijboer, T. C. W., Visser-Meily, J. M., Kappelle, L. J., Kant, N., … Dijkerman, H. C. (2015). Transcranial direct current stimulation to the parietal cortex in hemispatial neglect: A feasibility study. *Neuropsychologia, 74*, 152–161.

Stephen, L. J., & Brodie, M. J. (2000). Epilepsy in elderly people. *Lancet, 355*, 1441–1446.

Suemoto, C. K., Apolinario, D., Nakamura-Palacios, E. M., Lopes, L., Leite, R. E., Sales, M. C., … Fregni, F. (2014). Effects of a non-focal plasticity protocol on apathy in moderate Alzheimer's disease: A randomized, double-blind, sham-controlled trial. *Brain Stimulation, 7*, 308–313.

Sundaram, A., Stock, V., Cruciani, R. A., & Knotkova, H. (2009). Safety of transcranial direct current stimulation (tDCS) in protocols involving human subjects. *Journal of Pain Management, 2*, 285–293.

Tadini, L., El-Nazer, R., Brunoni, A. R., Williams, J., Carvas, M., Boggio, P., … Fregni, F. (2011). Cognitive, mood, and electroencephalographic effects of noninvasive cortical stimulation with weak electrical currents. *The Journal of ECT, 27*, 134–140.

Tahtis, V., Kaski, D., & Seemungal, B. M. (2014). The effect of single session bi-cephalic transcranial direct current stimulation on gait performance in sub-acute stroke: A pilot study. *Restorative Neurology and Neuroscience, 32*, 527–532.

Tippett, D. C., Hillis, A. E., & Tsapkini, K. (2015). Treatment of primary progressive aphasia. *Current Treatment Options in Neurology, 17*, 362.

Vestito, L., Rosellini, S., Mantero, M., & Bandini, F. (2014). Long-term effects of transcranial direct-current stimulation in chronic post-stroke aphasia: A pilot study. *Frontiers in Human Neuroscience, 8*, 785.

Wachter, D., Wrede, A., Schulz-Schaeffer, W., Taghizadeh-Waghefi, A., Nitsche, M. A., Kutschenko, A., … Liebetanz, D. (2011). Transcranial direct current stimulation induces polarity-specific changes of cortical blood perfusion in the rat. *Experimental Neurology, 227*, 322–327.

Wang, J., Wei, Y., Wen, J., & Li, X. (2015). Skin burn after single session of transcranial direct current stimulation (tDCS). *Brain Stimulation, 8*, 165–166.

Woods, A. J., Antal, A., Bikson, M., Boggio, P. S., Brunoni, A. R., Celnik, P., … Nitsche, M. A. (2015). A technical guide to tDCS, and related non-invasive brain stimulation tools. *Clinical Neurophysiology, 127*, 1031–1048.

Wu, D., Wang, J., & Yuan, Y. (2015). Effects of transcranial direct current stimulation on naming and cortical excitability in stroke patients with aphasia. *Neuroscience Letters, 589*, 115–120.

www.who.int/medicines/areas/quality_safety/safety_efficacy/.../definitions.pdf

Yook, S.-W., Park, S.-H., Seo, J.-H., Kim, S. J., & Ko, M. H. (2011). Suppression of seizure by cathodal transcranial direct current stimulation in an epileptic patient – a case report. *Annals of Rehabilitation Medicine, 35*, 579–582.

Young, S. J., Bertucco, M., Sheehan-Stross, R., & Sanger, T. D. (2013). Cathodal transcranial direct current stimulation in children with dystonia: A pilot open-label trial. *Journal of Child Neurology, 28*, 1238–1244.

Zhou, D., Zhou, J., Chen, H., Manor, B., Lin, J., & Zhang, J. (2015). Effects of transcranial direct current stimulation (tDCS) on multiscale complexity of dual-task postural control in older adults. *Experimental Brain Research, 233*, 2401–2409.

Part II
Transcranial Direct Current Stimulation Step-By-Step Practicum

Chapter 7
Methodological Considerations for Selection of Transcranial Direct Current Stimulation Approach, Protocols and Devices

Shapour Jaberzadeh, Donel Martin, Helena Knotkova, and Adam J. Woods

Evidence-Based tDCS Use

Appropriately selecting a transcranial direct current stimulation (tDCS) approach, design, protocol and specific device is a multifaceted process that requires careful and iterative consideration before the most suitable (and feasible) configuration is chosen. Practically speaking, the choice of an ideal or preferred selection is often a careful balance of available resources versus targeted outcomes. Thus, it is important to carefully consider how to balance the selection of tDCS approach, without compromising integrity and quality of the outcomes. Whether tDCS is used in research or non-research applications, the outcomes (or their segment, such as adverse event occurrence) become a part of the overall pool of evidence, which iteratively advances knowledge of the tDCS field and provides foundation for evidence-based tDCS practice. Building evidence-based tDCS practice (in the means of evidence-informed tDCS use) has the following implications:

S. Jaberzadeh
Department of Physiotherapy, School of Primary Health Care, Faculty of Medicine Nursing and Health Sciences, Monash University, Melbourne, Australia

D. Martin
Black Dog Institute, The University of New South Wales, Sydney, NSW, Australia

H. Knotkova
MJHS Institute for Innovation in Palliative Care, New York, NY, USA

Department of Family and Social Medicine, Albert Einstein College of Medicine, Bronx, NY, USA

A. J. Woods (✉)
Center for Cognitive Aging and Memory (CAM), McKnight Brain Institute, Department of Clinical and Health Psychology, College of Public Health and Health Professions, University of Florida, Gainesville, FL, USA
e-mail: ajwoods@phhp.ufl.edu

H. Knotkova et al. (eds.), *Practical Guide to Transcranial Direct Current Stimulation*, https://doi.org/10.1007/978-3-319-95948-1_7

1. tDCS users should be able to access and *critically interpret* available evidence
2. New tDCS studies or applications should be designed with consideration of their ability to *meaningfully contribute* to the existing pool of evidence
3. Standards or guidelines of tDCS use should be based on systematic review of evidence (and therefore periodically revised as the body of evidence is growing)

Clearly, all these points are highly relevant for the step-by-step process of determining the best approach, parameters or protocol. The decision-making process starts with defining the purpose of the intended tDCS application; "Why" tDCS will be used and "What" specifically should be achieved. Answers to these two questions, to a large extent, require selecting the right design, stimulation protocol or workflow for tDCS procedures. At the beginning of the planning process, the answers to Why and What are usually vague, embedded in a broader open question, issue, gap in knowledge, or need. At that stage of planning, a *critical* review of existing tDCS evidence is invaluable to help clarify the answers and prevent methodological mistakes or poor choices for the overall tDCS setup.

When critically reviewing and evaluating existing evidence, an "evidence ladder" (Fig. 7.1) can assist in navigating the process.

tDCS studies in animal models primarily provide evidence pertaining to tDCS mechanisms and safety, and association between animal models and human studies.

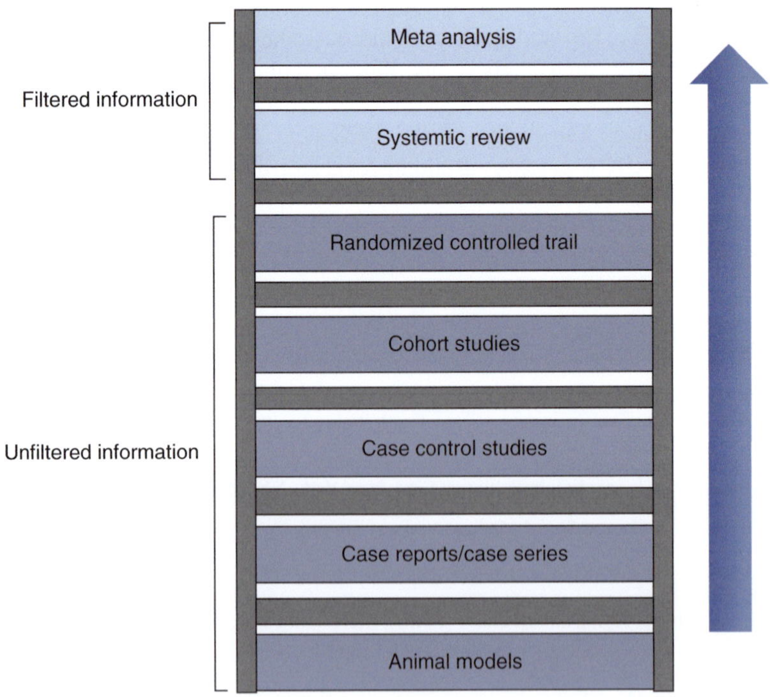

Fig. 7.1 Evidence Ladder

These studies supply evidence necessary for designing Randomized Controlled Trials (RCTs), such as initial evidence on effect size to properly power a study. The highest level of "unfiltered" evidence comes from RCTs, where the study design lacks methodological flaws. Alternatively, aggregate statistical evaluation of findings from a pool of RCT's, in the form of meta-analysis, then represents the "filtered evidence" at the top of the ladder. There are several systems available for evaluating the quality of the evidence. Although the evidence-scoring systems originate in health science/medical research, their principle fully applies to critical review of tDCS evidence as well. According to, for example, a "GRADE" scoring system (clinicalevidence.bmj.com), high quality evidence requires RCT's with only few methodological flaws. RCT GRADE quality is downgraded if RCT's have flaws, do not assess key elements, or the findings are inconsistent. Low quality evidence is usually produced by uncontrolled or observational studies; quality is upgraded if they include meticulous methods and produce moderate to large effects. Although uncontrolled studies and observations in general represent low-level evidence, they are essential as foundation for high-quality RCT's. Importantly, a carefully planned small-sample study may generate more meaningful evidence when implementing foundational support from preliminary studies. Moreover, in non-research settings, evidence-informed tDCS use may substantially facilitate progress in tDCS practice, while reckless tDCS applications not reflecting/ignoring the existing foundational knowledge may harm or set-back the field as a whole.

Practical Tips for Evidence Review

Meta-analysis:

- Review inclusion criteria – if the inclusion criteria are too broad, interpretation of the findings may be problematic. Although it is well known that tDCS outcomes are parameter specific, some published meta-analyses aggregate tDCS studies with other non-invasive neurostimulation modalities, or aggregate tDCS studies across brain targets or across delivered doses, (Lowe et al. 2017). In these cases, a careful interpretation is warranted. For example, results of meta-analysis evaluating studies of tDCS placing electrodes over the frontal lobes at F3 and F4 in 10 sessions over 10 consecutive days *and* studies placing the anode electrode over M1 and the cathode electrode over contralateral supraorbital area in once-a month regimen may be misleading and have little practical significance for planning of future applications, including selection of suitable approach or stimulation protocol.
- Evaluate bias – it is important to know not only if the included RCTs were biased, but also the source of the bias. The bias may originate from selection (systematic differences in baseline characteristics of the compared study groups), carry-over effect in cross-over RCTs, reporting (reported vs unreported findings), incomplete outcome data, unsuccessful/insufficient blinding, and other factors.

- Evaluate findings on the effects – What is the size and *direction* of the effect? What is the strength of evidence for the effect? Is the effect consistent across studies?

Critical review of clinical trials:

- Consider generalizability – findings may only be applicable to narrowly defined participant-population and may not be generalizable to other contexts.
- Consider power determination – Was the study adequately powered? How was the sample size determined? Interpretation of findings is especially problematic if the study is a non-inferiority trial that does not detect a significant difference between the study groups. It may be difficult to identify if the finding is really due to non-inferiority of the compared interventions or due to insufficient sample size.
- Consider overall quality of reporting of the study – clinical trial reporting should follow the CONSORT requirements (www.consort-statement.org).

Overall, a thorough review of published tDCS literature and other available evidence pertaining to the topic relevant for the planned tDCS use is a stepping-stone that helps progress through the tDCS approach, design, protocol and device decision-making process. Considerations, as discussed below, aim to assist the reader in selecting the most appropriate approach, design, protocol and specific tDCS device.

Experimental Versus Intervention Protocols

Non-invasive brain stimulation is a tool for modulation of brain physiological functions through alterations of brain activity, and excitability. It can be used as a: (1) research tool, (2) neuroenhancement tool and (3) therapeutic tool. As a research tool, it is applied to explore the role of different cortical and/or deeper areas of the brain in behavior (Filmer et al. 2014). The approach could potentially be used to shed light on the underlying mechanisms in different fields of neuroscience, as discussed in detail in Chap. 19. As a neuroenhancement tool, it is applied on healthy individuals to affect human motor control of movement and improve cognitive/sensory-motor learning capacity in a variety of tasks including sports, music, etc. (Furuya et al. 2014; Hendy et al. 2015; Moreau et al. 2015; Picazio et al. 2015; Zhu et al. 2015). As a therapeutic tool, it is used for management of pain, symptoms of aging, and reduction of clinical symptoms in neurological and psychiatric conditions (Anton et al. 2015; Fregni and Pascual-Leone 2007; George and Aston-Jones 2010; Nitsche et al. 2009).

tDCS as a Research Tool

Better understanding the brain-behavior relationship is a central goal in neuroscience research. A large number of studies focus on correlations between brain changes (Fig. 7.2) assessed by transcranial magnetic stimulation (TMS) and imaging techniques such as functional magnetic resonance imaging (fMRI), positron emission tomography (PET), magneto electroencephalography (MEG), electroencephalography (EEG), and near-infrared spectroscopy (NIRS) and behavioral

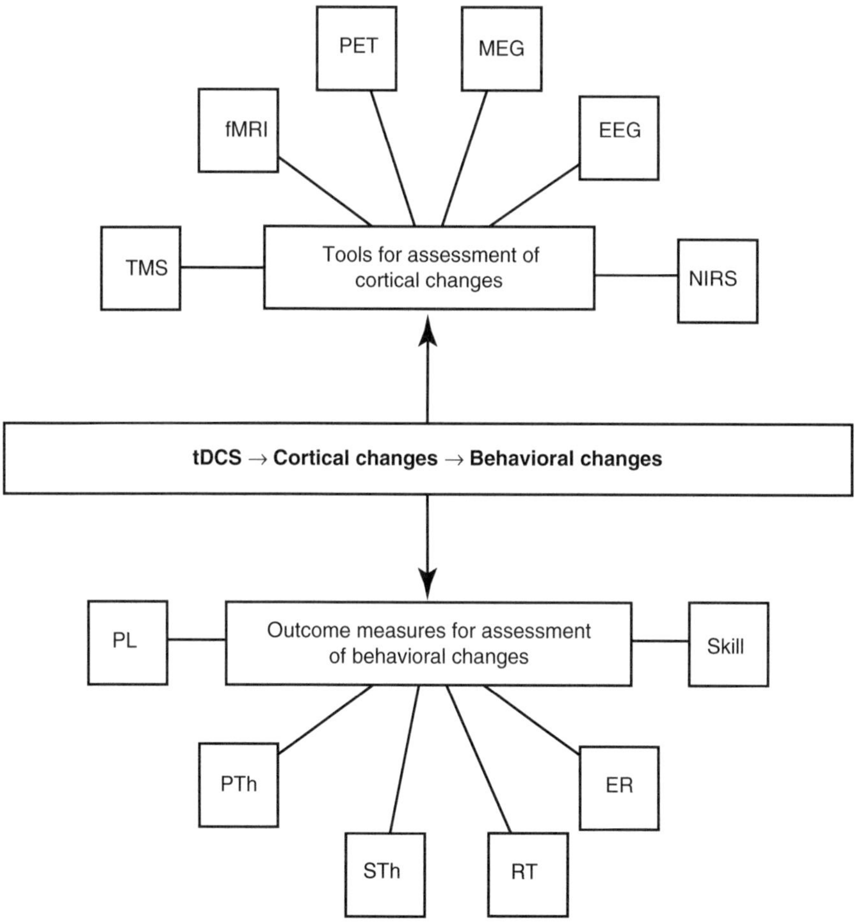

Fig. 7.2 Cortical and behavioral effects of tDCS. TMS transcranial magnetic stimulation, fMRI functional magnetic resonance imaging, PET positron emission tomography, MEG magneto electroencephalography, EEG electroencephalography, NIRS near infrared spectroscopy, PL Pain level, PTh pain threshold, STh sensory threshold, RT response time, ER error rate

changes assessed by a wide variety of outcome measures (Fig. 7.2) during sensory, motor or cognitive tasks. Combination of these methods and tDCS can convey significant insight for current basic and clinical research.

In this field of research, tDCS has been used to reduce or enhance the activity or excitability of cortical areas:

- To probe stimulation effects on near and far cortical regions (Vaseghi et al. 2015a, b), which helps to establish functional connectivity between different cortical areas.
- To measure stimulation effects on sensory, motor or cognitive functions (Apolinário-Souza et al. 2016; Nakagawa et al. 2016; Pope et al. 2015; Woods et al. 2014). This helps to establish the causal links between one specific cortical area and the task performed.
- To investigate hemispheric differences in processing of behavioral tasks (Bardi et al. 2013). When using certain parameters, the function of a cortical area in one side of the brain can be enhanced while the same area in the other side of brain is inhibited. The outcome of this interhemispheric imbalance can then be measured and used as evidence for communication and or rivalry between two hemispheres.
- To assess two or more behavioral outcomes to investigate if they are affected in the same way by tDCS to shed light on the functional organization of the brain (e.g., Iuculano and Cohen Kadosh 2013).
- To examine how it affects EEG power spectrum (Soekadar et al. 2014) and cortical excitability.

Blinding and Sham/Placebo Effects of tDCS

Blinding is a research procedural step for reduction of bias in modern RCTs. In double blinding, both participants and/or researchers are kept unaware of the allocation group. Without proper researcher blinding, they are more prone to bias during evaluation of the participants (Boutron et al. 2007; Brunoni et al. 2014). Lack of participants blinding is also problematic because it can increase the chance of placebo responses and treatment non-compliance (Noseworthy et al. 1994; Turner et al. 2012; Woods et al. 2016). Blinding integrity in any controlled trial or research study involves two main aspects: concealment allocation and a sham/placebo treatment.

Concealed allocation is not hard to achieve and technically is blinding during screening and separation of the candidates into two (or more) arms of a study. None the less, care should be taken in operator blinding including device options for coded programming (Alonzo et al. 2016; Russowsky Brunoni et al. 2015) and with subtle factors such as active-arm specific impedance changes or skin erythema considered (Ezquerro et al. 2017). On the other hand, it is not trivial to develop a reliable method of sham tDCS, as it should be very similar to the active tDCS condition (Fig. 7.3a), yet free of neuromodulatory effects (Boutron et al. 2007).

Literature suggests the following techniques for sham tDCS in randomized trials:

1. The fade in, short stimulation, fade out (FISSFO) approach (Fig. 7.3b). In this method, the Direct Current (DC) is initially increased incrementally over several seconds (e.g., 10 or 30 s) until reaching the current density of choice (Hummel et al. 2005; Iyer et al. 2005; Nitsche et al. 2003). In active tDCS, stimulation is

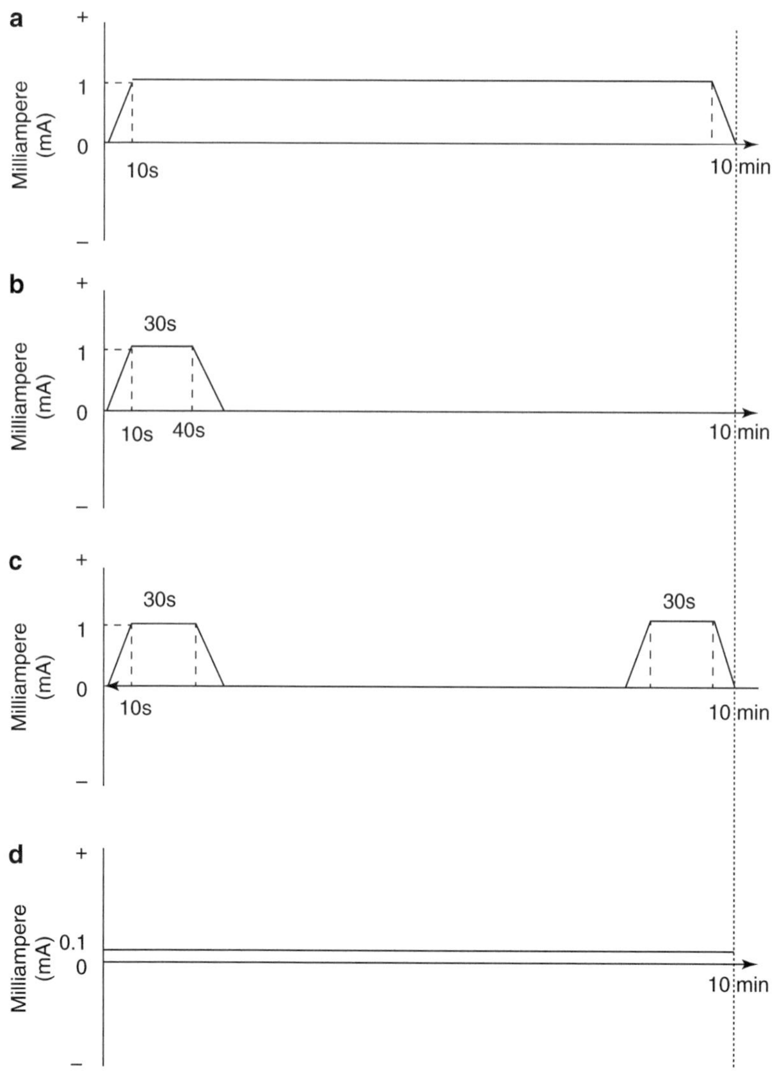

Fig. 7.3 Schematic diagram to simplify the techniques for application of sham tDCS (**a**) Active tDCS for 10 minutes with 10s fade in and 10s fade out at the beginning and end of the stimulation period. (**b**) The fade in, short stimulation, fade out (FISSFO) approach. (**c**) FISSFO at the beginning and FISSFO at the end of application time. (**d**) Low dose current (0.1mA) constant stimulation

maintained for the whole treatment time (e.g., between 10 and 20 min), while in sham tDCS it is ramped down after 30 s. The 30 s stimulation for sham tDCS was chosen based on previous reports that the perceived tingling sensations on the skin, usually fades during the start of tDCS (Nitsche et al. 2003). This method has been employed from the earliest tDCS studies. Gandiga et al. described similar rates of discomfort and adverse effects between active and sham tDCS (Gandiga et al. 2006). They also reported that none of the participants or investigators were able to distinguish between stimulation groups. This group concluded that tDCS can be used in double-blind sham controlled RCTs. In line with the findings in this study, other studies have also reported non-significant difference between the rate of common discomfort and adverse effects between the active vs. sham groups (Brunoni et al. 2011; Poreisz et al. 2007).

2. FISSFO at the beginning and FISSFO at the end of application time (Fig. 7.3c) (Caparelli-Daquer et al. 2012). In this approach, the current is ramped up and down at the beginning and end of the treatment time.
3. Maintaining a very low-dose current (e.g., 0.1 mA) during the stimulation session (Coffman et al. 2012; Fig. 7.3d).
4. For HD-tDCS, as the electrodes are smaller, a scalp-shunt sham is possible where electrodes are placed in close proximity (Richardson et al. 2014). The full current dose is provided (e.g. 2 mA for 20 min) even in the sham arm, but the proximity minimizes brain stimulation.

The tolerability (sensations) during any tDCS active or sham protocol is highly dependent on the electrodes use and preparation. Therefore, the internal validity of sham in any trial and the rationale for comparing sham reliability across trials is entirely depending on the reporting and controlled of electrode selection and preparation techniques (Woods et al. 2016).

It should be noted that the third sham technique (Fig. 7.3d), maintaining a very low-dose current during the stimulation session, is not used broadly by researchers. This may be partly due to the fact that lower intensities are also capable of inducing corticospinal changes (Bastani and Jaberzadeh 2013a, b), therefore this method is not a true 'sham' and it may confound interpretation of 'active' and 'sham' outcomes.

While the FISSFO procedure at 1 mA validated by Gandiga and colleagues (Gandiga et al. 2006) is followed in the majority of tDCS studies, results from a series of more recent studies questioned the reliability of this method. Ambrus and colleagues (Ambrus et al. 2010, 2012) have shown that experienced investigators were able to correctly distinguish between active and sham tDCS. Using higher current intensities (i.e. 2 mA instead of 1 mA) is considered as a key factor that is associated with detection of active tDCS (Ambrus et al. 2010; Dundas et al. 2007; O'Connell et al. 2012; Palm et al. 2013). Aforementioned examinations refer mainly to single-session studies. Integrity of blinding becomes more problematic in multiple-session tDCS studies, which refers to daily tDCS sessions for several days or weeks. This process may help participants to become more aware of the difference between their feelings during active and sham stimulation sessions, which may adversely affect the blinding process. In conclusion, compared to 2 mA, lower intensities (i.e. 1 mA) in single or multiple session tDCS studies represent a better approach to keep integrity of blinding. However, this is not in all cases the best functional solution and use of an "active" control (e.g., use of a behavioural task expected to not be influenced by stimulation of a given brain region) may provide greater clarity on tDCS specific effects.

tDCS as a Therapeutic Intervention

tDCS has been investigated as a therapeutic intervention for a large number of neurological and psychiatric conditions. In particular, tDCS has attracted a great deal of research attention in the areas of pain management, stroke rehabilitation, cognitive rehabilitation, and depression. There are a number of methodological considerations for selecting and designing tDCS protocols that should be taken into account depending on the method of intervention (i.e., as a stand-alone or adjunctive treatment). Considerations for both types of intervention are outlined below.

tDCS as a Stand-Alone Technique

Stand-alone tDCS, that is in the absence of a concomitant intervention, has promising therapeutic potential particularly for pain management and as a treatment for major depression. Additionally, it has been investigated for reducing symptoms in multiple other neurological and psychiatric conditions. These interventions typically involve the administration of repeated tDCS sessions over consecutive days, ranging from one to several weeks. The rationale is that the effects of tDCS on cortical excitability are cumulative when administered over repeated sessions (Alonzo et al. 2012; Galvez et al. 2013). There are several methodological considerations when designing a protocol for using tDCS as a stand-alone therapeutic technique.

First, both the number and spacing of treatments is potentially important for treatment outcomes. For example, for treatment of depression, greater number of sessions has been associated with increased treatment response (Brunoni et al. 2016). For management of neuropathic pain after spinal cord injury, however, shorter duration of treatment (i.e., <1 week) compared to longer duration of treatment (i.e., >1 week) was associated with better treatment effects (Mehta et al. 2015). The spacing of treatments also can affect physiological outcomes, with cumulative effects found with daily sessions, but not when sessions were spaced 1 day apart over a 5 day period (Alonzo et al. 2012). Choosing the optimal number and spacing of tDCS sessions therefore may be dependent on both the clinical condition and treatment outcome in question. Similar considerations should also be given to the duration of stimulation, current intensity and montage, as these factors may similarly affect outcomes differently for different clinical populations. This is the case as therapeutic outcomes for a particular clinical condition may depend on stimulation of different targeted regions. When investigating the therapeutic effects of tDCS in a new clinical condition, titration of stimulus parameters is therefore recommended, for example, in a clinical pilot.

A further consideration is standardization of subject's activity during the tDCS stimulation. This is potentially important as the relative activity levels within stimulated regions can interact with treatment outcomes. For example, the post stimulation physiological effects of tDCS have been shown to be dependent on whether subjects were sitting passively at rest during tDCS, paying attention to a cognitive task, or actively engaging the stimulated region with performance of a motor task (Antal et al. 2007; Fig. 7.4). The relative level of task-related activity may also affect treatment outcomes. Whilst performance of a slow motor task during stimulation of the motor cortex improved learning and increased cortical excitability, poorer learning and decreased cortical excitability occurred when subjects performed a fast motor task (Bortoletto et al. 2014). Due to these potential interactions dependent on

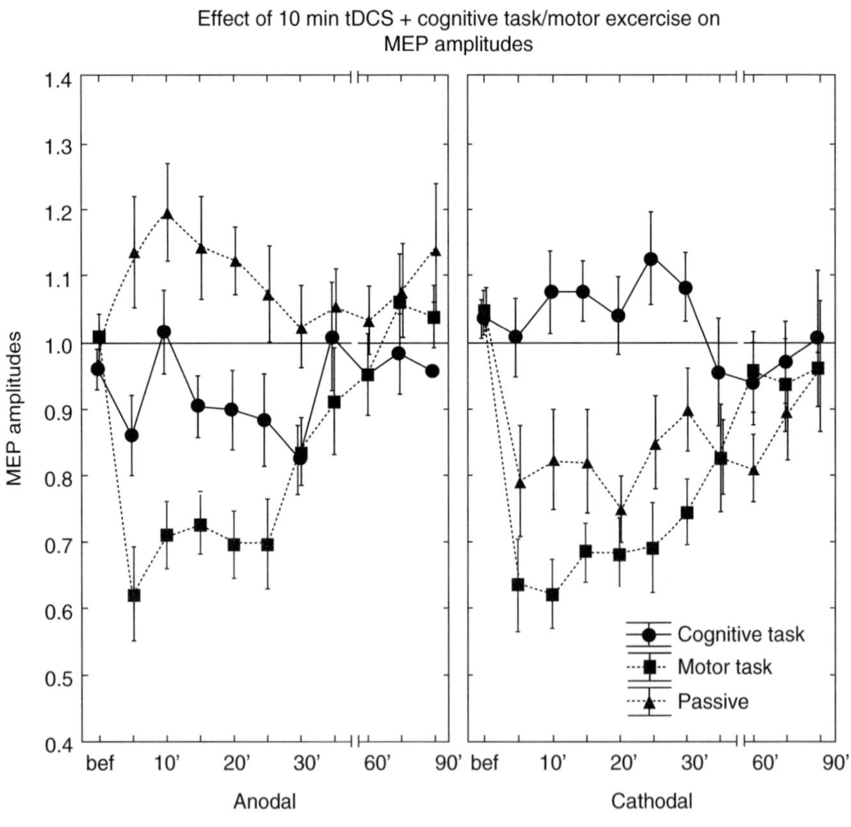

Fig. 7.4 Task related modulation of tDCS induced changes in cortical excitability within the motor cortex. (Reproduced with permission from Antal et al. (2007))

task activity during tDCS, attempts should be made to control for potential brain state effects during administration of tDCS as a stand-alone treatment. Implementing methods to either standardize or restrict behavioural activity, such as movement and talking, prior to, during and following stimulation is therefore recommended. Finally considering the interaction of placebo-related brain state changes with tDCS (Schambra et al. 2014), the patient experience (clinical ritual) including interaction with staff should be defined and controlled – especially in trials without concomitant intervention (explicit matched behavioural/cognitive therapy) as the case for most depression and pain trials.

For study design, the inclusion of a control condition that uses a different tDCS montage (e.g., actively stimulating an alternative target region) can also be considered. This could have potential utility for elucidating whether treatment effects are associated with neuromodulatory effects in particular brain regions. For example, Boggio et al. (2008) investigated the effects of stand-alone tDCS as a treatment for depression and randomized participants to receive either 10 sessions of active tDCS with the anode positioned either over the left dorsolateral prefrontal cortex (LDLPFC), or occipital cortex with the cathode positioned over the right supraorbital area, or sham. Results showed therapeutic effects only in the LDLPFC condition. This research thus formed the rationale for tDCS montages used in subsequent RCTs investigating tDCS for depression. Given limits on tDCS focality, computational models of current flow may be consulted in selecting the targeted intervention montage and active control montages (Truong et al. 2014).

tDCS as an Adjunctive Technique

Recently, there has been increased attention given to the investigation of tDCS as an adjunctive technique, through combining tDCS with other therapeutic interventions. These other therapeutic interventions could potentially be pharmacological, another form of brain stimulation, or behavioral. The rationale for using tDCS as an adjunct to pharmacological interventions is based on evidence that particular medications either potentiate or diminish tDCS neuromodulatory effects (Nitsche et al. 2012; Stagg and Nitsche 2011). tDCS may be used in combination with other forms of brain stimulation to prime, or precondition prior to administration of the second form of brain stimulation (Loo et al. 2009). Regarding combining tDCS with behavioral interventions, studies using animal models show that the presence of ongoing background activity is necessary for inducing lasting neuroplastic changes (i.e., Hebbian plasticity; Fritsch et al. 2010). In this regard, tDCS has been investigated as an adjunctive intervention to rehabilitative strategies in patients following stroke (Elsner et al. 2016), cognitive rehabilitation (Elmasry et al. 2015) and other interventions (e.g., cognitive behavioral therapy; D'Urso, Mantovani et al. 2013).

A potentially important methodological consideration for using tDCS as an adjunctive method with behavioral interventions is the timing of tDCS administration relative to intervention/task execution. Both behavioral and physiological outcomes have been shown to differ depending on whether tDCS is administered 'online' (i.e., during tDCS administration) or 'offline' (i.e., either immediately prior to or following stimulation). For example, while improvement in motor learning was found with 'online' tDCS, decreased learning occurred when the same task was performed 'offline' following tDCS stimulation (Stagg et al. 2011). Similarly, better performance on a cognitive training task was found during 'online' compared to 'offline' tDCS administration, with maintenance of performance benefits the following day (Martin et al. 2014). These effects could at least be partly attributed to relative differences in the effects of tDCS on regional blood flow (i.e., as an index of neuronal activity) between the two conditions, with widespread increased activity during 'online' stimulation, and decreased activity in the period immediately following stimulation (Stagg et al. 2013). Given that therapeutic outcomes are likely dependent on the nature of the intervention (e.g., the effect of cognitive behavioral therapy on tDCS neuromodulatory effects), careful consideration should therefore be given to the timing of tDCS administration.

A further consideration is study design. It is ideal to include stand-alone tDCS as a control condition when it is unclear whether there is a therapeutic, additive or synergistic effect of tDCS as a stand-alone treatment or when combined with a particular intervention. The SELECT DCS trial was conducted in patients with major depression (Brunoni et al. 2013). This study used a 2 × 2 factorial design which included the following conditions: sham tDCS + placebo, tDCS + placebo, sertraline + sham tDCS, and sertraline + tDCS conditions. Such a design thus enabled the investigation of whether tDCS as an adjunctive intervention combined with sertraline had additive or synergistic effects on treatment outcomes.

Selection of an appropriate tDCS protocol depends upon the nine parameters outlined in Fig. 7.5.

Physiologic/Therapeutic Goals

Physiologic Effects

Physiologic effects of tDCS can be polarity dependent (Priori et al. 1998; Rowny and Lisanby 2008; Wagner et al. 2007). Typically, it is considered in the literature that application of the positive polarity electrode (Anode) over the target brain area (a-tDCS), increases resting membrane potential (depolarization of soma of cortical neurons) which leads to increased cortical excitability (Nitsche and Paulus 2000). Instead, application of the negatively polarity electrode (cathode) over the target brain area (c-tDCS), decreases resting membrane potential (hyperpolarization of cortical neurons soma), and causes decreased cortical excitability. However, new literature indicates that the polarity dependent effect of tDCS on cortical excitability is protocol

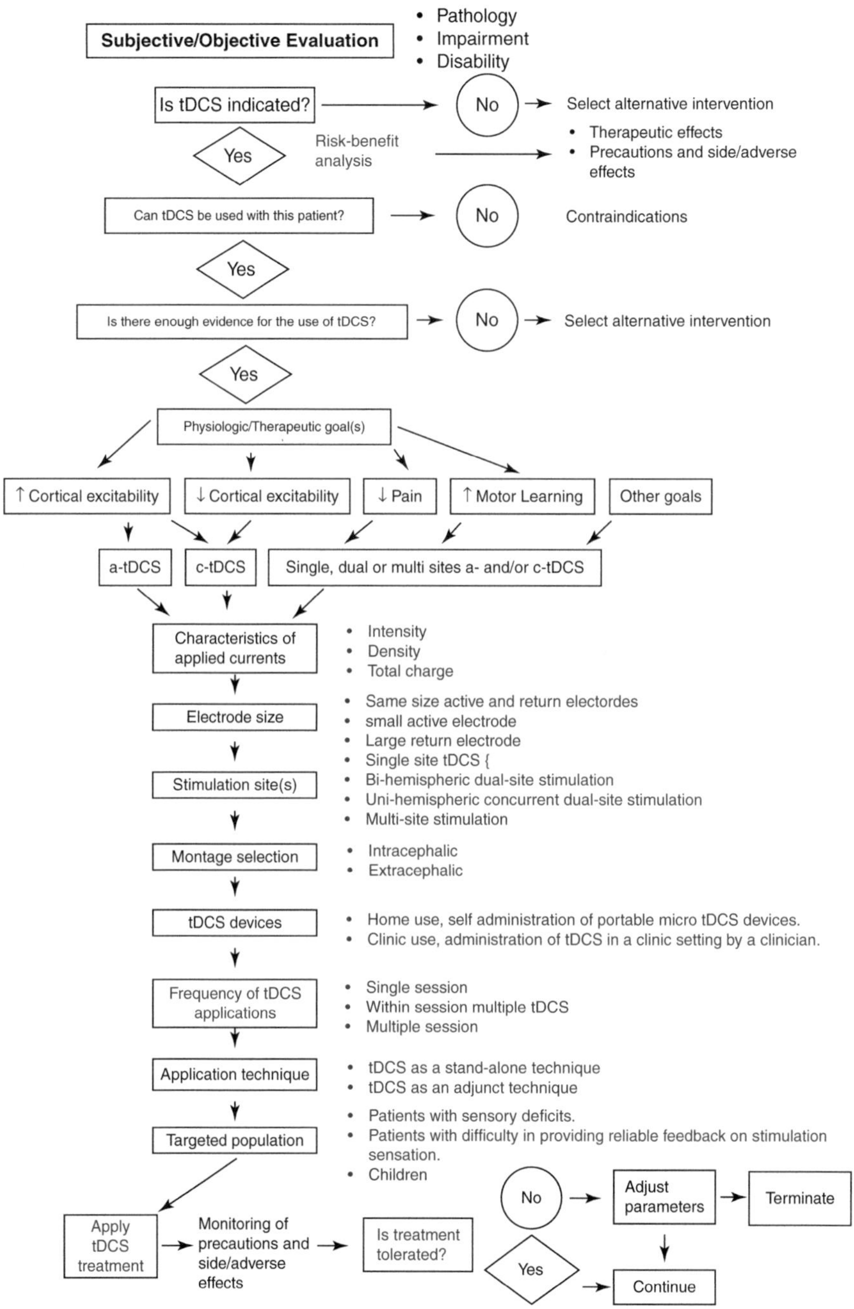

Fig. 7.5 Decision tree for selection of tDCS protocols

specific. This indicates that c-tDCS parameters, such as current intensity, duration of application, and site of stimulation, may determine its effects on corticospinal excitability (Batsikadze et al. 2013; Boros et al. 2008; Monte-Silva et al. 2010). Batsikadze et al. (2013) described a non-linear relationship between stimulation intensity and modulation of corticospinal excitability (Batsikadze et al. 2013). For example, one study showed that 20 min c-tDCS with intensity of 1 mA significantly *diminished* corticospinal excitability, while 20 min c-tDCS with intensity of 2 mA *increased* corticospinal excitability (Batsikadze et al. 2013). Recently, Vaseghi et al. showed that concurrent c-tDCS of M1 and DLPFC increased the corticospinal excitability, unlike separate stimulation of these two cortical centers (Vaseghi et al. 2016). These finding supports the notion that the effects of c-tDCS is protocol specific.

Therapeutic Effects

tDCS is a non-invasive technique that is considered to produce only transient and mild adverse effects (Aparício et al. 2016; Bikson et al. 2016, 2017; Russo et al. 2017). Its use in clinical research has significantly increased, particularly for neuropsychiatric disorders such as major depressive disorder, schizophrenia, rehabilitation after stroke, Parkinson's disease, drug addiction and other neurological and psychiatric conditions (Fregni and Pascual-Leone 2007; George and Aston-Jones 2010; Nitsche et al. 2009). In spite of heterogeneous results in some studies, typically due to differences in the methodological procedures and differing inclusion/exclusion criteria used in a given study, the findings are generally promising and further well controlled clinical studies are required to better address the therapeutic effects of tDCS.

Characteristics of Applied Currents

The extent of tDCS-induced corticospinal excitability changes depend on the current intensity/density (Nitsche and Paulus 2000) and duration of current application (Furubayashi et al. 2008; Nitsche et al. 2008; Nitsche and Paulus 2000; Nitsche and Paulus 2001). As reported in a systematic review (Bastani and Jaberzadeh 2012), tDCS with higher current densities induces larger corticospinal excitability changes. Nitsche and Paulus (2000) compared five current intensities between 0.2 and 1 mA (CDs between 0.006 and 0.029 mA/cm^2). They found that a stimulus intensity of at least 0.6 mA (electrode size 35 cm^2; CD: 0.017 mA/cm^2) for 5 min is required to induce a significant increase in corticospinal excitability (Nitsche and Paulus 2000).

Even though, literature indicates success in the use of 1–2 mA (10–20 min) for induction of different cortical and behavioral changes (Furubayashi et al. 2008; Nitsche and Paulus 2000; 2001; Nitsche et al. 2008), Bastani and Jaberzadeh (2013a, b) showed that lower intensities (i.e. 0.3 mA) induces larger corticospinal excitability changes than 0.7 mA or 1.4 mA. This indicates that effects of intensity may be non-linear. Thus, future research is required to further evaluate the modulatory effects of lower current intensities on the induction of corticospinal changes. Compared to higher intensities (1–2 mA), the 0.3 mA induces less side/adverse effects and therefore it is tolerated better by participants and could be safely used in protocols with multiple tDCS applications. However, the majority of current evidence in tDCS exists for stimulation intensities between 1 and 2 mA.

Electrode Size

Electrode size is a key factor in determination of current density and total charge density during application of tDCS, which also influences the relative spatial distribution of the applied current in the brain. Using smaller electrode sizes tends to increase the relative spatial focality, as measured by neurophysiological outcomes, of the induced cortical electric field during application of tDCS (Nitsche et al. 2007) though physical computational models (Datta et al. 2009; Dmochowski et al. 2011) and measurments (Antal et al. 2014; Huang et al. 2017; Jog et al. 2016) predict current must always flow in the brain regions between electrodes. Due to close proximity of cortical sites within the brain, larger electrodes can directly affect a number cortical sites affected by stimulation.

Nitsche et al. (2007) have manipulated the size of conventional pad electrodes and assessed its effects on modulation of corticospinal excitability. They found that a small (3.5 cm^2) anode placed over the abductor digiti minimi representation over M1 did not affect the excitability of the neighbouring representation of the first dorsal interosseus muscle, which located just outside the boundaries of the anode. Furthermore, computer modelling studies showed that larger electrodes resulted in more diffuse current flow between the electrodes (Datta et al. 2009; Wagner et al. 2007). Additionally, Bastani and Jaberzadeh (2013a, b) compared the effects of different electrode sizes over M1 and showed that using smaller electrodes with same current density induces larger corticospinal excitability changes. They concluded that the larger electrodes may also stimulate nearby cortical functional areas, which may have inhibitory effects on the M1. The relationship between electrode current density and resultant current density (electric field) in the brain is not simple, depending also in the position of the "return" electrode, and can be informed by computational current flow models (Bikson et al. 2010; Faria et al. 2011) (also see Chap. 9).

However, even the smallest brain regions can be functionally connected to other distal brain regions. Thus, it is not correct to assume that even more focal stimulation of a brain region, or even truly focal stimulation of a single gyrus (the latter of which is currently not possible with currently available methods – such as what we see during high definition tDCS), remains locally. Indeed, it may have downstream effects on the function of anatomically connected distal brain regions (Polanía et al. 2012). This fact highlights the critical importance for *not* over-interpreting the focality of tDCS results, even when using smaller electrodes such as 3.5 cm^2 or even 1 cm diameter high definition electrodes.

Stimulation Site(s)

The stimulation site should be selected carefully based on the desired effects of tDCS interventions. As discussed above, no brain region operates in true isolation. Different neural processes are carried out by a dynamic network of interacting brain regions (Baudewig et al. 2001; Lang et al. 2004, 2005). In addition, many behavioral indicators of neurological and psychiatric diseases are not merely the result of abnormality in one isolated brain region but represent alterations in different brain sites within brain networks. As a result, simultaneous or consecutive stimulation of different superficial sites in the brain networks may be central to optimizing tDCS outcomes.

Montage Selection

Traditional application of tDCS involves, placement of one electrode where current is delivered to the head over a cortical site of interest and one return electrode where that current is taken back up, over another area. This electrode arrangement is called a cephalic montage and is the most utilised montage for application of tDCS. If the return electrode is positioned over another region of the body (not over the cranium) the technique is called extracephalic. It should be noted that the size and the place of the return electrode determine the path of the penetrating current, which appears to influence the final effects of stimulation (Bikson et al. 2010; Kabakov et al. 2012). A common misconception in the literature is that the return electrode is passive (or inert). However, studies have shown that the return electrodes are not physiologically passive/inert and actively contribute (whether antagonistic or additive) based on return electrode position (Accornero et al. 2007; Antal et al. 2004).

tDCS Devices

Currently a limited set of certified tDCS-stimulators are available. All certified devices deliver constant current (Agnew and Mccreery 1987; Bronstein et al. 2015), are battery operated and can be broadly classified as either laboratory/clinic-based (DaSilva et al. 2011; Schestatsky et al. 2013; Villamar et al. 2013) or home-based (Kasschau et al. 2015) devices. Stimulators differ for specific features, such as suitability for other stimulation protocols (e.g., transcranial alternating current stimulation, transcranial random noise stimulation, etc.), programming capabilities, number of channels, size, weight, portability, suitability for magnetic resonance imaging (MRI), ramp features, and blinding options. All certified tDCS-stimulators provide the basic features required for tDCS. These basic features include the ability to produce constant current, the ability to ramp current up and down over a period of time (rather than on/off), a method for evaluating electrode contact quality (e.g., impedance), a method for setting stimulation intensity (e.g., 1 vs. 2 mA), and a method for setting stimulation duration (e.g., 10, 15, 20 min, etc.). As such, stimulator choice depends on planned application (e.g., need for blinding protocols, desired intensity level, number of electrodes, portability, wear-ability, home-use, lab/clinic-use, etc.). In contrast to lab/clinic stimulation devices, home-based devices are designed to simplify self- (or proxy-) administration to patients at home. In these home-based devices the stimulation parameters are usually set by the clinicians or researchers, and to avoid any un-authorized use, they are fitted with locking mechanisms (e.g., coded activation of device for single use, remote activation by clinician, etc.) (Charvet et al. 2015). In addition, exactness of delivered current delivered is of crucial importance, and should be tested (e.g., by aid of an oscilloscope), since minor deviances can result in prominent alterations of experimental or clinical outcomes.

Frequency of tDCS Applications

Earlier literature reported a monotonic relationship between the duration of tDCS application and its induced effects (Jaberzadeh et al. 2012; Nitsche and Paulus 2000, 2001). However, this notion was challenged by Monte-Silva et al. (2013). They concluded that the observed direct relationship between the duration of tDCS application, size and duration of the effect of stimulation may not exist during longer applications of tDCS. Neuronal counter-regulation, which prevents over-excitation of the involved neurons, is a possible mechanism for explanation of this observation (Monte-Silva et al. 2013). This finding suggests that increasing the duration of tDCS application is not the best strategy for induction of larger and longer lasting corticospinal excitability (Monte-Silva et al. 2013), but may not generalize to other outcomes (e.g., cognition, etc.). Within session repetition of shorter tDCS applications, could be considered as an alternative approach for induction of larger and more lasting effects (Bastani and Jaberzadeh 2014; Monte-Silva et al. 2013). Monte-Silva et al. (2013) showed that single-session repetition of 13 min of a-tDCS within certain time intervals induces M1 excitability alterations which lasted for 24 h. This finding was supported by Bastani and Jaberzadeh (2014), concluding that within-session repeated tDCS induces larger corticospinal excitability with day-long lasting effects. Multiple sessions of tDCS application appear to extend the size and duration of the effects (Goldsworthy et al. 2015; Meinzer et al. 2014).Stimulation repetition interval may also be relevant (Monte-Silva et al. 2013).

Application Technique

tDCS could be used as a stand-alone therapeutic intervention or as an adjunctive technique to prime the effects of other treatments (Hesse et al. 2007; Hummel and Cohen 2006). As a stand-alone therapeutic technique, tDCS has been used for modulation of pain (Mehta et al. 2015; Rostami et al. 2015), treatment of depression (Brunoni et al. 2016), and management of epileptic seizures (Assenza et al. 2014). As an adjunct technique it could be used to facilitate motor rehabilitation following stroke (Elsner et al. 2016), or to enhance learning with other interventions.

Targeted Population

tDCS can be used in both healthy and patient populations at different age levels. Differences in brain size and anatomy suggest that children and adult brains require different tDCS dosage (Kessler et al. 2013; Minhas, Bikson, Woods, Rosen, & Kessler, 2012). This is driven by a number of factors, including smaller overall head size, thinner cerebrospinal fluid space in children, thinner skulls in children, and a number of other physical factors. Likewise, compared to younger adults, the brain in elderly people, require special consideration for similar reasons (e.g., greater cerebrospinal space, etc.). This will be described further in Chap. 20. Population specific dosage calculations for these groups have not been established yet and should be considered as a priority for future tDCS research. Caution must be taken when selecting specific design criteria for populations yet unstudied or with limited prior study using tDCS. In addition, special consideration should be given to vulnerable populations or groups that may not clearly adhere to the study design considerations above (e.g., children). Ethical considerations regarding vulnerable populations and regarding protocol selection will be discussed in Chap. 14.

Conclusion

This chapter provided a framework for considering the factors relevant to make an informed choice about the appropriate tDCS approach, protocol and device for a given study or clinical trial. The necessary workspace that must be considered to reach an informed and appropriate decision is highly complex. Ranging from electrode size, stimulation intensity, online vs. offline application, stand-alone vs. adjunctive approaches, duration of stimulation, location of stimulation, or the additional factors covered in this chapter, each must be considered carefully before study initiation or clinical application. Many of the topics in this list deserve careful and detailed consideration in their own right. Other chapters in this book will serve to provide the detailed information necessary for full consideration of tDCS approach, protocol, and device in the design phase of clinical and research applications of tDCS. While the literature provides a primary point of reference for study protocols used in past studies, it is very often the case that incomplete methodological reporting limits our ability to fully replicate prior studies. The information provided in the current chapter will help the reader to identify critical considerations that should be attended to not only in their own study or trial design, but also in their evaluation of studies presented in the literature.

References

Accornero, N., Li Voti, P., & La Riccia, M. (2007). Visual evoked potentials modulation during direct current cortical polarization. *Experimental Brain Research, 178*(2), 261–266.

Agnew, W. F., & Mccreery, D. B. (1987). Considerations for safety in the use of extracranial stimulation for motor evoked potentials. *Neurosurgery, 20*, 143–147.

Alonzo, A., Aaronson, S., Bikson, M., Husain, M., Lisanby, S., Martin, D., … Loo, C. (2016). Study design and methodology for a multicentre, randomised controlled trial of transcranial direct current stimulation as a treatment for unipolar and bipolar depression. *Contemporary Clinical Trials, 51*, 65–71.

Alonzo, A., Brassil, J., Talyor, J., Martin, D., & Loo, C. K. (2012). Daily transcranial direct current stimulation (tDCS) leads to greater increases in cortical excitability than second daily transcranial direct current stimulation. *Brain Stimulation, 5*, 208–213.

Ambrus, G. G., Al-Moyed, H., & Chaieb, L. (2012). The fade-in--short stimulation – fade out approach to sham tDCS – reliable at 1 mA for naïve and experienced subjects, but not investigators. *Brain Stimulation, 5*(4), 499–504.

Ambrus, G. G., Paulus, W., & Antal, A. (2010). Cutaneous perception thresholds of electrical stimulation methods: Comparison of tDCS and tRNS. *Clinical Neurophysiology, 121*, 1908–1914.

Antal, A., Bikson, M., Datta, A., Lafon, B., Dechent, P., Parra, L. C., & Paulus, W. (2014). Imaging artifacts induced by electrical stimulation during conventional fMRI of the brain. *Neuroimage, 85 Pt 3*, 1040–1047.

Antal, A., Nitsche, M. A., & Kruse, W. (2004). Direct current stimulation over V5 enhances visuomotor coordination by improving motion perception in humans. *Journal of Cognitive Neuroscience, 16*(4), 521–527.

Antal, A., Terney, D., Poreisz, C., & Paulus, W. (2007). Towards unravelling task-related modulations of neuroplastic changes induced in the human motor cortex. *The European Journal of Neuroscience, 26*(9), 2687–2691.

Anton, S. D., Woods, A. J., Ashizawa, T., Barb, D., Buford, T. W., Carter, C. S., … Pahor, M. (2015). Successful aging: Advancing the science of physical independence in older adults. *Ageing Research Reviews, 24*, 304–327.

Aparício, L. V. M., Guarienti, F., Razza, L. B., Carvalho, A. F., Fregni, F., & Brunoni, A. R. (2016). A systematic review on the acceptability and tolerability of transcranial direct current stimulation treatment in neuropsychiatry trials. *Brain Stimulation, 9*, 671–681.

Apolinário-Souza, T., Romano-Silva, M. A., de Miranda, D. M., Malloy-Diniz, L. F., Benda, R. N., Ugrinowitsch, H., & Lage, G. M. (2016). The primary motor cortex is associated with learning the absolute, but not relative, timing dimension of a task: A tDCS study. *Physiology & Behavior, 160*, 18–25.

Assenza, G., Campana, C., Formica, D., Schena, E., Taffoni, F., Di Pino, G., & Di Lazzaro, V. (2014). Efficacy of cathodal transcranial direct current stimulation in drug-resistant epilepsy: A proof of principle. *Conference Proceedings: Annual International Conference of the IEEE Engineering in Medicine and Biology Society, 2014*, 530–533.

Bardi, L., Kanai, R., Mapelli, D., & Walsh, V. (2013). Direct current stimulation (tDCS) reveals parietal asymmetry in local/global and salience-based selection. *Cortex, 49*(3), 850–860.

Bastani, A., & Jaberzadeh, S. (2012). Does anodal transcranial direct current stimulation enhance excitability of the motor cortex and motor function in healthy individuals and subjects with stroke: A systematic review and meta-analysis. *Clinical Neurophysiology, 123*, 644–657.

Bastani, A., & Jaberzadeh, S. (2013a). Differential modulation of corticospinal plasticity by different current densities of anodal transcranial direct current stimulation. *PLoS One, 8*, e72254.

Bastani, A., & Jaberzadeh, S. (2013b). A-tDCS differential modulation of corticospinal excitability: The effects of electrode size. *Brain Stimulation, 6*(6), 932–937.

Bastani, A., & Jaberzadeh, S. (2014). Within-session repeated a-tDCS: The effects of repetition rate and inter-stimulus interval on corticospinal excitability and motor performance. *Clinical Neurophysiology, 125*(9), 1809–1818.

Batsikadze, G., Moliadze, V., & Paulus, W. (2013). Partially non-linear stimulation intensity-dependent effects of direct current stimulation on motor cortex excitability in humans. *The Journal of Physiology, 591*(7), 1987–2000.

Baudewig, J., Nitsche, M. A., & Paulus, W. (2001). Regional modulation of BOLD MRI responses to human sensorimotor activation by transcranial direct current stimulation. *Magnetic Resonance in Medicine, 45*, 196–201.

Bikson, M., Datta, A., Rahman, A., & Scaturro, J. (2010). Electrode montages for tDCS and weak transcranial electrical stimulation: Role of "return" electrode's position and size. *Clinical Neurophysiology, 121*, 1976–1978.

Bikson, M., Grossman, P., Thomas, C., Zannou, A. L., Jiang, J., Adnan, T., … Woods, A. J. (2016). Safety of transcranial direct current stimulation: Evidence based update 2016. *Brain Stimulation, 9*(5), 641–661.

Bikson, M., Grossman, P., Zannou, A. L., Kronberg, G., Truong, D., Boggio, P., … Woods, A. J. (2017). Response to letter to the editor: Safety of transcranial direct current stimulation: Evidence based update 2016. *Brain Stimulation, 10*(5), 986–987.

Boggio, P. S., Rigonatti, S. P., Ribeiro, R. B., Myczkowski, M. L., Nitsche, M. A., Pascual-Leone, A., & Fregni, F. (2008). A randomized, double-blind clinical trial on the efficacy of cortical direct current stimulation for the treatment of major depression. *The International Journal of Neuropsychopharmacology, 11*(2), 249–254.

Boros, K., Poreisz, C., Munchau, A., Paulus, W., & Nitsche, M. A. (2008). Premotor transcranial direct current stimulation (tDCS) affects primary motor excitability in humans. *The European Journal of Neuroscience, 27*, 1292–1300.

Bortoletto, M., Veniero, D., Thut, G., & Miniussi, C. (2014). The contribution of TMS–EEG coregistration in the exploration of the human cortical connectome. *Neuroscience and Biobehavioral Reviews, 49C*, 114–124.

Boutron, I., Guittet, L., Estellat, C., Moher, D., Hróbjartsson, A., & Ravaud, P. (2007). Reporting methods of blinding in randomized trials assessing nonpharmacological treatments. *PLoS Medicine, 4*(2), e61.

Bronstein, J. M., Tagliati, M., McIntyre, C., Chen, R., Cheung, T., Hargreaves, E. L., … Okun, M. S. (2015). The rationale driving the evolution of deep brain stimulation to constant-current devices. *Neuromodulation, 18*, 85–89.

Brunoni, A. R., Amadera, J., Berbel, B., Volz, M. S., Rizzerio, B. G., & Fregni, F. (2011). A systematic review on reporting and assessment of adverse effects associated with transcranial direct current stimulation. *The International Journal of Neuropsychopharmacology, 14*(8), 1133–1145.

Brunoni, A. R., Moffa, A. H., Fregni, F., Palm, U., Padberg, F., Blumberger, D. M., … Loo, C. K. (2016). Transcranial direct current stimulation for acute major depressive episodes: Meta-analysis of individual patient data. [Review]. *British Journal of Psychiatry.*

Brunoni, A. R., Schestatsky, P., Lotufo, P. A., Benseñor, I. M., & Fregni, F. (2014). Comparison of blinding effectiveness between sham tDCS and placebo sertraline in a 6-week major depression randomized clinical trial. *Clinical Neurophysiology, 125*(2), 298–305.

Brunoni, A. R., Valiengo, L., Baccaro, A., Zanão, T. A., de Oliveira, J. F., Goulart, A., … Fregni, F. (2013). The sertraline versus electrical current therapy for treating depression clinical study: Results from a factorial, randomized, controlled trial. *JAMA Psychiatry, 70*(4), 383–391.

Caparelli-Daquer, E. M., Zimmermann, T. J., Mooshagian, E., Parra, L. C., Rice, J. K., Datta, A., … Wassermann, E. M. (2012). A pilot study on effects of 4×1 high-definition tDCS on motor cortex excitability. *Conference Proceedings: Annual International Conference of the IEEE Engineering in Medicine and Biology Society.*

Charvet, L. E., Kasschau, M., Datta, A., Knotkova, H., Stevens, M. C., Alonzo, A., … Bikson, M. (2015). Remotely-supervised transcranial direct current stimulation (tDCS) for clinical trials: Guidelines for technology and protocols. *Frontiers in Systems Neuroscience, 9*, 26.

Coffman, B. A., Trumbo, M. C., & Clark, V. P. (2012). Enhancement of object detection with transcranial direct current stimulation is associated with increased attention. *BMC Neuroscience, 13*, 108.

D'Urso, G., Mantovani, A., Micillo, M., Priori, A., & Muscettola, G. (2013). Transcranial direct current stimulation and cognitive-behavioral therapy: Evidence of a synergistic effect in treatment-resistant depression. [Case Reports Letter]. *Brain Stimulation, 6*(3), 465–467.

DaSilva, A. F., Volz, M. S., Bikson, M., & Fregni, F. (2011). Electrode positioning and montage in transcranial direct current stimulation. *Journal of Visualized Experiments*. (51):e2744.

Datta, A., Bansal, V., Diaz, J., Patel, J., Reato, D., & Bikson, M. (2009). Gyri -precise head model of transcranial DC stimulation: Improved spatial focality using a ring electrode versus conventional rectangular pad. *Brain Stimulation, 2*, 201–207.

Dmochowski, J. P., Datta, A., Bikson, M., Su, Y., & Parra, L. C. (2011). Optimized multi-electrode stimulation increases focality and intensity at target. *Journal of Neural Engineering, 8*, 46011.

Dundas, J. E., Thickbroom, G. W., & Mastaglia, F. L. (2007). Perception of comfort during transcranial DC stimulation: Effect of NaCl solution concentration applied to sponge electrodes. *Clinical Neurophysiology, 118*(5), 1166–1170.

Elmasry, J., Loo, C., & Martin, D. (2015). A systematic review of transcranial electrical stimulation combined with cognitive training. *Restorative Neurology and Neuroscience, 33*(3), 263–278.

Elsner, B., Kugler, J., Pohl, M., & Mehrholz, J. (2016). Transcranial direct current stimulation (tDCS) for improving activities of daily living, and physical and cognitive functioning, in people after stroke. *Cochrane Database of Systematic Reviews.*

Ezquerro, F., Moffa, A. H., Bikson, M., Khadka, N., Aparicio, L. V. M., de Sampaio-Junior, B., … Brunoni, A. R. (2017). The influence of skin redness on blinding in transcranial direct current stimulation studies: A crossover trial. *Neuromodulation, 20*, 248–255.

Faria, P., Hallett, M., & Miranda, P. C. (2011). A finite element analysis of the effect of electrode area and inter-electrode distance on the spatial distribution of the current density in tDCS. *Journal of Neural Engineering, 8*, 66017.

Filmer, H. L., Dux, P. E., & Mattingley, J. B. (2014). Applications of transcranial direct current stimulation for understanding brain function. *Trends in Neurosciences, 37*(12), 742–753.

Fregni, F., & Pascual-Leone, A. (2007). Technology insight: Noninvasive brain stimulation in neurology-perspectives on the therapeutic potential of rTMS and tDCS. *Nature Clinical Practice. Neurology, 3*(7), 383–393.

Fritsch, B., Reis, J., Martinowich, K., Schambra, H. M., Ji, Y., Cohen, L. G., & Lu, B. (2010). Direct current stimulation promotes BDNF-dependent synaptic plasticity: Potential implications for motor learning. *Neuron, 66*(2), 198–204.

Furubayashi, T., Terao, Y., Arai, N., Okabe, S., Mochizuki, H., Hanajima, R., … Ugawa, Y. (2008). Short and long duration transcranial direct current stimulation (tDCS) over the human hand motor area. *Experimental Brain Research, 185*, 279–286.

Furuya, S., Klaus, M., Nitsche, M. A., Paulus, W., & Altenmüller, E. (2014). Ceiling effects prevent further improvement of transcranial stimulation in skilled musicians. *The Journal of Neuroscience, 34*(41), 13834–13839.

Galvez, V., Alonzo, A., & Martin, D. (2013). Transcranial direct current stimulation treatment protocols: Should stimulus intensity be constant or incremental over multiple sessions? *International Journal of Neuropsychopharmacology, 16*, 13–21.

Gandiga, P. C., Hummel, F. C., & Cohen, L. G. (2006). Transcranial DC stimulation (tDCS): A tool for double-blind sham-controlled clinical studies in brain stimulation. *Clinical Neurophysiology, 117*(4), 845–850.

George, M. S., & Aston-Jones, G. (2010). Noninvasive techniques for probing neurocircuitry and treating illness: Vagus nerve stimulation (VNS), transcranial magnetic stimulation (TMS) and transcranial direct current stimulation (tDCS). *Neuropsychopharmacology, 35*(1), 301–316.

Goldsworthy, M. R., Pitcher, J. B., & Ridding, M. C. (2015). Spaced noninvasive brain stimulation: Prospects for inducing long- lasting human cortical plasticity. *Neurorehabilitation and Neural Repair, 28*(8), 714–721.

Hendy, A. M., Teo, W. P., & Kidgell, D. J. (2015). Anodal transcranial direct current stimulation prolongs the cross-education of strength and corticomotor plasticity. *Medicine and Science in Sports and Exercise, 47*(9), 1788–1797.

Hesse, S., Werner, C., Schonhardt, E. M., Bardeleben, A., Jenrich, W., & Kirker, S. G. (2007). Combined transcranial direct current stimulation and robot-assisted arm training in subacute stroke patients: A pilot study. *Restorative Neurology and Neuroscience, 25*, 9–15.

Huang, Y., Liu, A. A., Lafon, B., Friedman, D., Dayan, M., Wang, X., … Parra, L. C. (2017). Measurements and models of electric fields in the in vivo human brain during transcranial electric stimulation. *Elife, 6*, e18834.

Hummel, F., Celnik, P., Giraux, P., Floel, A., Wu, W. H., Gerloff, C., & Cohen, L. G. (2005). Effects of non-invasive cortical stimulation on skilled motor function in chronic stroke. *Brain, 128*(3), 490–499.

Hummel, F. C., & Cohen, L. G. (2006). Non-invasive brain stimulation: A new strategy to improve neurorehabilitation after stroke? *Lancet Neurology, 5*(8), 708–712.

Iuculano, T., & Cohen Kadosh, R. (2013). The mental cost of cognitive enhancement. *The Journal of Neuroscience, 33*(10), 4482–4486.

Iyer, M. B., Mattu, U., Grafman, J., Lomarev, M., Sato, S., & Wassermann, E. M. (2005). Safety and cognitive effect of frontal DC brain polarization in healthy individuals. *Neurology, 64*(5), 872–875.

Jaberzadeh, S., Bastani, A., & Kidgell, D. (2012). Does the longer application of anodal-transcranial direct current stimulaton increase corticomotor excitability further? A pilot study. *Basic and Clinical Neuroscience, 3*, 28–35.

Jog, M. V., Smith, R. X., Jann, K., Dunn, W., Lafon, B., Truong, D., … Wang, D. J. J. (2016). In-vivo imaging of magnetic fields induced by transcranial direct current stimulation (tDCS) in human brain using MRI. *Scientific Reports, 6*, 34385.

Kabakov, A. Y., Muller, P. A., Pascual-Leone, A., Jensen, F. E., & Rotenberg, A. (2012). Contribution of axonal orientation to pathway-dependent modulation of excitatory transmission by direct current stimulation in isolated rat hippocampus. *Journal of Neurophysiology, 107*, 1881–1889.

Kasschau, M., Sherman, K., Haider, L., Frontario, A., Shaw, M., Datta, A., … Charvet, L. (2015). A protocol for the use of remotely-supervised transcranial direct current stimulation (tDCS) in multiple sclerosis (MS). *Journal of Visualized Experiments*. (106):e53542.

Kessler, S. K., Minhas, P., Woods, A. J., Rosen, A., Gorman, C., & Bikson, M. (2013). Dosage considerations for transcranial direct current stimulation in children: A computational modeling study. *PLoS One, 8*, e76112.

Lang, N., Nitsche, M. A., Paulus, W., Rothwell, J. C., & Lemon, R. N. (2004). Effects of transcranial direct current stimulation over the human motor cortex on corticospinal and transcallosal excitability. *Experimental Brain Research, 156*, 439–443.

Lang, N., Siebner, H. R., Ward, N. S., Lee, L., Nitsche, M. A., Paulus, W., … Frackowiak, R. S. (2005). How does transcranial DC stimulation of the primary motor cortex alter regional neuronal activity in the human brain? *The European Journal of Neuroscience, 22*, 495–504.

Loo, C., Martin, D., Pigot, M., Arul-Anandam, P., Mitchell, P., & Sachdev, P. (2009). Transcranial direct current stimulation priming of therapeutic repetitive transcranial magnetic stimulation: A pilot study. *Journal of ECT, 25*, 256–260.

Lowe, C. J., Vincent, C., & Hall, P. A. (2017). Effects of noninvasive brain stimulation on food cravings and consumption: A meta-analytic review. *Psychosomatic Medicine, 79*, 2–13.

Martin, D. M., Liu, R., Alonzo, A., Green, M., & Loo, C. K. (2014). Use of transcranial direct current stimulation (tDCS) to enhance cognitive training: Effect of timing of stimulation. *Experimental Brain Research, 232*, 3345–3351.

Mehta, S., McIntyre, A., Guy, S., Teasell, R. W., & Loh, E. (2015). Effectiveness of transcranial direct current stimulation for the management of neuropathic pain after spinal cord injury: A meta-analysis. *Spinal Cord, 53*(11), 780–785.

Meinzer, M., Lindenberg, R., Sieg, M. M., Nachtigall, L., Ulm, L., & Floel, A. (2014). Transcranial direct current stimulation of the primary motor cortex improves word-retrieval in older adults. *Frontiers in Aging Neuroscience, 6*.

Minhas, P., Bikson, M., Woods, A. J., Rosen, A. R., & Kessler, S. K. (2012). Transcranial direct current stimulation in pediatric brain: A computational modeling study. *Conference Proceedings: Annual International Conference of the IEEE Engineering in Medicine and Biology Society, 2012*, 859–862.

Monte-Silva, K., Liebetanz, D., Grundey, J., Paulus, W., & Nitsche, M. A. (2010). Dosage-dependent non-linear effect of L-dopa on human motor cortex plasticity. *The Journal of Physiology, 588*, 3415–3424.

Monte-Silva, K., Kuo, M. F., Hessenthaler, S., Fresnoza, S., Liebetanz, D., Paulus, W., & Nitsche, M. A. (2013). Induction of late LTP-like plasticity in the human motor cortex by repeated non-invasive brain stimulation. *Brain Stimulation, 6*, 424–432.

Moreau, D., Wang, C. H., Tseng, P., & Juan, C. H. (2015). Blending transcranial direct current stimulations and physical exercise to maximize cognitive improvement. *Frontiers in Psychology, 22*(6), 678.

Nakagawa, K., Mochizuki, H., Koyama, S., Tanaka, S., Sadato, N., & Kakigi, R. (2016). A transcranial direct current stimulation over the sensorimotor cortex modulates the itch sensation induced by histamine. *Clinical Neurophysiology, 127*(1), 827–832.

Nitsche, M. A., & Paulus, W. (2000). Excitability changes induced in the human motor cortex by weak transcranial direct current stimulation. *The Journal of Physiology, 527*(3), 633–639.

Nitsche, M. A., & Paulus, W. (2001). Sustained excitability elevations induced by transcranial DC motor cortex stimulation in humans. *Neurology, 57*, 1899–1901.

Nitsche, M. A., Muller-Dahlhaus, F., Paulus, W., & Ziemann, U. (2012). The pharmacology of neuroplasticity induced by non-invasive brain stimulation: Building models for the clinical use of CNS active drugs. *The Journal of Physiology, 590*, 4641–4662.

Nitsche, M. A., Boggio, P. S., Fregni, F., & Pascual-Leone, A. (2009). Treatment of depression with transcranial direct current stimulation (tDCS): A review. *Experimental Neurology, 219*(1), 14–19.

Nitsche, M. A., Cohen, L. G., Wassermann, E. M., Priori, A., Lang, N., Antal, A., & Pascual-Leone, A. (2008). Transcranial direct current stimulation: State of the art 2008. *Brain Stimulation, 1*, 206–223.

Nitsche, M. A., Fricke, K., Henschke, U., Schlitterlau, A., Liebetanz, D., Lang, N., … W. (2003). Pharmacological modulation of cortical excitability shifts induced by transcranial direct current stimulation in humans. *The Journal of Physiology, 553*.(Pt 1, 293–301.

Nitsche, M. A., Doemkes, S., Karaköse, T., et al. (2007). Shaping the effects of transcranial direct current stimulation of the human motor cortex. *Journal of Neurophysiology, 97*(4), 3109–3117.

Noseworthy, J. H1., Ebers, G. C., Vandervoort, M. K., Farquhar, R. E., Yetisir, E., & Roberts, R. (1994). The impact of blinding on the results of a randomized, placebo-controlled multiple sclerosis clinical trial. *Neurology, 44*(1), 16–20.

O'Connell, N. E., Cossar, J., Marston, L., Wand, B. M., Bunce, D., Moseley, G. L., & De Souza, L. H. (2012). Rethinking clinical trials of transcranial direct current stimulation: Participant and assessor blinding is inadequate at intensities of 2mA. *PLoS One, 7*(10), e47514.

Palm, U., Reisinger, E., & Keeser, D. (2013). Evaluation of sham transcranial direct current stimulation for randomized, placebo-controlled clinical trials. *Brain Stimulation, 6*, 690–695.

Picazio, S., Granata, C., Caltagirone, C., Petrosini, L., & Oliveri, M. (2015). Shaping pseudoneglect with transcranial cerebellar direct current stimulation and music listening. *Frontiers in Human Neuroscience, 26*(9), 158.

Polanía, R., Paulus, W., & Nitsche, M. A. (2012). Modulating cortico-striatal and thalamo-cortical functional connectivity with transcranial direct current stimulation. *Human Brain Mapping, 33*, 2499–2508.

Pope, P. A., Brenton, J. W., & Miall, R. C. (2015). Task-specific facilitation of cognition by anodal transcranial direct current stimulation of the prefrontal cortex. *Cerebral Cortex, 25*(11), 4551–4558.

Poreisz, C., Boros, K., Antal, A., & Paulus, W. (2007). Safety aspects of Tran-scranial direct current stimulation concerning healthy subjects and patients. *Brain Research Bulletin, 72*(4–6), 208–214.

Priori, A., Berardelli, A., Rona, S., Accornero, N., & Manfredi, M. (1998). Polarization of the human motor cortex through the scalp. *Neuroreport, 9*, 2257–2260.

Richardson, J. D., Fillmore, P., Datta, A., Truong, D., Bikson, M., & Fridriksson, J. (2014). Toward development of sham protocols for high- definition transcranial direct current stimulation (HD-tDCS). *NeuroRegulation, 1*(1), 62–72.

Rostami, R., Badran, B. W., & Kazemi, R. (2015). Long-lasting analgesic effect of transcranial direct current stimulation in treatment of chronic endometriosis pain. *The Journal of Obstetrics and Gynaecology Research, 41*(12), 1998–2001.

Rowny, S., & Lisanby, S. H. (2008). Brain stimulation in psychiatry. Wiley-Blackwell, West Sussex, England: In *Psychiatry* (3rd ed., pp. 2354–2371).

Russo, C., Souza Carneiro, M. I., Bolognini, N., & Fregni, F. (2017). Safety review of transcranial direct current stimulation in stroke. *Neuromodulation, 20*, 215–222.

Russowsky Brunoni, A. I., Sampaio-Junior, B. I., Henrique Moffa, A., III, Borrione, L. I., Schwair Nogueira, B., III, Vanessa Marotti Aparício, L. V., … Martins Benseñor, I. (2015). The escitalopram versus electric current therapy for treating depression clinical study (ELECT-TDCS): Rationale and study design of a non-inferiority, triple-arm, placebo-controlled clinical trial. *São Paulo Medical Journal, 133*, 252–263.

Schambra, H. M., Bikson, M., Wager, T. D., Dossantos, M. F., & Dasilva, A. F. (2014). It's all in your head: Reinforcing the placebo response with tDCS. *Brain Stimulation, 7*, 623–624.

Schestatsky, P., Morales-Quezada, L., & Fregni, F. (2013). Simultaneous EEG monitoring during transcranial direct current stimulation. *Journal of Visualized Experiments, 76*, 1–11.

Soekadar, S. R., Witkowski, M., & Cossio, E. G. (2014). Learned EEG-based brain self-regulation of motor-related oscillations during application of transcranial electric brain stimulation: Feasibility and limitations. *Frontiers in Behavioral Neuroscience*. eCollection 2014.

Stagg, C. J., Jayaram, G., Pastor, D., Kincses, Z. T., Matthews, P. M., & Johansen-Berg, H. (2011). Polarity and timing-dependent effects of transcranial direct current stimulation in explicit motor learning. [Research Support, Non-U.S. Gov't]. *Neuropsychologia, 49*(5), 800–804.

Stagg, C. J., Lin, R. L., Mezue, M., Segerdahl, A., Kong, Y., Xie, J., & Tracey, I. (2013). Widespread modulation of cerebral perfusion induced during and after transcranial direct current stimulation applied to the left dorsolateral prefrontal cortex. [Research Support, Non-U.S. Gov't]. *The Journal of Neuroscience, 33*(28), 11425–11431.

Stagg, C. J., & Nitsche, M. A. (2011). Physiological basis of transcranial direct current stimulation. *The Neuroscientist, 17*(1), 37–53.

Truong, D. Q., Hüber, M., Xie, X., Datta, A., Rahman, A., Parra, L. C., … Bikson, M. (2014). Clinician accessible tools for GUI computational models of transcranial electrical stimulation: BONSAI and SPHERES. *Brain Stimulation, 7*, 521–524.

Turner, L., Shamseer, L., Altman, D. G., Schulz, K. F., & Moher, D. (2012). Does use of the CONSORT statement impact the completeness of reporting of randomised controlled trials published in medical journals? A Cochrane review. *Cochrane Database Systematic Review.*

Vaseghi, B., Zoghi, M., & Jaberzadeh, S. (2015a). How does anodal transcranial direct current stimulation of the pain neuromatrix affect brain excitability and pain perception? A randomised, double-blind, sham-control study. *PLoS One, 10*(3), e0118340. eCollection 2015.

Vaseghi, B., Zoghi, M., & Jaberzadeh, S. (2015b). Differential effects of cathodal transcranial direct current stimulation of prefrontal, motor and somatosensory cortices on cortical excitability and pain perception – a double-blind randomised sham-controlled study. *The European Journal of Neuroscience, 42*(7), 2426–2437.

Vaseghi, B., Zoghi, M., & Jaberzadeh, S. (2016). Unihemispheric concurrent dual-site cathodal transcranial direct current stimulation: The effects on corticospinal excitability. *The European Journal of Neuroscience, 43*, 1161–1172.

Villamar, M. F., Volz, M. S., Bikson, M., Datta, A., Dasilva, A. F., & Fregni, F. (2013). Technique and considerations in the use of 4x1 ring high-definition transcranial direct current stimulation (HD-tDCS). *Journal of Visualized Experiments.* (77):e50309.

Wagner, T., Fregni, F., Fecteau, S., Grodzinsky, A., Zahn, M., & Pascual-Leone, A. (2007). Transcranial direct current stimulation: A computer-based human model study. *NeuroImage, 35*, 1113–1124.

Woods, A. J., Antal, A., Bikson, M., Boggio, P. S., Brunoni, A. R., Celnik, P., … Nitsche, M. A. (2016). A technical guide to tDCS, and related non-invasive brain stimulation tools. *Clinical Neurophysiology, 127*, 1031–1048.

Woods, A. J., Hamilton, R. H., Kranjec, A., Minhaus, P., Bikson, M., Yu, J., & Chatterjee, A. (2014). Space, time, and causality in the human brain. *NeuroImage, 92*, 285–297.

Zhu, F. F., Yeung, A. Y., Poolton, J. M., Lee, T. M., Leung, G. K., & Masters, R. S. (2015). Cathodal transcranial direct current stimulation over left dorsolateral prefrontal cortex area promotes implicit motor learning in a golf putting task. *Brain Stimulation, 8*(4), 784–786.

Chapter 8
Stimulation Parameters and Their Reporting

Adam J. Woods, Helena Knotkova, Alexa Riggs, Dennis Q. Truong, and Marom Bikson

Following the proposal of Peterchev et al. (2012), transcranial direct current stimulation (tDCS) dose is defined "by all parameters of the stimulation device that affect the electromagnetic field generated in the body." tDCS dose therefore includes the stimulation waveform (i.e. DC), intensity and duration, and the number of electrodes and their surface area (size/shape). For electrode surface area, it is specifically the surface where the electrolyte contacts the skin that defines electrode size/shape. For example, for an electrode design where a conductive rubber electrode is inserted into a saline-saturated sponge-pocket, it is the surface area of the sponge (when saturated), but not the conductive rubber that defines electrode area. Not strictly part of dose, but also critical for reproducibility, are complete details of the electrode assembly including electrode material, coupling medium, electrode

A. J. Woods
Center for Cognitive Aging and Memory (CAM), McKnight Brain Institute, Department of Clinical and Health Psychology, College of Public Health and Health Professions, University of Florida, Gainesville, FL, USA

H. Knotkova
MJHS Institute for Innovation in Palliative Care, New York, NY, USA

Department of Family and Social Medicine, Albert Einstein College of Medicine, Bronx, NY, USA

A. Riggs
MJHS Institute for Innovation in Palliative Care, New York, NY, USA

D. Q. Truong
Department of Biomedical Engineering, The City College of the City University of New York, New York, NY, USA

M. Bikson (✉)
Department of Biomedical Engineering, The City College of New York, New York, NY, USA
e-mail: bikson@ccny.cuny.edu

H. Knotkova et al. (eds.), *Practical Guide to Transcranial Direct Current Stimulation*, https://doi.org/10.1007/978-3-319-95948-1_8

thickness, and any relevant details of electrode specifics, such as if they are designed for a single or repeated use. These must be provided or referenced through a unique make/model number (Woods et al. 2016).

A single tDCS session is conceived as the period from initiation of current flow (start of ramp up) to end of current flow (end of ramp down). However, conventionally the "duration" of a tDCS session is exclusive of the ramp up or ramp up period and thus refers to the period when tDCS is at the target sustained current (e.g. 2 mA). Ideally, to avoid ambiguity, description of "duration" should clearly identify if ramping is in- or excluded. For example, one could state that "the overall duration of the current flow and the duration of the ramp up/down was 21 min including both ramp up and ramp down period for 30 s each". Or, "the overall duration of the stimulation was 20 min, with an additional 30 s ramp up and ramp down."

All tDCS devices produce an imperfect signal, resulting in a fractional superimposed non-DC component (noise). At what level does this fractional non-DC component become significant enough to not meet the definition of tDCS (Salimpour et al. 2016a, b)? It is hard to set a specific threshold for noise on the direct current based simply on output (e.g. 1% noise of DC, 0.1% noise of DC). A simple rule of thumb may be: when a high quality tDCS source does not reproduce the tolerability or efficacy of a noisy tDCS source, then the outcomes of the noisy tDCS rely on a non-DC component and, per our definition, it is not strictly tDCS. To avoid such ambiguity, the performance of any tDCS stimulator should be independently verified by the trial site. It is also recommended that stimulation intensity and polarity are independently verified (e.g. using an ammeter) before any new device is used.

Transcranial direct current stimulation must involve at least one electrode on the scalp. The anode is defined as any electrode where current (positive quantity) enters the body and the cathode is defined as any electrode where the current (positive quantity) exits the body. tDCS must have at least one anode and at least one cathode. As such, the terms "anodal-tDCS" (a-tDCS) and "cathodal-tDCS" (c-tDCS), though common, should be used with caution. There is no pure unipolar tDCS (effects exerted under one electrode), as may be implied by these terms. The terms "anodal" and "cathodal" in this context thus reflect the *intended* outcome of stimulation at the electrode of interest to the operators and should be understood as only an expected outcome (or hypothesis). However, the extent to which the inevitable concurrent anodal and cathodal sources produce net effects on brain excitability, especially in the context of brain processing and behavior, are complex and unresolved. In any case, since electrical field orientation relative to neuronal orientation determines the neuronal effects of tDCS, and the former depends on the placement of both the anode and the cathode, referral to just one electrode is misleading. The preferred language should thus be descriptive and refer to physical aspects of electrode placement, such as "the anode electrode *over* brain region X" (Clemens et al. 2014) or "anode electrode at scalp coordinate Z defined by the EEG 10-20 positioning system" rather than "anodal tDCS *of* brain region X" since the latter incorrectly implies current delivered to just that brain region (Datta et al. 2009) and moreover oversimplistic intended outcomes. Similarly, the terms "active", "reference", and "return" electrode have no specific physical meaning and again refer to an operator fixation on one electrode with a hypothesis of action (see below).

Transcranial direct current stimulation produces current flow though brain regions not just under, but spanning between the electrodes (Antal et al. 2014; Datta et al. 2009), including theoretical influence of current reaching subcortical regions (Dasilva et al. 2012). The region of potential influence of tDCS (brain regions whose stimulation may explain outcomes) is thus significantly wider than the typically assumed "under" one electrode (Lang et al. 2005). Just because there are well established montage specific effects on bio-markers (e.g. TMS evoked MEPs) or behaviors (e.g. change in reaction time or performance) associated with brain regions nominally targeted by tDCS, this does not imply that current was restricted to one brain area (e.g. "under" the "active" electrode) (Fig. 8.1).

Early forms of tDCS dating before 2000 used a wide range of intensities, durations, and montages (Esmaeilpour et al. 2017). In contemporary tDCS, post 2000, most conventional efforts used current intensities spanning between 1.0 and 2.5 mA; though higher current (3–4 mA) has been tested (Chhatbar et al. 2017). Some exploratory studies tested durations spanning 4 s (used only for transient changes; Nitsche and Paulus 2000) but the majority of trials used stimulation lasting several

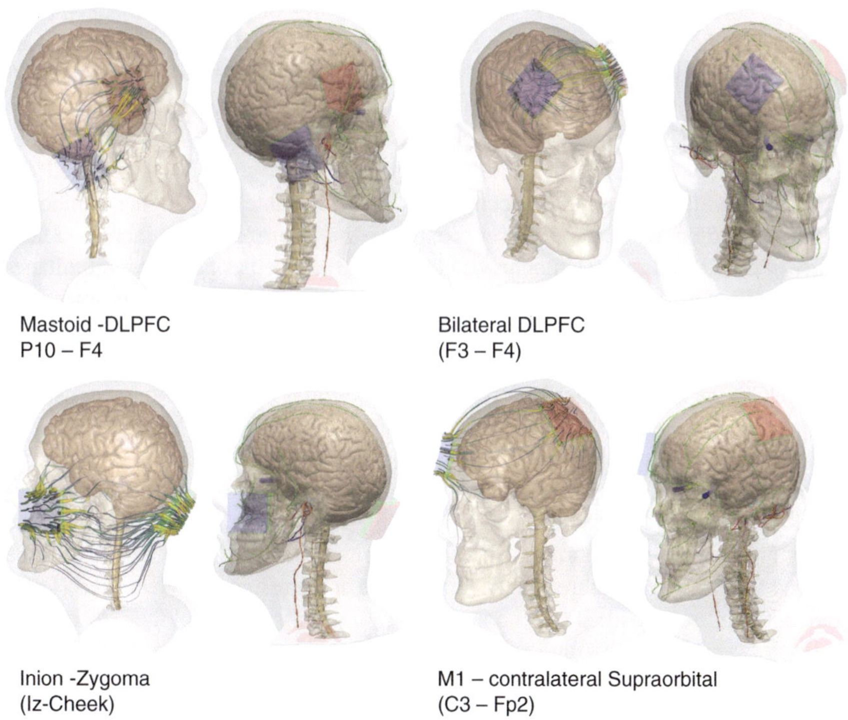

Fig. 8.1 Example of conventional tDCS montages. For four montages (clockwise from top left: DLPFC-mastoid, Bilateral DLPFC, Inion-Zygoma, M1-SO) the electrode position (right panel), along with resulting predicted current flow (left panel)

minutes (typically 10–40 min used for durable changes; (Acler et al. 2013; D'Urso et al. 2013; Ferrucci et al. 2014; Kühnl et al. 2008; Sandrini et al. 2014). tDCS limited to a few mA which, when proper technologies and protocols are used (Fertonani et al. 2015; Minhas et al. 2010; Moliadze et al. 2015; Paneri et al. 2016) is well tolerated.

Contemporary tDCS uses rectangular electrode assemblies of 5x5 cm to 5x7 cm skin-electrolyte contact area, though both smaller and larger electrode assemblies have been explored (Nitsche et al. 2007). Common tDCS electrodes assemblies use either metal or conductive rubber electrodes (Kronberg and Bikson 2012). Electrolytes or more commonly isotonic saline (saturated in a sponge) but gels and/or creams have also been used. The details of electrode assembly design and preparation (including operator training) are considered important for tolerability. For example, it is important to maintain a minimal distance between the electrode and skin (Kronberg and Bikson 2012). The details of electrode design and preparation protocols are also critical for dose reproducibility. Excessive saturation leading to leakage across the scalp or insufficient saturation (including drying during use) will change the electrolyte-skin contact area, which is the electrode area as defined in dose. Poorly controlled dose, even in a minority of subjects, can undermine the reproducibility of any effort.

Conventional tDCS commonly uses 2 electrodes, though 3- or 4-electrode montages are conceivable (Sellers et al. 2015). tDCS limits of feasible number of electrodes is related to the conventional size of electrodes, since using large electrodes limits the number that can be positioned on the scalp. High-definition tDCS (HD-tDCS) is defined as any tDCS montage using electrodes with a compact (e.g. <5 cm^2 total electrode contact area) skin-electrolyte that is defined by a rigid holder (e.g. comparable to EEG designs). Two or more electrodes may be used for HD-tDCS. A feature of smaller electrodes is the potential to use a higher number of electrodes and/or electrodes in closer proximity; this in turn provides increased flexibility in montage design (Dmochowski et al. 2013) as well as facilitates simultaneous recording of EEG during tES Roy et al. (2014). HD-tDCS may be optimized for focality with targeted current flow or for intensity with broad current flow (Dmochowski et al. 2012).

In tDCS, the terms "return" or "reference" electrodes have been typically used to describe an electrode with *presumed* "physiological inertness" or perceived lack of importance—for example as a consequence of not being in proximity to the brain regions of interest for a particular intended use. However, all electrodes are functional (even if they are not related to the hypothesis tested) in the engineering sense if they are used to carry current. The physiological "activity" of electrodes can be reduced for example by increasing electrode size or using a ring of electrodes (Datta et al. 2008; Nitsche et al. 2007); none-the-less, the configuration of these electrodes needs to be made explicit and their polarity and configuration must be indicated. The configuration and position of the "return" electrode has in any case a profound effect on current flow near the "active" electrode including current direction and strength – the use of an extra-cephalic electrode evidently does not cancel the role of this electrode in brain current flow (Bikson et al. 2010; Truong et al. 2014).

The term "active" or "stimulating" electrode has been typically used to refer to those electrodes presumed to be physiologically active – or more specifically that the physiological / behavioral outcome of interest is due to current passing through these electrodes. "Active", "Stimulating", "Return", and "Reference" are thus terms that typically relate to the "intent" of stimulation and if they are used it should be (i) with the recognition that despite intent, the physiological actions of stimulation may be unexpected and (ii) with the complete documentation of the stimulation dose (e.g. it is never appropriate to not provide details of reference electrode size, placement, and materials).

In summary, the essential stimulation parameters for tDCS, also called dose, are in principle simple to define, control, and reproduce. These are stimulation intensity (typically a few mA), the duration during with that intensity is maintained (typically tens of minutes), and the electrode montage (the skin-electrolyte contact area of all electrodes). Yet as explained above, lack of attention to detail or appreciation of the technology can lead to ambiguity (e.g. are ramps part of duration?) and irreproducibility (e.g. undefined level of saline). In addition, it is necessary to appreciate terminology which is loaded with assumptions (hypothesis) such as "anodal/cathodal tDCS" or "active/return" electrode, and that during tDCS all electrodes are active and current travels through brain regions spanning between the electrodes. These issues, along with the rational for selecting a given dose for a given application, are expounded on throughout this book.

References

Acler, M., Bocci, T., Valenti, D., Turri, M., Priori, A., & Bertolasi, L. (2013). Transcranial direct current stimulation (tDCS) for sleep disturbances and fatigue in patients with post-polio syndrome. *Restorative Neurology and Neuroscience, 31*(5), 661–668.

Antal, A., Bikson, M., Datta, A., Lafon, B., Dechent, P., Parra, L. C., & Paulus, W. (2014). Imaging artifacts induced by electrical stimulation during conventional fMRI of the brain. *NeuroImage, 85*(3), 1040–1047.

Bikson, M., Datta, A., Rahman, A., & Scaturro, J. (2010). Electrode montages for tDCS and weak transcranial electrical stimulation: role of "return" electrode's position and size. *Clinical Neurophysiology, 121*(12), 1976–1978.

Chhatbar, P. Y., Chen, R., Deardorff, R., Dellenbach, B., Kautz, S. A., George, M. S., & Feng, W. (2017). Safety and tolerability of transcranial direct current stimulation to stroke patients – A phase I current escalation study. *Brain Stimulation, 10*(3), 553–559.

Clemens, B., Jung, S., Mingoia, G., Weyer, D., Domahs, F., & Willmes, K. (2014). Influence of anodal transcranial direct current stimulation (tDCS) over the right angular gyrus on brain activity during rest. *PLoS One, 9*(4), e95984.

Dasilva, A. F., Mendonca, M. E., Zaghi, S., Lopes, M., Dossantos, M. F., Spierings, E. L., … Fregni, F. (2012). tDCS-induced analgesia and electrical fields in pain-related neural networks in chronic migraine. *Headache, 52*(8), 1283–1295.

Datta, A., Bansal, V., Diaz, J., Patel, J., Reato, D., & Bikson, M. (2009). Gyri-precise head model of transcranial direct current stimulation: improved spatial focality using a ring electrode versus conventional rectangular pad. *Brain Stimulation, 2*(4), 201–207.

Datta, A., Elwassif, M., Battaglia, F., & Bikson, M. (2008). Transcranial current stimulation focality using disc and ring electrode configurations: FEM analysis. *Journal of Neural Engineering, 5*(2), 163–174.

Dmochowski, J. P., Datta, A., Huang, Y., Richardson, J. D., Bikson, M., Fridriksson, J., & Parra, L. C. (2013). Targeted transcranial direct current stimulation for rehabilitation after stroke. *NeuroImage, 75*, 12–19.

Dmochowski, J. P., Bikson, M., Datta, A., Richardson, J., Fridriksson, J., & Parra, L. C. (2012). On the role of electric field orientation in optimal design of transcranial current stimulation. *Conference Proceedings: Annual International Conference of the IEEE Engineering in Medicine and Biology Society, 6426*, 9.

D'Urso, G., Mantovani, A., Micillo, M., Priori, A., & Muscettola, G. (2013). Transcranial direct current stimulation and cognitive- behavioral therapy: evidence of a synergistic effect in treatment-resistant depression. *Brain Stimulation, 6*(3), 465–467.

Esmaeilpour, Z., Schestatsky, P., Bikson, M., Brunoni, A. R., Pellegrinelli, A., Piovesan, F. X., … Fregni, F. (2017). Notes on human trials of transcranial direct current stimulation between 1960 and 1998. *Frontiers in Human Neuroscience, 11*, 71.

Ferrucci, R., Vergari, M., Cogiamanian, F., Bocci, T., Ciocca, M., Tomasini, E., … Priori, A. (2014). Transcranial direct current stimulation (tDCS) for fatigue in multiple sclerosis. *Neuropsychological Rehabilitation, 34*(1), 121.

Fertonani, A., Ferrari, C., & Miniussi, C. (2015). What do you feel if I apply transcranial electric stimulation? Safety, sensations and secondary induced effects. *Clinical Neurophysiology, 126*(11), 2181–2188.

Kronberg, G., & Bikson, M. (2012). Electrode assembly design for transcranial Direct Current Stimulation: a FEM modeling study. *Conference Proceedings: Annual International Conference of the IEEE Engineering in Medicine and Biology Society, 2012*, 891–895.

Kühnl, S., Terney, D., Paulus, W., & Antal, A. (2008). The effect of daily sessions of anodal tDCS on chronic pain. *Brain Stimulation, 3*, 281.

Lang, N., Siebner, H. R., Ward, N. S., Lee, L., Nitsche, M. A., Paulus, W., … Frackowiak, R. S. (2005). How does transcranial DC stimulation of the primary motor cortex alter regional neuronal activity in the human brain? *The European Journal of Neuroscience, 22*(2), 495–504.

Minhas, P., Bansal, V., Patel, J., Ho, J. S., Diaz, J., Datta, A., & Bikson, M. (2010). Electrodes for high-definition transcutaneous DC stimulation for applications in drug delivery and electrotherapy, including tDCS. *Journal of Neuroscience Methods, 190*(2), 188–197.

Moliadze, V., Andreas, S., Lyzhko, E., Schmanke, T., Gurashvili, T., Freitag, C. M., & Siniatchkin, M. (2015). Ten minutes of 1 mA transcranial direct current stimulation was well tolerated by children and adolescents: Self-reports and resting state EEG analysis. *Brain Research Bulletin, 119*, 25–33.

Nitsche, M. A., Doemkes, S., Karaköse, T., Antal, A., Liebetanz, D., Lang, N., … Paulus, W. (2007). Shaping the effects of transcranial direct current stimulation of the human motor cortex. *Journal of Neurophysiology, 97*(4), 3109–3117.

Nitsche, M. A., & Paulus, W. (2000). Excitability changes induced in the human motor cortex by weak transcranial direct current stimulation. *The Journal of Physiology, 527*(3), 633–639.

Paneri, B., Adair, D., Thomas, C., Khadka, N., Patel, V., Tyler, W. J., … Bikson, M. (2016). Tolerability of repeated application of transcranial electrical stimulation with limited outputs to healthy subjects. *Brain Stimulation, 9*(5), 740–754.

Peterchev, A. V., Wagner, T. A., & Miranda, P. C. (2012). Fundamentals of transcranial electric and magnetic stimulation dose: definition, selection, and reporting practices. *Brain Stimulation, 5*(4), 435–453.

Roy, A., Baxter, B., & He, B. (2014). High-definition transcranial direct current stimulation induces both acute and persistent changes in broadband cortical synchronization: a simultaneous tDCS-EEG study. *IEEE Transactions on Biomedical Engineering, 61*(7), 1967–1978.

Salimpour, Y., Mills, K. A., Wei, Z., Duy, P. Q., & Anderson, W. S. (2016a). Does transcranial direct current stimulation actually deliver DC stimulation: response to letter to the editor. *Brain Stimulation, 9*(4), 627–628.

Salimpour, Y., Wei, Z., Duy, P. Q., & Anderson, W. S. (2016b). Does transcranial direct current stimulation actually deliver DC stimulation? *Brain Stimulation, 9*(4), 623–624.

Sandrini, M., Brambilla, M., Manenti, R., Rosini, S., Cohen, L. G., & Cotelli, M. (2014). Noninvasive stimulation of prefrontal cortex strengthens existing episodic memories and reduces forgetting in the elderly. *Frontiers in Aging Neuroscience, 6*, 289.

Sellers, K. K., Mellin, J. M., Lustenberger, C. M., Boyle, M. R., Lee, W. H., Peterchev, A. V., & Fröhlich, F. (2015). Transcranial direct current stimulation (tDCS) of frontal cortex decreases performance on the WAIS-IV intelligence test. *Behavioural Brain Research, 290*, 32–44.

Truong, D. Q., Hüber, M., Xie, X., Datta, A., Rahman, A., Parra, L. C., … Bikson, M. (2014). Clinician accessible tools for GUI computational models of transcranial electrical stimulation: BONSAI and SPHERES. *Brain Stimulation, 7*(4), 521–524.

Woods, A. J., Antal, A., Bikson, M., et al. (2016). A technical guide to tDCS, and related non-invasive brain stimulation tools. *Clinical Neurophysiology, 127*(2), 1031–1048.

Chapter 9
Role of Computational Modeling for Dose Determination

Ricardo Salvador, Dennis Q. Truong, Marom Bikson, Alexander Opitz, Jacek Dmochowski, and Pedro C. Miranda

Computational Forward Models in Transcranial Direct Current Stimulation

Introduction to Dose Definition and Selection

Dose, as defined in the context of transcranial stimulation with magnetic or electrical fields (E-fields), includes all the controllable parameters of the stimulation device that affect the electromagnetic field induced in the body (Peterchev et al. 2012). In the case of tDCS, this includes parameters such as the size, geometry, position, orientation and number of electrodes, the current intensity and polarity in each electrode, the duration of the applied current and the duration of the ramp-up/down period. Other parameters related to the experimental protocol and the skin preparation techniques

R. Salvador
Neuroelectrics, Barcelona, Spain

D. Q. Truong
Department of Biomedical Engineering, The City College of the City University of New York, New York, NY, USA

M. Bikson
Department of Biomedical Engineering, The City College of New York, New York, NY, USA

A. Opitz
Department of Biomedical Engineering, University of Minnesota, Minneapolis, MN, USA

J. Dmochowski
Neural Engineering Laboratory, Department of Biomedical Engineering, Grove School of Engineering, The City College of the City University of New York, New York, NY, USA

P. C. Miranda (✉)
Instituto de Biofísica e Engenharia Biomédica, Faculdade de Ciências, Universidade de Lisboa, Lisbon, Portugal
e-mail: pcmiranda@fc.ul.pt

H. Knotkova et al. (eds.), *Practical Guide to Transcranial Direct Current Stimulation*, https://doi.org/10.1007/978-3-319-95948-1_9

used can also be included in this definition of dose to the extent they influence electromagnetic fields in the body – though they are always important in the broader content of protocol reproducibility. Replicating all of these dose parameters across subjects does not guarantee, however, that the subjects' response will be the same. This has become increasingly evident by studies indicating that the responses to tDCS can vary substantially across subjects within the same protocol (Lopez-Alonso et al. 2014; Wiethoff et al. 2014). One cause for this difference is the fact that the E-field distribution in the head during tDCS can be substantially different across subjects due to individual differences in head geometry. Since direct *in vivo* measurement of the E-field distribution during tDCS is not possible, except in special cases where implanted electrodes are present (Datta et al. 2016; Dymond et al. 1975; Opitz et al. 2016), computational models remain the only practical tool available to predict E-field in the brain for a given tDCS dose. Information from these models can be used to adjust dose parameters to induce comparable E-field across subjects, or it can be used to optimize these parameters to maximize the effects in a specific target cortical region (Dmochowski et al. 2011; Ruffini et al. 2014).

Methods for Generation of Computational Models

The first models to predict the E-field in brain stimulation techniques relied on analytical solutions of the underlying physical equations (Eaton 1992; Rush and Driscoll 1968). The complexity of such approaches often demanded drastic simplifications at the level of head geometry, number of tissues involved and electrode/coil geometry. Numerical computational approaches were soon identified as promising alternatives, but the limited computational resources available at first imposed similar limitations to the models (Roth et al. 1991; Tofts 1990). As such, many of the first computational studies of E-field distribution induced in tDCS adopted spherical head models (Miranda et al. 2006) or computer-aided design (CAD) generated simplified geometries (Wagner et al. 2007). The advent of powerful computational resources has made it possible to build increasingly realistic head and electrode models (Datta et al. 2009a; Oostendorp et al. 2008).

Table 9.1 summarizes several published studies that have employed computational models of tDCS. Most of the recent studies have used realistic head models, and they employ similar techniques to generate such models. A generalized pipeline to create computational models is shown in Fig. 9.1. It should be mentioned that although the studies usually employ the same steps as those highlighted in the figure, the methods employed at each step can be substantially different across studies. The description of the studies presented in Table 9.1 shows the wide variety of electrode configurations and geometries that has been studied (see columns 'Electrodes' and 'Montages'). It also shows that the studies can be used in a variety of applications, such as investigating the fundamental properties of the induced E-field, studying the distribution of the E-field in montages typically used in clinical settings, optimizing montages to target specific cortical areas and/or studying the

Table 9.1 List of all studies involving computational models in tDCS

Reference	Tissues represented	Electrodes	Montages	Study description / Additional comments
Spherical head models				
1. Miranda et al. (2006)	$\sigma_{Scalp} = 0.45\ S/m$ $\sigma_{Skull} = 0.006\ S/m$ $\sigma_{Brain} = 0.45\ S/m$ Isotropic.	Rectangular: $5 \times 5\ cm^2$ $6.5 \times 15\ cm^2$. Homogeneous conductivity: 2 S/m.	4 electrode montages.	Type (1).
2. Datta et al. (2008)	$\sigma_{Scalp} = 0.465\ S/m$ $\sigma_{Skull} = 0.01\ S/m$ $\sigma_{CSF} = 1.65\ S/m$ $\sigma_{Brain} = 0.2\ S/m$ Isotropic.	Cylindrical $0.5\ cm^2$. Ring (variable diameters) Homogeneous conductivity: $5.9 \times 10^7\ S/m$.	6 electrode montages.	Type (1) and (2). Concentric ring electrodes induced a field with the highest focality and directionality.
3. Faria et al. (2011)	$\sigma_{Scalp} = 0.465\ S/m$ $\sigma_{Skull} = 0.0083\ S/m$ $\sigma_{CSF} = 1.79\ S/m$ $\sigma_{Brain} = 0.332\ S/m$ Isotropic.	Cylindrical with areas between $1 - 35\ cm^2$. Homogeneous conductivity: 0.332 S/m.	Various bipolar configurations.	Type (1).
4. Rampersad et al. (2012)	$\sigma_{Scalp} = 0.435\ S/m$ $\sigma_{Brain} = 0.333\ S/m$ Isotropic. The skull was given several different properties: Isotropic, three-layers, anisotropic.	Rectangular: $35\ cm^2$. Homogeneous conductivity: 1.4 S/m.	Several bipolar configurations with electrodes separated by 180°, 90° and 45°.	Type (1). Single layer anisotropic skull or a single layer isotropic skull with a conductivity equal to that of the conductivity in the radial direction of the anisotropic model, gives similar results to 3-layered model.
CAD generated models				
5. Wagner et al. (2007)	$\sigma_{Scalp} = 0.465\ S/m$ $\sigma_{Skull} = 0.01\ S/m$ $\sigma_{CSF} = 1.654\ S/m$ $\sigma_{GM} = 0.276\ S/m$ $\sigma_{WM} = 0.126\ S/m$ Isotropic.	Rectangular: $5 \times 5\ cm^2$ $7 \times 5\ cm^2$ $1 \times 1\ cm^2$ $7 \times 7\ cm^2$.	7 bipolar montages.	Type (1), (3) and (4). Implemented 3 stroke models.
Models generated from segmentation of MR images				
6. Oostendorp et al. (2008)	$\sigma_{Scalp} = 0.33\ S/m$ $\sigma_{Skull} = 0.102\ S/m$ $\sigma_{CSF} = 1.79\ S/m$ $\sigma_{GM} = 0.33\ S/m$ $\sigma_{WM} = 0.14\ S/m$ Isotropic. For WM and skull, anisotropy was also included.	Rectangular: $5 \times 9\ cm^2$ (patch projected into scalp).	Anode over LM1 and cathode over RSO.	Type (1).

(continued)

Table 9.1 (continued)

Reference	Tissues represented	Electrodes	Montages	Study description / Additional comments
7. Datta et al. (2009a)	$\sigma_{Scalp} = 0.465\ S/m$ $\sigma_{Skull} = 0.01\ S/m$ $\sigma_{CSF} = 1.65\ S/m$ $\sigma_{GM} = 0.2\ S/m$ $\sigma_{WM} = 0.2\ S/m$ Isotropic.	Rectangular: $5 \times 7\ cm^2$. Cylindrical $0.5\ cm^2$. Modelled with a copper layer ($5.9 \times 10^7\ S/m$) on top of a layer of gel ($0.3\ S/m$).	Rectangular anode over LM1 and cathode over RSO. 4×1 cylindrical electrode configuration (1 anode over LM1 and 4 cathodes surrounding it).	Type (1), (2) and (3).
8. Datta et al. (2009b)	Same as (7).			Type (1). No significant temperature increases were reported in any tissue including the scalp during tDCS.
9. Sadleir et al. (2010)	$\sigma_{Scalp} = 0.43\ S/m$ $\sigma_{Skull} = 0.0015\ S/m$ $\sigma_{CSF} = 1.8\ S/m$ $\sigma_{GM} = 0.1\ S/m$ Isotropic. σ_{WM}: Anisotropic Other tissues were included (total of 11).	Rectangular: $22\ cm^2$. Homogeneous conductivity: 1 S/m.	Anode over F3 and cathode over RSO. Anode over F4 and cathode over LSO.	Type (1) and (2).
10. Datta et al. (2010)	Same as (7). Skull holes were modelled (either filled with CSF or scar tissue).	Rectangular: $5 \times 7\ cm^2$. Modelled as in (7).	Anode over C3 and cathode over RSO. Anode over O1 and cathode over RSO.	Type (1) and (4). Placing electrode over skull hole significantly affects the E-field distribution, but if the hole is midway between the two electrodes, no significant effects occur.
11. Parazzini et al. (2011)	$\sigma_{Scalp} = 0.012147\ S/m$ $\sigma_{Skull} = 0.020028\ S/m$ $\sigma_{CSF} = 2\ S/m$ $\sigma_{GM} = 0.027512\ S/m$ $\sigma_{WM} = 0.027656\ S/m$ Isotropic. Many other tissues were considered (total of 26).	Rectangular: Anode: $3.5 - 35\ cm^2$ Cathode: $25 - 100\ cm^2$ Electrodes modelled as perfect conductors.	Anode over C3 and cathode over Fp2.	Type (1), (2) and (3).

Table 9.1 (continued)

Reference	Tissues represented	Electrodes	Montages	Study description / Additional comments
12. Mendonca et al. (2011)	$\sigma_{Scalp} = 0.465\ S/m$ $\sigma_{Skull} = 0.01\ S/m$ $\sigma_{CSF} = 1.65\ S/m$ $\sigma_{GM} = 0.276\ S/m$ $\sigma_{WM} = 0.126\ S/m$ Isotropic. Many other tissues were considered (total of 8). A synthetic neck and shoulder region was added with an isotropic conductivity of 0.17 S/m.	Rectangular: $4 \times 4\ cm^2$ and $8 \times 10\ cm^2$. Modelled as in (7).	Anode over C3 and the cathode over cervical/ thoracic transition dorsal midline. Anode over RSO and cathode unchanged. Anode over C3 and cathode over RSO.	Type (1), (3) and (5). Effects of extracephalic return electrodes and application to fibromyalgia.
13. Halko et al. (2011)	Same as (12) (without "synthetic" neck-shoulder region). Includes a stroke lesion modelled as CSF.	Rectangular: $5 \times 7\ cm^2$. Modelled as in (7).	Anode over Cz and the cathode over Oz.	Type (4) and (5). Patient specific model of a patient with a stroke lesion.
14. Datta et al. (2011)	Same as (12) but with synthetic neck-shoulder region with a conductivity of 0.35 S/m. Includes a stroke lesion modelled as CSF.	Rectangular: $5 \times 5\ cm^2$. Modelled as in (7).	Anode over C3 and cathode over: (a) Right shoulder (b) Right mastoid (c) Right orbitofrontal Anode over C4 and cathode over left shoulder	Type (4) and (5). Position of return electrode significantly affected E-field distribution.
15. Dmochowski et al. (2011)	Same as (7) but with muscle and air cavities segmented as well.	Cylindrical $1.1\ cm^2$. Modelled as in (7).	64 possible positions according to the 10/10 international system.	Type (6). Algorithms to determine current intensity and polarity in pre-defined grid of electrodes to optimize E-field in target region.
16. Suh et al. (2012)	$\sigma_{Scalp} = 0.33\ S/m$ $\sigma_{Skull} = 0.0132\ S/m$ $\sigma_{CSF} = 1.79\ S/m$ $\sigma_{GM} = 0.33\ S/m$ $\sigma_{WM} = 0.14\ S/m$ Isotropic. Skull and WM anisotropy was also modelled.	Cylindrical $0.5\ cm^2$. Modelled as homogeneous.	Anode over C3 and cathode over C4.	Type (1). Skull anisotropy significantly affects the E-field distribution whereas the WM anisotropy has a smaller effect (except on deeper regions).
17. Dasilva et al. (2012)	Same as (12), but more tissues were segmented (total of 15).	Rectangular: $5 \times 7\ cm^2$ Modelled as in (7).	Anode over C3 and cathode over RSO.	Type (3) and (5). Application to chronic migraine.
18. Turkeltaub et al. (2012)	Same as (12).	Rectangular: $5 \times 5\ cm^2$. Modelled as in (7).	Anode over RpTC (midway between T7 and TP7) and cathode placed over LpTC (midway between T8 and TP8).	Type (3) and (5). Application to dyslexia study.

(continued)

Table 9.1 (continued)

Reference	Tissues represented	Electrodes	Montages	Study description / Additional comments
19. Datta et al. (2012)	Same as (12) (without "synthetic" neck-shoulder region).	Rectangular: $5 \times 7\ cm^2$. Cylindrical $1.1\ cm^2$. Modelled as in (7).	Same as (7).	Type (1) and (3). Compares E-field distribution across 3 different subjects. Reports the need to incorporate subject specific models.
20. Minhas et al. (2012)	Same as (19).			Type (1) and (4). Compares E-field distribution in an adult model and a model of a child (12 years old).
21. Sadleir et al. (2012)	Same as (9).		19 possible locations selected from the 10 to 20 system.	Type (6). Algorithms to determine current intensity and polarity in pre-defined grid of electrodes to optimize E-field's magnitude in target region.
22. Parazzini et al. (2012)	Same as (11).	Rectangular: $5 \times 7\ cm^2$. Modelled as perfect conductors.	1 electrode over LTA (halfway between C3 and T5) and another one over Fp2. Electrodes over F3 and F4.	Type (3) and (6). Study of electrode montages used in the treatment of tinnitus.
23. Truong et al. (2013)	Same as (19). Includes fat as a separate tissue.	Same as (19).	Same as in (7) Anode over F8 and cathode over LSO.	Type (1), (3) and (4). Compares E-field distribution in individualized models of 5 subjects with various body-mass indexes (ranging from normal to obese).
24. Shahid et al. (2013)	$\sigma_{Scalp} = 0.43\ S/m$ $\sigma_{Skull} = 0.015\ S/m$ $\sigma_{CSF} = 1.79\ S/m$ $\sigma_{GM} = 0.32\ S/m$ $\sigma_{WM} = 0.15\ S/m$ Isotropic. WM anisotropy was also modelled. Other tissues were also segmented (total of 15).	Rectangular: $5 \times 5\ cm^2$. Homogeneous conductivity: 1.4 S/m.	Anode over C3 and cathode over Fp2.	Type (1) and (3). Reports significant effects of anisotropy in current density distribution.

Table 9.1 (continued)

Reference	Tissues represented	Electrodes	Montages	Study description / Additional comments
25. Miranda et al. (2013)	$\sigma_{Scalp} = 0.33\ S/m$ $\sigma_{Skull} = 0.008\ S/m$ $\sigma_{CSF} = 1.79\ S/m$ $\sigma_{GM} = 0.32\ S/m$ $\sigma_{WM} = 0.15\ S/m$ Isotropic.	Rectangular $5 \times 7\ cm^2$, $3 \times 3\ cm^2$. Cylindrical $\pi\ cm^2$. Homogeneous conductivity: 2 S/m.	Anode over C3 and cathode over right SO. The rectangular anodes were rotated 45° so that their edge is approximately parallel to the central sulcus.	Type (1) and (3). Reports E-field maxima at the bottom of the sulci under the electrodes.
26. Dmochowski et al. (2013)	Same as (12) (without "synthetic" neck-shoulder region). Includes stroke lesions modelled as CSF.	Cylindrical $1.1\ cm^2$. Modelled as in (7).	74 possible positions according to the 10/10 international system.	Type (4) and (6). "Optimized" electrode positions increased E-field strength, as compared to conventional montages, at stroke lesion sites in 8 patients.
27. Kessler et al. (2013)	Same as (19).	Rectangular: $25\ cm^2$. Cylindrical $0.95\ cm^2$. Modelled as in (7).	Rectangular electrodes: Anode/cathode over C3/C4. Anode/cathode over the posterior left/ right STG. Anode/cathode over F3/F4. Anode cathode over left M1/ RSO 4 × 1 cylindrical electrode configuration (1 anode over LM1 and 4 cathodes surrounding it). Two distances from cathodes to anode were modelled	Type (1), (3) and (4). 4 models of healthy adults and 2 models of children (ages 8 and 12) were created. For the same currents, the E-field in the children models is stronger.

(continued)

Table 9.1 (continued)

Reference	Tissues represented	Electrodes	Montages	Study description / Additional comments
28. Parazzini et al. (2013a)	Same as (11).	Anodes: Rectangular $5 \times 7.5\ cm^2$ copper conductor ($5.9 \times 10^7\ S/m$) on top of a $7 \times 8\ cm^2$. "Sponge" (0.3 S/m). Cathode: Same as before but with different dimensions for the copper $5 \times 9.5\ cm^2$ and sponge $7 \times 10\ cm^2$.	Anode over Fz and cathode over the right tibia. Anode over T3 and cathode over right deltoid. Two anodes over C3 and C4 and a cathode over right deltoid.	Type (1) and (3). Reports current density magnitude in the midbrain, pons and medulla. Data suggests that interference of the extracephalic reference electrodes with the brainstem should be limited.
29. Parazzini et al. (2013b)	Same as (11).		Anode/cathode over F3/F4. Same as the last two configurations in (28).	Type (1) and (3). Reports current density magnitude in the heart. The induced current density in the heart is lower than reported values for ventricular fibrillation threshold.
30. Wagner et al. (2014a, b)	$\sigma_{Scalp} = 0.43\ S/m$ $\sigma_{Skull\ Compacta} = 0.007\ S/m$ $\sigma_{Skull\ Spongiosa} = 0.025\ S/m$ $\sigma_{CSF} = 1.79\ S/m$ $\sigma_{GM} = 0.33\ S/m$ $\sigma_{WM} = 0.14\ S/m$ Isotropic. WM was also modelled as anisotropic.	Rectangular $5 \times 7\ cm^2$. Homogeneous conductivity: 1.4 S/m.	Anode over left M1 and cathode over RSO. Anode and cathode place bilaterally over the area of TP9/10, P7/8, T7/8 and CP5/6.	Type (1) and (3). Reports moderate changes due to WM anisotropy in current density direction in GM. In the WM bigger differences are observed.
31. Rampersad et al. (2014)	$\sigma_{Scalp} = 0.465\ S/m$ $\sigma_{Skull\ Compacta} = 0.007\ S/m$ $\sigma_{Skull\ Spongiosa} = 0.025\ S/m$ $\sigma_{CSF} = 1.65\ S/m$ Isotropic. GM/WM, cerebellar GM/WM and brainstem: Anisotropic with volume normalized approach. Other tissues were considered (total of 9).	Rectangular $5 \times 7\ cm^2$. Homogeneous conductivity: 1.4 S/m.	Anode-cathode: LM1-RSO LDLPFC-RSO LDLPFC-RDLPFC LIFG-RSO Oz-Cz Right cerebellum – right cheek.	Type (1) and (3). Reports sub-optimal field strengths in the target regions for each electrode configuration.

Table 9.1 (continued)

Reference	Tissues represented	Electrodes	Montages	Study description / Additional comments
32. Shahid et al. (2014)	Same as (24). WM, GM and skull anisotropy was included as well. Other tissues were also represented (total of 19).	Rectangular: 5 × 5 cm^2. Homogeneous conductivity: 1.4 S/m. Cylindrical 1.1 cm^2. Modelled as in (7).	Rectangular anode over C3 and cathode over Fp2. Cylindrical anode over C3 and cathodes over C1, FC3, CP3 and C5. Cylindrical anode over C1 and cathodes over Cz, C3, FC1 and CP1.	Type (1) and (3). The effects of anisotropy would not affect the clinical decision in the examples analyzed. However, they are of importance if cellular model predictions are to be made.
33. Ruffini et al. (2014)	Same as (25).	Cylindrical π cm^2, 25 cm^2. Homogeneous conductivity: 2 S/m.	π electrodes: Any one of 27 positions in the 10–20 system. 25 cm^2 electrodes: Several bipolar montages based on literature.	Type (3) and type (6).
34. Parazzini et al. (2014a)	Same as (11) but with skin conductivity set to 0.1 S/m.	Rectangular 5 × 7 cm^2 copper conductor (5.9 × 10^7 S/m) on top of sponge (1.4 S/m).	Cathode over the midpoint between C3 and F3 and anode over: RSO area; Right shoulder area.	Type (3) and (4). Determines the E-field distribution in children models. The cathode was placed in the most common epileptogenic focus in children.
35. Parazzini et al. (2014b)	Same as (11).	Rectangular 5 × 7 cm^2 copper conductor (5.9 × 10^7 S/m) on top of 7 × 8 cm^2 sponge (0.3 S/m).	Anode/cathode centered over cerebellum and reference electrode over the right arm.	Type (3). Reports current density distribution in tDCS of the cerebellum.
36. Gillick et al. (2014)	No details provided.	Rectangular 5 × 7 cm^2. No details provided regarding modelling.	Anode/cathode over C3/C4. Anode/cathode over LM1/RSO.	Type (3) and (5). Shows results of E-field modelling in a child brain model with a stroke.

(continued)

Table 9.1 (continued)

Reference	Tissues represented	Electrodes	Montages	Study description / Additional comments
37. Brunoni et al. (2014)	Same as (12) (without "synthetic" neck-shoulder region).	Rectangular: $5 \times 7\ cm^2$. Modelled as in (7).	Anode over left DLPFC and cathode either over occipital area or left TPJ.	Type (3). Shows E-field distribution in montages typically used in schizophrenia.
38. Metwally et al. (2015)	$\sigma_{Scalp} = 0.33\ S/m$ $\sigma_{Skull} = 0.0132\ S/m$ $\sigma_{CSF} = 1.79\ S/m$ $\sigma_{GM} = 0.33\ S/m$ $\sigma_{WM} = 0.14\ S/m$ Isotropic. WM and skull were also modelled as anisotropic.	Rectangular: $5 \times 7\ cm^2$. Cylindrical $0.5\ cm^2$. Homogeneous conductivity: $5.8 \times 10^7\ S/m$.	Rectangular anode over C3 and cathode over RSO. 4×1 cylindrical electrode configuration (1 anode over LM1 and 4 cathodes surrounding it). Cylindrical anode over C3 and cathode over C4.	Type (1) and (3). The presence of WM anisotropy leads to significant differences in the E-field direction, especially within the sulci.
39. Opitz et al. (2015)	$\sigma_{Scalp} = 0.25\ S/m$ $\sigma_{Skull\ Compacta} = 0.008\ S/m$ $\sigma_{Skull\ Spongiosa} = 0.025\ S/m$ $\sigma_{CSF} = 1.79\ S/m$ Isotropic. The GM and WM were considered anisotropic. Other tissues were considered (total of 8 tissues).	Rectangular: $5 \times 7\ cm^2$. Homogeneous conductivity: 1.79 S/m, but other values were considered as well.	Same as (25).	Type (1) and (3). Studies the influence of several parameters such as skull thickness, sulcal depth and CSF thickness on E-field distribution.
40. Saturnino et al. (2015)	$\sigma_{Scalp} = 0.25\ S/m$ $\sigma_{Skull\ Compacta} = 0.008\ S/m$ $\sigma_{Skull\ Spongiosa} = 0.025\ S/m$ $\sigma_{CSF} = 1.654\ S/m$ $\sigma_{GM} = 0.275\ S/m$ $\sigma_{WM} = 0.126\ S/m$ Isotropic. Other tissues were considered (total of 8 tissues).	Rectangular: $5 \times 7\ cm^2$. Ring: Outer/ inner diameters: 5 cm/ 2.5 cm. Cylindrical 1.1 cm^2 or $\pi\ cm^2$. Electrodes modelled with increasing degrees of complexity.	Rectangular/ring anode over C3 and cathode over RSO. 4 + 1 cylindrical electrode configuration (1 anode over C3 and 4 cathodes surrounding it).	Type (1) and (3). The way the electrodes are modelled can significantly affect the E-field distribution. Important parameters include the location of the metal connector and the conductive rubber's conductivity.

Table 9.1 (continued)

Reference	Tissues represented	Electrodes	Montages	Study description / Additional comments
41. Laakso et al. (2015)	$\sigma_{Scalp} = 0.08\ S/m$ $\sigma_{Skull\ Compacta} = 0.013\ S/m$ $\sigma_{Skull\ Spongiosa} = 0.06\ S/m$ $\sigma_{CSF} = 1.8\ S/m$ $\sigma_{GM} = 0.1\ S/m$ $\sigma_{WM} = 0.1\ S/m$ Isotropic. Other tissues were considered (total of 10 tissues).	Cylindrical 25 cm^2. Homogeneous conductivity: 0.3 S/m.	Anode over C3 and cathode over Fp2.	Type (1) and (3). Studies E-field distribution in 24 head models. Reports significant differences in magnitude and E-field distribution across subjects. States that CSF and brain geometry are factors that explain these differences and that age is the only external factor that had a significant effect on results.
42. Salvador et al. (2015)	Same as (25). GM-WM anisotropy was included.	Rectangular: 5 × 7 cm^2. Cylindrical $\pi\ cm^2$. Homogeneous conductivity: 2 S/m.	Anode (rectangular or cylindrical) over C3 and rectangular cathode over right SO. The rectangular anode was oriented as in (25).	Type (1) and (3). Compares the E-field distribution of tDCS and TMS of the motor cortex. Reports significant E-field differences in direction, magnitude and location of maxima.
43. Schmidt et al. (2015)	Does a sensitivity analysis varying the conductivities of 4 of the 5 represented tissues: $\sigma_{Scalp} = 0.280 - 0.575\ S/m$ $\sigma_{Skull} = 0.0016 - 0.0173\ S/m$ $\sigma_{CSF} = 1.79\ S/m$ $\sigma_{GM} = 0.220 - 0.445\ S/m$ $\sigma_{WM} = 0.090 - 0.190\ S/m$ Isotropic.	No details provided.	74 possible electrode positions (extended 10/10 system). An optimization scheme was used for auditory cortex stimulation.	Type (1), (3) and (6). Optimization scheme to induce a field radial to the cortical target in the auditory cortex. The influence of tissue conductivity in this optimization scheme was studied.
44. Galletta et al. (2015)	Same as (12) (without "synthetic" neck-shoulder region). Includes stroke lesions modelled as CSF.	Rectangular: 5 × 7 cm^2. Modelled as in (7).	Anode over CP5/F5 and cathode over RSO. Anode over CP6/F6 and cathode over LSO. Anode over F5 and cathode over F6.	Type (3) and (4). Study of tDCS montages used to promote recovery of post-stroke aphasia.

(continued)

Table 9.1 (continued)

Reference	Tissues represented	Electrodes	Montages	Study description / Additional comments
45. Parazzini et al. (2016)	$\sigma_{Scalp} = 0.43\ S/m$ $\sigma_{Skull} = 0.015\ S/m$ $\sigma_{CSF} = 1.79\ S/m$ $\sigma_{GM} = 0.32\ S/m$ $\sigma_{WM} = 0.15\ S/m$ Isotropic.	17.5 cm long electrode (area of 35 cm^2) that follows approximately the trajectory of the central sulcus. 17.5 cm long electrode (area of 35 cm2) rounded crown. Rectangular 10x7 cm^2 pad. Modelled as in (34).	The long 17.5 cm electrodes were positioned either over M1 or S1. The rectangular electrode was placed over Oz.	Type (1), (2) and (3). Investigates the use of a personalized electrode to modulate the entire extension of the motor / somato-sensitive area.
46. Bortoletto et al. (2016)	Same as (25).	Rectangular: $5 \times 7\ cm^2$. Ring with inner/outer radius of 3.5 cm/4.0 cm. Homogeneous conductivity: 2 S/m.	Same as (25). Central cylindrical anode placed over the FDI region in the LM1. Ring cathode was surrounding it.	Type (2), (3) and (5). Reports higher focality of the radial component of the E-field with the concentric ring configuration.

A priority was given to papers published in international peer reviewed journals, so conference proceedings were ignored unless the work they reported was not found published elsewhere. For notes regarding the classification of the study and the positions of the electrodes, please refer to the bottom of the table

Legend: R/LM1 Right/Left motor cortex, RSO/LSO Right/Left supra-orbital area, L/RDLPFC Left/Right dorsolateral prefrontal cortex, LIFG Left inferior frontal gyrus, STG Superior temporal gyrus, FDI First dorsal interosseous, TPJ Temporoparietal junction, C1, C3/4, Cz, Fp2, FC1, FC3, O1, Oz, T5, T7/8, TP7/8, F3/4, F8, CP1, CP3, CP5/6, P7/8 Positions of the 10–10 international system

Classification:

Type (1): Basic principles of E-field distribution in tDCS: influence of tissue dielectric properties (including anisotropy), electrode modelling, tissue thickness, tissue heating…

Type (2): Study of electrode design: study of a particular electrode design for improving focality of field for a specific application

Type (3): Study of E-field distribution in well-known montages for specific applications

Type (4): Study of tDCS in possible susceptible populations: stroke, obese, children, subjects with skull openings, …

Type (5): Modelling study integrated in study involving trials with subjects

Type (6): Electrode montage optimization

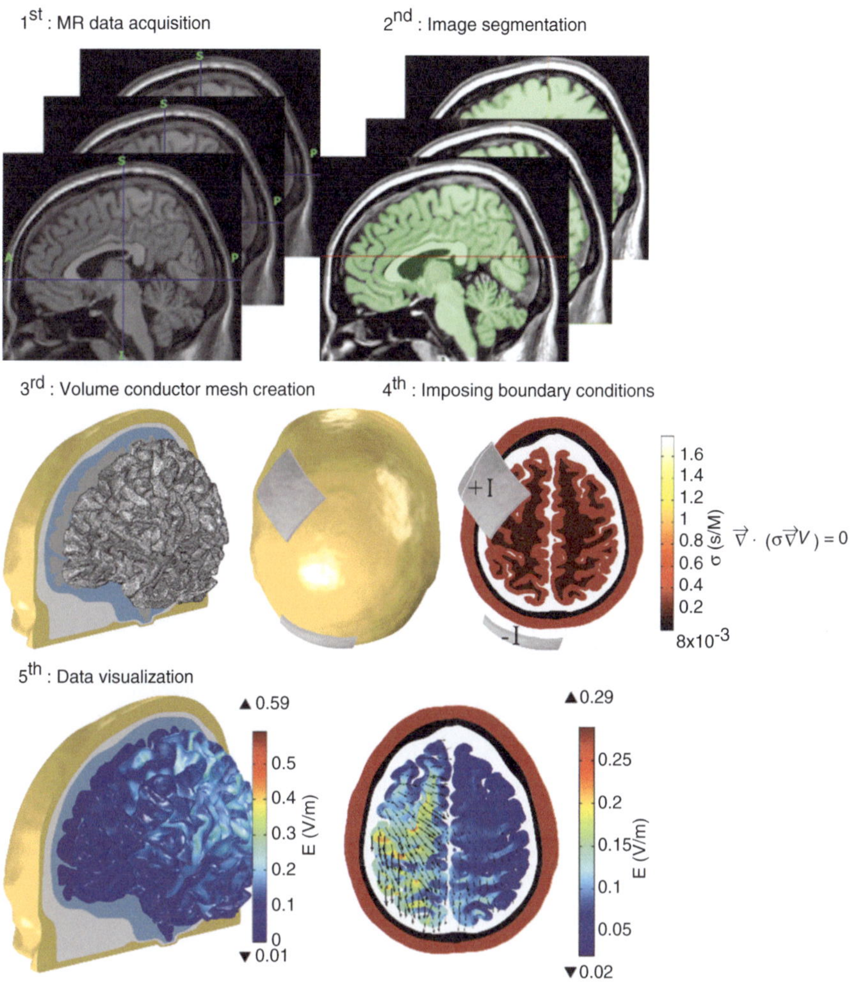

Fig. 9.1 Modeling steps involved in the creation of a computational high-resolution model of the E-field induced in tDCS

properties of the E-field induced in susceptible populations (more on this in section "Use of Computational Models in Clinical Practice").

The majority of studies shown in Table 9.1 employ a numerical technique known as the finite element method (FEM) to solve the governing physical equations that determine the E-field induced in tDCS (i.e., Laplace's equation) (Johnson 1997). The FEM yields an approximate numerical solution to a specific equation (or set of equations) that specifies a physical problem in a geometry. In the FEM, the geometry is subdivided into a number of finite elements of a specific shape that are connected by nodes. The latter comprise the finite element's mesh. Within each element of the mesh, the solution to the equation can be written in terms of an interpolation function whose parameters depend on the values of the dependent variable in the nodes of each element. In the case of tDCS, the dependent variable is V, the electrostatic potential, and its gradient yields the electric field vector, E. By approximating the solution to the equation with an interpolation function in every element of the mesh, the original equation can be rewritten as a linear equation of the form **AV** = **b**, where **A** is a matrix (whose values depend on the geometry of the mesh and the type of elements used), **V** is the column vector with the values of the dependent variable (electrostatic potential) in each node of the mesh and **b** is another column vector whose values depend on the boundary conditions of the problem (for instance the current injected at each electrode). In order to obtain the column vector **V**, it is necessary to invert matrix **A**, which can be performed using a number of numerical algorithms.

The first step for creating computational tDCS models is the specification of the geometry of the volume conductor, i.e., the head and electrodes. In most recent studies this is achieved by segmentation of structural magnetic resonance (MR) images, thus obtaining masks, i.e., the set of voxels labeled as belonging to a specific tissue. The choice of MR over other image modalities, such as computed tomography (CT), is mainly related to the fact that it does not involve ionizing radiation. It also offers a higher contrast between soft tissues, such as grey matter (GM) and white matter (WM) and the possibility for molecular phenomena to be observed (e.g. diffusion weighted imaging) (Bashir et al. 2015). MR also has some limitations, however, like the fact that the skull emits a very weak MR signal, therefore making its reconstruction difficult (Windhoff et al. 2013). Most studies use T1-weighted MR images with an isotropic resolution of 1 mm (lower resolutions are sometimes used), although other studies have employed T2 and even PD-weighted images to allow for a better segmentation of the CSF and skull (Miranda et al. 2013; Windhoff et al. 2013). A variety of algorithms and software are described in the literature in order to perform the automatic segmentation of the images. However, manual inspection of the resulting masks and manual segmentation of some structures is often reported as well. The majority of studies produce segmentation masks for the skin, skull, CSF compartments, GM and WM, but others include many more tissues such as muscle, subdermal fat, and eye sclera (Shahid et al. 2013). A number of studies segment the skull into compact and spongy bone (Laakso et al. 2015; Opitz et al. 2015; Rampersad et al. 2012; Saturnino et al. 2015; Wagner et al. 2014a, b). MR images do not usually allow for these two tissues to be segmented, so manual methods (Opitz et al. 2015) or custom MR sequences (Rampersad et al. 2014) are employed.

Generation of the finite element mesh from the segmentation masks is performed using several possible software and algorithms. Three aspects related to the mesh are noteworthy. The first one is its resolution, i.e. the mean distance between the nodes in the mesh. The mesh must have sufficient resolution to accurately predict the spatial distribution of the E-field. The second aspect is the type of element, i.e. the geometry of the finite element. Tetrahedra are often used because they allow for easier compliance to complex curved geometries. However, meshes with hexaedra are described in some studies (Laakso et al. 2015; Sadleir et al. 2010). Tetrahedral meshes are more time consuming to produce, since they require that smooth triangulated surfaces be built for each mask. These surfaces are then used to generate the volume meshes. Hexahedral meshes can be built directly from the masks, but they do not allow for smooth tissue boundaries to be represented. The only study that was found that compares these two types of meshes (Indahlastari and Sadleir 2015), focused on differences between mean values of the current density in predefined volumes. The differences on the direction of the E-field, however, remain unclear. The third aspect is the quality of the elements in the mesh, which is related to the shape of the elements. Elements with low quality, i.e. elongated elements with very small or very large angles (Windhoff et al. 2013), may lead to numerical instabilities in the FEM. The impact of mesh size and quality is of paramount importance to the obtained E-field results, but remains largely unaddressed in studies published up until now. This is in part due to the complexity of the head geometry, which makes a systematic study of the impact of the mesh challenging.

The stimulating electrodes are accommodated in the model by modifying the scalp's volume mesh. The latter can have different geometries and can be modeled with different degrees of complexity (see Table 9.1). Most models represent the electrodes as homogeneous patches with uniform conductivities (Miranda et al. 2013; Sadleir et al. 2010; Wagner et al. 2007) or as two layers of materials with different conductivities (metal on top of conductive gel) (Datta et al. 2009a). However, recent studies have shown the importance of accurately modeling the geometry of the electrodes, including the presence of a rubber pad inside the saline soaked sponge (sock-electrodes) and accounting for the position of the metal connector in the electrode (Saturnino et al. 2015).

Once the finite element mesh is obtained, the electric conductivity of each tissue and the boundary conditions must be set. The skin and CSF compartments are usually modeled as homogeneous and isotropic. In most models, the GM, WM and cerebellum are also modeled as such, but several studies use diffusion weighted (DW) MR to estimate the diffusion tensor and assign a conductivity tensor for these tissues (Metwally et al. 2015; Oostendorp et al. 2008; Opitz et al. 2015; Rampersad et al. 2014; Sadleir et al. 2010; Salvador et al. 2015; Schmidt et al. 2015; Shahid et al. 2013, 2014; Suh et al. 2012; Wagner et al. 2014a, b), thus allowing for the anisotropy to be taken into account. The skull can either be modeled as isotropic (single layer or three layers, when spongy bone and compact bone are segmented) or as anisotropic (with a single layer) (Rampersad et al. 2012). Conductivity values for DC or low frequencies can be found in a number of recent studies in the literature (Gabriel et al. 1996; Wagner et al. 2014a, b). However, the results are sometimes in disagreement with older data (more on this in the next section). The conductivity of the electrodes/conductive gel/conductive rubber in the electrode models is also often unknown. For homogeneous electrodes this seems to have a limited effect on the results (Opitz et al. 2015), but for more complex electrode models, this can significantly affect the E-field distribution (Saturnino et al. 2015). Other important boundary conditions specify the currents injected by each electrode. This is performed by adjusting the difference between the electric potential of the electrodes (upper boundary of the electrodes in simple electrode models or the metal connector in more realistic models), until the desired current is obtained.

The next step in these models involves inverting the matrix **A,** therefore obtaining the values of the potential at each node of the mesh. Since these models can have more than ten million degrees of freedom (nodes), iterative procedures are usually employed (Barrett et al. 1993). These have been shown to provide solutions that have a small error with respect to analytical solutions (Faria et al. 2011). This form of validation, i.e. comparing the results of models with the numerical solution of the E-field, can only be performed in simpler geometrical models, when analytical solutions can be obtained (Ferdjallah et al. 1996; Rush and Driscoll 1968). It also does not allow for a validation of the model *per se*, since many simplifications are introduced related to the geometry of the volume conductor (head) and the electric properties of the tissues. The latter likely affect the predictions of these models much more than numerical inaccuracies.

The final step of the pipeline illustrated in Fig. 9.1 involves the visualization of the E-field distribution and its analysis. This is a crucial step as it will directly influence any clinical decision made about dose. These types of models allow for volume or surface data to be analyzed. Volume data can be processed to yield mean/maximum E-field magnitude values in regions of interest (ROI). Mean E-field values are preferred because they are less sensitive to variations in element size or low-quality elements in the mesh. Surface data can be used to extract information regarding the orientation of the field, particularly in directions perpendicular to the surface (normal component) and tangential to it (tangential component). Analysis of surface data must be performed with care, as the normal component of the E-field is discontinuous across interfaces between tissues (Miranda et al. 2013). In order to further aid the visualization of the results, methods of cortical surface inflation have also been proposed (Laakso et al. 2015; Opitz et al. 2015), since they allow for an easier identification of the E-field maxima at the bottoms of sulci (Miranda et al. 2013). Another challenge lies in the comparison of E-field distributions across subjects, as inter-individual anatomical variability render direct comparisons non-trivial. One interesting solution that has been proposed is to register the individual models to a common atlas (Laakso et al. 2015).

Limitations of State-of-the-Art Computational Models

Computational models based on segmented structural MR images remain the only viable alternative to predict the E-field as a function of the dose parameters. However, they present limitations that can significantly affect the accuracy of their predictions. The first limitation is related to the inherent difficulties associated with segmentation of certain tissues in MR images. As mentioned previously, the skull and the CSF are particularly difficult to segment from T1/T2 images, and thus require manual corrections, or the use of specific image acquisition parameters that are not commonly used in a clinical setting. However, correctly modeling these tissues is critical to achieving accurate predictions, particularly because the largest change in electrical conductivity occurs precisely at the skull-CSF border. Many studies have shown the impact of the skull modeling (Opitz et al. 2015; Rampersad et al. 2012) and of the thickness of the CSF layer on the electric field in the brain (i.e., cortical regions where the CSF is thin have a significantly higher E-field magnitude, (Opitz et al. 2015)).

The geometry of the head models is usually obtained from MR images of a single individual. This can significantly bias the obtained E-field distribution, since great anatomical variations can exist between individuals (Huang et al. 2016). The effects of these differences have been addressed in a number of studies (Datta et al. 2012; Laakso et al. 2015). One alternative is to create individualized models for each participant in a given study, but this is difficult due to the high computational resources and specific know-how required to build such models. One other option is to use a volume conductor geometry that is obtained from averaged MR images of a number of individuals (Huang et al. 2016). This makes the particular features of the geometry of the volume conductor less susceptible to individual features of a single head but might be less representative for a specific individual (i.e., patients or research subjects).

One large difference between studies lies in the way the electrical conductivity of tissues is modeled, and which values are assigned to it. This can be clearly seen by the sometimes great disparity between the conductivity values assigned to the different tissues (see the second column of Table 9.1). Since this greatly affects the predictions of computational models, some studies have conducted sensitivity analyses on the values of the isotropic conductivities or the effects of the presence of skull and/or WM anisotropy (Laakso et al. 2015; Metwally et al. 2015; Schmidt et al. 2015; Shahid et al. 2013, 2014; Suh et al. 2012; Wagner et al. 2014a, b). No "gold standard" exists nowadays for a way to model the electrical properties of tissues in the DC range of frequencies, so care must be taken when comparing predictions between studies that employ different settings.

Another important limitation of computational models is that the information they provide is hampered by the lack of knowledge about the precise mechanisms of interaction of the E-field with the neurons. In other words, much is still unclear about how the information obtained from these computational models about the magnitude and direction of the E-field translates into modulation of the electrical activity of neurons. At first this may sound paradoxical, since the fundamentals of the E-field interaction with single neurons have been known for a long time (see Chap. 2 and (Roth 1994) for a review). In summary, polarization will occur in regions of maximum value of the activation function (gradient along the neuron of the E-field parallel to the neuron's trajectory) (Rattay 1986). At the scale of cortical neurons, the gradient of the E-field along the neuron is small, but strong polarizations can occur in regions where the axon or dendritic tree processes bend or terminate (Amassian et al. 1992; Nagarajan et al. 1993) as well as on the soma (Rahman et al. 2013).

The existence of several potential interaction mechanisms, together with the fact that the actual geometry of the neurons is rather complex, makes predictions about sites of activation and the components of the E-field more likely to influence them hard to make. One generally adopted approximation that has been proposed to solve this is to assume that the polarization of the neurons will be proportional to the

E-field's magnitude. This is termed the "quasi-uniform" assumption (Bikson et al. 2013) and similar approximations have been proposed before in other forms of stimulation, such as TMS (Ruohonen 1998). The E-field's component in a direction either perpendicular (radial) or tangential to the cortical sheet may also be explicitly computed (Faria et al. 2011) and might be the relevant factor in determining the field's interaction with neurons. The radial component of the E-field optimally polarize pyramidal cells in the cortex with dendrites that extend normal to the surface (Bikson et al. 2004; Datta et al. 2008). It also easily explains the polarity dependent nature of the neuro-modulatory effects elicited by tDCS that is observed up to a certain value of current intensity (Merlet et al. 2013; Nitsche and Paulus 2000). Tangential E-fields would optimally polarize axon afferents projecting along the surface (Rahman et al. 2013). The quasi-uniform assumption does not model neuron specific effects (Radman et al. 2009) or consider the role of changes in electric fields, as notably occurs across the grey-white matter interface (Miranda et al. 2003, 2007; Salvador et al. 2011).

Use of Computational Models in Clinical Practice

Optimizing Efficacy

Since the early days of tDCS, many options regarding dose parameters have been chosen on a trial-and-error basis. As an example, consider the original study by Nitsche and Paulus (Nitsche and Paulus 2000), which demonstrated that tDCS could elicit long lasting excitability changes in the motor cortex, by placing one electrode over the primary motor cortex and the other over the contralateral supraorbital area (M1-SO montage). In that study, the authors reported several other bipolar electrode configurations that were tested and that failed to elicit the same results. While in some follow-up studies these canonical results were interpreted as suggesting that current flow in the M1-SO montage affected mostly the motor region- and by extension that tDCS could be focalized to any region by placing a large pad electrode over it – it is import to recognize that such an interpretation was not implied by the authors of the original study.

The recent computational studies that have emerged provide useful insights into the E-field distribution in the brain that can aid in optimizing the efficacy in clinical applications of tDCS. Many of the initial computational studies aimed at clarifying the E-field distribution in realistic representations of electrode montages used in clinical practice in a series of applications (Datta et al. 2009a; Miranda et al. 2013; Sadleir et al. 2010). In contrast to earlier models based on concentric spheres (Miranda et al. 2006; Rush and Driscoll 1968) or abstracted geometry (CAD, (Wagner et al. 2007)), a critical feature of models applied since ~2009 is the incorporation of "gyri-precise" resolution based on precise anatomical MRI scans, and attention to continuity of CSF involving smoothing beyond scan resolution. This level of detail resulted in several key predictions that challenged prevailing views on dose design: (1) significant current flow occurs between (rather than simply under) electrodes; (2) current is clustered in hot-spots whose locations depend on idiosyncratic anatomy; (3) both electrodes are functional regardless of position (including extracephalic or "supra-orbital) and current under each electrode is influenced by the position of the others (Bikson et al. 2010). It should be noted that even as modeling technology has continued to evolve (e.g. addition of anisotropy; (Oostendorp et al. 2008; Suh et al. 2009)), and despite variation in methods (e.g. conductivity, (Opitz et al. 2015)), these basic predictions remain largely intact over the last 7 years of intensive modeling studies. In fact, is it precisely because current flow is not intuitive that models are important tools in the interpretation and design of tDCS studies.

These high-resolution studies proved useful in determining which regions were targeted by these configurations and what was the direction of the induced E-field in different regions. Based on the latter, a newer batch of studies has appeared geared towards optimizing multi-electrode montages to achieve a target E-field distribution and orientation in pre-defined cortical regions of interest (Dmochowski et al. 2011; Ruffini et al. 2014; Sadleir et al. 2012). They use the superposition principle, i.e., the principle that the E-field distribution in the head induced by a given set of electrodes can be obtained by the weighted sum of the E-fields induced by bipolar electrode configurations with a common return electrode. The weights used to sum the bipolar induced E-field configurations are the currents set in each electrode of the multi-electrode configuration. These types of models then determine the current intensity applied at each electrode (placed in a predefined array of positions) such that the induced E-field best approximates a pre-defined target E-field distribution in the brain. This optimization procedure can be further constrained by imposing maximum values for the current on each electrode and the total injected current.

The main difference between the implementations in each study is related to the components of the E-field which were optimized (pre-determined E-field with any desired direction, as specified by the user (Dmochowski et al. 2011), E-field component radial to the cortical sheet in (Ruffini et al. 2014) or magnitude of the E-field (Sadleir et al. 2012)). Other differences are the algorithms used to minimize the difference between the induced E-field and the target field, and the type of electrodes and pre-defined electrode positions. These studies have shown that it is possible to induce E-fields in target regions with higher focality and/or magnitude that those using conventional approached (i.e. bipolar "pad-like" electrodes) (Dmochowski et al. 2011). Moreover, they suggest the possibility of using data from functional imaging techniques (electroencephalography, positron emission tomography and functional magnetic resonance imaging) to derive cortical activation maps that may serve as the target E-field distribution that served as input to these studies (Ruffini et al. 2014). Finally, they offer the possibility of avoiding unwanted stimulation of certain regions by minimizing the E-field induced in the latter (Sadleir et al. 2012).

In spite of the usefulness of computational models, their implementation can be a complex task for research groups, particularly those with clinical applications. Working in close collaboration with a computational modeling group might be an alternative, and indeed, many studies nowadays seek to incorporate the information from these models as a rationale to dose parameter decisions and/or as support for some of the conclusions of the study (see references marked as type (5) in Table 9.1). The creation of tools to allow for easier implementation of these models (Jung et al. 2013; Windhoff et al. 2013) and of databases of models (Truong et al. 2014) can also allow for a wider implementation of computational models as part of the pipeline for experiment design.

Safety and Tolerability Considerations

It is not trivial to translate the predictions of computational E-field calculations to statements about safety or tolerability of a specific dose selection in tDCS. This occurs because, while the E-field distribution in tDCS can be predicted from these models in different tissues, the relation between the field and potential unwanted side-effects are not well known. None-the-less, under the assumption that increasing the E-field in a given target increases the theoretical risk of injury, even by providing comparative electric field across montages and subject populations (e.g. pediatric, stroke, injury), models are a valuable tool to assess risk.

One aspect related to tolerability, for instance, are the reported tingling and itching sensations under the electrodes and the acute erythema that has been associated with vasodilation (Woods et al. 2016). Computational models allow for the E-field in the skin-electrode interface to be calculated, and complex electrode models incorporating the gel and conductive rubber pads within saline soaked electrodes have been produced (Saturnino et al. 2015). These calculations, however, are of limited application since no model exists at the moment to relate the E-field to the reported undesired effects.

Regarding safety issues, attention has focused on predicting the electric field (current density) threshold at which injury may occur in the brain, skin or other structures. This work has, in turn, relied on injury thresholds proposed by animal models – which generally suggest thresholds more than one order of magnitude above clinical tDCS intensities. Computational models are essential to make scaling of intensities between animal models and humans more precise for this purpose, because for the same applied current or current density at electrodes, the resulting electric fields in rodent are much higher than those in human. For instance, injuries linked to possible tissue damage caused by heating (joule heating) may be relevant to tDCS. This has been addressed in a study (Datta et al. 2009b) which has shown that application of tDCS with a current to electrode area ratio of 142.9 A/m^2, a value that has been shown to lead to lesions in *in vivo* rat models (Liebetanz et al. 2009), caused a small maximum temperature increase in the brain (0.55 °C) but a significant scalp temperature increase (14.68 °C). However, these models require validation and many important factors, like sweat gland response in the scalp, were not modeled.

Another important safety issue is related to the usage of extracephalic return electrodes, which have been proposed to avert unwanted effects of tDCS in cortical areas away from the target region (Moliadze et al. 2010). However, modeling studies showed that use of extracephalic electrodes does not "cancel" the role of the return electrode, but rather creates extensive current flow through the foramen magnum, thereby affecting deep and mid-brain structures (Datta et al. 2011). It was speculated that current flow produced by extracephalic electrodes might interfere with other excitable tissues in the brainstem or the heart, which can lead to severe complications. Studies addressing this (Parazzini et al. 2013a, b) calculated current density magnitudes in these tissues and compared them to reported threshold values for cardiac fibrillation or with values induced in the brainstem during conventional bipolar montages, as these do not show unwanted brainstem neuromodulatory effects. These approaches to assess the lack of unwanted effects of the induced E-field still have some potential shortcomings, however, since the direction of the E-field is also a factor influencing neuronal stimulation and this aspect is not taken into account when analyzing only the magnitude of the field. One alternative to the use of extracephalic electrodes is the use of the multi-electrode optimization approaches that were mentioned in the last section, which may allow for a reduction of the unwanted secondary activations in unwanted brain areas. The latter also allows for the current in each electrode and the total overall current to be limited to specified maximum values.

The use of tDCS in subjects with skull defects (Datta et al. 2010) or in children (Gillick et al. 2014; Kessler et al. 2013; Minhas et al. 2012; Parazzini et al. 2014a) is also a matter that warrants caution, since the E-field distribution in these populations may be significantly different from that in healthy adult subjects. The presence of skull holes, for instance, was found to significantly increase the E-field if the electrode is placed directly on top of it. Regarding pediatric tDCS applications, the E-field induced in the child brain was found to be on average higher than that induced in adult brain using the same dose parameters. These results support the importance of carefully studying the E-field distribution in these models and leveraging them as a means to adjust dose parameters.

Dose Selection on an Individual Basis

Currently, the technical sophistication required to generate high-resolution computational models make implementation on a subject specific basis a very time-consuming process. Recent efforts have aimed to automate the individual segmentation process in a manner that does not compromise model precision (Huang and Parra 2015). Typically, however, computational studies involve the creation of one head model and the generalization of the results to other head geometries. This approach works well when the study's goal is to determine basic principles of the spatial distribution of the E-field in tDCS. A few modeling studies have studied the impact of intersubject variability in the E-field distribution in tDCS (Datta et al. 2012; Laakso et al. 2015). These studies report significant differences arising from details in the geometry of the cortical sheet. One of these studies reports that the E-field in the hand motor area across 24 individual subjects followed a normal distribution with a standard deviation of about 20% of the mean (Laakso et al.

2015). Recently, a standardized head based on the MNI has been developed specifically for tDCS modeling, and has been show to provide reasonable predictions of individualized subject response (Huang et al. 2016).

Other examples of cases warranting individualized head models are studies involving stroke patients, for which the size of the lesion and its location and shape can significantly affect the distribution of the induced E-field (Datta et al. 2011). Other examples are the already mentioned studies involving children (Minhas et al. 2012) or studies involving obese subjects (Truong et al. 2013). In those cases, individualized models remain the only viable way to provide a realistic E-field distribution and thus optimize dose parameters (Dmochowski et al. 2013).

Examples of Application of Computational Modeling in Case Studies

Computational models of tDCS can be performed proactively or retroactively. Proactive modeling can influence montage selection by informing researchers of stimulation focality and intensity for a region of interest. In atypical case studies, safety concerns can be assessed and mitigated by proactively modeling the stimulation protocol and comparing to a typical subject. Examples of this strategy include pediatrics, stroke, and subjects with cranial defects (Bikson et al. 2016; Minhas et al. 2012). In Fig. 9.2, tDCS is simulated in a subject with and without idealized Deep Brain Stimulation (DBS) leads. As an extreme case, the burrhole defect typical in subthalamic nucleus DBS is allowed to be fluid filled and relatively conductive. Common sponge (conventional) and HD-tDCS montages for motor and cerebellar stimulation are compared. Fluid filled burrholes draw a greater amount of current density than what would normally exist with healthy tissue (dashed images). However, peak current density and electric field are minimally affected (less than twofold). In general, HD configurations exhibit lower electric field intensities in deep brain structures while exhibiting more focal field patterns.

While tDCS modeling tools are becoming more accessible (COMETS, Bonsai, SimNIBS) (Jung et al. 2013; Thielscher et al. 2015; Truong et al. 2014) many transcranial stimulation studies have been and are performed without the guidance of modeling. Retroactive modeling of a specific study's stimulation parameters can help to resolve mechanisms of action or explain variance within or between studies. Fig. 9.3 represents a post-hoc analysis of common tDCS montages used in schizophrenia (Brunelin et al. 2012; Shiozawa et al. 2013). The electric field magnitude on the cortical surface depicts regions of maximum stimulation regardless of field orientation (A). The radial component of the electric field predicts the effects of stimulation on layer V pyramidal neurons aligned perpendicular to the cortical surface (B). Field orientation, anodal (red) or cathodal (blue), is commonly postulated to have excitatory or inhibitory effects on local regions (B). Meanwhile, tangential electric field magnitude is predicted to affect local connections oriented along the cortical surface (C).

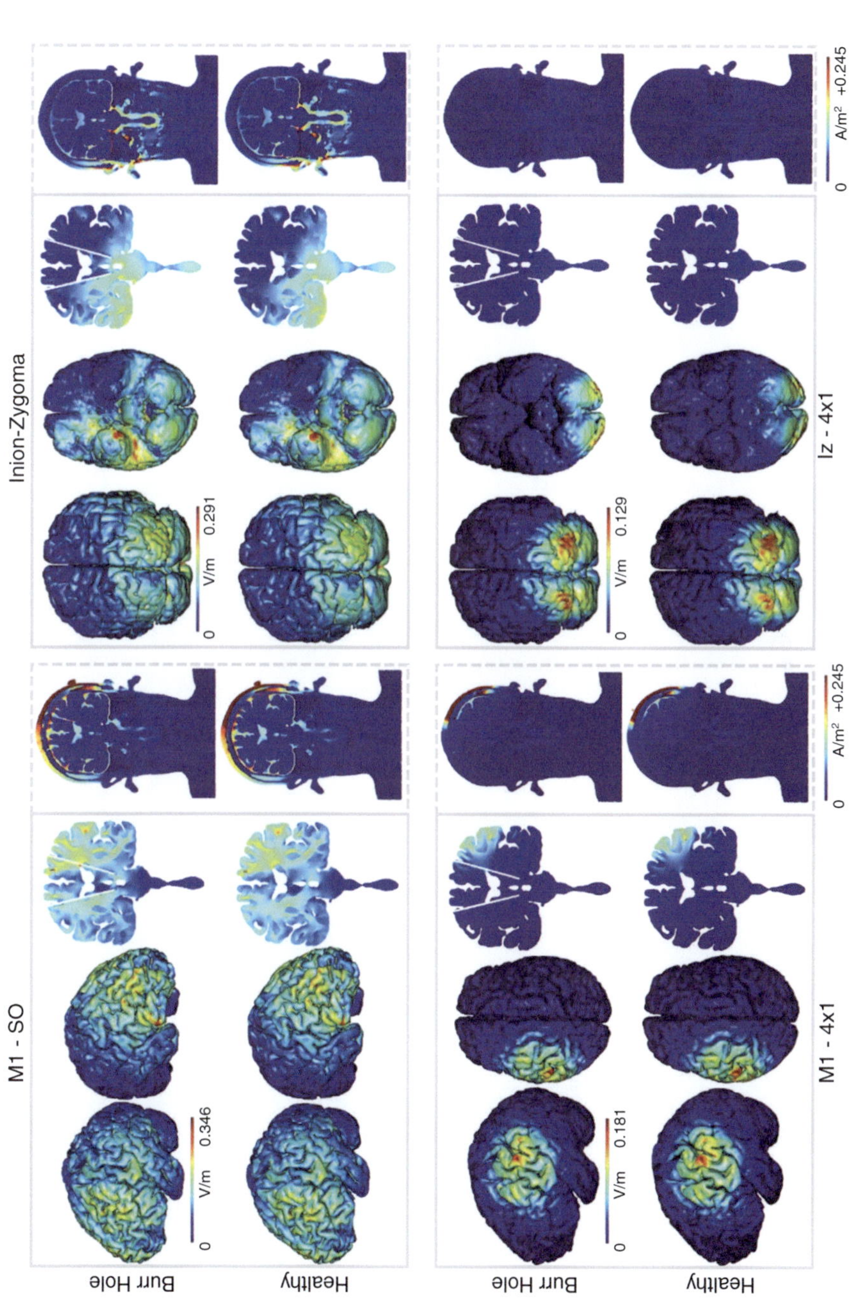

Fig. 9.2 Simulation of tDCS in subjects with idealized Deep Brain Stimulation (DBS) leads using conventional 5 × 7 cm sponge and HD (4 × 1) montages

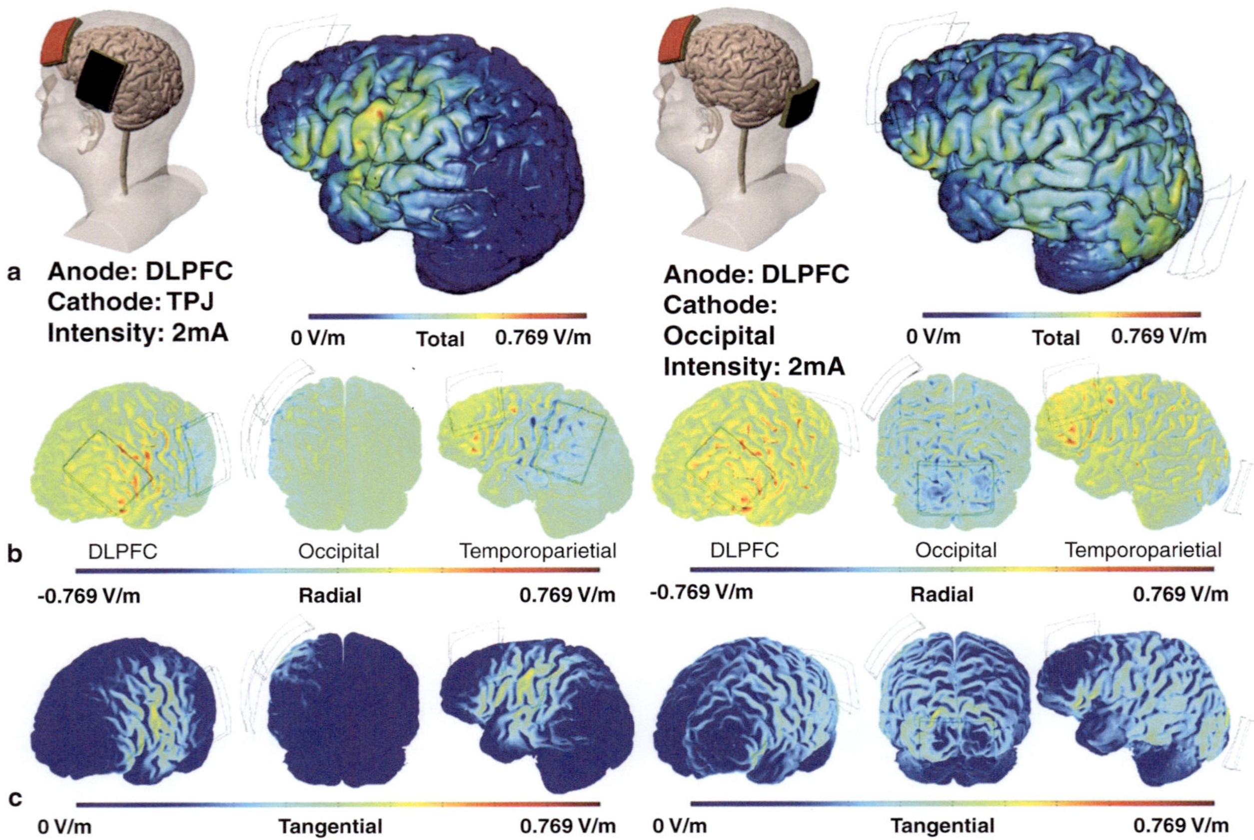

Fig. 9.3 Posthoc analysis of common tDCS montages used in schizophrenia. (**a**) electric field magnitude; (**b**) electric field normal to the cortical surface; (**c**) electric field tangential to the cortical surface (Brunelin et al. 2012; Shiozawa et al. 2013). (Adapted from Brunoni et al. (2014); with permission)

References

Amassian, V. E., Eberle, L., Maccabee, P. J., & Cracco, R. Q. (1992). Modelling magnetic coil excitation of human cerebral cortex with a peripheral nerve immersed in a brain-shaped volume conductor: The significance of fiber bending in excitation. *Electroencephalography and Clinical Neurophysiology, 85*(5), 291–301.

Barrett, R., Berry, M., Chan, T. F., Demmel, J., Donato, J. M., Dongarra, J., … Van der Vorst, H. (1993). *Templates for the solution of linear systems: Building blocks for iterative methods* (2nd ed.). Philadelphia, PA: Society for Industrial and Applied Mathematics.

Bashir, U., Mallia, A., Stirling, J., Joemon, J., MacKewn, J., Charles-Edwards, G., … Cook, G. J. (2015). PET/MRI in oncological imaging: State of the art. *Diagnostica, 5*(3), 333–357.

Bikson, M., Datta, A., Rahman, A., & Scaturro, J. (2010). Electrode montages for tDCS and weak transcranial electrical stimulation: Role of "return" electrode's position and size. *Clinical Neurophysiology, 121*(12), 1976–1978.

Bikson, M., Dmochowski, J., & Rahman, A. (2013). The "quasi-uniform" assumption in animal and computational models of non-invasive electrical stimulation. *Brain Stimulation, 6*(4), 704–705.

Bikson, M., Grossman, P., Thomas, C., Zannou, A..L., Jiang, J., Adnan, T., … Woods, A. J. (2016). Safety of transcranial direct current stimulation: Evidence based update 2016. *Brain Stimulation, 9*(5), 641–661.

Bikson, M., Inoue, M., Akiyama, H., Deans, J. K., Fox, J. E., Miyakawa, H., & Jefferys, J. G. (2004). Effects of uniform extracellular DC electric fields on excitability in rat hippocampal slices in vitro. *The Journal of Physiology, 557.*(Pt 1, 175–190.

Bortoletto, M., Rodella, C., Salvador, R., Miranda, P. C., & Miniussi, C. (2016). Reduced current spread by concentric electrodes in transcranial electrical stimulation (tES). *Brain Stimulation, 9*(4), 525–528.

Brunelin, J., Mondino, M., Gassab, L., Haesebaert, F., Gaha, L., Suaud-Chagny, M. F., … Poulet, E. (2012). Examining transcranial direct-current stimulation (tDCS) as a treatment for hallucinations in schizophrenia. *The American Journal of Psychiatry, 169*(7), 719–724.

Brunoni, A. R., Shiozawa, P., Truong, D., Javitt, D. C., Elkis, H., Fregni, F., … Bikson, M. (2014). Understanding tDCS effects in schizophrenia: A systematic review of clinical data and an integrated computation modeling analysis. *Expert Review of Medical Devices, 11*(4), 383–394.

Dasilva, A. F., Mendonca, M. E., Zaghi, S., Lopes, M., Dossantos, M. F., Spierings, E. L., … Fregni, F. (2012). tDCS-induced analgesia and electrical fields in pain-related neural networks in chronic migraine. *Headache, 52*(8), 1283–1295.

Datta, A., Baker, J. M., Bikson, M., & Fridriksson, J. (2011). Individualized model predicts brain current flow during transcranial direct-current stimulation treatment in responsive stroke patient. *Brain Stimulation, 4*(3), 6.

Datta, A., Bansal, V., Diaz, J., Patel, J., Reato, D., & Bikson, M. (2009a). Gyri-precise head model of transcranial direct current stimulation: Improved spatial focality using a ring electrode versus conventional rectangular pad. *Brain Stimulation, 2*(4), 201–207.

Datta, A., Bikson, M., & Fregni, F. (2010). Transcranial direct current stimulation in patients with skull defects and skull plates: High-resolution computational FEM study of factors altering cortical current flow. *NeuroImage, 52*(4), 1268–1278.

Datta, A., Elwassif, M., Battaglia, F., & Bikson, M. (2008). Transcranial current stimulation focality using disc and ring electrode configurations: FEM analysis. *Journal of Neural Engineering, 5*(2), 163–174.

Datta, A., Elwassif, M., & Bikson, M. (2009b). *Bio-heat transfer model of transcranial DC stimulation: Comparison of conventional pad versus ring electrode.* Paper presented at the 31st annual international conference of the IEEE engineering in medicine and biology society (EMBC), Minneapolis.

Datta, A., Krause, M. R., Pilly, P. K., Choe, J., Zanos, T. P., Thomas, C., & Pack, C. C. (2016). *On comparing in vivo intracranial recordings in non-human primates to predictions of optimized transcranial electrical stimulation.* Paper presented at the 36th Annual International Conference of the IEEE Engineering in Medicine and Biology Society (EMBC), Orlando.

Datta, A., Truong, D., Minhas, P., Parra, L. C., & Bikson, M. (2012). Inter-individual variation during transcranial direct current stimulation and normalization of dose using MRI-derived computational models. *Frontiers in Psychiatry, 3*, 91.

Dmochowski, J. P., Datta, A., Bikson, M., Su, Y. Z., & Parra, L. C. (2011). Optimized multi-electrode stimulation increases focality and intensity at target. *Journal of Neural Engineering, 8*(4), 046011.

Dmochowski, J. P., Datta, A., Huang, Y., Richardson, J. D., Bikson, M., Fridriksson, J., & Parra, L. C. (2013). Targeted transcranial direct current stimulation for rehabilitation after stroke. *NeuroImage, 75*, 12–19.

Dymond, A. M., Coger, R. W., & Serafetinides, E. A. (1975). Intracerebral current levels in man during electrosleep therapy. *Biological Psychiatry, 10*(1), 101–104.

Eaton, H. (1992). Electric field induced in a spherical volume conductor from arbitrary coils: Application to magnetic stimulation and MEG. *Medical & Biological Engineering & Computing, 30*(4), 433–440.

Faria, P., Hallett, M., & Miranda, P. C. (2011). A finite element analysis of the effect of electrode area and inter-electrode distance on the spatial distribution of the current density in tDCS. *Journal of Neural Engineering, 8*(6), 066017.

Ferdjallah, M., Bostick, F. X., Jr., & Barr, R. E. (1996). Potential and current density distributions of cranial electrotherapy stimulation (CES) in a four-concentric-spheres model. *IEEE Transactions on Biomedical Engineering, 43*(9), 939–943.

Gabriel, C., Gabriel, S., & Corthout, E. (1996). The dielectric properties of biological tissues: I. Literature survey. *Physics in Medicine and Biology, 41*(11), 2231–2249.

Galletta, E. E., Cancelli, A., Cottone, C., Simonelli, I., Tecchio, F., Bikson, M., & Marangolo, P. (2015). Use of computational modeling to inform tDCS electrode montages for the promotion of language recovery in post-stroke aphasia. *Brain Stimulation, 8*(6), 1108–1115.

Gillick, B. T., Kirton, A., Carmel, J. B., Minhas, P., & Bikson, M. (2014). Pediatric stroke and transcranial direct current stimulation: Methods for rational individualized dose optimization. *Frontiers in Human Neuroscience, 8*, 739.

Halko, M. A., Datta, A., Plow, E. B., Scaturro, J., Bikson, M., & Merabet, L. B. (2011). Neuroplastic changes following rehabilitative training correlate with regional electrical field induced with tDCS. *NeuroImage, 57*(3), 885–891.

Huang, Y., & Parra, L. C. (2015). Fully automated whole-head segmentation with improved smoothness and continuity, with theory reviewed. *PLoS One, 10*(5), e0125477.

Huang, Y., Parra, L. C., & Haufe, S. (2016). The New York head-a precise standardized volume conductor model for EEG source localization and tES targeting. *NeuroImage, 140*, 150–162.

Indahlastari, A., & Sadleir, R. J. (2015). *A comparison between block and smooth modeling in finite element simulations of tDCS.* Paper presented at the 37th annual international conference of the IEEE engineering in medicine and biology society (EMBC), Milan.

Johnson, C. R. (1997). Computational and numerical methods for bioelectric field problems. *Critical Reviews in Biomedical Engineering, 25*(1), 1–81.

Jung, Y.-J., Kim, J.-H., & Im, C.-H. (2013). COMETS: A MATLAB toolbox for simulating local electric fields generated by transcranial direct current stimulation (tDCS). [journal article]. *Biomedical Engineering Letters, 3*(1), 39–46.

Kessler, S. K., Minhas, P., Woods, A. J., Rosen, A., Gorman, C., & Bikson, M. (2013). Dosage considerations for transcranial direct current stimulation in children: A computational modeling study. *PLoS One, 8*(9), e76112.

Laakso, I., Tanaka, S., Koyama, S., De Santis, V., & Hirata, A. (2015). Inter-subject variability in electric fields of motor cortical tDCS. *Brain Stimulation, 8*(5), 8.

Liebetanz, D., Koch, R., Mayenfels, S., Konig, F., Paulus, W., & Nitsche, M. A. (2009). Safety limits of cathodal transcranial direct current stimulation in rats. *Clinical Neurophysiology, 120*(6), 1161–1167.

Lopez-Alonso, V., Cheeran, B., Rio-Rodriguez, D., & Fernandez-Del-Olmo, M. (2014). Inter-individual variability in response to non-invasive brain stimulation paradigms. *Brain Stimulation, 7*(3), 372–380.

Mendonca, M. E., Santana, M. B., Baptista, A. F., Datta, A., Bikson, M., Fregni, F., & Araujo, C. P. (2011). Transcranial DC stimulation in fibromyalgia: Optimized cortical target supported by high-resolution computational models. *The Journal of Pain, 12*(5), 610–617.

Merlet, I., Birot, G., Salvador, R., Molaee-Ardekani, B., Mekonnen, A., Soria-Frisch, A., … Wendling, F. (2013). From oscillatory transcranial current stimulation to scalp EEG changes: A biophysical and physiological modeling study. *PLoS One, 8*(2), e57330.

Metwally, M. K., Han, S. M., & Kim, T. S. (2015). The effect of tissue anisotropy on the radial and tangential components of the electric field in transcranial direct current stimulation. *Medical & Biological Engineering & Computing, 53*(10), 1085–1101.

Minhas, P., Bikson, M., Woods, A. J., Rosen, A. R., & Kessler, S. K. (2012). *Transcranial direct current stimulation in pediatric brain: A computational modeling study.* Paper presented at the 34th annual international conference of the IEEE engineering in medicine and biology society (EMBC), San Diego.

Miranda, P. C., Correia, L., Salvador, R., & Basser, P. J. (2007). Tissue heterogeneity as a mechanism for localized neural stimulation by applied electric fields. *Physics in Medicine and Biology, 52*(18), 5603–5617.

Miranda, P. C., Hallett, M., & Basser, P. J. (2003). The electric field induced in the brain by magnetic stimulation: A 3-D finite-element analysis of the effect of tissue heterogeneity and anisotropy. *IEEE Transactions on Biomedical Engineering, 50*(9), 1074–1085.

Miranda, P. C., Lomarev, M., & Hallett, M. (2006). Modeling the current distribution during transcranial direct current stimulation. *Clinical Neurophysiology, 117*(7), 1623–1629.

Miranda, P. C., Mekonnen, A., Salvador, R., & Ruffini, G. (2013). The electric field in the cortex during transcranial current stimulation. *NeuroImage, 70*, 48–58.

Moliadze, V., Antal, A., & Paulus, W. (2010). Electrode-distance dependent after-effects of transcranial direct and random noise stimulation with extracephalic reference electrodes. *Clinical Neurophysiology, 121*(12), 2165–2171.

Nagarajan, S. S., Durand, D. M., & Warman, E. N. (1993). Effects of induced electric-fields on finite neuronal structures – A simulation study. *IEEE Transactions on Biomedical Engineering, 40*(11), 1175–1188.

Nitsche, M. A., & Paulus, W. (2000). Excitability changes induced in the human motor cortex by weak transcranial direct current stimulation. *The Journal of Physiology London, 527*(3), 633–639.

Oostendorp, T. F., Hengeveld, Y. A., Wolters, C. H., Stinstra, J., van Elswijk, G., & Stegeman, D. F. (2008). *Modeling transcranial DC stimulation.* Paper presented at the 30th annual international conference of the IEEE engineering in medicine and biology society (EMBC), Vancouver.

Opitz, A., Falchier, A., Yan, C. G., Yeagle, E. M., Linn, G. S., Megevand, P., … Schroeder, C. E. (2016). Spatiotemporal structure of intracranial electric fields induced by transcranial electric stimulation in humans and nonhuman primates. *Scientific Reports, 6*, 31236.

Opitz, A., Paulus, W., Will, S., Antunes, A., & Thielscher, A. (2015). Determinants of the electric field during transcranial direct current stimulation. *NeuroImage, 109*, 140–150.

Parazzini, M., Fiocchi, S., Cancelli, A., Cottone, C., Liorni, I., Ravazzani, P., & Tecchio, F. (2016). A computational model of the electric field distribution due to regional personalized or non-personalized electrodes to select transcranial electric stimulation target. *IEEE Transactions on Biomedical Engineering, 64*, 184–195.

Parazzini, M., Fiocchi, S., Liorni, I., Priori, A., & Ravazzani, P. (2014a). Computational modeling of transcranial direct current stimulation in the child brain: Implications for the treatment of refractory childhood focal epilepsy. *International Journal of Neural Systems, 24*(2), 1430006.

Parazzini, M., Fiocchi, S., & Ravazzani, P. (2012). Electric field and current density distribution in an anatomical head model during transcranial direct current stimulation for tinnitus treatment. *Bioelectromagnetics, 33*(6), 476–487.

Parazzini, M., Fiocchi, S., Rossi, E., Paglialonga, A., & Ravazzani, P. (2011). Transcranial direct current stimulation: Estimation of the electric field and of the current density in an anatomical human head model. *IEEE Transactions on Biomedical Engineering, 58*(6), 1773–1780.

Parazzini, M., Rossi, E., Ferrucci, R., Liorni, I., Priori, A., & Ravazzani, P. (2014b). Modelling the electric field and the current density generated by cerebellar transcranial DC stimulation in humans. *Clinical Neurophysiology, 125*(3), 577–584.

Parazzini, M., Rossi, E., Rossi, L., Priori, A., & Ravazzani, P. (2013a). Evaluation of the current density in the brainstem during transcranial direct current stimulation with extra-cephalic reference electrode. *Clinical Neurophysiology, 124*(5), 1039–1040.

Parazzini, M., Rossi, E., Rossi, L., Priori, A., & Ravazzani, P. (2013b). Numerical estimation of the current density in the heart during transcranial direct current stimulation. *Brain Stimulation, 6*(3), 457–459.

Peterchev, A. V., Wagner, T. A., Miranda, P. C., Nitsche, M. A., Paulus, W., Lisanby, S. H., … Bikson, M. (2012). Fundamentals of transcranial electric and magnetic stimulation dose: Definition, selection, and reporting practices. *Brain Stimulation, 5*(4), 435–453.

Radman, T., Ramos, R. L., Brumberg, J. C., & Bikson, M. (2009). Role of cortical cell type and morphology in subthreshold and suprathreshold uniform electric field stimulation in vitro. *Brain Stimulation, 2*(4), 215–228.

Rahman, A., Reato, D., Arlotti, M., Gasca, F., Datta, A., Parra, L. C., & Bikson, M. (2013). Cellular effects of acute direct current stimulation: Somatic and synaptic terminal effects. *Journal of Physiology London, 591*(10), 2563–2578.

Rampersad, S., Stegeman, D., & Oostendorp, T. (2012). Single-layer skull approximations perform well in transcranial direct current stimulation modeling. *IEEE Transactions on Neural Systems and Rehabilitation Engineering, 1*(3), 8.

Rampersad, S. M., Janssen, A. M., Lucka, F., Aydin, U., Lanfer, B., Lew, S., … Oostendorp, T. F. (2014). Simulating transcranial direct current stimulation with a detailed anisotropic human head model. *IEEE Transactions on Neural Systems and Rehabilitation Engineering, 22*(3), 441–452.

Rattay, F. (1986). Analysis of models for external stimulation of axons. *IEEE Transactions on Biomedical Engineering, 33*(10), 974–977.

Roth, B. J. (1994). Mechanisms for electrical-stimulation of excitable tissue. *Critical Reviews in Biomedical Engineering, 22*(3–4), 253–305.

Roth, B. J., Cohen, L. G., & Hallett, M. (1991). The electric field induced during magnetic stimulation. *Electroencephalography and Clinical Neurophysiology, 43*, 268–278.

Ruffini, G., Fox, M. D., Ripolles, O., Miranda, P. C., & Pascual-Leone, A. (2014). Optimization of multifocal transcranial current stimulation for weighted cortical pattern targeting from realistic modeling of electric fields. *NeuroImage, 89*, 216–225.

Ruohonen, J. (1998). *Transcranial magnetic stimulation: Modelling and new techniques.* Unpublished PhD, Helsinki University of Technology, Espoo.

Rush, S., & Driscoll, D. A. (1968). Current distribution in the brain from surface electrodes. *Anesthesia and Analgesia, 47*(6), 717–723.

Sadleir, R. J., Vannorsdall, T. D., Schretlen, D. J., & Gordon, B. (2010). Transcranial direct current stimulation (tDCS) in a realistic head model. *NeuroImage, 51*(4), 1310–1318.

Sadleir, R. J., Vannorsdall, T. D., Schretlen, D. J., & Gordon, B. (2012). Target optimization in transcranial direct current stimulation. *Frontiers in Psychiatry, 3*, 90.
Salvador, R., Silva, S., Basser, P. J., & Miranda, P. C. (2011). Determining which mechanisms lead to activation in the motor cortex: A modeling study of transcranial magnetic stimulation using realistic stimulus waveforms and sulcal geometry. *Clinical Neurophysiology, 122*(4), 748–758.
Salvador, R., Wenger, C., & Miranda, P. C. (2015). Investigating the cortical regions involved in MEP modulation in tDCS. [original research]. *Frontiers in Cellular Neuroscience, 9*: 405 (11 pages).
Saturnino, G. B., Antunes, A., & Thielscher, A. (2015). On the importance of electrode parameters for shaping electric field patterns generated by tDCS. *NeuroImage, 120*, 25–35.
Schmidt, C., Wagner, S., Burger, M., Rienen, U., & Wolters, C. H. (2015). Impact of uncertain head tissue conductivity in the optimization of transcranial direct current stimulation for an auditory target. *Journal of Neural Engineering, 12*(4), 046028.
Shahid, S., Wen, P., & Ahfock, T. (2013). Numerical investigation of white matter anisotropic conductivity in defining current distribution under tDCS. *Computer Methods and Programs in Biomedicine, 109*(1), 48–64.
Shahid, S. S., Bikson, M., Salman, H., Wen, P., & Ahfock, T. (2014). The value and cost of complexity in predictive modelling: Role of tissue anisotropic conductivity and fibre tracts in neuromodulation. *Journal of Neural Engineering, 11*(3), 036002.
Shiozawa, P., da Silva, M. E., Cordeiro, Q., Fregni, F., & Brunoni, A. R. (2013). Transcranial direct current stimulation (tDCS) for the treatment of persistent visual and auditory hallucinations in schizophrenia: A case study. *Brain Stimulation, 6*(5), 831–833.
Suh, H. S., Kim, S. H., Lee, W. H., & Kim, T. S. (2009). *Realistic simulation of transcranial direct current stimulation via 3-D high-resolution finite element analysis: Effect of tissue anisotropy.* Paper presented at the 29th annual international conference of the IEEE engineering in medicine and biology society (EMBC), Minneapolis.
Suh, H. S., Lee, W. H., & Kim, T. S. (2012). Influence of anisotropic conductivity in the skull and white matter on transcranial direct current stimulation via an anatomically realistic finite element head model. *Physics in Medicine and Biology, 57*(21), 6961–6980.
Thielscher, A., Antunes, A., & Saturnino, G. B. (2015). Field modeling for transcranial magnetic stimulation: A useful tool to understand the physiological effects of TMS? *Conference Proceedings: Annual International Conference of the IEEE Engineering in Medicine and Biology Society, 2015*, 222–225.
Tofts, P. S. (1990). The distribution of induced currents in magnetic stimulation of the nervous-system. *Physics in Medicine and Biology, 35*(8), 1119–1128.
Truong, D. Q., Huber, M., Xie, X., Datta, A., Rahman, A., Parra, L. C., … Bikson, M. (2014). Clinician accessible tools for GUI computational models of transcranial electrical stimulation: BONSAI and SPHERES. *Brain Stimulation, 7*(4), 521–524.
Truong, D. Q., Magerowski, G., Blackburn, G. L., Bikson, M., & Alonso-Alonso, M. (2013). Computational modeling of transcranial direct current stimulation (tDCS) in obesity: Impact of head fat and dose guidelines. *NeuroImage Clinical, 2*, 759–766.
Turkeltaub, P. E., Benson, J., Hamilton, R. H., Datta, A., Bikson, M., & Coslett, H. B. (2012). Left lateralizing transcranial direct current stimulation improves reading efficiency. *Brain Stimulation, 5*(3), 201–207.
Wagner, T., Eden, U., Rushmore, J., Russo, C. J., Dipietro, L., Fregni, F., … Valero-Cabré, A. (2014a). Impact of brain tissue filtering on neurostimulation fields: A modeling study. *NeuroImage, 85*(Pt 3), 1048–1057.
Wagner, T., Fregni, F., Fecteau, S., Grodzinsky, A., Zahn, M., & Pascual-Leone, A. (2007). Transcranial direct current stimulation: A computer-based human model study. *NeuroImage, 35*(3), 1113–1124.

Wagner, S., Rampersad, S. M., Aydin, U., Vorwerk, J., Oostendorp, T. F., Neuling, T., … Wolters, C. H. (2014b). Investigation of tDCS volume conduction effects in a highly realistic head model. *Journal of Neural Engineering, 11*(1), 016002.

Wiethoff, S., Hamada, M., & Rothwell, J. C. (2014). Variability in response to transcranial direct current stimulation of the motor cortex. *Brain Stimulation, 7*(3), 468–475.

Windhoff, M., Opitz, A., & Thielscher, A. (2013). Electric field calculations in brain stimulation based on finite elements: An optimized processing pipeline for the generation and usage of accurate individual head models. *Human Brain Mapping, 34*(4), 923–935.

Woods, A. J., Antal, A., Bikson, M., Boggio, P. S., Brunoni, A. R., Celnik, P., … Nitsche, M. A. (2016). A technical guide to tDCS, and related non-invasive brain stimulation tools. *Clinical Neurophysiology, 127*(2), 1031–1048.

Chapter 10
Transcranial Direct Current Stimulation Electrodes

Niranjan Khadka, Adam J. Woods, and Marom Bikson

Importance of tDCS Electrodes

Significant contributors to the broad adaption of transcranial direct current stimulation (tDCS) are the portability and ease-of-use along with the tolerability profile of tDCS – adverse events limited to transient cutaneous sensations (e.g. perception of warmth, itching, and tingling) and erythema (Aparício et al. 2016; Bikson et al. 2016; Dundas et al. 2007; Fertonani et al. 2015). Therefore, the design and preparation of tDCS electrodes are central to tolerability, and design increasingly emphasizes ease and robustness of use. Conversely, when established electrode protocols are not followed or poor electrode design used, tDCS can produce unnecessary significant skin irritation and burns (Dundas et al. 2007). Thus, tDCS electrode design is central to understand the proper preparation of stimulation and prevent avoidable adverse events. Given that cutaneous sensation and irritation are the primary risks of tDCS, proper electrode uses and essential care at electrode preparation are vital to enhance tolerability and maximize reproducibility (Dundas et al. 2007; Minhas et al. 2011; Turi et al. 2014). Since sensations also determine effective

N. Khadka
Department of Biomedical Engineering, The City College of New York, CUNY,
City College Center for Discovery and Innovation, New York, NY, USA

A. J. Woods
Center for Cognitive Aging and Memory (CAM), McKnight Brain Institute,
Department of Clinical and Health Psychology, College of Public Health and Health Professions, University of Florida, Gainesville, FL, USA

M. Bikson (✉)
Department of Biomedical Engineering, The City College of New York, New York, NY, USA
e-mail: bikson@ccny.cuny.edu

H. Knotkova et al. (eds.), *Practical Guide to Transcranial Direct Current Stimulation*, https://doi.org/10.1007/978-3-319-95948-1_10

blinding, tDCS electrodes are critical for blinding reliability. Finally, to the extent tDCS electrodes design shaped the current flow through the brain, electrode selection and preparation is critical for the reproducibility of efficacy.

The conventional tDCS electrode configuration utilizes two electrodes – one anode and one cathode – of comparable size (e.g. 5 × 5 cm^2) positioned around the head. However, strategies scaling bipolar electrode size or increasing number of electrodes (using High-Definition electrodes) have been investigated to address concerns about tDCS spatial focality (Galletta et al. 2015; Minhas et al. 2012; Monte-Silva et al. 2010). This chapter does not address the question on montage design to target specific brain regions (instead see Chap. 9) or achieve specific neuromodulation outcomes, but only focus on the fundamental issue of electrode selection and preparation. Background on the design of electrodes is needed to guide users on electrode selection and proper application.

Technically, an "electrode" refers only to the surface of metal or conductive rubber that makes a proper contact with an electrolyte such saline or conductive gel (Merrill et al. 2005). However, in the tDCS literature, an electrode conventionally refers to the totality of entire assembly that includes (1) an actual electrode (metal snaps, pin, pellet, disk, sheet, mesh or conductive rubber); (2) a conductive electrolyte such as the saline, conductive paste, or conductive gel that serves as the contact between the electrode and the skin; (3) a sponge material, if used, has a function of holding a liquid electrolyte in place; (4) any non-conductive mechanical support material either adhesive or non-adhesive (for e.g. rubber straps, headgear, electrode holder/adapter, HD-electrode casing, adhesive layer) used to hold the assembly in place or support its shape; (5) any conductive material supporting electrical connections such as wires or metal snaps that are integrated with the electrode assembly (with some elements like a metal snap connector serving both a mechanical and electrical connection role).

An essential function of the sponge and/or other support materials (such as the HD case) is to prevent direct contact between metal/conductive rubber electrode and skin. The reason is that electrochemical reactions (including changes in pH) occur right at the metal/rubber and electrolyte interface (Merrill et al. 2005) such that a "thick" electrolyte (e.g. realized by a thick sponge, or rigid shape) minimizes these reactions from reaching the skin. Thus, the saline, conductive paste, or conductive gel is used to maintain good contact quality at the skin but also serves as a buffer between the metal/rubber and the skin surface (Minhas et al. 2010). If as result of poor electrode design (e.g. conductive metal/rubber not fully protected from the skin) or preparation (e.g. a metal/rubber electrode pushed through paste) the metal/rubber contacts the skin, these electrochemical changes then directly impact the skin and skin irritation is likely.

An important function of electrodes used in tDCS is to protect the skin from electrochemical reactions occurred at the surface of the metal/rubber. Therefore, all electrodes designed for tDCS include some mechanism to separate the metal/rubber from the skin. As explained in the following sections, this separation can be generally facilitated by:

1. Sponge-electrode: A sponge which is saturated with the electrolyte, typically saline;
2. Self-adhesive electrode or Dry electrode: An electrolyte, typically gel, that itself has sufficient rigidity and which can either include an adhesive (self-adhesive electrode) or does not include an adhesive (dry electrode); or
3. HD electrode: A stiff mechanical support material that contains the electrolyte, typically gel and controls the position of the metal.

These choices between these general design approach also create restrictions on the size of the electrode (e.g. small HD vs large sponge) and how it is applied (e.g. self-adhesive gel or not adhesive with saline).

Sponge-Electrode

This electrode type is the most common electrode design used in conventional tDCS (Fig. 10.1, (Dasilva et al. 2011)), largely due to its apparent simplicity and historical norms – starting with the canonical tDCS studies circa 2000 (Nitsche and Paulus 2000). However, there are significant details in both the optimization of sponge-electrode design and techniques in sponge-electrode preparation (Woods et al. 2016) – especially as in their most basic form, sponge-electrode requires component assembly at every use. Most commonly in current tDCS protocols, a conventional sponge-electrode pad has a skin contact area of either 25 cm^2 or 35 cm^2 with the scalp. For sponge electrodes, selection and positioning of the conductive carbon rubber sheath or metal can be varied. For example, Soterix Medical (EasyPad, Soterix Medical Inc., NY, USA) provides rubber electrode embedded inside a rectangular sponge pocket and uses plastic rivets to hold the rubber in place. In the Neuroconn sponge-electrode (neuroCare, Munich, Germany), the rubber sheath is similarly inserted into a sawn rectangular sponge pocket. In both cases, the rubber electrode is smaller than the outer dimensions of the sponge. In the Amrex-style sponge electrode (Caputron, NY, USA) a metal electrode is placed behind the rectangular sponge, and an insulating rubber encases the metal and sponge, except on the skin contact side. These conductive rubber electrodes typically include a female port which is connected to a male banana clip or pin terminated wire from the stimulator.

There are updated variants on the sponge-electrode design. The conductive rubber may be (semi) permanently embedded into a circular (Sponstim, Neuroelectrics, Spain) or rectangular (EasyPad-2, Soterix Medical Inc., NY, USA) sponge with a male metallic connector attached to the rubber and emerging through the sponge (on the side opposite the skin contact). The male connector can be affixed to a female connector on the head-gear directly. As with other sponge electrodes, the electrodes can be re-used or are single-use – for a single-use, electrodes are further available as pre-saturated so requiring no preparation (Soterix EasyPad-2). A recent innovation is a more rigid sponge with bristles that enhances preparation through hairs and uses

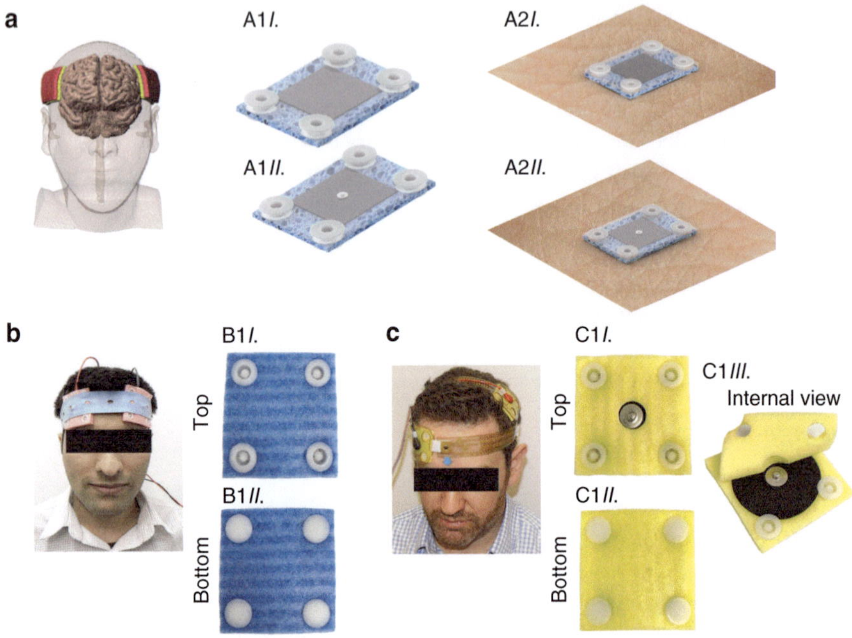

Fig. 10.1 The architecture of sponge-electrode and its variations. (**a**) An exemplary FEM model of sponge pad positioning over left and right dorsolateral prefrontal cortex (dlPFC) in a head model. (**a1I**, **a1II**) CAD exemplars of sponge assembly variations wherein both variations rubber electrode is placed in between two layers of sponges, except the later has metal snap on top of the rubber (see **c1III**) to facilitate connection with customized headgear (head strap). Both variations of sponges have rivets to minimize edge effects, hence, maximizing tolerability. (**a2I**, **a2II**) shows the computational model of the above- mentioned sponges positioned over the skin surface. (**b**) Bifrontal placement of riveted sponge electrode (as in **a1I**) on a subject forehead. (**b1I**, **b1II**) Images of actual sponge electrode (5 × 5 cm) as used in **b1**. (**c**) illustrates the positioning of updated snap-in sponge-electrode assembly on a fixed montage specific headgear, in this case, M1-SO. (**c1I**, **c1II**) depict different views of the snap-in sponge electrodes (5 × 5 cm) as in **A1II**. The shape of the rubber electrode doesn't influence the total current delivery to the brain region. (**c1III**) illustrates an internal view of the snap-in sponge electrode where the circular rubber electrode is placed exactly at the center of the sponge pad

sponge material embedded with salt in a manner that only water can be added over multiple uses (Halo Neuroscience, San Francisco, CA). Along with new types of associated head-gear (e.g. home-use; (Kasschau et al. 2015)) and connectors (e.g. magnetic), these examples illustrate that even with the conventional sponge-electrode paradigm, there is an ongoing innovation often focused on ease-of-use (e.g. pre-assembled and saturated) or reliability (e.g. sponge shape).

Sponge electrodes are intended to increase the contact quality even in the areas of the scalp with thick hairs because the electrolyte (saline) may penetrate under the hair and saturate the skin surface. Theoretically, the saturation of skin may also reduce inhomogeneity in current flow through the skin (Kronberg and Bikson,

2012). In some designs, where the sponges are readily accessible during the treatment session, sponge hydration must be carried out with care: oversaturated sponges with saline has indicted changes in impendence or reported tolerability (Woods et al. 2016). Some disadvantages of using sponges are that sponge is prone to leaking which distorts the "effective" electrode size making stimulation not reproducible – for this reason the volume of saline added to the sponges should be carefully calibrated (to the sponge model, size, and application) and a cap (e.g. neoprene) may be avoided since both obscure and support fluid spread.

Sponge electrode of various sizes have been used for tDCS (including 3 × 3, 5 × 5, 5 × 7, 10 × 10 cm) but smaller sizes are not practical or necessarily tolerated (but see HD electrodes). Neither changing sponge-skin contact shape from square to circular (Ambrus et al. 2011; Minhas et al. 2011) nor changing sponges-skin contact size within the conventional range (with larger electrode potentially producing slightly *more* irritation (Turi et al. 2013)) had significant effect on tolerability (Aparício et al. 2016; Fertonani et al. 2015). Potentially, more important than electrode-skin contact area/shape is the electrode design, such as material thickness and use of rivets (Kronberg and Bikson 2012) and electrolyte salinity (Dundas et al. 2007). However, changes in electrode shape and size (Nitsche et al. 2007), and even design (Opitz et al. 2015), may influence brain current flow even in the absence of significant changes in reported tolerability. Sponge electrode requires a head-gear to hold them in place (but see self-adhesive electrodes). In general, sponge-electrodes are easy to set up preferred by many researchers and clinicians worldwide (Fig. 10.1).

Self-Adhesive Electrode

Relatively uncommon but of interest for wearable technologies, self-adhesive electrodes adhere to the skin surface and require minimal preparation – making them easiest to use at a location without significant hair (Paneri et al. 2016). The bottom of the electrode has a layer of conductive hydrogel along with an adhesive material, over this layer is a conductive wire, rubber or metal, and over either of them is a layer of insulation (see Fig. 10.2d2). The metal may be connected to a short cable with a female pin connection and the cable from the stimulator can be connected to this female pin or the metal may be connected to a snap connector that protrudes through the insulation layer. Adhesive electrodes have been used in a limited number of tDCS trials (Paneri et al. 2016) but are common in other applications where pulses and AC stimulation are used such as cranial nerve electrical stimulation (Feusner et al. 2012). Although self-adhesive electrodes are easy to apply, their use is limited as they are not practical for stimulating areas of the head with hairs. Moreover, while they are many brands and designs of self-adhesive electrodes, most are not suitable for direct current stimulation and may produce skin lesions.

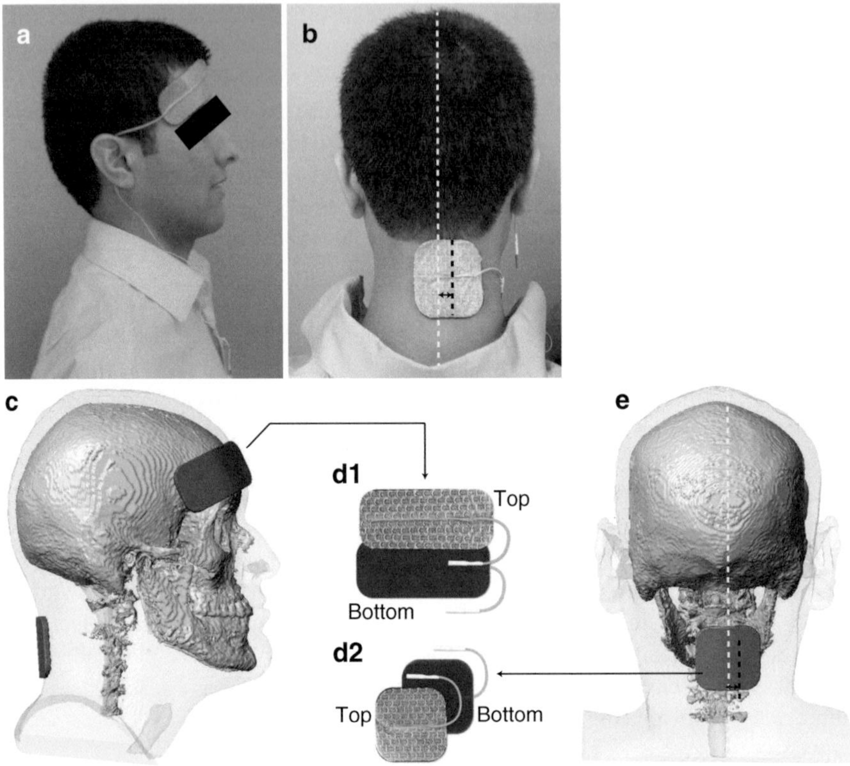

Fig. 10.2 Illustration of adhesive hydrogel electrode (left and right). (**a**) Placement of rectangular anode on the subject's right temples. (**b**) A square cathode electrode positioned about 1 cm to the right of the subject's midline on the back of the neck. (**c**, **e**) representation of analogous electrode positioning as A and B on a realistic head model. (**d1, d2**) An actual image of the anode and cathode adhesive electrode. The bottom of the electrode has an adhesive hydrogel to enhance adherence with the skin whereas, at the top, there is a mesh of fabric used to hold the conductive in place

High Definition Electrode (HD-Electrode)

High definition (HD) electrodes are another variant of the tDCS electrode assembly with a skin contact area of fewer than 5 cm^2. The HD electrode includes a cup that sits on the skin and determines the skin contact area. The cup is filled with conductive gel or paste (Minhas et al. 2010). Suspended inside the gel is a metal ring, disk or pellet made from Ag/AgCl. The gel and metal are thus positioned by the interior dimensions of HD cup. The design of the HD cup controls the important factors of gel contact area with the skin and the distance between the metal and the skin (Fig. 10.3). As with conventional tDCS using sponge electrodes, there are different montages of HD-tDCS but HD electrodes, by the virtue of being smaller, can be deployed in significantly higher number and/or precision of placement (Borckardt et al. 2012; Dmochowski et al. 2011; Kuo et al. 2013). A common HD montage is the

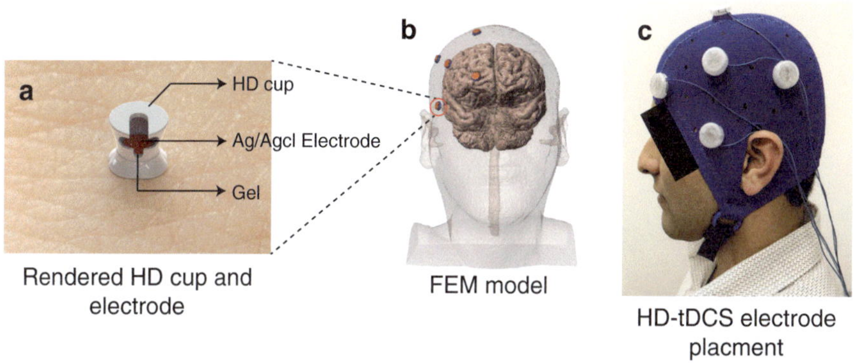

Fig. 10.3 Positioning of high definition (HD) electrode on a head model. (**a**) HD-cup with an electrode submerged in a conductive gel. (**b**) 4 × 1-ring configuration of electrode placement where four cathode electrodes are positioned around a central anode. (**c**) Illustration of HD-electrode assembly on a subject head. Electrodes are secured in a 4 × 1 configuration using a specialized head cap that follows EEG standard electrode position nomenclature

4 × 1-ring montage where a ring/circular fashion using four "return" (cathode) disk electrodes arranged around an "active" (anode) electrode at the center (Datta et al. 2009; Alam et al. 2016; Shen et al. 2016; Hill et al. 2017). The active electrode is positioned over the scalp (coinciding with the center of the active tDCS sponge pad) and surrounded by four return electrodes: each at a disk distance (from center to center of the disk) of ~3 cm from the active electrode). The HD electrodes are held in place using a cap headgear and a conductive electrolytic gel is filled into the electrode holders. Note that in contrast to sponge-electrodes, here a cap does not introduce issues related to electrolyte spread since the gel is well confined by the HD cup (Fig. 10.3).

Electrode Preparation

The preparation and placement of tDCS electrodes remain the most critical and hence prone-to-error step in tDCS (Dasilva et al. 2011). Materials required for conventional tDCS (Fig. 10.4) are simple but the safety and tolerability of the treatment require the administrator to firmly follow standard protocols.

Monitoring of electrode resistance before and during tDCS is considered important for tolerability (Dasilva et al. 2011; Khadka et al. 2015a) where an unusually high electrode resistance is indicative of undesired electrochemical changes and/or poor skin contact conditions. However, monitoring of electrode impedance in no way reduces the need and importance of proper electrode selection and set-up- in the sense that poor electrodes conditions may be associated with a low resistance and, conversely, in some cases (e.g. subjects with high resistance scalp) good contact may be associated with a moderately high resistance. Skin irritation and discomfort may

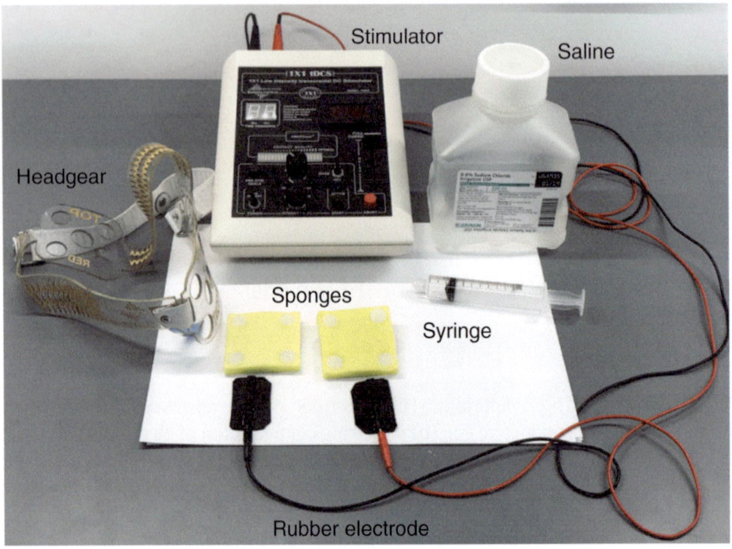

Fig. 10.4 Lists of material used for conventional tDCS sessions with sponge electrodes. Generally, conventional sponges are soaked with saline using a syringe and the rubber electrodes are placed inside the sponge pockets. Sponge-electrodes are then secured over the brain target using customized headgear or head-strap. Finally, the rubber electrodes are energized using corresponding anode and cathode wires connected to the stimulator

be associated with high resistance, but not necessarily. Thus, monitoring of resistance is an adjunct tool to detect not only ideal conditions at the electrode-skin interface but also a substitute for quality electrode design and strict protocol adherence (Khadka et al. 2015a; Woods et al. 2016).

As noted, direct poor contact between the metal or conductive rubber electrode (site for electrochemical reaction) and the skin can trigger skin irritation (Merrill et al. 2005). Hence, sufficient electrolytic gel, cream or saline should be used as a buffer in between. However, oversaturation of saline in the sponge-electrode is a concern. Oversaturated sponges will be leaky and can impact the reproducibility of the treatment. Sufficiently, saturated sponges maintain good contact quality between the electrode and enhance the tolerability of the treatment. Since the saline soaked sponges are exposed to the ambient room temperature and are in contact with the human body surface (convection), saline will evaporate, and dehydration will be an issue. Therefore, it is imperative to obtain good contact quality directly under the electrode while maintaining an adequate saline saturation at the sponge-electrode. For sponge-electrodes, simple methods of quantifying saline saturation (e.g. use of medical grade syringes to dispense saline) can assist in achieving a consistent and appropriate amount of contact medium.

Consistent with the issues introduced by oversaturation of sponges, the shape or size of tDCS electrodes significantly alter the distribution of current delivered to the brain (Khadka et al. 2015b; Kronberg and Bikson 2012; Minhas et al. 2011). Variation in the electrode assemblies or particularly electrode size results in differences in the distribution of the current across the surface area of the scalp and to the brain (Kronberg and Bikson 2012; Minhas et al. 2011). Thus, it is critical for investigators to consistently report not only the current intensity applied and the amount of contact medium used but also the shape and size of the electrode assembly.

Inter-individual variation in the head size and shape demands subject-specific headgears or head straps (Bikson et al. 2010). Often elastic straps are used to fasten the conventional saline-soaked tDCS electrodes over the desired location. However, the force applied to secure the electrodes over the skin might induce pressure under the electrode and thus pressure-induced erythema either under or around the edges of the electrode as observed during sham stimulation (Ezquerro et al. 2017). Moreover, excess force can cause leakage of saline from the sponge-electrode causing unnecessary mess or hindrance in current distribution over the scalp and requires frequent hydration of the sponge-electrode.

Electrode Placement

A central consideration for tDCS is determining where to place electrodes on the head (montage). Studies monitoring neuro-physiological changes following tDCS and current flow FEM prediction have demonstrated that the relative location of electrodes result in significant differences in where and how much current is delivered to the brain (Kessler et al. 2013; Minhas et al. 2012; Woods et al. 2015). For example, Nitsche and Paulus (2000) demonstrated that relative differences in electrode locations alter tDCS impacted TMS generated motor-evoked potentials (MEPs). Numerous modeling studies have demonstrated significant differences between relative locations of electrodes, with results varying from stimulation of the whole brain to selective brain targets (Kessler et al. 2013; Minhas et al. 2012; Woods et al. 2015). Hence, even a small variation in electrode location (distance between the anode electrode and the cathode electrode) significantly alters overall distribution of predicted field intensity in the brain. This chapter addresses proper electrode selection and placement, but these issues impact the control and reproducibility of dose (Woods et al. 2015). Generally, the importance of electrode location also highlights yet another critical consideration, preparation of a stable electrode placement on the head.

As head size and shape vary from person to person, it is important to use a method for common localization of electrode position. Few methods/techniques for addressing this issue includes: (1) International 10–20 (or 10–10 or 10–5) Electrode Placement System (Klem et al. 1999; Oostenveld and Praamstra 2001) or another gross anatomical coordinate system (Seibt et al. 2015); (2) neuro-navigation systems (e.g., MRI guided; (Feurra et al. 2011a, b; Santarnecchi et al. 2014); (3) physiology-based placement (e.g., TMS generated MEPs). At present, physiology-based placement can only be performed for motor and other primary cortices (e.g., sensory). However, further options may become available in the future (e.g., TMS-EEG methods). Use of EEG to guide (HD) tDCS electrode placement is investigated (Fernández-Corazza et al. 2016). Any positioning technique should specify the center of each electrode along with electrode orientation. If any special accommodations are made for individual subjects, beyond those already inherent to the positioning technique (e.g. EEG 10-10) dosage must be noted (Kessler et al. 2013). In essence, any positioning method selected must be clearly documented and reproducible allowing the study to be reproduced.

Once desired locations are identified, the electrode assembly must be affixed to the head for delivery of current. Non-conductive headgear used to position the electrodes on the body or scalp (e.g. elastic straps) are critical for appropriate electrode placement (Woods et al. 2016). For tDCS using sponge-electrodes, elastic straps or other head-gear is used to secure electrodes in place during the entire tDCS session. Pressure-induced erythema even during sham stimulation has been previously reported by Ezquerro et al. (2017). Furthermore, if electrode straps are over-tightened, there is an increased probability of saline leakage. Especially with rubber bands (elastic strips) or poorly designed caps, there is a risk with the increasing tightening of drift toward the vertex (Woods et al. 2015). Specific head-gear designs prevent drift and can provide more reliable pressure across subjects and operators (Fig. 10.5).

With conventional rubber straps, various techniques exist to mitigate the above-mentioned issues. For example, the contour at the base of the skull below the inion

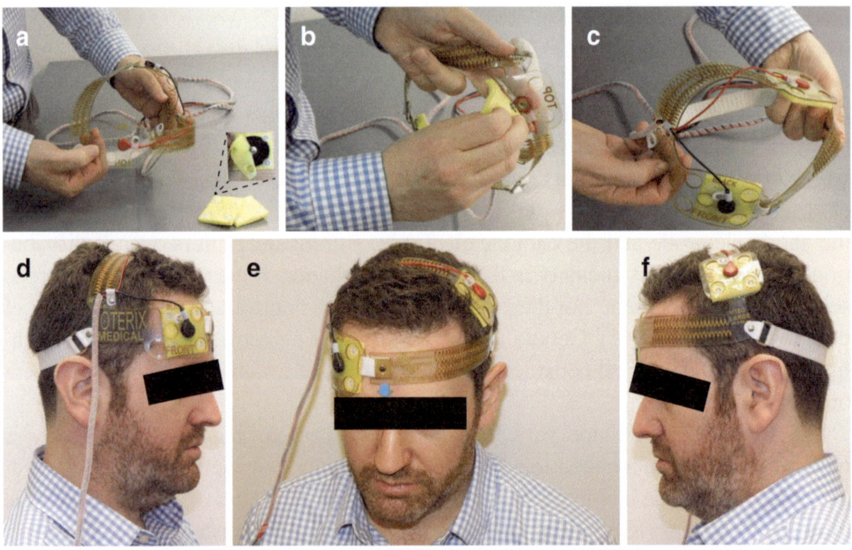

Fig. 10.5 An updated method for electrode placement using fixed position head-gear and pre-saturated snap sponge-electrode. (**a**) Example of a headgear with a build-in anode and cathode snap-in wire terminals at a fixed position (M1-SO montage). (**b**) Pre-saline-soaked sponges with snap connected are affixed to the anode or cathode terminal. (**c**) Complete assembly of sponges-electrode and a headgear. (**d–f**) Different views of head-strap placement on a subject head

and the flat of forehead provide stable placement of a strap around the head. For participants with long hair, placement of the back of the strap under the hairline also improves the stability of the strap preparation, whereas placement over the hair leads to a high probability of upward drift of the strap and the electrodes placed on the head. Use of cross straps over the head should also avoid over-tightening of the cross-strap to avoid this same issue. However, the use of a cross-strap under the chin can counteract this tendency but may be uncomfortable to participants. If under-chin straps are used, these should be used for all participants to maintain consistency of participant experience in the study. In totality, an advancement in the electrode assembly, particularly electrode straps can enhance the reproducibility of tDCS. One exemplar of updated snap-in sponge electrode headgear with a fixed montage (Knotkova et al. 2017) is shown above.

Further Consideration for Electrode Design and Selection

Erythema May Be Important for Blinding But Not Injurious

Skin redness (erythema) during or after tDCS is one of the most evident side-effects in tDCS trials. The causes of tDCS erythema may include but not limited to exposure to saline, iontophoresis, pressure by headgear, and the stimulation current itself. Redness resolves spontaneously after stimulation and is not injurious. Electrode design and thickness, gender, skin type, nature of stimulation (anodal or cathodal), and intensity of stimulation may mediate its strength (Dundas et al. 2007; Guarienti et al. 2014; Guleyupoglu et al. 2014). Recent studies have been conducted to characterize and control tDCS-induced erythema. Brunoni and colleagues previously reported that skin pretreatment with ketoprofen reduces tDCS-induced erythema (Guarienti et al. 2014), although such an approach inconveniently increases the preparation time. Erythema induced during tDCS varies from mild to moderate. Rater based evaluation of erythema can be overestimated which is solely based on visual inspection of the skin. Hence, a novel approach is to use the collected images for estimating a probability heat map on the skin area, which presumably represents the erythema distribution under the electrode. This model also corroborates the investigators' observation of skin redness after sham stimulation which might have occurred for some reasons such as (1) the brief period of active stimulation at the session onset; (2) pressure of the pad, depending on how it is fixed; and (3) irritation of the skin due to the saline solution.

Skin redness (erythema) compared between rater-based and software-based data has demonstrated a very mild erythema occurred after sham stimulation although it was significantly higher after active stimulation, and even higher for the thick compared to thin sponge-electrodes (Fig. 10.6). In the stimulation groups: stimulation using both thin and thick electrode of the same size, erythema was comparable between the groups. Moreover, redness did not concentrate around the pad edges but it was rather diffuse under the electrode (Ezquerro et al. 2017). Assuming that

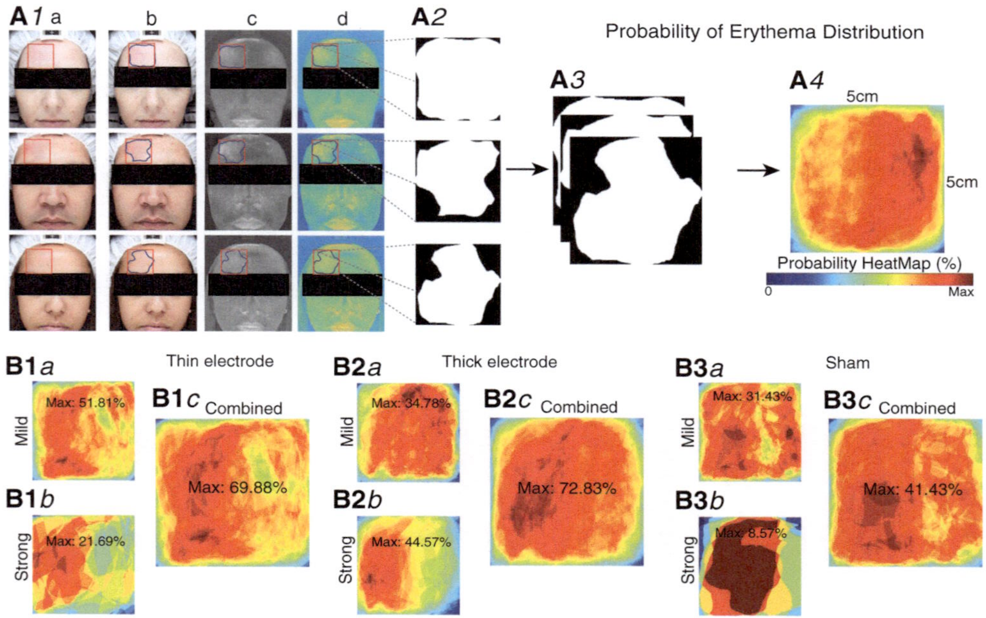

Fig. 10.6 Erythema distribution analysis in the ROI (site of stimulation) for active (using thin and thick sponges) and sham stimulation. (**A1a**) An Illustration of high definition images of the subject photographed before and after the stimulation. (**A1b**) represents ROI and traced erythema distribution. (**A1c**, **A1d**) Representation of filtered Images to isolate erythema from regular skin color tone. (**A2**) illustrates the binary image of erythema traces in the ROI. (**A3**) Illustration of the probability of erythema distribution calculation via stacking equi-dimensional binary images. (**A4**) Probability heatmap of erythema distribution (in percentage) across the ROI. Max represents 100% probability in the color bar. (**B1a**) Graphical illustration of the calculated mild erythema distribution for the "thin" sponge. Mild erythema distribution had a higher probability than strong (**B1b**). The calculated maximum combined probability (B1c) was diffused across the ROI. Strong erythema distribution (**B2b**) was slightly higher than mild (**B2a**) for "thick" sponges. (**B2c**) represents a maximum combined probability of erythema distribution. For sham, mild erythema (**B3a**) had a higher probability than strong erythema (**B3b**). (**B3c**) illustrates the maximum combined probability of erythema distribution. The probability of the erythema distribution in sham compared to the active stimulation sponge types was significantly lower

the electric current causes redness, it seems that current density is fairly homogeneous below the pad, and redness would be caused by an increase in blood perfusion among the tissue. This contrasts with a previous modeling study that showed that a thin sponge would have the current concentrated in the center of the sponge and a thick sponge, on the edges (Wagner et al. 2007). However, that model did not fully capture the inhomogeneity and anisotropy within the skin; for instance, skin/scalp was considered a combined mass of muscle, skin, fat and connective tissues.

The implications of erythema results in informing tDCS trial design should be taken with caution. First, the results can be specific to the headgear (e.g., presuming sham erythema reflects pressure), electrode technologies, electrolyte (gel/saline/cream) used, subject demographics, and waveforms tested. In fact, a prior study has shown dependence on electrode design and skin type. Trial-specific considerations would determine the need and value to mitigate erythema-related sham concerns. At a minimum, researchers should be rigorous in controlling and reporting the relevant headgear and electrode, as well as other factors that could induce erythema. Simple methods to conceal exposed skin areas can be implemented. If appropriate, erythema intensity can be reduced by treating skin with 2% ketoprofen before stimulation (Guarienti et al. 2014). Importantly, a protocol that involves either trained operators or quantified segmentation, with optimal lighting and image capture, and with the targeted intention to identify erythema difference across arms, is something impractical for regular use in tDCS trials. The finding from the respective tDCS erythema study (Ezquerro et al. 2017), therefore, do not necessarily contradict conventional experience in tDCS trials where sham was found effective by operator and subject reports, but rather raise a need for more detailed report of procedures used in future research to conceal stimulation group allocation, since it is now well documented that erythema is an independent factor for breaking investigator blinding in within-subjects design.

Technical Comments on Resistance (Impedance) in tDCS

The simplest way to minimize skin irritation is through limiting current applied (e.g. peak current, total charge per session), use of well-designed electrodes (e.g. designed for tDCS), and following protocols for electrode and skin preparation. None-the-less, none ideal conditions can arise. Subject reporting of sensation, general observation of electrode/skin conditions, and the monitoring of "electrode resistance" during stimulation (Wagner et al. 2007) are the only methods to monitor electrode conditions – and of these, electrode resistance is the only device controlled and objective measures. Electrode resistance is thus, universally relied on tDCS. However, the "electrode resistance" is, in fact, the voltage at the current stimulator output (as the voltage is adjusted to maintain a constant current) divided by the applied current. This voltage reflects many non-linear processes at both electrodes and the tissue (shown as Rt and RE in Fig. 10.7). While valuable in tDCS monitoring, since large excursions in voltage are indicative of non-ideal electrode conditions, this is not a first measure of "skin conditions" nor a measure of single

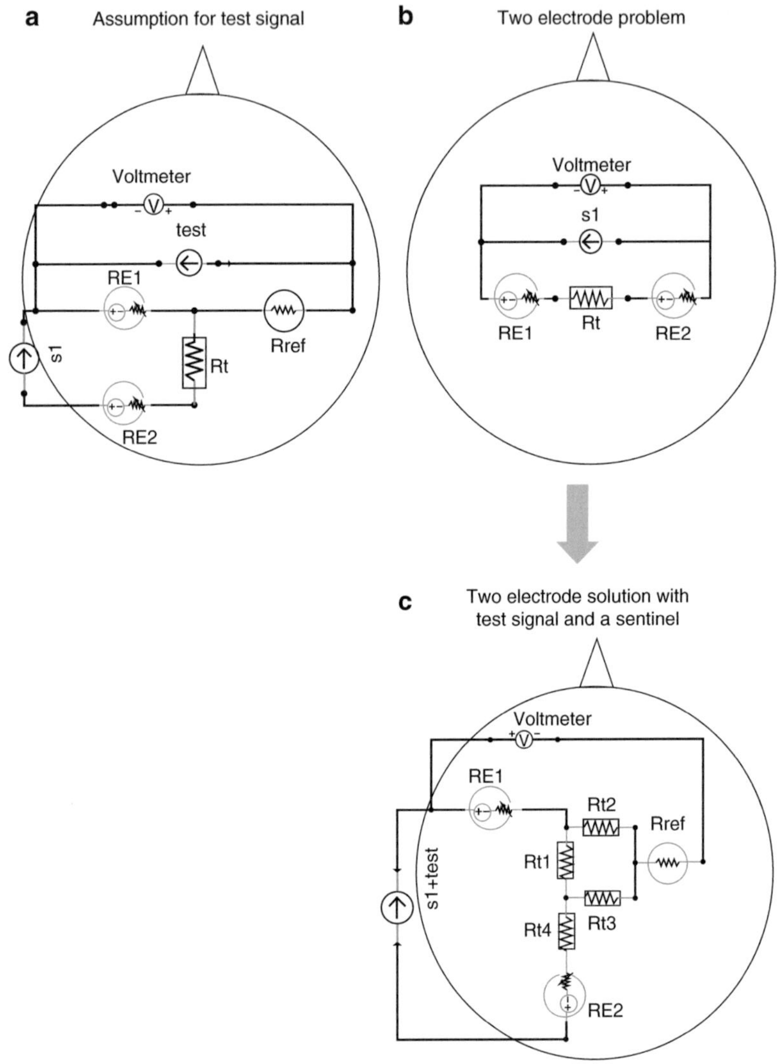

Fig. 10.7 Lumped circuit analysis of tDCS using two electrodes with an additional sentinel electrode (not carry direct current). (**a**) represents an exemplary circuit using a test signal (test) and a sentinel (R_{ref}) to predict DC voltage. This example includes two sources, S1 (DC) and a test AC signal, two active electrodes used for DC simulation: RE1 and RE2, and a sentinel electrode (R_{ref}) to test the assumption that the AC voltage detected across RE1 and R_{ref} can predict the DC voltage (hence, DC-resistance) of RE1. (**b**) Illustrates methodology to detect single electrode resistance changes. The schematic has two electrodes (RE1 & RE2) and a DC source (S1). The resulting voltage across these electrodes is the function of tissue impedance (Rt) and the resistance of both electrodes. (**c**) Presents a solution for the problem indicated in B based on the assumptions outlined in A, where a sentinel electrode (R_{ref}) is used to selectively monitor a stimulating electrode (in this case RE1) of interest. Here, a single source produces a combined direct current with superimposed test AC signal and the sentinel electrode (not used for DC stimulation) is required, but not additional current sources

electrode resistance, or even strictly resistance – since electrode over-potentials contribute as well. Rational development of tDCS can benefit from recognizing the non-triviality of this "electrode resistance" measurement.

Before and after tDCS, measurement of resistance requires the application of a low-intensity test current. Even prior to stimulation, the resistance reported by a device will speak about the properties of the test current used. Minor variations in the waveform of the test current (e.g. pulses vs DC test waveform, 10 vs 20 μA test current) can significantly change the calculated resistance (Hahn et al. 2013). Therefore, the pre/post resistance reported by different tDCS devices, even under exactly identical electrode and skin contact conditions may vary. Since resistance during stimulation is measured under relatively high current (e.g. 1 mA), the pre/post resistance also does not simply predict resistance during stimulation, though a general correlation is expected (e.g. very high pre-resistance is associated with high during resistance). None of this diminishes the value of testing resistance in tDCS, but compounded by the issues discussed next, raises cautions about interpreting resistance values in strictly absolute terms.

A relevant outcome of tDCS is that the passage of current itself across the skin may lower the skin resistance. This means that the effective resistance measured during tDCS is less than before tDCS. This feature can be taken advantage of in a situation where it is desired to limit the voltage (energy) generated by a tDCS device (Hahn et al. 2013). It also has important consequences for blinding. If the active tDCS arm produces a distinct current-dependent change in resistance that is absent in the sham arm, then devices that report resistance to the operator during stimulation are not strictly blinded. However, one does not want to remove resistance reporting since its value is warning of non-optimal conditions. One solution is to replace resistance measured during stimulation with more categorical indicators of resistance (e.g. "Good", "Moderate" or "Poor"), that can further be calibrated to be even across active and sham conditions (Alonzo et al. 2016; Russowsky Brunoni et al. 2015). The source of this resistance drop is likely a decrease in skin impedance (Hahn et al. 2013).

The electrochemical performance of electrodes under DC, as well as tissue, has been addressed elsewhere (Merrill et al. 2005). None-the-less, context is necessary to inform rational design. tDCS is current controlled with the voltage output (total source-voltage) of the stimulator adjusted to maintain a controlled current application. The electrode and tissue have complex non-linear impedances. For example, the impedance may change over time and both electrodes and tissue may generate internal potentials. For electrodes, this is the overpotential from the electrode interface (Minhas et al. 2010) and for tissue, this includes skin potentials (Nitsche and Paulus 2000). How then does this complex system of impedance inform monitoring of "electrode resistance" for tDCS safety? It is accepted that during tDCS, significantly increased voltage (at the current source output), which is associated with increased cell impedance, suggests non-optimal conditions at the electrode or electrode-skin interface. This is biophysically justified since maintaining a low electrode over-potential voltage (Minhas et al. 2010) for a detailed discussion) at the electrodes and high conductivity (e.g. good gel/saline contact with the electrode and skin) are associated with minimized chemical reactions and good contact. These, in turn promote, but do not guarantee, tolerated stimulation. In multiple electrode scenarios, the challenges in measuring single electrode resistance still exist where electrode impedances are confounded through crosstalk. Measurements of "electrode resistance" (as extrapolated from the voltage as one of the current sources) may be misleading such that poor electrode conditions are not detected (false negative) or good electrode conditions as reported as poor (false positive). Thus, individual electrode impedance measurement is valuable for two electrode tDCS, for multi-electrode tDCS it becomes essential (Fig. 10.7).

Isolation of individual electrode resistance has been previously demonstrated, based on tested fundamental assumptions: (1) passage of a low-intensity and low-frequency sinusoid current (test signal) across a tDCS electrode produces a sinusoid voltage across an electrode that predicts the DC voltage across that same electrode. Hence, the sinusoid test impedance should predict the DC impedance of the electrode (Fig. 10.8a1, b1), (2) electrode resistance (for both DC and test signal) is greater than tissue impedance. Rational to this assumption is that poor electrode conditions will result in high electrode resistance and therefore will be detected. High electrode resistance is indicative of poor electrode conditions whereas a low or comparable tissue resistance is not a matter of concern, (3) administration of test current (Fig. 10.7 "test") does not itself confound either tolerability of tDCS or electrode performance (Fig. 10.8a2, b2). This assumption appears to be valid as physiological actions on the skin or peripheral nerves could be resulting from a change in sensation or resistance. Moreover, current densities at the brain are much lower than skin (Dasilva et al. 2011) where changes could not be detected, and experimentally, it has been validated by prior observations (Antal et al. 2008; Nitsche and Paulus 2000) that a low amplitude and frequency test signal as used in this study do not influence brain function (Fig. 10.8).

Fig. 10.8 Demonstration of failures to detect single electrode impedance changes (electrode faults) with specificity and methods to correct (**a1**, **b1**) Type A error and method of correction using a sentinel electrode and test signal in *in vitro*. A constant source (S1) energizes an anode and cathode with 2 mA whereas a second source (S2) delivers a test sinusoidal current (38 μA peak-peak at 10 Hz) across the anode (shared) and a sentinel electrode (not used for direct current). At any instance (in above illustration around 100–120 s of stimulation; **a1**) when the anode electrode becomes faulty – here, intentionally made defective through reduced electrode gel contact area – the voltage/resistance increases across the DC current source and at the time the AC voltage/impedance increases across the second test source. In contrast, when a fault is created at the cathode, DC-resistance across the first source again increases but AC-impedance at the second course is unaffected. (**a2**, **b2**) Type B error and method for correction using a sinusoidal test signal. Two independent sources pass direct current (DC) across independent pairs of electrodes. S1 generates a superimposed test signal (38 μA) on top of a DC (0.5 mA) while S2 generates 2 mA DC. S2 is activated transiently (around 100–150 s) whereas the DC voltage/ resistance across S1 is contaminated by the voltage produced when S2 is energized, the AC voltage/impedance is not affected

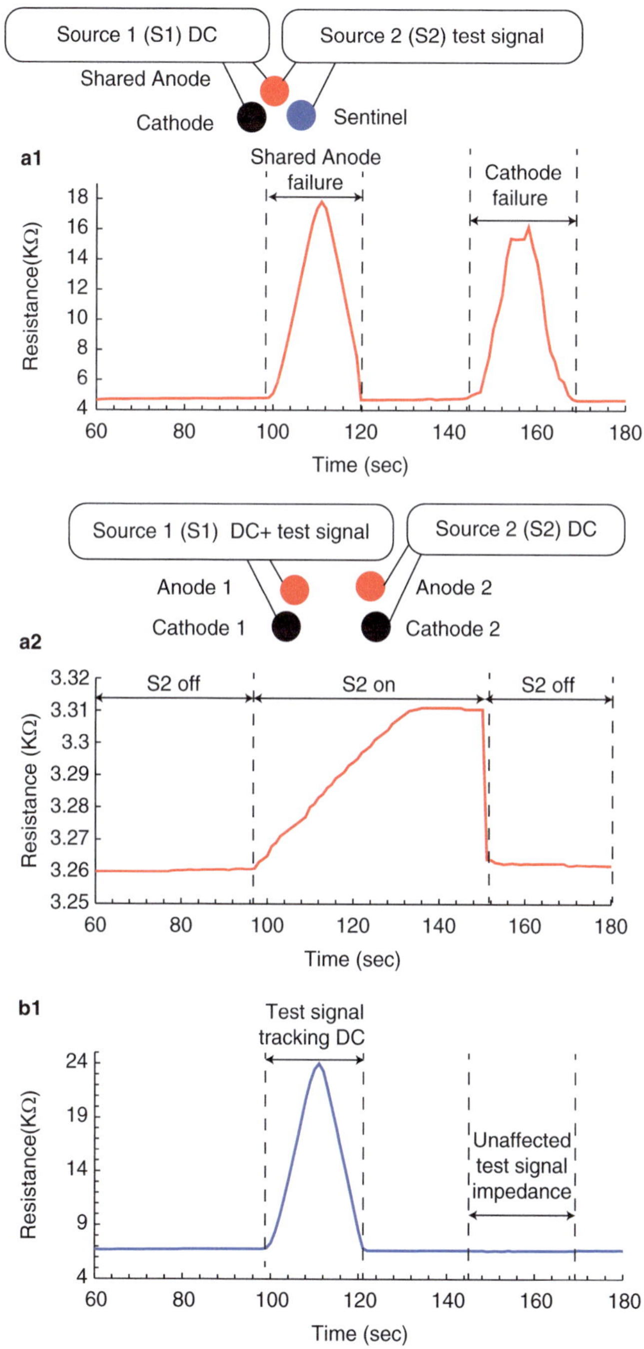
Source 1 (S1) DC
Source 2 (S2) test signal
Shared Anode
Cathode
Sentinel
a1
Shared Anode failure
Cathode failure
Resistance(KΩ)
Time (sec)
Source 1 (S1) DC+ test signal
Source 2 (S2) DC
Anode 1
Cathode 1
Anode 2
Cathode 2
a2
S2 off
S2 on
S2 off
Resistance (KΩ)
Time (sec)
b1
Test signal tracking DC
Unaffected test signal impedance
Resistance(KΩ)
Time (sec)

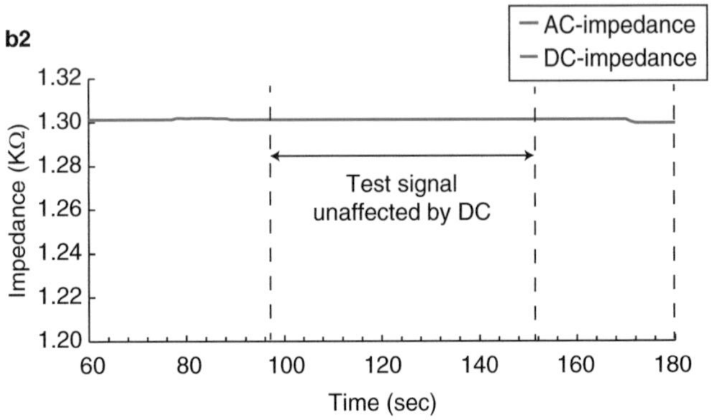

Fig. 10.8 (continued)

Tingling, Itching, and Related Sensations

Tingling is yet another common adverse effect reported in tDCS studies, observed in almost 3 out of 4 subjects (Kessler et al. 2012; Poreisz et al. 2007). Generally, the severity of adverse events is low across all condition (Brunoni et al. 2012), however, the frequency of tingling is significantly higher under thin vs. thick sponge stimulation (88% vs. 64% incidence, respectively) (Minhas et al. 2010). As discussed above, electrode size and salinity of sponge-electrodes may influence sensation (Dundas et al. 2007). In principle, electrode design must be optimized to reduce the frequency and intensity of tingling and related sensations in clinical trials, which enhances blinding effectiveness. For this same reason, studies which have focused on the effectiveness of tDCS blinding technique but provide little attention to the electrode design and preparation techniques (including document operator training), are of limited generalized value. There is a dissociation between erythema and tingling – tingling being higher under thin sponge stimulation than thick electrodes (Ezquerro et al. 2017). A potential reason may be that the thick sponge produces more uniform current density at the skin surface, resulting in evenly diffused erythema distribution and hence, lower tingling sensation.

Heating, No Evidence in tDCS

One of the concerns to be addressed during tDCS is the change in temperature at the skin surface. These changes might be stimulation polarity (anode or cathode) specific, contributed due to passive heating, or due to a change in blood perfusion. Small non-injurious changes in skin temperature during tDCS may influence cutaneous sensation (Lagopoulos and Degabriele 2008) and even influence current flow patterns to the brain (Dasilva et al. 2011; Gholami-Boroujeny et al. 2015). Such changes may also confound blinding of subjects (e.g., a sensation of warmth that is based on real temperature changes) or operators (e.g., in the active case sponges are warmer). Although higher temperature changes may be injurious and contribute to less tolerable treatment, prior experimental and FEM modeling studies have curtailed a role for significant temperature increases during tDCS. Datta et al. (2009) predicted no significant temperature rise at the sponge-electrode and the scalp interface deploying 4 × 1 ring HD-tDCS and conventional tDCS, however, this temperature increase phenomenon was not reported using experimental measures. A recent study conducted by Khadka et al. (2017b) indicated a moderate and non-hazardous increase in temperature (~1 °C) at the skin surface during 2 mA tDCS that was independent of polarity and resulted from stimulation induced blood flow rather than passive heating (Fig. 10.9).

Any electrical stimulation might produce temperature changes; reflecting complex interactions between joule heat due to applied current across the resistive tissue, changes in metabolism (neuronal activation) or perfusion (flare), and heat conduction (Abram et al. 1980; Elwassif et al. 2006). Temperature changes in the body are typically considered insignificant in the efficacy or safety of neuromodulation technologies (Balogun et al. 1996; Cramp et al. 1999). Skin surface temperature changes of 1 °C are none injurious and within normal variation (e.g., due to exercise, environment; (Elwassif et al. 2006; Scudds et al. 1995)). Moreover, as this small increment is, in fact, compensating for a reduction in surface temperature following application of room-temperature sponges, and since the core body temperature of the blood limits perfusion-based heating, this mechanism is not hazardous. Warmth sensation felt under the tDCS electrode can be attributed to electrical nerve activation rather than heating, and any significant skin irritation (that occurs only when standard protocols are not followed) being electrochemical in nature (Minhas et al. 2010). Any warming of sponges observed by subjects or operators touching the electrode surface would reflect passive heating from the body and it is unlikely that the difference between active and sham can be resolved, hence, not a confound to blinding.

Future Electrode Advancement

Within Electrode Current Steering (WECS)

Conventionally, tDCS employs rectangular saline-soaked sponge pads (25–35 cm^2) placed on the scalp, with an internal electrode (carbon rubber electrode) connected to the direct current source. In many cases, impedance measurement across the current source output may fail to recognize any non-uniform conditions at the electrode-skin interface such as an uneven content or saturation. Hence, there is a need to have a technology that enhances the sophistication of electrode design, and further augments tolerability and promote broad use (for e.g., remotely supervised use or in-house use). Within electrode current steering (WECS), a novel method by Khadka et al. (2015b), is distinct from across electrode current steering as developed for implanted devices technology such as deep brain stimulation (DBS), where current is steered between electrodes that are in contact with the deeper brain tissues with the goal of changing desired brain regions that are activated. In WECS, current is adjusted between electrodes, not in contact with tissue but rather embedded in an electrolyte on the body surface (Fig. 10.10a2). The goal here is 'not' to alter brain current flow (Fig. 10.10e), but rather compensate for non-ideal conditions (Fig. 10.10b) at the electrode-skin interface. This technology also leverages methods for independently isolating electrode impedance and over potential during multichannel stimulation (Khadka et al. 2015a). Having presented this novel idea through an exemplary case, WECS supports the need of future studies in the optimization of tDCS electrode design, automation of algorithms to control current (including using impedance measurement), and ultimately validation using experimental measures.

In principle, WECS applies to noninvasive electrical stimulation with two or more electrodes (metal-rivets) embedded in an electrolyte (saline or gel)) on the skin (Poreisz et al. 2007). Each electrode is independently powered by a current source. Success in the implementation of WECS depends on geometry and material of each component of the assembly and an algorithm for current steering between electrodes. Changing the diameter and distance between the electrodes, the distance between the electrodes and skin, or electrolyte conductivity will discriminate how

Fig. 10.9 Skin surface temperature increases under tDCS electrodes during pre-stimulation, stimulation, and post-stimulation phases in the phantom, *in vivo* studies, and FEM simulations. (**a1**) An architecture of a skin model showing three skin layers (epidermis, dermis, and subcutaneous layers) and an electrode positioned on the skin surface. (**a2**) illustrates uniformly seeded current density flow streamlines inside the different skin tissue layers from the top surface of the anode electrode. (**b**) represents an average temperature change in subjects (*in vivo* testing) and phantom (*in vitro* testing) normalized to a temperature at $t = 0$. In the phantom, ΔT was approximately identical across test samples and mode of stimulation, whereas in the subject testing, maximum ΔT was measured under the active electrode (max. under cathode) during stimulation. (**c1**) Analysis of normalized average ΔT in the phantom study ($p < 0.01$). No significant difference in ΔT was found in the control, compared to the anode and the cathode. (**c2**) shows predicted ΔT for the non-stimulation (control) and stimulation cases in the phantom FEM model. Predicted findings indicated no significant effect of stimulation on the phantom. (**d1**) *In vivo* analysis of temperature difference over time within subjects during pre-stimulation, stimulation, and post-stimulation. Red and green asterisks symbolize a statistical significant difference ($p < 0.01$) between anode and control, and cathode and control, respectively. There was a significant difference in ΔT under the anode ($p < 0.01$) and the cathode ($p < 0.01$), compared to the control. Temperature under both anode and cathode gradually increased due to stimulation. (**d2**) FEM representation of the predicted ΔT in the skin model. A maximum ΔT of 1.36 °C was predicted by the computational model during direct current simulation

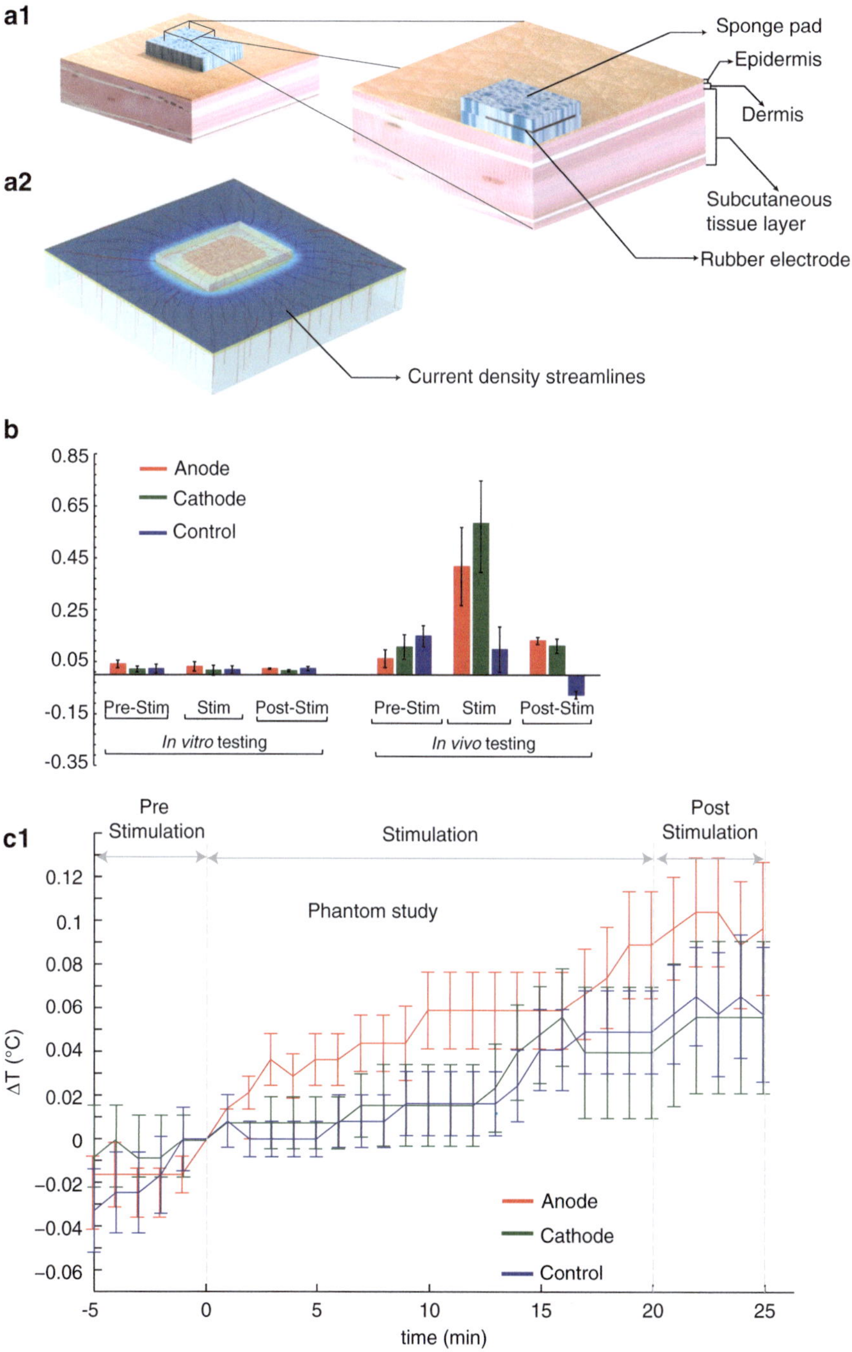
a1
Sponge pad
Epidermis
Dermis
Subcutaneous tissue layer
Rubber electrode
a2
Current density streamlines
b
0.85
0.65
0.45
0.25
0.05
-0.15
-0.35
Anode
Cathode
Control
Pre-Stim
Stim
Post-Stim
In vitro testing
In vivo testing
c1
Pre Stimulation
Stimulation
Post Stimulation
Phantom study
ΔT (°C)
0.12
0.1
0.08
0.06
0.04
0.02
0
−0.02
−0.04
−0.06
-5
5
10
15
20
25
time (min)

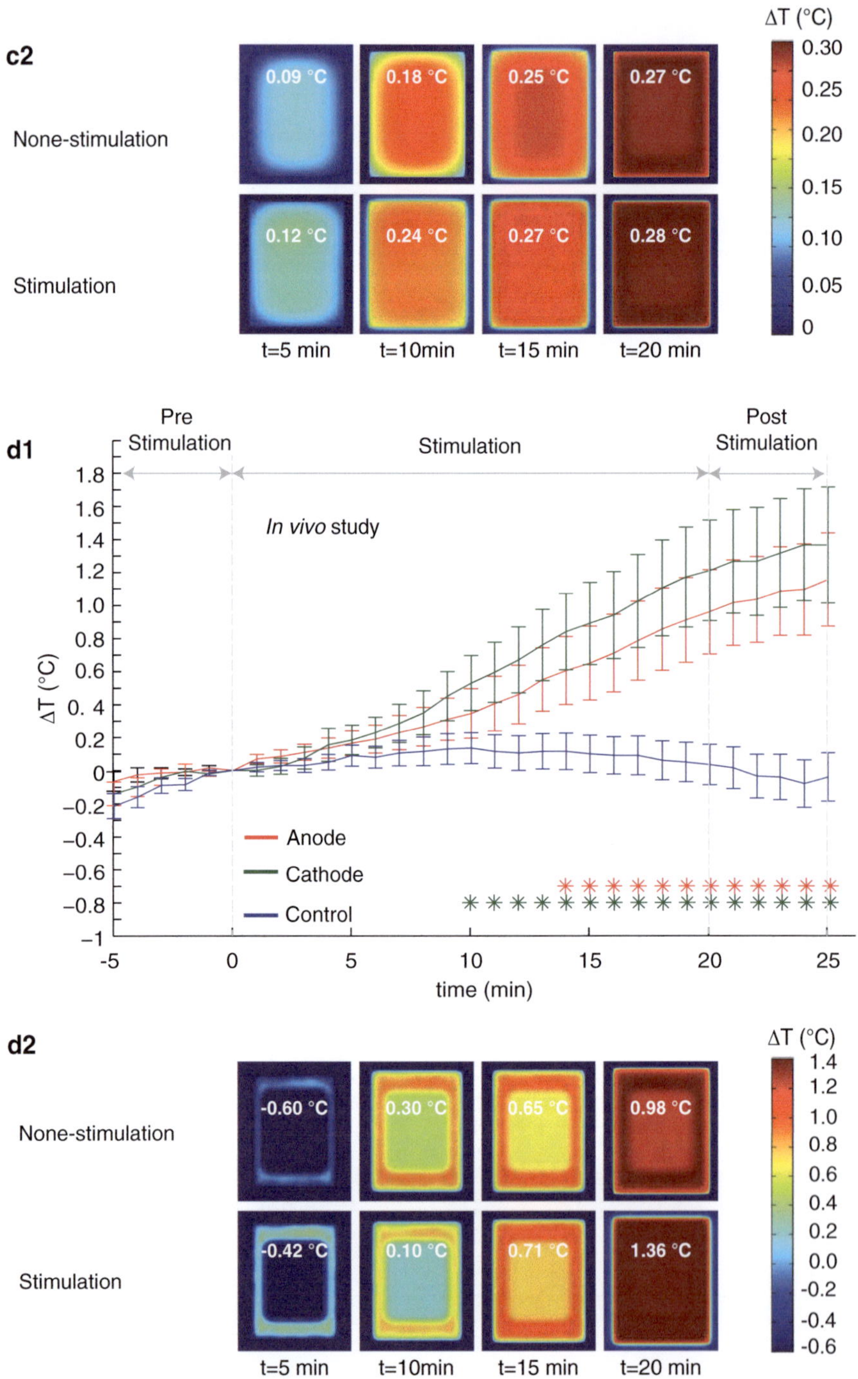

Fig. 10.9 (continued)

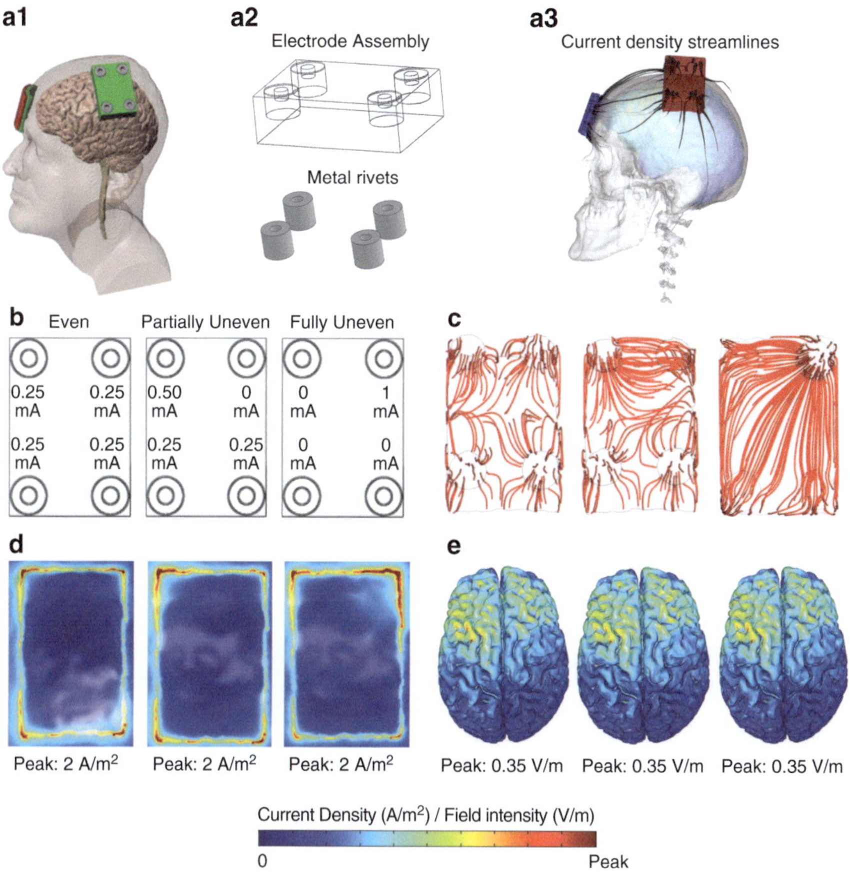

Fig. 10.10 Validation of the underlying assumption of within electrode current steering (WECS) using FEM simulation. (**a1**) represents a realistic head model with an electrode assembly. (**a2**) illustration of an exemplary electrode assembly for WECS. (**a3**) Uniformly seeded current density streamlines originated from within electrodes to the head tissues. (**b**) An "Even", "Partially Uneven", and "Fully Uneven" current administration mode through metal rivets of an electrode assembly keeping total current constant was considered. (**c**) Current flow isolines from each energized metal rivets. (**d**) Predicted current density at the electrode-scalp interface. (**e**) Presents an even electric field distribution in the brain target, even under different current administration conditions

current from the electrode reaches the skin (Kronberg and Bikson 2012), however, the total brain current flow remains unaltered and is independent of electrode configuration (Fig. 10.10e). In WECS technique, an entire electrode assembly receives a fixed total current (intensities vary based on application). Current is evenly divided across the electrodes within the electrode assembly. For example, if an assembly has four electrodes, under an "even" current split of 2 mA, each electrode receives 0.50 mA current (Fig. 10.10b).

WECS can be generalized to other noninvasive electrical stimulation techniques and potentially invasive techniques where an artificial or natural electrolyte barrier

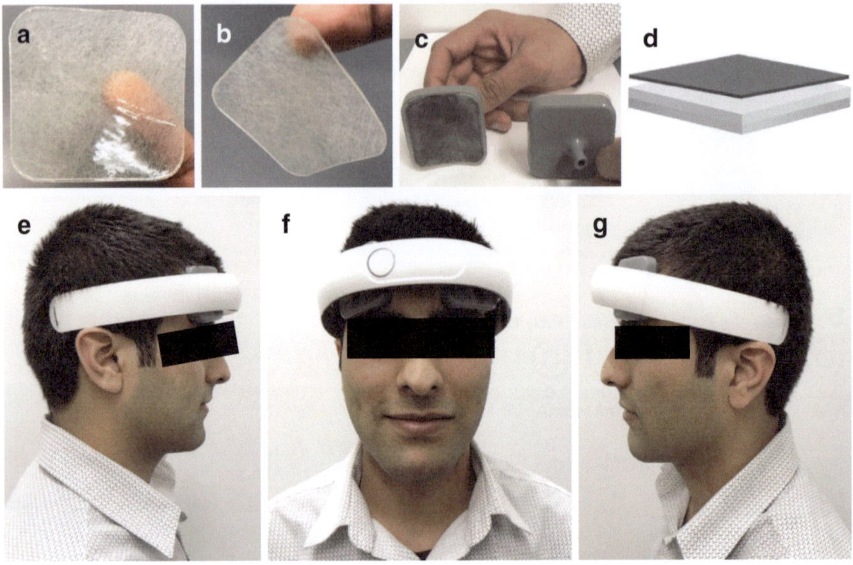

Fig. 10.11 Future electrode advancement in tDCS, multilayer hydrogel composite (MHC) dry electrode. (**a**, **b**) Images of actual MHC dry electrode. (**c**) illustrates placement of the dry electrode over the specialized rubber electrode with the adhesive layer facing the rubber while the non-adhesive layer on the opposite side (skin side). The rubber holder is encapsulated in a flexible insulated holder. (**d**) shows an electrode assembly (CAD model render) – rubber electrode positioned over the MHC electrode. (**e**–**g**) Images of MHC dry electrode secured over the brain region through the specialized headgear (wearable built-in stimulator)

exists between the electrode and the tissue. For invasive techniques, WECS may complement traditional current steering but be used to protect electrode and tissue from injury. A further consideration is how current flow at the skin (scalp) is altered. On the one hand, current steering should avoid significant increases in current density at the skin, maintaining as uniform a current density at the skin as practical. On the other hand, when non-ideal conditions at the electrode or skin arise, including increasingly non-uniform current flow or electrode failure, current steering may be used to compensate. For example, if a given electrode fails and a high overpotential at the electrode is detected, current may be steered to other electrodes to minimize electrochemical hazard (Kessler et al. 2012) or if one region of the sponge becomes dry during use, current may be diverted to the most distant electrodes. Inherent to the above concept is the ability to detect non-ideal conditions and program appropriate corrective measures. The simplest feedback is the voltage at each current source, which using signal processing and "test signals" (superimposed currents not used for neuromodulation) or a "sentinel electrode" (not used for DC) may be used to calculate single electrode impedance (Khadka et al. 2015a). Additional information can be derived by using test signals to isolate the impedance of the sponge/electrolyte between the electrodes, generating a prediction for current density patterns that can be corrected.

Multilayer Hydrogel Composite (MHC) Dry Electrode

Dry electrodes are defined as electrodes that exclude: (1) any saline or other conductive hydrogel based paste or gel, that is prone to leaking; (2) an adhesive at the electrode-skin interface or 3) any electrode preparation steps. The Multilayer Hydrogel Composite (MHC) electrode design fulfills these criteria. A dual layer structure of the MHC dry electrode was adopted by independently optimizing mechanical, electrical, and chemical properties of each layer to get some novel characteristics. First, in order to attain a dry surface, a non-adhesive bio-compatible polymer hydrogel containing Poly-Vinyl Alcohol (PVA) was used as a bottom surface layer (thickness 1 mm) and an adhesive polymer hydrogel was used in an inner layer (top layer, thickness 0.6 mm) (Fig. 10.11). The top layer was optimized to have a low impedance to redistribute the current within the electrode, whereas the bottom layer was optimized to have a high impedance to avoid current clustering at the skin defect sites. Further pH changes at the non-ionic/ionic conduction interfaces within the electrodes were optimized by using the top layer as a diffusion barrier and the rubber electrode/top layer interface was designed to avoid skin surface exposure.

Preliminary analysis of the performance of this MHC electrode using experimental measures on skin-phantom and FEM predictions has shown a comparable voltage and current/current density distribution under the MHC dry electrode when compared to the state-of-the-art conventional sponge-electrode, however, the FEM model of the former predicted more homogeneous current density distribution at the electrode-skin interface. tDCS using MHC dry electrode and conventional sponge-electrode was equally tolerated with comparable VAS ratings and adverse event reporting (Khadka et al. 2017a). In general, this study reveals a potential alternative of saline-soaked sponge-electrode in wearable devices with comparable performance.

Summary

Electrodes represent a critical component of tDCS application. In this chapter, we have described technical and practical considerations for electrode preparation, design, and application. While, at present, sponge-covered electrodes and Ag/AgCl electrodes are the most commonly applied variety, this too will change with material science and engineering advances. We also described the state-of-the-art work in this domain as well as appropriate practices for the common electrode types. Regardless of an electrode type, careful consideration must be given in preparation and application procedures to maximize safety and reproducibility. Common mistakes in electrode preparation and placement can significantly alter outcomes and in the worst cases (e.g., over-saturation leading to the distribution of saline beyond the electrode, bridging of electrodes, etc.) interfere with the ability to deliver tDCS that penetrates the skull. However, appropriate use of electrodes can provide safe and effective delivery of tDCS in a variety of study designs and application settings.

References

Abram, S. E., Asiddao, C. B., & Reynolds, A. C. (1980). Increased skin temperature during transcutaneous electrical stimulation. *Anesthesia and Analgesia, 59*, 22–25.

Alam, M., Truong, D. Q., Khadka, N., & Bikson, M. (2016). Spatial and polarity precision of concentric high-definition transcranial direct current stimulation (HD-tDCS). *Physics in Medicine and Biology, 61*, 4506–4521.

Alonzo, A., Aaronson, S., Bikson, M., Husain, M., Lisanby, S., Martin, D., … Loo, C. (2016). Study design and methodology for a multicentre, randomised controlled trial of transcranial direct current stimulation as a treatment for unipolar and bipolar depression. *Contemporary Clinical Trials, 51*, 65–71.

Ambrus, G. G., Antal, A., & Paulus, W. (2011). Comparing cutaneous perception induced by electrical stimulation using rectangular and round shaped electrodes. *Clinical Neurophysiology, 122*, 803–807.

Antal, A., Boros, K., Poreisz, C., Chaieb, L., Terney, D., & Paulus, W. (2008). Comparatively weak after-effects of transcranial alternating current stimulation (tACS) on cortical excitability in humans. *Brain Stimulation, 1*, 97–105.

Aparício, L. V. M., Guarienti, F., Razza, L. B., Carvalho, A. F., Fregni, F., & Brunoni, A. R. (2016). A systematic review on the acceptability and tolerability of transcranial direct current stimulation treatment in neuropsychiatry trials. *Brain Stimulation, 9*, 671–681.

Balogun, J. A., Tang, S., He, Y., Hsieh, J. M., & Katz, J. S. (1996). Effects of high-voltage galvanic stimulation of ST36 and ST37 acupuncture points on peripheral blood flow and skin temperature. *Disability and Rehabilitation, 18*, 523–528.

Bikson, M., Datta, A., Rahman, A., & Scaturro, J. (2010). Electrode montages for tDCS and weak transcranial electrical stimulation: Role of "return" electrode's position and size. *Clinical Neurophysiology, 121*, 1976–1978.

Bikson, M., Grossman, P., Thomas, C., Zannou, A. L., Jiang, J., Adnan, T., … Woods, A. J. (2016). Safety of transcranial direct current stimulation: Evidence based update 2016. *Brain Stimulation, 9*, 641–661.

Borckardt, J. J., Bikson, M., Frohman, H., Reeves, S. T., Datta, A., Bansal, V., … George, M. S. (2012). A pilot study of the tolerability and effects of high-definition transcranial direct current stimulation (HD-tDCS) on pain perception. *The Journal of Pain, 13*, 112–120.

Brunoni, A. R., Nitsche, M. A., Bolognini, N., Bikson, M., Wagner, T., Merabet, L., … Fregni, F. (2012). Clinical research with transcranial direct current stimulation (tDCS): Challenges and future directions. *Brain Stimulation, 5*, 175–195.

Cramp, A. F., Gilsenan, C., Lowe, A. S., & Walsh, D. M. (1999). The effect of high- and low-frequency transcutaneous electrical nerve stimulation upon cutaneous blood flow and skin temperature in healthy subjects. *Clinical Physiology, 20*, 150–157. doi: cph240 [pii].

Dasilva, A. F., Volz, M. S., Bikson, M., & Fregni, F. (2011). Electrode positioning and montage in transcranial direct current stimulation. *Journal of Visualized Experiments*, e2744.

Datta, A., Elwassif, M., Bikson, M. (2009). Bio-heat transfer model of transcranial DC stimulation: Comparison of conventional pad versus ring electrode. *Annual International Conference of the IEEE Engineering in Medicine and Biology Society, 2009. EMBC 2009*, 2009, pp. 670–673.

Dmochowski, J. P., Datta, A., Bikson, M., Su, Y., & Parra, L. C. (2011). Optimized multi-electrode stimulation increases focality and intensity at target. *Journal of Neural Engineering, 8*, 46011.

Dundas, J. E., Thickbroom, G. W., & Mastaglia, F. L. (2007). Perception of comfort during transcranial DC stimulation: Effect of NaCl solution concentration applied to sponge electrodes. *Clinical Neurophysiology, 118*, 1166–1170.

Elwassif, M. M., Kong, Q., Vazquez, M., & Bikson, M. (2006). Bio-heat transfer model of deep brain stimulation-induced temperature changes. *Journal of Neural Engineering, 3*, 306–315.

Ezquerro, F., Moffa, A. H., Bikson, M., Khadka, N., Aparicio, L. V., de Sampaio-Junior, B., … AR, B. (2017). The influence of skin redness on blinding in transcranial direct current stimulation studies: A crossover trial. *Neuromodulation, 20*, 248–255.

Fernández-Corazza, M., Turovets, S., Luu, P., Anderson, E., & Tucker, D. (2016). Transcranial electrical neuromodulation based on the reciprocity principle. *Frontiers in Psychiatry, 7.*

Fertonani, A., Ferrari, C., & Miniussi, C. (2015). What do you feel if I apply transcranial electric stimulation? Safety, sensations and secondary induced effects. *Clinical Neurophysiology, 126*, 2181–2188.

Feurra, M., Bianco, G., Santarnecchi, E., Del Testa, M., Rossi, A., & Rossi, S. (2011a). Frequency-dependent tuning of the human motor system induced by transcranial oscillatory potentials. *The Journal of Neuroscience, 31*, 12165–12170.

Feurra, M., Paulus, W., Walsh, V., & Kanai, R. (2011b). Frequency specific modulation of human somatosensory cortex. *Frontiers in Psychology, 2*, 13.

Feusner, J. D., Madsen, S., Moody, T. D., Bohon, C., Hembacher, E., Bookheimer, S. Y., & Bystritsky, A. (2012). Effects of cranial electrotherapy stimulation on resting state brain activity. *Brain and Behavior: A Cognitive Neuroscience Perspective, 2*, 211–220.

Galletta, E. E., Cancelli, A., Cottone, C., Simonelli, I., Tecchio, F., Bikson, M., & Marangolo, P. (2015). Use of computational modeling to inform tDCS electrode montages for the promotion of language recovery in post-stroke aphasia. *Brain Stimulation, 8*, 1108–1115.

Gholami-Boroujeny, S., Mekonnen, A., Batkin, I., & Bolic, M. (2015). Theoretical analysis of the effect of temperature on current delivery to the brain during tDCS. *Brain Stimulation, 8*, 509–514.

Guarienti, F., Caumo, W., Shiozawa, P., Cordeiro, Q., Boggio, P. S., Benseñor, I. M., … Brunoni, A. R. (2014). Reducing transcranial direct current stimulation-induced erythema with skin pretreatment: Considerations for sham-controlled clinical trials. *Neuromodulation, 18*, 261–265.

Guleyupoglu, B., Febles, N., Minhas, P., Hahn, C., & Bikson, M. (2014). Reduced discomfort during high-definition transcutaneous stimulation using 6% benzocaine. *Frontiers in Neuroengineering, 7*, 28.

Hahn, C., Rice, J., Macuff, S., Minhas, P., Rahman, A., & Bikson, M. (2013). Methods for extra-low voltage transcranial direct current stimulation: Current and time dependent impedance decreases. *Clinical Neurophysiology, 124*, 551–556.

Hill, A. T., Rogasch, N. C., Fitzgerald, P. B., & Hoy, K. E. (2017). Effects of prefrontal bipolar and high-definition transcranial direct current stimulation on cortical reactivity and working memory in healthy adults. *NeuroImage, 152*, 142–157.

Kasschau, M., Sherman, K., Haider, L., Frontario, A., Shaw, M., Datta, A., … Charvet, L. (2015). A protocol for the use of remotely-supervised transcranial direct current stimulation (tDCS) in multiple sclerosis (MS). *Journal of Visualized Experiments*. (106):e53542. .

Kessler, S. K., Minhas, P., Woods, A. J., Rosen, A., Gorman, C., & Bikson, M. (2013). Dosage considerations for transcranial direct current stimulation in children: A computational modeling study. *PLoS One, 8*, e76112.

Kessler, S. K., Turkeltaub, P. E., Benson, J. G., & Hamilton, R. H. (2012). Differences in the experience of active and sham transcranial direct current stimulation. *Brain Stimulation, 5*, 155–162.

Khadka, N., Borges, H., Paneri, B., Boateng, A., Jang, J., Kim, B., … Bikson, M. (2017a). Dry electrodes for transcranial direct current stimulation (tDCS). *Brain Stimulation, 10*, e32.

Khadka, N., Rahman, A., Sarantos, C., Truong, D. Q., & Bikson, M. (2015a). Methods for specific electrode resistance measurement during transcranial direct current stimulation. *Brain Stimulation, 8*, 150–159.

Khadka, N., Truong, D. Q., & Bikson, M. (2015b). Principles of within electrode current steering. *Journal of Medicine Devices, 9*, 020947–020947-2.

Khadka, N., Zannou, A. L., Zunara, F., Truong, D. Q., Dmochowski, J., & Bikson, M. (2017b). Minimal heating at the skin surface during transcranial direct current stimulation. *Neuromodulation Technol Neural Interface*.

Klem, G. H., Lüders, H. O., Jasper, H. H., & Elger, C. (1999). The ten-twenty electrode system of the international federation. The International Federation of Clinical Neurophysiology. *Electroencephalography and Clinical Neurophysiology Supplement, 52*, 3–6.

Knotkova, H., Riggs, A., Patel, V., Truong, D., Arce, D., Bernstein, H., … Bikson, M. (2017). Proceedings #24. A novel approach to determining M1 tDCS montage without Neuronavigational measurements, suitable for patients in home settings. *Brain Stimulation, 10*, e78–e80.

Kronberg, G., & Bikson, M. (2012). Electrode assembly design for transcranial direct current stimulation: A FEM modeling study. *Conference Proceedings of Annual Intenational Conference on IEEE Engineering Medicine and Biology Society. IEEE Engineering in Medicine and Biology Society. Annual Conference, 2012*, 891–895.

Kuo, H. I., Bikson, M., Datta, A., Minhas, P., Paulus, W., Kuo, M. F., & Nitsche, M. A. (2013). Comparing cortical plasticity induced by conventional and high-definition 4 ?? 1 ring tDCS: A neurophysiological study. *Brain Stimulation, 6*, 644–648.

Lagopoulos, J., & Degabriele, R. (2008). Feeling the heat: The electrode–skin interface during DCS. *Acta Neuropsychiatrica, 20*, 98–100.

Merrill, D. R., Bikson, M., & Jefferys, J. G. R. (2005). Electrical stimulation of excitable tissue: Design of efficacious and safe protocols. *Journal of Neuroscience Methods, 141*, 171–198.

Minhas, P., Bansal, V., Patel, J., Ho, J. S., Diaz, J., Datta, A., & Bikson, M. (2010). Electrodes for high-definition transcutaneous DC stimulation for applications in drug delivery and electrotherapy, including tDCS. *Journal of Neuroscience Methods, 190*, 188–197.

Minhas, P., Bikson, M., Woods, A. J., Rosen, A. R., & Kessler, S. K. (2012). Transcranial direct current stimulation in pediatric brain: A computational modeling study. *Conference Proceedings: Annual International Conference of the IEEE Engineering in Medicine and Biology Society, 2012*, 859–862.

Minhas, P., Datta, A., & Bikson, M. (2011). Cutaneous perception during tDCS: Role of electrode shape and sponge salinity. *Clinical Neurophysiology, 122*, 637–638.

Monte-Silva, K., Kuo, M.-F., Liebetanz, D., Paulus, W., & Nitsche, M. A. (2010). Shaping the optimal repetition interval for cathodal transcranial direct current stimulation (tDCS). *J Neurophysiol, 103*, 1735–1740.

Nitsche, M. A., Doemkes, S., Karaköse, T., Antal, A., Liebetanz, D., Lang, N., … Paulus, W. (2007). Shaping the effects of transcranial direct current stimulation of the human motor cortex. *Journal of Neurophysiology, 97*, 3109–3117.

Nitsche, M. A., & Paulus, W. (2000). Excitability changes induced in the human motor cortex by weak transcranial direct current stimulation. *The Journal of Physiology, 527*(Pt 3), 633–639. doi: PHY_1055 [pii].

Oostenveld, R., & Praamstra, P. (2001). The five percent electrode system for high-resolution EEG and ERP measurements. *Clinical Neurophysiology, 112*, 713–719.

Opitz, A., Paulus, W., Will, S., Antunes, A., & Thielscher, A. (2015). Determinants of the electric field during transcranial direct current stimulation. *NeuroImage, 109*, 140–150.

Paneri, B., Adair, D., Thomas, C., Khadka, N., Patel, V., Tyler, W. J., … Bikson, M. (2016). Tolerability of repeated application of transcranial electrical stimulation with limited outputs to healthy subjects. *Brain Stimulation, 9*, 740–754.

Poreisz, C., Boros, K., Antal, A., & Paulus, W. (2007). Safety aspects of transcranial direct current stimulation concerning healthy subjects and patients. *Brain Research Bulletin, 72*, 208–214.

Russowsky Brunoni, A. I., Sampaio-Junior, B. I., Henrique Moffa, A., III, Borrione, L., Nogueira, B. S., Aparício, L. V., … Benseñor, I. M. (2015). The escitalopram versus electric current therapy for treating depression clinical study (ELECT-TDCS): Rationale and study design of a non-inferiority, triple-arm, placebo-controlled clinical trial. *São Paulo Medical Journal, 133*, 252–263.

Santarnecchi, E., Feurra, M., Barneschi, F., Acampa, M., Bianco, G., Cioncoloni, D., ... Rossi, S. (2014). Time course of corticospinal excitability and autonomic function interplay during and following monopolar tDCS. *Frontiers in Psychiatry, 5*, 86.

Scudds, R. J., Helewa, A., & Scudds, R. A. (1995). The effects of transcutaneous electrical nerve stimulation on skin temperature in asymptomatic subjects. *Physical Therapy, 75*, 621–628.

Seibt, O., Brunoni, A. R., Huang, Y., & Bikson, M. (2015). The pursuit of DLPFC: Non-neuronavigated methods to target the left dorsolateral pre-frontal cortex with symmetric bicephalic transcranial direct current stimulation (tDCS). *Brain Stimulation, 8*, 590–602.

Shen, B., Yin, Y., Wang, J., Zhou, X., Mcclure, S. M., & Li, J. (2016). High-definition tDCS alters impulsivity in a baseline-dependent manner. *NeuroImage, 143*, 343–352.

Turi, Z., Ambrus, G. G., Ho, K. A., Sengupta, T., Paulus, W., & Antal, A. (2014). When size matters: Large electrodes induce greater stimulation-related cutaneous discomfort than smaller electrodes at equivalent current density. *Brain Stimulation, 7*, 460–467.

Turi, Z., Ambrus, G. G., Janacsek, K., Emmert, K., Hahn, L., Paulus, W., & Antal, A. (2013). Both the cutaneous sensation and phosphene perception are modulated in a frequency-specific manner during transcranial alternating current stimulation. *Restorative Neurology and Neuroscience, 31*, 275–285.

Wagner, T., Fregni, F., Fecteau, S., Grodzinsky, A., Zahn, M., & Pascual-Leone, A. (2007). Transcranial direct current stimulation: A computer-based human model study. *NeuroImage, 35*, 1113–1124.

Woods, A. J., Antal, A., Bikson, M., Boggio, P. S., Brunoni, A. R., Celnik, P., ... Nitsche, M. A. (2016). A technical guide to tDCS, and related non-invasive brain stimulation tools. *Clinical Neurophysiology, 127*, 1031–1048.

Woods, A. J., Bryant, V., Sacchetti, D., Gervits, F., & Hamilton, R. (2015). Effects of electrode drift in transcranial direct current stimulation. *Brain Stimulation, 8*, 515–519.

Chapter 11
Transcranial Direct Current Stimulation Integration with Magnetic Resonance Imaging, Magnetic Resonance Spectroscopy, Near Infrared Spectroscopy Imaging, and Electroencephalography

Adam J. Woods, Marom Bikson, Kenneth Chelette, Jacek Dmochowski, Anirban Dutta, Zeinab Esmaeilpour, Nigel Gebodh, Michael A. Nitsche, and Charlotte Stagg

A. J. Woods (✉)
Center for Cognitive Aging and Memory (CAM), McKnight Brain Institute, Department of Clinical and Health Psychology, College of Public Health and Health Professions, University of Florida, Gainesville, FL, USA
e-mail: ajwoods@phhp.ufl.edu

M. Bikson
Department of Biomedical Engineering, The City College of New York, New York, NY, USA

K. Chelette
ANT Neuro North America, Philadelphia, PA, USA

J. Dmochowski
Neural Engineering Laboratory, Department of Biomedical Engineering, Grove School of Engineering, The City College of the City University of New York, New York, NY, USA

A. Dutta
Neuroengineering and Informatics for Rehabilitation Laboratory, Jacobs School of Medicine & Biomedical Sciences, Department of Biomedical Engineering, University at Buffalo SUNY, Buffalo, NY, USA

Z. Esmaeilpour · N. Gebodh
Department of Biomedical Engineering, The City College of the City University of New York, New York, NY, USA

M. A. Nitsche
Department of Psychology and Neurosciences, Leibniz Research Centre for Working Environment and Human Factors, Dortmund, Germany

University Medical Hospital Bergmannsheil, Bochum, Germany

C. Stagg
Oxford Centre for fMRI of the Brain, Nuffield Department of Clinical Neurosciences, University of Oxford, Oxford, UK

Oxford Centre for Human Brain Activity, Department of Psychiatry, University of Oxford, Oxford, UK

H. Knotkova et al. (eds.), *Practical Guide to Transcranial Direct Current Stimulation*, https://doi.org/10.1007/978-3-319-95948-1_11

Introduction

Transcranial direct current stimulation (tDCS) is a non-invasive brain stimulation technique that involves application of low intensity direct currents at the scalp for the modulation of central nervous system excitability in humans (Woods et al. 2016). tDCS is an increasingly important tool, being used in a wide range of human neuroscience applications, as well as a potential adjunct therapy for a range of neurological and psychiatric disorders including chronic stroke recovery, depression and migraine. However, despite its obvious promise, the potential of tDCS cannot as yet be fully exploited as there is still a lack of understanding of the neural mechanisms underpinning stimulation. A key methodological advance toward bridging the gap in our understanding of the neural mechanisms of tDCS effects involves integration of tDCS with modern clinical and cognitive neuroscience techniques. This chapter will discuss integration of tDCS with three major neuroscience techniques: magnetic resonance imaging/spectroscopy (MRI/MRS), near infrared spectroscopy (NIRS) imaging, and human electroencephalography (EEG).

MRI provides a high degree of spatial resolution regarding both brain structure and function, with the ability to assess brain-behaviour questions across the entire brain. However, the temporal resolution of magnetic resonance methods is limited. In contrast, EEG provides a high degree of temporal resolution for neural processes, but overall poor spatial resolution. NIRS provides both spatial and temporal resolution for brain activity, but typically only for tissue near the cortical surface. Each method has both strengths and weaknesses regarding the types of hypotheses that can be tested. From an observational perspective, these techniques provide novel insight into the relationship between brain structure/function and behaviour. However, when combined with tDCS, a wide variety of novel questions and hypotheses can be tested. tDCS provides a method for directly intervening on brain tissue, altering the resting membrane potential of stimulated neurons. Thus, integration of tDCS with these methods provides the ability to evaluate not only correlations between brain function and behaviour, but also experimentally manipulate brain activity in stimulated brain regions and assess how these observational relationships between the brain and behaviour change. Thus, integration of tDCS with modern neuroscience methods has the potential to providing greater causal insight into the brain-behaviour relationship in contrast to observational studies using these methods in isolation. In addition, these integrated methods may also provide critical insight for understanding how, where and when stimulation is most effective in the context of tDCS treatment studies (e.g., pain, cognitive aging, dementia, etc.). This information may prove critical in optimizing treatment efficacy and outcome.

The chapter will review the current state of the art in efforts to integrate MRI/MRS, NIRS, and EEG methodologies and discuss technical challenges commonly faced with integration. In addition, the chapter will give the reader a better understanding of experimental design concerns that should be considered prior to undertaking integration of tDCS with these methods. We will first describe the integration of tDCS with MRI and MRS methods, also covering arterial spin labelling (ASL). We will then turn to integration of tDCS with NIRS. Finally, we will discuss integration with EEG. In each case, careful considerations must be taken to acquire quality data in the presence of tDCS. This chapter will help the reader to understand what considerations must be made, as well as methods for addressing these issues.

Integration with MRI

To date, the neural effects of tDCS have been primarily studied through experiments utilizing transcranial magnetic stimulation (TMS), sometimes in combination with pharmacological agents (Stagg and Nitsche 2011) which have added greatly to our understanding of the local physiological effects of stimulation. However, in recent years, there has been an increasing interest in using advanced neuroimaging techniques to study the effects of tDCS – both in healthy controls and clinical populations. Once technical difficulties are overcome, the combination of tDCS with Magnetic Resonance (MR) provides a powerful tool that allows us to study not only brain regions directly stimulated by tDCS, but unlike most TMS approaches, also how tDCS modulates activity in the rest of the brain.

It is important to note at this point that the neural effects of tDCS are probably dependent, at least to some extent on a number of parameters of the stimulation paradigm, including the duration of stimulation; the site of stimulation; and the electrode configuration used. The majority of studies investigating the mechanistic underpinnings of tDCS using MR approaches have studied the "conventional" electrode placement as first described by Nitsche and Paulus (Nitsche and Paulus 2000), with one 5 × 7 cm electrode over the primary motor cortex (M1) and one 5 × 7 cm electrode over the contralateral supraorbital ridge, with a current of 1–2 mA applied for up to 20 min. This section will therefore focus on studies using these stimulation parameters, important studies using other electrode placements are included where these shed important light on the mechanisms of tDCS.

It is important to note that while some of the findings from studies involving an M1 montage will be applicable to other sites, it cannot be assumed that this is always the case, and therefore the results from these studies should not be assumed to be directly relevant for other stimulation montages. While it is still not clear exactly what facets of neural anatomy have significant effects on tDCS, the distinctive layers in M1and its position on the anterior bank of the large central sulcus, as well as its anatomical connectivity, may well mean that tDCS effects cortical excitability in this region differently to other cortical areas.

MR Approaches

Functional Magnetic Resonance Imaging (fMRI)

Functional magnetic resonance imaging (fMRI) is a versatile and non-invasive tool that has been used for a number of years to study many aspects of neural activity. The first paper to highlight that fMRI can be used to inform our understanding of how tDCS can modulate activity within the brain was published in 2001 by Baudewig et al. (2001b), since when the literature has been rapidly increasing. The majority of the studies discussed here rely on the quantification of the blood oxygen level dependent (BOLD) contrast, the most widely used fMRI technique, although other fMRI techniques are available, of which Arterial Spin Labelling (see later) is perhaps the most relevant in the context of studying the effects of tDCS.

BOLD Functional MRI

The BOLD signal relies on changes in the relative concentrations of deoxygenated haemoglobin (DeoxyHb) and oxygenated haemoglobin (OxyHb) caused by local changes in brain activity, and is therefore an indirect measure of neuronal activity. The BOLD signal is reliant on the magnetic properties of these two compounds. In brief, DeoxyHb contains an iron molecule making it paramagnetic; meaning it has a significant interaction with the applied magnetic field during MRI. By contrast, OxyHb is diamagnetic, so has little effect on the magnetic field. Therefore, if the ratio of OxyHb:DeoxyHb changes within a localized region of tissue, then this can be detected using BOLD fMRI. However, the precise relationship between changes in neuronal activity and a detectable change in the BOLD signal is complex and not yet fully understood (Aroniadou and Keller 1995; Castro-Alamancos et al. 1995; Hess et al. 1996; Logothetis 2008; Trepel and Racine 1998, 2000). FMRI is currently used in two major approaches to study the effects of tDCS either in the presence or absence of a task.

Task-Based fMRI

Task-based fMRI is the classical brain imaging approach, and is a versatile tool that can be used to inform our understanding of how tDCS can modulate activity within the brain while a task is being performed. Task-based fMRI can be done using a number of paradigms, but broadly the BOLD signal from each brain area is compared during task and rest, where the difference in signal reflects changes resulting from changing neural activity in task-based areas of the brain (Woods et al. 2014). This approach usually results in the acquisition of data across the whole brain with a high spatial (in the order of 2–3 mm) and reasonably high temporal resolution.

Resting State fMRI

Functional MRI acquired while the subject is lying in the scanner at rest, and commonly following the instruction "not to think of anything in particular" is an increasingly used method to studying brain connectivity. Without a super-imposed task to perform, the on-going physiological fluctuations in the BOLD signal associated with quiet wakefulness can be recorded. In any given brain region the BOLD signal will vary across time as a function of on-going neural activity. By studying the relationship of the BOLD signal from one brain region to that of others, regions where the time course of fluctuations are highly correlated can be identified, and these regions are said to be "functionally connected". Studies of functional connectivity can be made using a wide array of statistical methods including those utilizing graph theory and independent component analysis (ICA) approaches (for more detail see, for example (Beckmann et al. 2005; Cole et al. 2010; Fornito et al. 2013).

"Resting State Networks" (RSNs) are robust distributed networks identified from ICA that show coordinated and highly reproducible fluctuations in activity between spatially distinct but anatomically closely connected areas while subjects lie at rest (Fox and Raichle 2007; Raichle et al. 2001; Snyder and Raichle 2012). RSNs are being widely investigated due to observed differences during different cognitive and clinical states. They are thought to reflect intrinsic functional architecture in the brain, and separable networks can be identified within resting fMRI data which closely reflect brain regions that are active during task performance (Beckmann et al. 2005; Smith et al. 2009; Stagg and Nitsche 2011). While the physiological underpinnings of changes in RSN connectivity are are still very much the focus of investigation and open to often complex interpretation (Johansen-Berg 2013; Nitsche and Paulus 2000), it is clear that RSNs are highly sensitive to changes in connectivity in a wide range of diseases (Baudewig et al. 2001a; Filippini et al. 2009; Pievani et al. 2011, 2014), and that resting state fMRI is a potentially powerful approach for the study of a wide range of clinical conditions as it removes the confound of task performance (Aroniadou and Keller 1995; Castro-Alamancos et al. 1995; Fornito et al. 2013; Hess et al. 1996; Logothetis 2008; Trepel and Racine 1998, 2000).

Arterial Spin Labelling (ASL)

Although BOLD fMRI is the most common method of assessing neural activity changes during or following tDCS, it has some limitations. BOLD has a relatively high signal-to-noise ratio, meaning that data can be acquired over relatively short timescales, making is highly suitable for studying the effects of non-invasive brain stimulation, the physiological underpinnings of the BOLD effect are complex and currently relatively poorly understood. This may be of particular importance when studying the effect of tDCS in clinical populations, where changes in blood supply or neurovascular coupling may be expected.

An alternative approach is that of Arterial Spin Labelling (ASL). ASL is a relatively novel fMRI technique that is able to quantify changes in tissue perfusion directly in the brain. It has a much lower signal to noise ratio than BOLD fMRI but has two significant advantages over the BOLD signal: (1) It is primarily sensitive to low-frequency signals and is therefore the ideal modality to detect blood flow changes induced by the minutes-long tDCS protocols commonly used and (2) the physiological basis of the contrast is inherently simpler to understand than BOLD.

Magnetic Resonance Spectroscopy

As well as utilising advances in functional MR Imaging to understand the activity changes induced by tDCS, MR can also be used to investigate how tDCS affects the neurochemicals underpinning these plastic changes via magnetic resonance spectroscopy (MRS); a technique that enables us to detect and quantify concentrations of different metabolites within a volume of tissue.

MRS was first performed in the human brain in 1985 (Beckmann et al. 2005; Bottomley et al. 1985; Cole et al. 2010; Fornito et al. 2013), and since then has been primarily used to investigate metabolic changes in pathological states. MRS measures signals are produced by the behaviour of certain diamagnetic molecules within a magnetic field. While MRI focuses on the variations in signal across space, MRS most commonly examines signals produced from only one volume of tissue. A number of atomic nuclei have diamagnetic properties, including 1H, 31P and 13C MRS, of which 1H MRS is used most widely. The ability of MRS to discriminate between different molecules relies on the fact that the structure of the molecules within which these atoms are bound, and the environment surrounding these molecules, influence the behaviour of the atoms within the magnetic field. MRS focuses on very small differences in the signals produced by the atoms contained within different metabolites within a predetermined volume of interest (VOI) or voxel (a 3 dimensional pixel).

The characteristic peaks and frequencies of many neurochemicals are well described, meaning that the resonances produced from these metabolites can be identified from sample spectra. The amplitudes of the peaks derived from a given metabolite are directly proportional to the concentration of that compound within the target volume of tissue, therefore allowing accurate quantification.

There are a number of limitations to MRS approaches. The most relevant of these relates to the inherently low signal-to-noise of the technique. Signals in MRS are typically summed across a large volume in comparison with other forms of MR imaging (e.g. in the order of 3 cm × 3 cm × 3 cm in 1H MRS compared with 3 mm × 3 mm × 3 mm in MRI); this creates an increase in the signal produced by given metabolites relative to the background noise. However even summing across a large area, only metabolites present in millimolar concentrations are detectable. Fortunately, many neurochemicals involved in neurotransmission and metabolism are present in concentrations above this threshold, but others (for example Dopamine) are not, making their detection and quantification impossible with current MRS methods.

MRS lacks some of the flexibility of functional imaging – it requires a large number of options to be pre-specified: volumes of interest must be decided in advance; as must the acquisition parameters, which determine which molecule signals can be resolved. Traditionally MRS only allowed spectra to be obtained of one volume of interest at a time, but recent developments, both for MR Spectroscopic Imaging (MRSI) at 3 T and the advent of ultra-high field 7 T MR scanners have demonstrated robust spectra from multiple brain regions simultaneously (e.g. Fox and Raichle 2007; Lemke et al. 2015; Maudsley et al. 2006; Raichle et al. 2001; Snyder and Raichle 2012). This is of particular importance when considering the use of MRS to study the effects of tDCS, where a control VOI, placed in an anatomically distant site, is important to understand the anatomical limits of any described relationships, often requiring an additional experimental session.

Considerations When Combining tDCS and MRI

To date, tDCS has been integrated with functional magnetic resonance imaging (fMRI), both in terms of Blood Oxygen Level Dependent (BOLD) fMRI (Amadi et al. 2014; Antal et al. 2011; Baudewig et al. 2001b; Stagg et al. 2009b) and Arterial Spin Labelling (ASL) (Stagg et al. 2013; Zheng et al. 2011); as well as proton and non-proton MR Spectroscopy (MRS) (Binkofski et al. 2011; Clark et al. 2011; Stagg et al. 2009a).

tDCS may be combined with MR using two approaches. The techniques may be used sequentially, where the stimulation is delivered outside of the scanner with the participant placed in the scanner before and immediately following the stimulation period. Alternatively, stimulation can be delivered within the bore of the scanner (concurrently) either at the same time as collecting MR data, or during rest.

Both approaches have been used successfully in the literature. A concurrent acquisition is often more advantageous due to the logistical and timing issues associated with removing and replacing the participant before subsequent MR data can be collected. Concurrent acquisition also has the advantage that pre- and post-stimulation data can be controlled for reproducibility (in terms of placement for spectroscopy voxels or high-resolution fMRI slices). However, while there are obvious advantages to concurrent stimulation, integration of tDCS to MRI requires multiple extra considerations including MR specific kit, additional setup criteria and potential adverse effects on MR acquisitions which need to be considered when taking this approach.

The following should be seen only as a summary of the most significant risks of the approach, and given the inherent risks of the technique, tDCS should only be used in the scanner environment by trained individuals.

Practical Considerations When Combining tDCS and MR

Prior to the advent of MR compatible tDCS systems, studies were limited to sequential acquisition. This presents logistical and analytical issues for BOLD fMRI and MRS data, most significantly in terms of accurate subject placement and the need to acquire data as soon as possible after stimulation has ceased, although neither of these are insurmountable. However, with the advent of MR-compatible tDCS system it became possible to stimulate subjects in the bore of the magnet. Thus, participants can undergo baseline scans prior to stimulation, simultaneous acquisition of data during stimulation, and/or post-stimulation scanning immediately after stimulation has ceased while remaining in the same position throughout the scan. This has obvious advantages for studies where the reproducibility of the subject is important, for example for MRS voxel placement or high-resolution fMRI. However, integration of the tDCS device into an MRI system is not without complications, and a number of technical aspects need to be considered carefully.

It perhaps goes without saying that when tDCS is integrated with MRI, standard subject safety standards for both MRI and tDCS (for example, no metal on or in the head, no implants susceptible to electrical current or magnetic fields, etc.) should be adhered to. In addition, standard tDCS acquisition considerations including the accurate localization of electrodes, careful preparation and placement of electrodes, and methods to ensure that electrodes, once sited, remain in a stable location on the head remain critical in order to acquire good quality data.

Concurrent tDCS/MRI requires a specialist kit that is MR compatible and rigorously tested. The use of tDCS within the bore of the MR scanner requires the placement of specially designed MRI-compatible (non-ferrous or appropriately shielded) tDCS electrodes with cables passed from the stimulator, through the magnet suite waveguide, and into the magnet bore. The electrodes used should be fitted with high-ohmic (commonly 10 KOhm) resistors to prevent induction of eddy currents within the stimulating leads. It is vital to ensure that electrodes are not in contact with the head coil, or headphones, to prevent electrode displacement and, also, unexpected interactions between the stimulator and the scanner.

Care should also be taken to keep the leads away from the subject to prevent burns and run parallel to the bore without loops to prevent eddy currents. The tDCS stimulator should be kept in the control room as it is not magnet safe and stimulation, as with tDCS outside the scanner, should be monitored closely by a researcher for the entire duration of the stimulation. Careful monitoring of the subject is particularly necessary as the subject is at a distance and, if engaged in a task during stimulation, verbal communication is impossible.

Electrodes should be carefully prepared with high conductance electrical paste (such as that used for EEG) as the saline-soaked sponges which are often used for tDCS applied outside the scanner will dry out over time, making them unsuitable for use in MRI scans that ordinarily last around 60–90 min. This is particularly the case where often a baseline scan or scans lasting tens of minutes are acquired before tDCS is applied. Dry sponges result in poor conductance of the electrical current, which can be uncomfortable or even painful for the participant and might result in skin burning in severe cases. A thick, even, coating ($\geq$3 mm) of paste should be applied to the electrode to provide sufficient distance between the electrode and scalp, ensuring that stimulation is delivered evenly across the electrode.

As with all tDCS experiments, care should be taken to ensure that the electrodes do not move. However, most tDCS electrodes are not visible using standard MRI acquisition, so they electrodes are often marked with oil-capsules to confirm their position on the resulting MR images. The adhesive quality of the paste often assists in maintaining the electrode placement, but also requires additional straps for fully secure placement. The entire montage can be covered by a relatively loose-fitting cap, which has the dual roles of protecting the electrodes from accidental movement during subject placement in the MR and protecting the scanner from the electrode paste.

Data Quality Considerations When Combining tDCS and MR

The constant electrical current which constitutes tDCS interacts with the magnetic field generated by the MR scanner, resulting in warping of the images acquired. This artifact is of critical concern for BOLD fMRI protocols, as it has the potential to result in false positive changes in the BOLD signal. The magnitude and nature of any artefacts are likely to depend on the exact experimental setup and therefore will vary from centre to centre. This variability is reflected by the published studies: one study demonstrated evidence of BOLD signal within the brains of two cadavers during a concurrent tDCS and fMRI protocol (Antal et al. 2014), strongly suggesting that tDCS is capable of inducing significant BOLD signal, although it is worth noting that in most situations the timecourse of this "activation" is likely to be distinct from the task performed and will most likely follow the stimulation period. Another study demonstrated visual evidence of change in EPI field maps, but this was limited to the scalp and cortical tissue near to the electrode site (Holland et al. 2011). Other sites also observe artefacts directly under the electrodes, but these are limited to the scalp and soft tissues (unpublished data, CJS). However, to date, very few studies have provided explicit data on change in the magnetic field in relation to concurrent tDCS/fMRI, in terms, for example, of visible artefacts, change in signal to noise or non-physiological signal change. The contrasting evidence from the literature demonstrates the need for careful consideration of concurrent data and acquisition of appropriate field map data to allay concerns over false positive functional results from perturbation of the magnetic field.

fMRI Studies of tDCS

The relative ease with which resting-state fMRI experiments can be performed and the absence of the confound of task performance has meant a relatively large number of studies utilizing the combination of tDCS and rs-fMRI have been published. A number of studies have demonstrated that tDCS is capable of modulating the resting functional connectivity between a number of brain regions, although to date no clear consensus across the literature has emerged as to the specific pattern of stimulation-induced changes (Amadi et al. 2014; Bachtiar et al. 2015; Polanía et al. 2011a, b, 2012; Sehm et al. 2012, 2013). This lack of agreement between studies as to the effects of tDCS probably reflects the likely sensitivities of different analysis approaches as well as differences in MR acquisition and stimulation parameters, but makes interpretation of the literature as it stands somewhat difficult.

Task-Based Studies in Healthy Controls

Behaviourally, tDCS applied with anode over M1 concurrently with a motor task has been shown to improve performance in a variety of domains, including motor speed and dexterity (Nitsche et al. 2003; Stagg et al. 2011b), and motor learning and adaptation (Boggio et al. 2006; Nitsche et al. 2003; Reis et al. 2009). In prior studies, tDCS under the cathode electrode has been shown to either impair (Stagg et al. 2011b) or to have no effect on learning (Nitsche et al. 2003; Reis et al. 2009) or simple reaction times (Nitsche et al. 2003). A number of studies have employed task-based fMRI to understand not only the activity changes underlying these behavioural effects within the stimulated cortex, but also in more anatomically distant regions.

Baudewig and colleagues initially confirmed the feasibility of combining functional MRI and tDCS (Baudewig et al. 2001a). In this study, the BOLD signal was recorded in a group of six subjects before and after 5 min of tDCS. The authors reported small stimulation-induced changes in activation in the supplementary motor area (SMA), an effect still noticeable 15 min after the end of stimulation.

Since this work, a number of imaging studies in healthy controls have investigated the effects of tDCS on motor-related activity (Antal et al. 2011; Kwon et al. 2008; Lindenberg et al. 2013; Meinzer et al. 2014; Stagg et al. 2009b). Of these, one investigated the effects of a conventional electrode montage (left M1 and the right supraorbital ridge) and a stimulation period of 10 min, on the performance of a simple explicit sequence learning task (Stagg et al. 2009b). The expected increase in activation after stimulation with the anode over M1 compared to sham was observed in the stimulated M1, ipsilateral dorsal premotor cortex (dPMC) and SMA. After stimulation with cathode over M1, an increase in BOLD signal was observed under the stimulating electrode (left M1), as well as in the contralateral (right) M1, dPMC and SMA.

ASL Studies

The first study to combine tDCS with ASL was performed by Zheng and colleagues, which showed an increase in perfusion after short periods of both anode over M1 and cathode over M1 (Zheng et al. 2011). A subsequent ASL study during concurrent tDCS to the left dorsolateral prefrontal cortex (DLPFC) demonstrated an increase in perfusion during and after stimulation with the anode over left DLPFC and a decrease in perfusion during and after stimulation with the cathode over left DLPFC (Stagg et al. 2013), a finding in line with animal models (Wachter et al. 2011). This study also went on to analyse the tDCS-induced changes in perfusion across the whole brain and demonstrated significantly increased perfusion during the anode over DLPFC condition in those areas anatomically connected to the DLPFC (Stagg et al. 2013).

Combining tDCS with MRS

The majority of studies investigating the effects of tDCS on 1H MRS-measured neurochemistry have focused on applying anode or cathode electrodes over M1. Stimulation with anode over M1 leads to a decrease in MRS measured GABA levels in the stimulated area of cortex (Bachtiar et al. 2015; Kim et al. 2014; Stagg et al. 2009a, 2011a). Studies in parietal cortex have demonstrated a concurrent increase in glutamate/glutamine (Clark et al. 2011; Hunter et al. 2015), though this has not been demonstrated in M1 (Stagg et al. 2009c, 2011a). This lack of consistency between studies raises an interesting question about whether the location of brain stimulation alters its effects on neurochemistry, or whether this is a facet of the different MRS approaches used, but it is not possible to draw global conclusions as neither of these parietal cortex studies examined GABA changes.

Integration with NIRS Imaging

Beyond effects on neuronal excitability, after-effects of tDCS on regional cerebral blood flow (rCBF) have been demonstrated (Zheng et al. 2011). Changes in rCBF can be related to the local neuronal activation, which is termed neurovascular coupling (NVC) (Girouard and Iadecola 2006). NVC is defined by neural activity closely related, spatially and temporally, to rCBF. Although the proposition of a correlation between neuronal activity and the increment of vascular supply due to the brain's energy demand increase is a long-standing concept (Roy and Sherrington 1890): "…the brain possesses an intrinsic mechanism by which its vascular supply can be varied locally in correspondence with local variations of functional activity," the exact cellular mechanism of NVC is still elusive (Girouard and Iadecola 2006).

The importance of NVC to the health of the normal brain has been highlighted in a review by Girouard and Iadecola (2006) that suggested it as a therapeutic target in pathologies associated with cerebrovascular dysfunction. Pulgar (2015) has proposed tDCS for improvement of cerebrovascular dysfunction, based on findings showing that it modulates cerebral vasomotor reactivity (VMR), and heart rate variability (Vernieri et al. 2010). Also, tDCS can influence downstream metabolic systems regulated by the brain (Binkofski et al. 2011). However, the effects depend on the tDCS electrode montage, e.g., List et al. (2015) showed with a double-blind crossover within-subject design that 20 min of stimulation did not affect cerebral autoregulation assessed by low-frequency oscillations (LFO) of cerebral blood flow where VMR was measured by transcranial Doppler sonography. Therefore, they hypothesized that the extracephalic return electrode in the study by Vernieri et al. (2010) may have stimulated the brainstem autonomic centers which can be confirmed with the calculations of electric field (and current density) induced by the tDCS montage (Noetscher et al. 2014).

The neurovascular unit (NVU) consists of the endothelium, glia, neurons, pericytes, and the basal lamina where computational models can capture NVU dynamics (Dutta 2015; Huneau et al. 2015). Simple low-dimensional models can describe NVU as a lumped system to relate neural activity with an "energy" variable (analogous to ATP) as output (Chhabria and Chakravarthy, 2016). ATP is required for neuronal metabolic processes like synapto-vescicular recycling and maintenance of the gradient potential (Attwell et al. 2010; Hamel 2006). Specifically, tDCS-evoked increases of neuronal activity might result in aerobic glycolysis (Vaishnavi et al. 2010) and associated lactate surge (Mintun et al. 2004) which can modulate spatiotemporal activity of primary cortical neurons through a receptor-mediated pathway (Bozzo et al. 2013). Besides the role of lactate in energy metabolism, a signaling molecule inducing calcium influx and the expression of long-term plasticity-related genes in neurons has recently been identified (Yang et al. 2014). Also, glial involvement in tDCS-induced plasticity in mouse brain has been shown using calcium imaging (Monai et al. 2016) where a minimum current of ~50 μA (current density, ~2.5 mA/cm^2) at the anode was required to induce cortex-wide calcium surge. However, at lower current intensity of ~14 μA (current density, ~0.7 mA/cm^2), the calcium surge was local at the anode. Such local effects can be due to subthreshold shift of neuronal resting membrane potentials by tDCS that may alter the spontaneous activity with no effects on synaptic plasticity (Stagg and Nitsche 2011). Alterations in spontaneous activity can affect rCBF via various metabolites like K+, adenosine, NO, or CO2 (Dutta 2015). Four kinds of potassium channels, namely ATP-sensitive potassium channels, calcium-activated potassium channels, delayed rectifier potassium channels, and inward rectifier potassium channels play the major role in maintenance of vascular tone of cerebral blood vessels. Via activation of these channels, efflux of K+ causes closure of voltage-dependent calcium channels leading to vascular relaxation (Bonnet et al. 1991; Brayden 1996; Edwards and Weston 1993; Kitazono et al. 1995; Nelson et al. 1990). Also, neuronal nitric oxide synthase (NOS) plays a significant role in maintenance of cerebral blood flow (Attwell et al. 2010). The aftereffects of stimulation following sufficient duration of stimulation depend on the modulation of both GABAergic and glutamatergic synapses and are calcium-dependent (Giordano et al. 2017; Stagg and Nitsche, 2011) where activation of neuronal NMDA receptors via glutamate causes an influx of calcium that activates NOS and can further increase blood flow (Attwell et al. 2010). At higher current density, glial involvement in tDCS-induced plasticity is possible (Monai et al. 2016) that can be powerful regulators of neuronal spiking, synaptic plasticity and brain blood flow (Bazargani and Attwell, 2016), and are involved in the generation of calcium waves between neighbored neurons via metabotropic glutamate receptors (Leybaert et al. 1998) leading to cortex-wide calcium surge (Monai et al. 2016). Within NVU, glial-cells astrocytes regulate increased local blood-flow during neuronal activation (high energy demand) by secretion of vasoactive substances like NO, and Prostaglandin E2 that are involved in synaptic plasticity (Leybaert et al. 1998; Oomagari et al. 1991). Anatomical connections between the vascular system and astrocytes at the functional level are well known (Mathiisen et al. 2010). Astrocytes express a surface protein required to detect neuronal activation and facilitate the gated efflux of K+ that causes vasodilation (Paulson and Newman 1987). Astrocytic network has extensive connectivity via gap junctions and direct tDCS effects on the astrocytic network (Dutta 2015) will cause widespread changes in the cerebral blood flow, as shown by a recent study (Takai et al. 2016). Moreover, direct effects on the astrocytic network can facilitate neural efficiency by its priming effects on the NVU (Dutta et al. 2015). Stimulation of astrocytes raises calcium in the end-feet that can have a vasoactive effect on parenchymal arterioles. Dilation or constriction depends on the level of calcium (Mulligan and MacVicar 2004). Here, a transition between vasoconstriction and vasodilatation was observed in single vessels by varying the stimulation intensity (Tsytsarev et al. 2011). Indeed, differences of calcium dynamics are proposed to result in different effects of specific tDCS protocols (Stagg and Nitsche 2011) where astrocytic Ca2+/IP3 signaling has been implicated in the metaplasticity changes of the cortex with tDCS (Monai et al. 2016). Our current understanding of glial involvement in tDCS (Monai et al. 2016) and its relation to neuronal function (Bazargani and Attwell 2016) lends to the possibility of bidirectional interactions between neuronal and hemodynamic responses to tDCS (Dutta 2015). This can lead to multi-timescale cross-talk and resulting complex non-linear spatiotemporal dynamics (Jolivet et al. 2015) that may not remain limited to the area immediately under the stimulation electrode (Takai et al. 2016).

The primary purpose of NVU is to maintain homeostasis of the brain's microenvironment (Abbott et al. 2006) where the hemodynamic component of the tDCS response can be captured by functional magnetic resonance imaging (fMRI) as well as functional near-infrared spectroscopy (fNIRS) neuroimaging. MRI can have a high resolution (up to isotropic resolution of 140 μm (Stucht et al. 2015) with full coverage of human brain but with relatively slow sampling rate (e.g., ASL scan taking approximately 3.5 min (Zheng et al. 2011), and MRI suffers from potentially confounding interference from current flow during tDCS (Antal et al. 2014). Therefore, fNIRS is better suited being an optical functional neuroimaging using NIRS technique (Obrig 2014). NIRS can noninvasively and continuously measure cerebral hemoglobin oxygenation, which is widely used for monitoring of cerebral vascular status under various clinical conditions. The photons in the near-infrared (NIR) spectral range (650–950 nm) are able to penetrate human tissue. NIR wavelengths can be selected such that the change in concentration of oxy-hemoglobin (O2Hb) and deoxy-hemoglobin (HHb) in the brain tissue can be detected. NIR light spectrum between 700 and 900 nm is mostly transparent to skin, tissue, and bone, while O2Hb and HHb are stronger absorbers of this spectrum. Differences in the absorption spectra of O2Hb and HHb enable us to measure relative changes in hemoglobin concentration through the use of light attenuation at multiple wavelengths (Scholkmann et al. 2014). Two or more wavelengths can be selected, with one wavelength above and one below the isobestic point of 810 nm at which HHb and O2Hb have identical absorption coefficients. Using the modified Beer-Lambert Law (mBLL), relative concentration can be calculated as a function of total photon path length. Typically, the light emitter and detector are placed ipsilaterally on the subjects skull so recorded measurements are due to back-scattered (reflected) light following elliptical pathways. NIRS instrumentation works on different measuring principles, e.g., continuous wave (CW) (Scholkmann et al. 2014), frequency domain (FD) (Fantini 2014), and time domain (TD) (Torricelli et al. 2014). Absolute concentration measurements may be possible with more expensive TD and FD techniques (Scholkmann et al. 2014), but quantification is not a crucial factor when one needs to detect a relative change in O2Hb and HHb in cerebral hemodynamic response to tDCS rather than to quantify the hemodynamic response in absolute terms. CW fNIRS signal is strongly contaminated with systemic interference of superficial origin where more expensive TD fNIRS can discriminate between intra- and extra-cerebral signals (Torricelli et al. 2014). Nevertheless, CW fNIRS offers a relatively inexpensive, non-invasive, safe, and portable method of monitoring microvascular hemodynamics in parallel to tDCS in a neurorehabilitation setting. However, CW fNIRS imaging during tDCS requires identification of systemic interference to avoid measuring fNIRS hemodynamic responses that are not due to neurovascular coupling (Tachtsidis and Scholkmann 2016), e.g., by the means of a regression analysis (Kirilina et al. 2012) using short-separation NIRS measurements (Sood et al. 2015) to explicitly sample the extra-cerebral tissue response.

NIRS Probe Development for Imaging of tDCS Responses

The 4 × 1 HD-tDCS montage allows precise targeting of cortical structures (Villamar et al. 2013). Anode centered HD-tDCS increases cortical excitability and is postulated to induce local neuronal and hemodynamic response during focal stimulation (Sood et al. 2016) that can be captured with NIRS-EEG joint imaging, as shown in Fig. 11.1a, b. Freely available SimNIBS software pipeline (Windhoff et al. 2013) was used to develop a subject-specific head model based on MRI data. SimNIBS incorporates FreeSurfer tools (Fischl 2012) to segment the brain and FSL (Jenkinson et al. 2012) BET/BETsurf tools to segment the rest of the head. Developers of the SimNIBS software pipeline recommend MPRAGE acquisitions with selective water excitation for fat suppression for FreeSurfer tools to work well (http://simnibs.de/version2/mri_sequences). For FSL BET/BETsurf tools, they recommend high bandwidths both for the T1- and T2-weighted images and thin slices with gaps in-between for the T2-weighted images. Therefore, ideally four sets of images should be acquired, two with fat suppression and two without fat suppression, but with high bandwidth and thin slices. The SimNIBS software pipeline (Windhoff et al. 2013) can use the fat-suppressed T1 as input for FreeSurfer, the fat-suppressed T1- and T2-weighted images to reconstruct the inner skull boundary, and the normal T1- and T2-weighted images to reconstruct the outer skull boundary and the skin surface with FSL (Jenkinson et al. 2012) BET/BETsurft tools. This software pipeline was applied on the Colin27 average brain, which is based on 27 times on an individual, and linear registration of the images to create an average with high SNR and structure definition (Holmes et al. 2015). The tetrahedral head meshes from the Colin27 average brain MRI data were generated using the 'mri2mesh' tool in the SimNIBS software pipeline (Windhoff et al. 2013). The tDCS electrode positions in the SimNIBS software pipeline was defined using MNI coordinates of 10–20 scalp positions given by Okamoto et al. (2004) for the finite element analysis (FEA) using GetDP – a freely available finite element solver (http://getdp.info/). The FEA model used electrostatic volume conductor physics with default (in SimNIBS) material conductivities (in S/m): white matter = 0.126; gray matter = 0.275; CSF = 1.654; bone = 0.01; scalp = 0.465; spongy bone = 0.025; compact bone = 0.008; eye balls = 0.5; eye region = 0.25. The electric field magnitude can be used (Datta et al. 2011) to determine tDCS-affected brain areas as shown in Fig. 11.1c.

The open-source software package AtlasViewer (Aasted et al. 2015) was used to design NIRS probes to cover tDCS-affected (based on electric field magnitude (Datta et al. 2011)) brain areas using NIR sources and detectors. AtlasViewer provides tools for spatial registration, probe sensitivity computation, and reconstruction of images. The NIRS forward model (and probe sensitivity) can be computed by the Monte-Carlo photon transport software, 'tMCimg', available in the AtlasViewer package that computes the probabilistic path of photons from the optode source located at the scalp through the head model tissues to the re-emission at the scalp located optode detectors. Colin27 head model (Holmes et al. 2015) with the International 10–20 system as the reference points for the NIRS probe design. AtlasViewer also provides 'iso2mesh' – an image-based 3D surface and volumetric mesh generator comparable to 'mri2mesh' tool in the SimNIBS software pipeline (Windhoff et al. 2013) – to generate individual MRI-based head models. The AtlasViewer package allows a probe to be designed, amended, and assessed prior to probe fabrication (Aasted et al. 2015). Increasing the source-detector (SD) separation past 2 cm monotonically increases sensitivity to brain tissue; diminishing returns appear to begin at around 4–5 cm (Strangman et al. 2013). The probe sensitivity can be found using the Monte-Carlo (MC) photon transport software 'tMCimg' (Boas et al. 2002) available in the AtlasViewer package. Initial rapid assessment of the probe placement and sensitivity was performed with 1e6 photons and more accu-

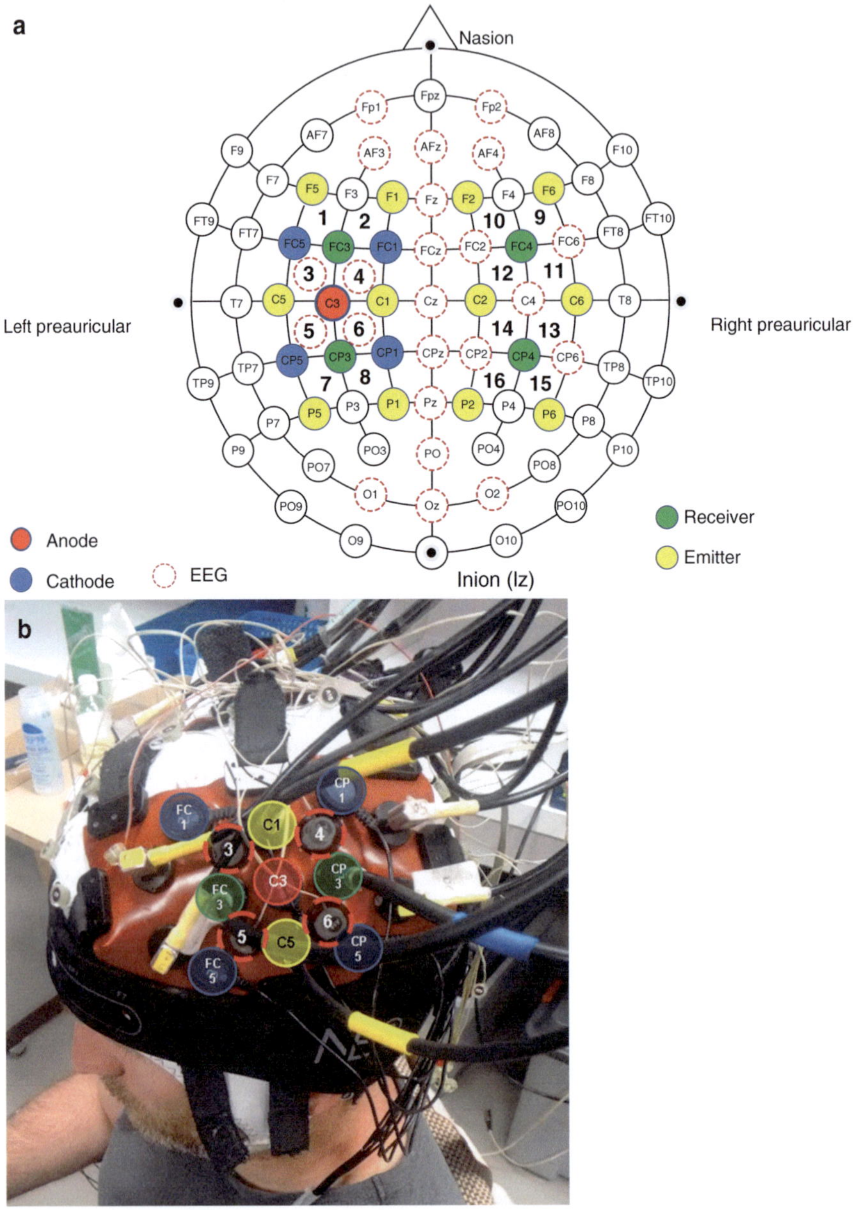

Fig. 11.1 (**a**) An illustrative NIRS-EEG/HD-tDCS montage with NIRS channels, 1–16, according to the standard EEG 10–10 at the ipsilateral and contralateral sensorimotor areas (**b**) The experimental set-up of the HD-tDCS electrodes and local NIRS-EEG channels, 3–6, (**c**) Electric field magnitude due to HD-tDCS in the gray matter surface, (**d**) Sensitivity distribution of NIRS probe at gray matter surface. (Pictures adapted from Sood et al. (2016) with permission)

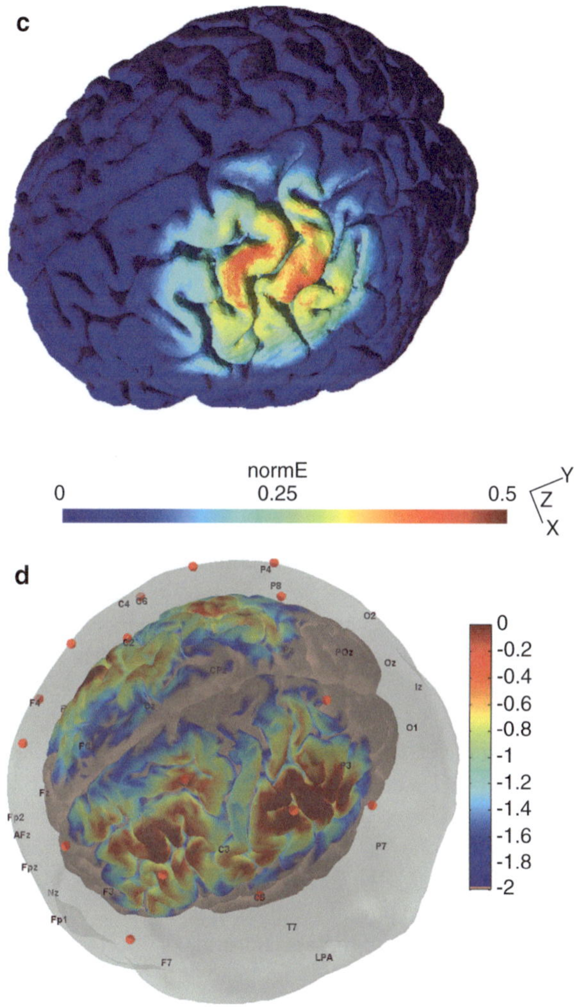

Fig. 11.1 (continued)

rate results were obtained with 1e8 photons to evaluate the final probe design. This time-consuming MC simulation generates the forward matrix that represents the spatial sensitivity profile of each measurement channel to cortical absorption changes. A graphical processor unit can substantially speed up the simulation by more than 100× using mesh-based MC simulation (Fang 2010). The NIRS forward model was identified for the head volume where AtlasViewer projects the volumetric sensitivity in the gray matter onto the surface of the pial matter and implements the AAL atlas (Tzourio-Mazoyer et al. 2002) for localizing the brain region of interest. In fact, NIRS signals in adult humans are strongly biased towards the outermost 1–1.5 cm of the intracranial space (Strangman et al. 2013). Registration of this head model to a subject can be achieved using affine transformation in the AtlasViewer with fiducials 3D digitized at Nz, Iz, Cz, right and left preauricular points. It is also essential to incorporate optical properties representing heterogeneously lesioned individual brains to build realistic individual head models, especially, for the reconstruction of images of the measured brain activation patterns in stroke survivors.

Preliminary Results

The set-up of the HD-tDCS electrodes and NIRS optodes was formed on the surface of the skull according to the standard used EEG 10–20 (Jasper 1958) at the ipsilateral and contralateral primary sensorimotor cortex (SMC), as shown in Fig. 11.1a, b. The HD-tDCS (Starstim®, Neuroelectrics NE, Barcelona) cathodes were placed on FC1, FC5, CP5 and CP1 with the anode in the center, C3, in a 4 × 1 ring configuration (Fig. 11.1a). The corresponding electric field magnitude at the gray matter surface is shown in Fig. 11.1c. Measurements of hemodynamic changes were made from 16-channel CW NIRS system (Oxymon MkIII, Artinis, Netherlands) at a sampling frequency of 10 Hz. Pathlength Differential Factor was calculated based on the age of the subject in order to know the variations in concentration of O2Hb and HHb (Delpy et al. 1989). The receiver-transmitter distance of 3 cm was chosen based on computational modeling; the respective measurement sensitivity distribution of the NIRS probe at the gray matter surface is shown in Fig. 11.1d. The receivers (Rx) were placed on FC3 and CP3 for the left hemisphere and FC4 and CP4 for the right hemisphere (Fig. 11.1a). Transmitters (Tx) were placed diagonally, i.e., at P1, P5, C1, C5, F5 and F1 for the left hemisphere and at P6, P2, C6, C2, F2 and F6 for the right hemisphere. These Rx and Tx fibres were held in place with a plastic ring on a 1 mm thick silicone-based band and the bands were held together with Velcro® tape (see Fig. 11.1b). The experiment was divided into three sessions: 10 min before (pre), at 10 min during ("online"), and 3 min after ("offline") anode centered HD-tDCS of the SMC (2 mA: 20 min), the subject performed a self initiated simple finger sequence (SFS) task with their right and left hand in an alternating block design (30-s task and 30-s rest, repeated 5 times). The fNIRS results showed that anodal HD-tDCS induced a significant reduction in bilateral SMC activation (i.e., smaller decrease in HHb) for a similar SFS frequency (i.e., motor output) (Muthalib et al. 2016) that is shown for NIRS channels 4 and 12 (left and right SMC respectively) in Fig. 11.2a. Muthalib and colleagues (2016) postulated that anodal HD-tDCS induced a "greater efficiency" of neuronal transmission in the bilateral SMC to perform the same SFS task where "greater efficiency" can be related to anodal HD-tDCS "priming" the NVU with evoked hemodynamic response (Guhathakurta and Dutta 2016). Indeed, the resting state fNIRS data showed focal hemodynamic responses as a correlate of the electrical field distribution (see Fig. 11.1c) in the stimulated hemisphere during HD-tDCS (Muthalib et al. 2016). Figure 11.2b shows that online HD-tDCS at rest induced a gradual increase in the concentration of O2Hb (red line) at the left hemisphere peaking after 5 min at the fNIRS channels located adjacent to the 4 × 1 HD-tDCS electrode montage (e.g.,

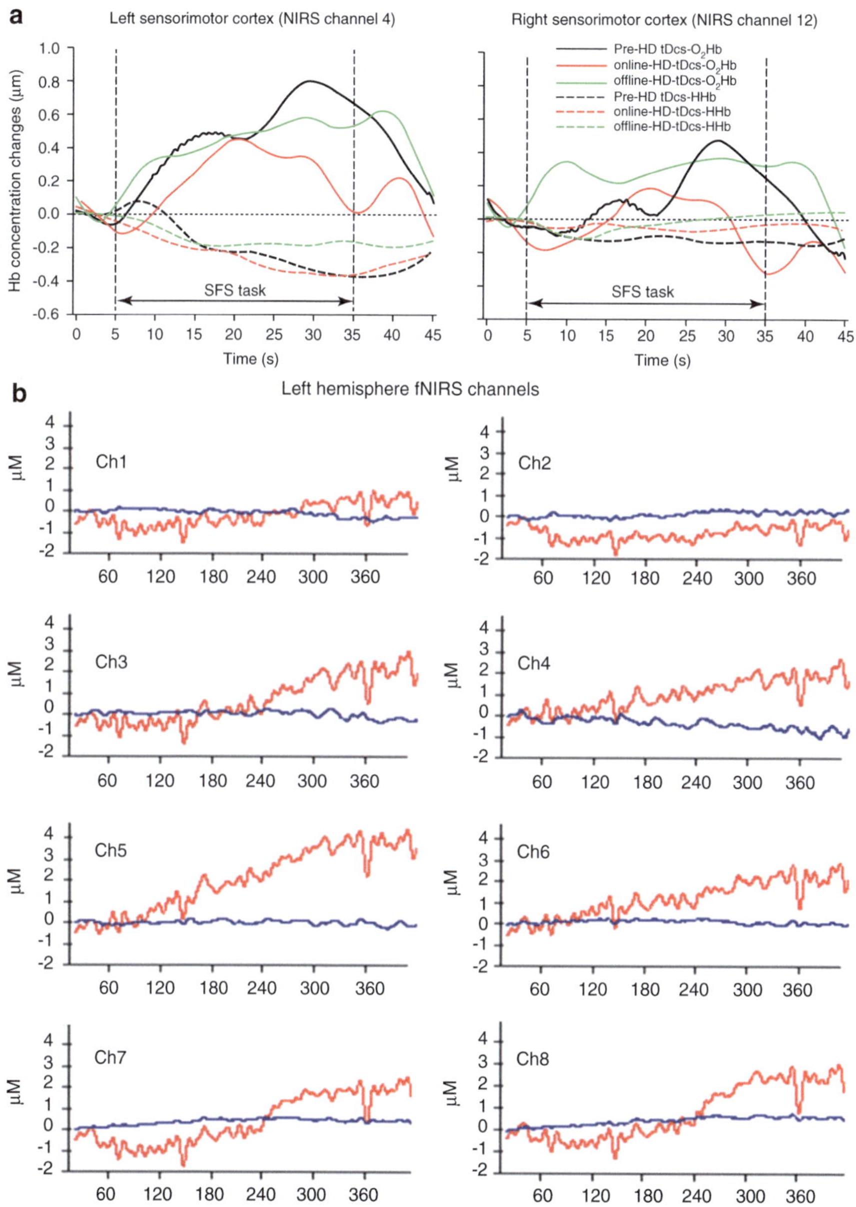

Fig. 11.2 Illustrative fNIRS result in healthy humans. (Adapted from Muthalib et al. (2016), (Muthalib et al. 2017)). (**a**) fNIRS changes of left SMC (left panel: channel 4) and right SMC (right panel: channel 12) during the right hand simple finger sequence (SFS) task before "Pre", during "Online" and after "Offline" anode centered HD-tDCS. (**b**) Online HD-tDCS at rest induced a gradual increase in the concentration O2Hb (red line peaking after 5 min, x-axis shows the number of the datapoint sampled at 10 Hz) in the left hemisphere fNIRS channels (3, 4, 5, 6) located adjacent to the 4 × 1 HD-tDCS electrode montage. The concentration of HHB (blue line) did not show a significant change during HD-tDCS

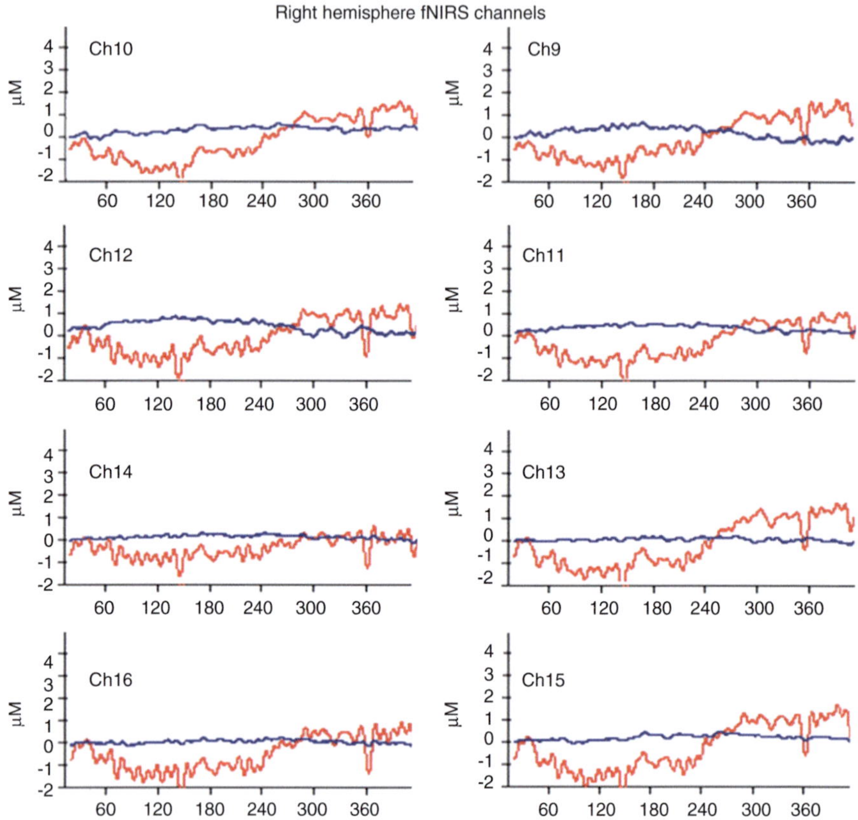

Fig. 11.2 (continued)

channels 3, 4, 5, 6). Also, online HD-tDCS at rest induced a decrease in the concentration of O2Hb (red line) at the right (contralateral) hemisphere (e.g., channels 9–15) peaking after 2 min which may be related to inter-hemispheric inhibition. However, the concentration of HHB (blue line) did not show a significant change during HD-tDCS where tDCS can have direct effects on glial cells (Monai et al. 2016) and smooth muscles of blood vessels (Pulgar 2015) without affecting oxygen utilization leading to alterations in rCBF (and O2HB). Therefore, an analysis of the resting-state NVC was conducted based on local NIRS-EEG channels adjacent to the 4 × 1 HD-tDCS electrode montage (i.e., channels 3, 4, 5, 6). An autoregressive (ARX) model was developed to track the transient coupling relation between log (base-10) transformed EEG band-power (0.5–11.25 Hz) and NIRS O2Hb signal in the low frequency ($\leq$0.1 Hz) range (Sood et al. 2016), as shown in Fig. 11.3. This transient coupling fluctuated between in-phase and out-of-phase during anodal HD-tDCS which may be due to the dynamics within NVU. A stroke case-series demonstrated an impaired NVC functionality during anodal tDCS in chronic (>6 months) ischemic stroke survivors (Dutta et al. 2015) that revealed the lesioned hemisphere with impaired circulation (Jindal et al. 2015). Therefore, we postulate

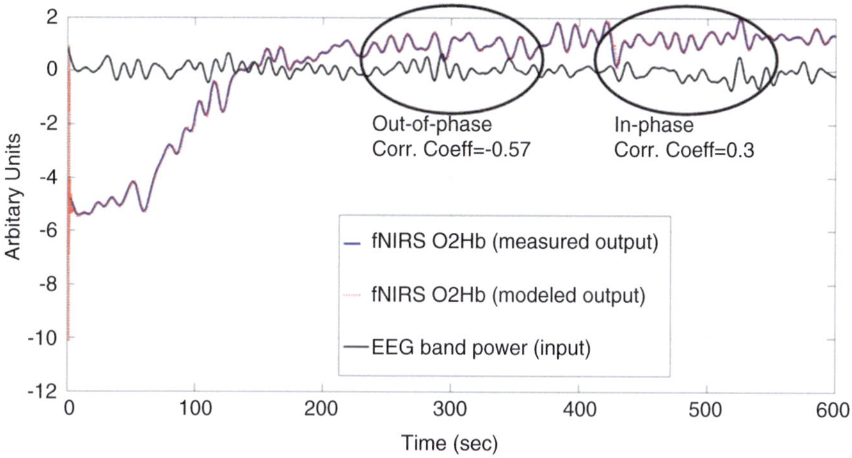

Fig. 11.3 Transient coupling in the low frequency (≤0.1 Hz) range between the electrophysiological (EEG band power within 0.5–11.25 Hz) and the hemodynamic (fNIRS O2Hb) signals representing resting-state spontaneous brain activation during anodal HD-tDCS in healthy humans. (Picture adapted from Sood et al. (2016) with permission)

that portable NIRS-EEG joint imaging of tDCS responses incorporated into brain computer interfaces may be used to identify, assess, and customize dosing of tDCS in cerebrovascular diseases (Dutta 2015).

Integration with EEG

Recent technological advances in the field of EEG and tDCS have allowed for increasingly seamless integration of tDCS and EEG. Combining non-invasive brain stimulation with imaging, especially concurrent online integration, provides objective outcome measures and allows for optimization of the interventions (Baudewig et al. 2001a; Hunter et al. 2013; Komssi et al. 2002). These optimizations can be done using the concept of reciprocity, which suggests that EEG electrical recordings can be inverted to guide electrical stimulation (tDCS) to specific targets within the brain (Cancelli et al. 2016; Fernández-Corazza et al. 2016; Wagner et al. 2016). Similar to other integrated modalities though, the integration of EEG and tDCS does come with some limitations. These can include the type of integration, hardware limitations, as well as several types of artifacts that can occur with integration.

Both EEG and tDCS (Minhas et al. 2010) use conductive interfaces between electrodes and scalp across the head, are portable and low-cost (Charvet et al. 2015), and have broad applications spanning the cognitive and neuropsychiatric domains (Al-Kaysi et al. 2016; Brunoni et al. 2012; Buch et al. 2017). In the case of EEG, electrolyte gel is used between the scalp and recording electrodes, whereas with tDCS saline soaked sponges or electrolyte gel can be used, specifically in

HD-tDCS. The use of HD-tDCS when combined with EEG is advantageous compared to traditional tDCS, due to its increased focality, small area required to apply stimulation as well as its gel interface with the scalp, which is similar that of EEG. Analogous to EEG, with HD-tDCS small stimulation electrodes holders are used to hold externally applied stimulating electrodes, alternatively these cups can incorporate both stimulation and recording electrode options. With the integration of EEG with tDCS protocols, high resolution real time scalp voltage monitoring can be achieved as well as voltage dynamics and frequency shifts prior to, during, and after tDCS. These features, combined with the perception that tDCS produces only DC artifacts in the EEG that are readily filtered, have encouraged human trials of concurrent (online) EEG recording during tDCS (Cunillera et al. 2015; Faehling and Plewnia 2016; Faria et al. 2012; Mancini et al. 2015; Mangia et al. 2014; Roy et al. 2014).

Previous studies that have reported on concurrent tDCS and EEG have used signal processing of varying complexity to remove what are presumed "non-physiologic stimulation artifacts" – namely artifacts that arise from non-ideal stimulation and recording amplifier performance (Cunillera et al. 2015; Faehling and Plewnia 2016; Faria et al. 2012; Mancini et al. 2015; Mangia et al. 2014; Roy et al. 2014). Studies reporting effects of tDCS on EEG have made varied assumptions about the nature of the stimulation artifact such as: the artifact is narrowband in the frequency domain (DC at 0 Hz), allowing for simple high-pass filtering; or the artifact is time invariant, supporting stationary artifact removal techniques (e.g. ICA); the artifact is montage independent, supporting the use of control tDCS montages (i.e. montage/polarity/current specific); and/or the artifacts do not outlast stimulation, supporting pre/post (offline) comparisons without need for corrections. In light of new and emerging evidence though, these assumptions warrant further testing (Noury et al. 2016).

EEG Integration Approaches: Practical Aspects

With the integration of EEG and tDCS technologies several approaches can be taken. These approaches can be structured upon practical limitations with experimental design, hardware limitations, or regions of interest on the scalp. Experimental design is a key component that should be considered when designing EEG –tDCS protocols. This can influence the type of hardware used as well as quality of data acquired. For example, if comparisons of offline (no stimulation) and online (stimulation) EEG are to be compared, understanding what type of baseline measures to compare to and when to acquire proper baseline measures would be important. Improper experimental designs including inadequate tDCS washout periods, missing study arms, etc. can introduce detrimental confounds that can detract from meaningful study outcomes and should be avoided. Specific regions of interest on the scalp (i.e. standard sites C3 commonly associated with motor cortex stimulation) may influence the selected EEG electrode density and placement, relative to stimulation sites. It can also dictate the number of head caps used (i.e. one solely for acquiring EEG and one solely for applying stimulation).

Hardware limitations, including the lack of bandwidth or encoding bit depth to record large voltages produced by stimulation, can greatly influence the types of EEG amplifiers used. Amplifiers that cannot accommodate large voltages produced during stimulation can produce nonlinear artifacts when voltages approach the limit of the amplifier's dynamic range. When voltages go beyond the dynamic range of the amplifier non-recoverable saturation occurs, leaving unusable EEG data.

Offline EEG-tDCS

In cases where EEG data during stimulation is not required (or "offline" stimulation) the hardware options are to utilize (1) a single cap with overlapping stimulation and acquisition sites where EEG data acquisition sites are shared with stimulation sites; (2) a single cap with non-overlapping stimulation and acquisition sites where EEG data acquisition sites are interleaved with stimulation sites; or (3) two caps, one for EEG data acquisition with designated EEG electrode positioning and one for HD-tDCS with designated sites for delivering stimulation. With a single cap containing overlapping sites, stimulation sites can be digitally selected and changed from recording to stimulation sites over the course of an experiment. When utilizing a single cap with non-overlapping, interleaved stimulation sites; the option of stimulation at specific data acquisition sites is not available; instead stimulation is delivered to neighboring sites. For example, with an M1SO (motor to contralateral supraorbital) stimulation montage, data can be acquired over the motor cortex from standard site C3 and stimulation can be delivered at standard site C5 (centimeters away from C3) with a contralateral supraorbital return electrode at F8. Utilizing two different caps, involves acquiring data then swapping caps to one that holds stimulation sites then applying stimulation (or vice versa). In this case, if data acquisition and stimulation are done in close temporal proximity to each other, technical issues like gel smearing can arise. This smearing of gel can lead to electrical bridging with EEG data acquisition or current shunting with stimulation and is typically not recommended.

Online EEG-tDCS

If EEG data acquisition during stimulation (or "online" stimulation) is of interest and amplifier bandwidth can accommodate large voltages, then several options, similar to offline stimulation, are available with the use of a single cap. Single or integrated caps can have (1) overlapping stimulation and acquisition sites where at each scalp location electrodes can acquire EEG data or be used to deliver stimulation; or (2) non-overlapping stimulation and acquisition sites where there are sites dedicated solely to data acquisition and additional interleaved scalp locations dedicated to stimulation

(Fig. 11.4a); or (3) selectively removed acquisition sites. When using a cap with overlapping sites, locations for stimulation and data acquisition can be digitally selected and EEG data can be derived from the same points of stimulation during the stimulation. When utilizing online stimulation with non-overlapping sites, acquired data are in close proximity (centimeters away) to stimulation sites but do not overlap with them. With selective removal of acquisition sites, selected EEG recording sites are mechanically removed at some point over the course of an experiment and replaced with stimulating electrodes. They can either be removed during the course of both data acquisition and stimulation or just over the course of stimulation.

Stimulation Device Selection

When designing stimulation protocol, the choice of stimulation device is of great importance. With tDCS, devices that specifically deliver a direct current should be used. Ideally devices that adhere to circuit architectures that utilize current controlled, current sources should be utilized for DC delivery. In many cases, studies performing tDCS have resorted to utilizing iontophoresis devices, which in essence do deliver an averaged desired DC output, but have voltage outputs that are oscillatory. When acquiring online stimulation EEG data with devices such as iontophoresis devices, large oscillatory voltage artifacts can be introduced in acquired EEG data (Fig. 11.5a). These oscillating artifacts can be difficult to attenuate in post processing and can significantly decimate signal quality. For these reasons stimulation devices should be tested to ensure they deliver a stable DC, prior to incorporating them into integrated online stimulation and EEG protocols (see also section "Inherent Stimulator Artifacts").

Characteristics of the DC Voltage

During HD-tDCS, the application of an external direct current strongly influences the recorded voltages at all EEG electrodes (Fig. 11.4b–e). Across protocols (application routines, montages, currents), the largest deviations in voltage track the applied current, increasing to a value during the tDCS ramp up, generally maintaining the value (the "DC offset") during the sustained current phase, and decreasing along with the tDCS ramp down (Fig. 11.5a). The largest positive and negative voltage deviations are observed near the anode and cathode, respectively. These polarity specific offsets indicate that DC offset is montage specific. This indicates that the EEG voltage profile for an M1SO stimulation montage will be different from that of a Bifrontal stimulation montage. Applying 2 mA of current during tDCS produces a DC offset that is up to 1000 fold larger than baseline neural EEG signals (Fig. 11.5a). This large voltage offset is also consistent across all different types of stimulation devices that deliver a DC.

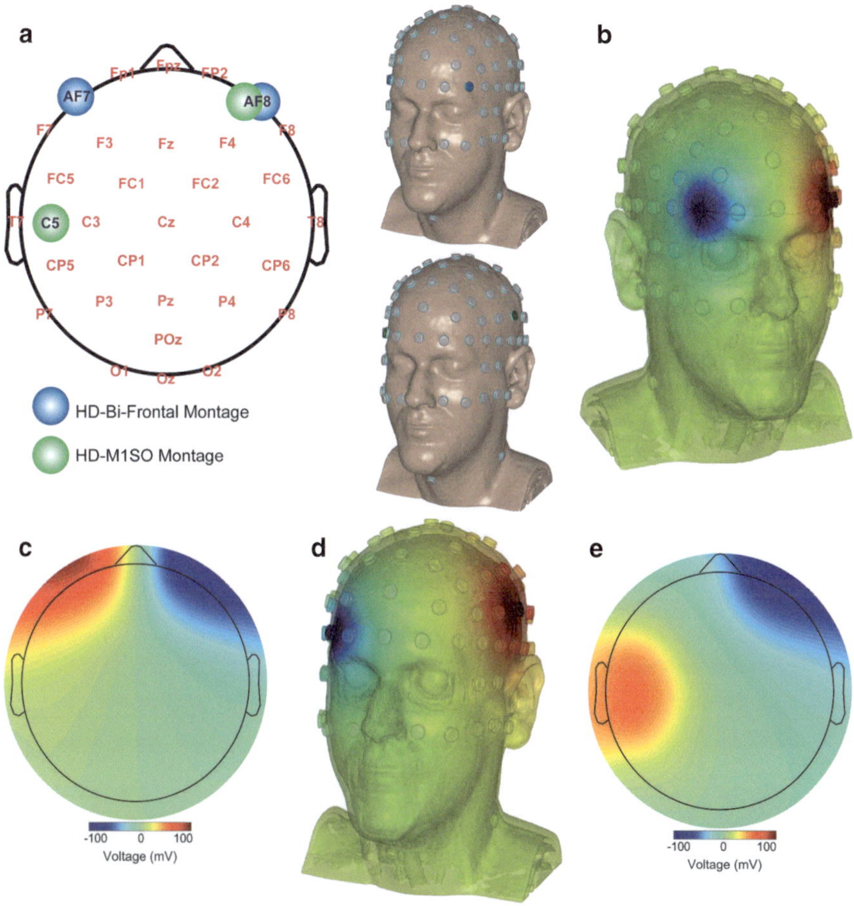

Fig. 11.4 (**a**) EEG cap layout with the locations of the integrated stimulation sites indicated at sites AF7, AF8, and C5. The HD-Bifrontal stimulation montage is demonstrated (blue pairs) where electrodes are placed over standard sites AF7 and AF8. The HD-M1SO montage is demonstrated (green pairs) where electrodes are placed over standard sites AF8 and C5. In both cases polarities can be interchanged within each montage. MRI derived head model indicating scalp locations of stimulating electrodes for HD-Bifrontal stimulation (top, blue disks), HD-M1SO stimulation (bottom, green disks), and some EEG recording electrodes (gray disks). (**b**) Skin voltage distribution predicted by computational models for 2 mA of HD-Bifrontal stimulation where the anode is placed at AF8 and the cathode is placed at AF7. Flux lines (black) indicate direction of current flow across the skin, with maximal voltages near the anode and cathode as well as in frontal EEG electrodes. (**c**) Topographic voltage distribution for 2 mA of HD-Bifrontal stimulation from model predictions. Model scalp voltages were sampled at EEG recording sites for HD-Bifrontal stimulation. (**d**) Skin voltage distribution predicted by computational models for HD-M1SO stimulation where the anode is placed at C5 and the cathode is placed at AF8. Flux lines (black) indicate direction of current flow across the skin, with maximal voltages near the anode and cathode as well as in frontal and left parietal EEG electrodes. (**e**) Topographic voltage distribution for HD-M1SO stimulation from model predictions. Model scalp voltages were sampled at EEG recording sites for HD-M1SO stimulation. With both montages, colorbars indicate voltages for both computational models' skin voltage and scalp topographic distributions

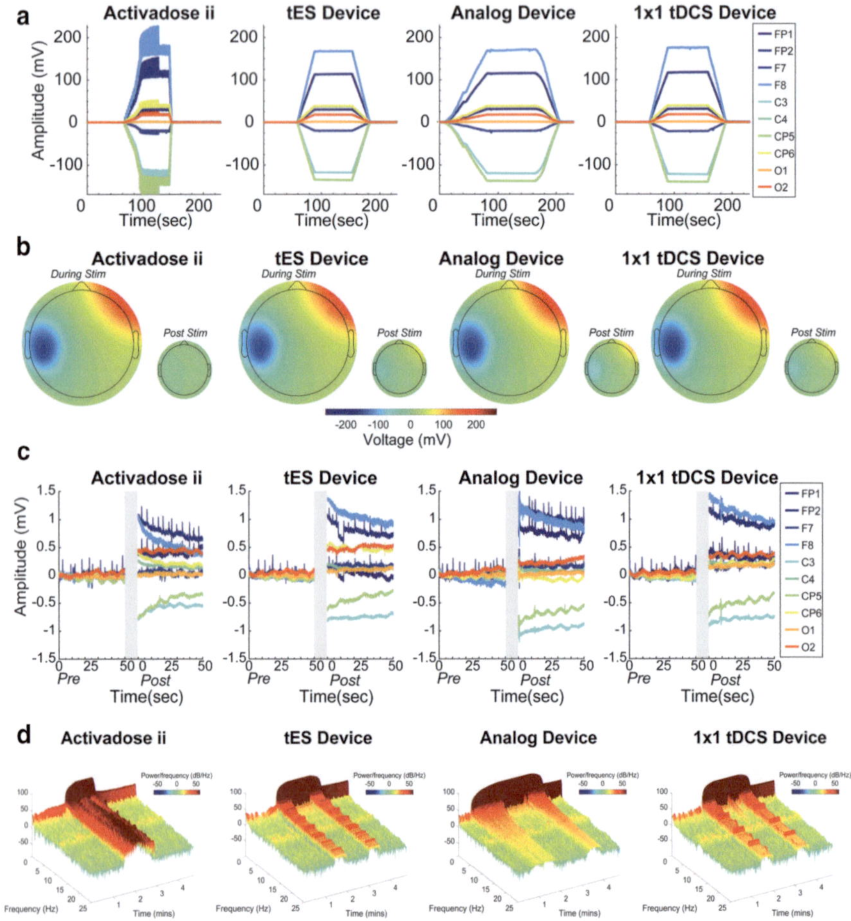

Fig. 11.5 (**a**) Voltage over time across different stimulation devices. The largest voltage offsets or DC voltage is seen at electrodes closest to the stimulation sites (anode: AF8, cathode: C5). The linear ramp-up and ramp-down periods can also be observed at the beginning and end of the stimulation period. (**b**) Mean voltage topographies across stimulation devices where the largest voltage negativity is observed near the cathode (C5) and the largest voltage positivity is observed near the anode (AF8). During the post stimulation period mean voltage topographies show the presence of residual scalp voltage across devices. The spatial distribution of the post stimulation voltage topographies is identical those during stimulation. (**c**) Post stimulation, electrodes exhibit a decay in voltage. Electrodes that are closest to the stimulation sites show the largest residual voltage after stimulation ends. (**d**) Spectrograms over time show the broadband distortion produced during the ramp-up and ramp-down periods. They also show the low-frequency spectral density offset produced during stimulation as well as post stimulation. Physiologically related frequency bands can be seen between 8 and 12 Hz across the pre, during, and post stimulation periods. (**e**) Across devices, the frequency distribution across electrodes differed. Electrodes near the anode show larger power offsets than those near the cathode at lower frequencies (0–10 Hz). (**f**) Compared to baseline conditions electrodes near the cathode (C5) show pronounced peaks between 1 and 1.2 Hz

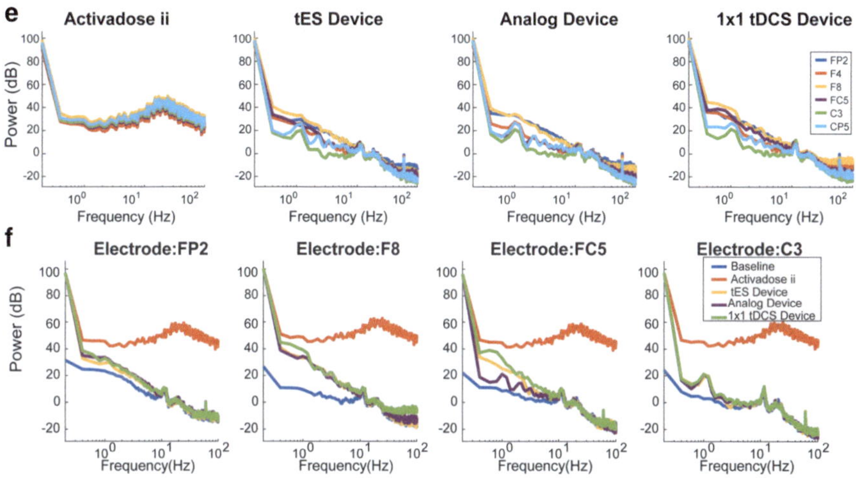

Fig. 11.5 (continued)

The DC offset can sometimes change incrementally ("drift") while stimulation is sustained (Hahn et al. 2013), this fractional change (up to ~ 3 mV or 2% of the DC offset over 50 secs with 2 mA of current) is still larger than EEG signals in general. Residual DC offset post stimulation can also be evident for up to approximately 1 min after the end of the ramp down (Fig. 11.2c). These residual voltages are significantly less than the peak DC offset during stimulation (~1.5 mV) but are on the order of magnitude of drift in the DC offset during stimulation. The spatial distribution of the scalp topography of the residual DC offset (scalp voltage after stimulation) is comparable to that of the DC offset during stimulation (scalp voltage during stimulation), where it has the largest positive and negative values near the anode and cathode electrodes, respectively (See Fig. 11.5b Post Stim).

Characteristics of the Spectral Profile

By utilizing spectrograms, the broadband harmonic distortions created during the ramp-up/ramp-down periods of the stimulators as a result of the stepwise escalation/de-escalation of current and resultant stepwise voltage offset can be easily illustrated (Fig. 11.5d). The distortions created during the ramp-up/ramp-down periods introduce broadband noise that contaminate these period of online stimulation EEG data and can be difficult to attenuate during post processing. After ramp-up though, this broadband step-wise contamination is eliminated during the delivery of the DC. During stimulation, significant power at low frequency (~0 Hz) reflect the DC offset. Overall low frequency activity (<10 Hz), also has increased power compared to no stimulation conditions. The reduced but significant DC offset post stimulation is also apparent and should be noted (See period after ramp-down in Fig. 11.5d).

With online stimulation, EEG features like inherent alpha activity (8–12 Hz) can be resolved with proper frequency windowing. In some cases, spectrograms can reveal increased low frequency activity (1–1.2 Hz) during but not pre or post stimulation, with higher power near stimulation electrodes (see also Fig. 11.5e). For example, clear 1–1.2 Hz peaks are observed at electrode C3, nearest the cathode (C5), whereas at electrodes FP2 and F8 such prominent peaks are not evident (possibly due to blink interference at frontal channels; Fig. 11.5f).

Linearity of DC Voltage

With Bifrontal stimulation (anode:AF7, cathode: AF8), EEG electrodes closest to the anode exhibit a positive voltage offset and those near the cathode exhibit a negative voltage offset; whereas the opposite polarities can be seen at the aforementioned electrodes when the stimulation polarities are switched (anode:AF8, cathode:AF7; Fig. 11.6a). In this case electrodes F7 and F8 exhibited the highest voltage changes, whereas those further away from the stimulating electrodes exhibited a smaller change in voltage during stimulation (Fig. 11.6b).

When the current intensity is increased (from 0.5 to 2.0 mA), scalp topographies show increases in the area of the high voltage offsets (both negative and positive depending on the montage used; Fig. 11.6b). When applying a series of different current intensities (i.e. 0.5, 1.0 1.5, 2.0 mA) over the course of one EEG recording, the mean voltage offset for repeated current intensities are linearly correlated across the majority of EEG electrodes (Fig. 11.6c). This is true for different current polarities as well (i.e. switching the anode and cathode). In other words, the voltage offset changes linearly between applied current intensities. Although electrodes further away from the stimulation sites do not exhibit large voltage offsets, they do show a linear relationship across applied stimulation intensities. Taking the topographic difference between stimulation intensities results in a slope computation across the scalp and shows that the change in voltage between current intensities has identical spatial patterning across the scalp (Fig. 11.6d). This demonstrates that although there is a large voltage change between stimulation intensities the slope or increase in voltage (mV/mA) remains similar between stimulation intensities.

Inherent Physiologic Artifacts

Inherent physiological artifacts can be characterized as artifacts that are independent of stimulators as well as EEG devices and that result from physiologic integration with the overall DC artifact produced by stimulation (see Fig. 11.5a). These physiologic artifacts that occur during stimulation can range over a broad spectrum of physiologic processes, however here we highlight four types of physiological distortions that are seen during concurrent EEG and tDCS. These include cardiac

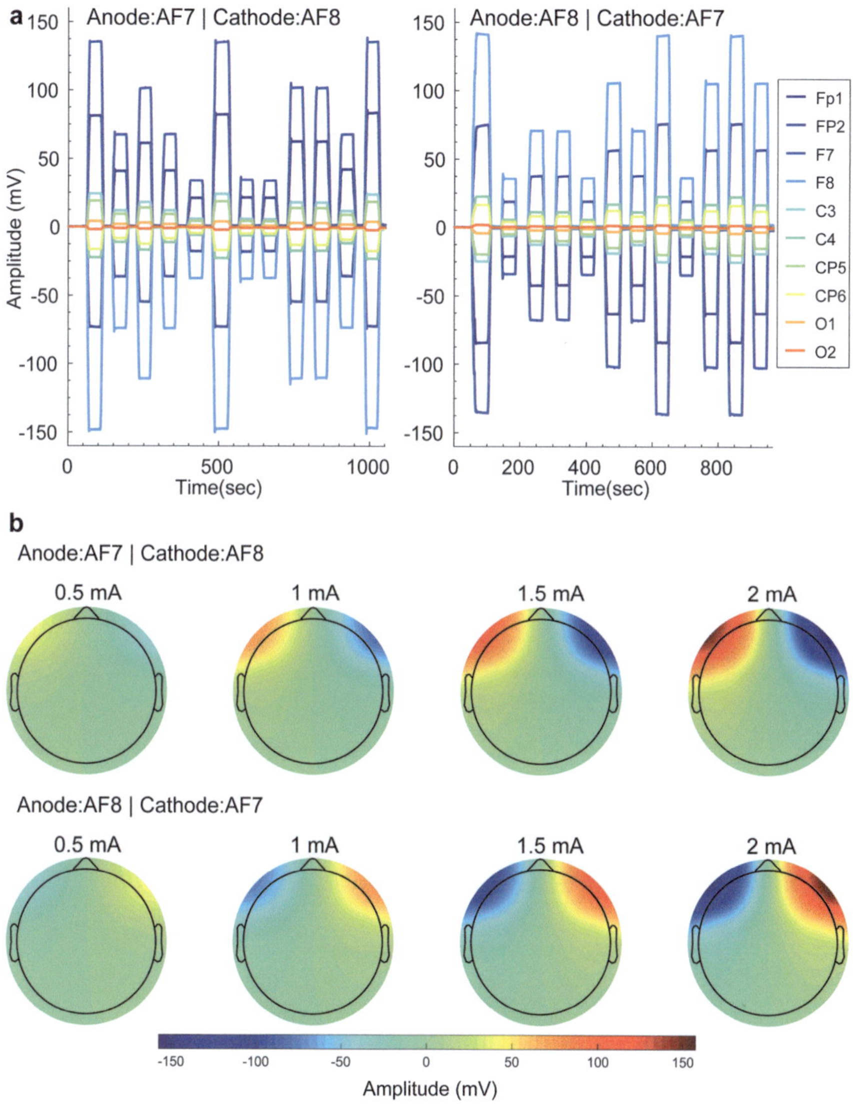

Fig. 11.6 (**a**) EEG voltage over time with online stimulation and EEG. The DC voltage offset can be seen when randomized current intensities between 0.5–2.0 mA are applied and removed over time. The largest DC voltage offset is seen at electrodes closest to the anode and cathode. (**b**) For Bifrontal stimulation frontal EEG electrodes have the largest increase (negatively and positively) with increasing current intensity. Areas under the anode have large positive offsets whereas those under the cathode have larger negative offsets. (**c**) The mean voltage offset across applied current intensities for both stimulation polarities are linearly correlated across the majority of EEG electrodes. (**d**) The change in voltage between current intensities (mV/mA) have identical spatial patterning across the scalp for different current intensities. This spatial patterning is consistent across current intensities applied for both stimulation polarities

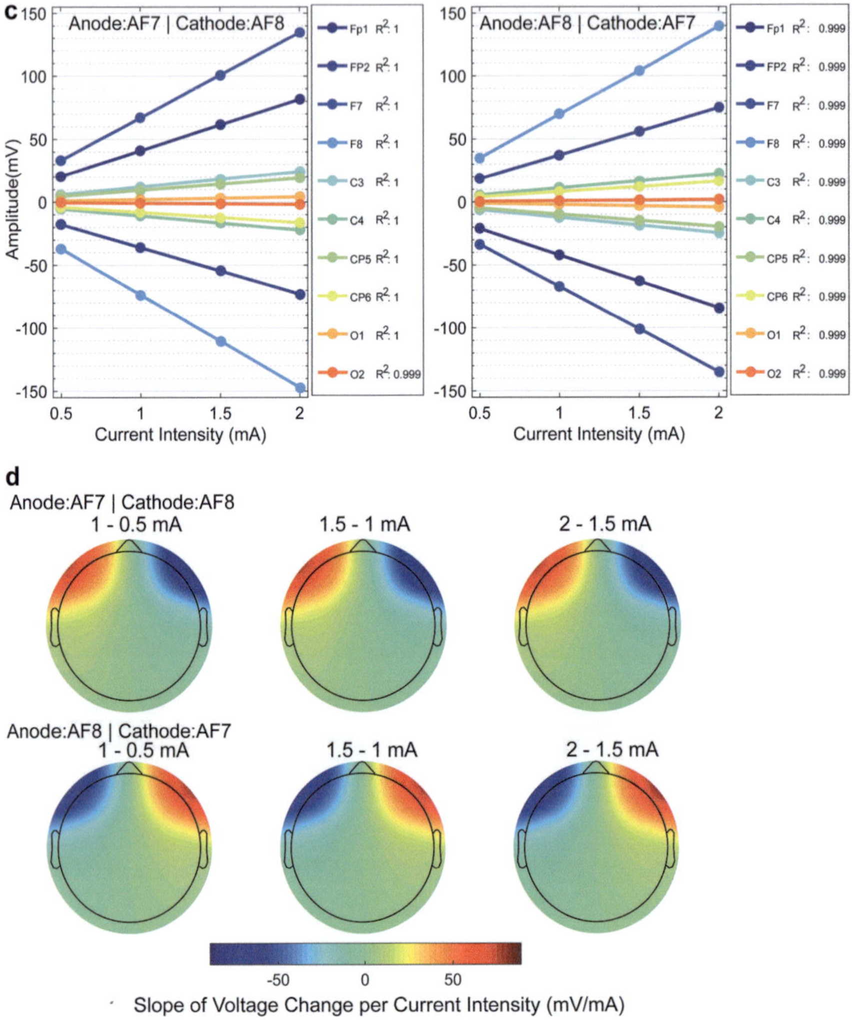

Fig. 11.6 (continued)

artifacts, oculomotor artifacts, myogenic artifacts, and DC drift artifacts. We also talk about the use of computational head models, which can be used to model and understand the dynamics and sources of these artifacts.

We define “physiologic stimulation artifacts” as real changes in the voltage on scalp that reflect physical interaction of applied current with the body – by definition these artifacts are then inherent (or unavoidable) to any stimulation or recording hardware. Of particular concern is if such physiologic artifacts, by failing to meet the assumptions above, may not be removed or properly attenuated by conventional signal processing techniques, leading to spurious conclusions. Identifying the mechanisms and features of physiologic artifacts allows for identifying and applying suitable signal processing and having greater confidence in outcomes.

Physiological Artifact: Cardiac Artifact

The cardiac artifact, sometimes referred to as a ballistocardiographic artifact or ballistocardiogram (Rubin and Daube 2016; Schmitt 2017), can be observed consistently during stimulation and is highly disruptive to acquired data. The artifact, which can sometimes resemble and be mistaken for stimulator shifts in voltage (Roy et al. 2014), is stimulation device independent (Fig. 11.7a, b), montage specific (see Fig. 11.7b, f), narrowband (Fig. 11.7c), and stimulation intensity specific (Fig. 11.7e).

When paired with concurrent electrocardiogram (ECG) the oscillatory cardiac artifact shows consistent peaks following the QRS complex but preceding the T-wave of the ECG (Fig. 11.7a). These cardiac related peaks can be observed across different types of DC stimulators, excluding iontophoresis devices which can introduce device related artifacts obscuring the cardiac artifact. The artifacts' peaks are also polarity dependent and montage specific indicating that it is strongest near stimulation electrodes (Fig. 11.7b). In the frequency domain, the cardiac artifact's activity is seen as a low frequency, heartbeat-locked peak at approximately 1 Hz (depending on subjects' heart rate; Fig. 11.7c). This activity is seen during but not before or after stimulation. Analogous to the DC offsets, this activity is present in electrodes closest to the stimulating electrodes in a montage specific manner. Since the cardiac artifact exhibits a slow rise and fall that is time locked relative to the R-wave of ECG signals and is montage specific; it is believed to be a mechanical cardiac signal amplified with local changes in skin impedance during stimulation (Noury et al. 2016).

The artifact can also be easily produced with currents as low as 0.5 mA and increases as more current is introduced during stimulation (Fig. 11.7e–g). The montage specificity is seen with the spatial scalp distribution of the cardiac artifact; a maximal negative deflection is present nearest the cathode and maximal positive deflection is present nearest the anode (Fig. 11.7b, f). EEG electrodes further away from the stimulating electrodes however do not exhibit significant voltage modulations resulting from the cardiac artifact.

Assuming a skin impedance change of 0.01% during stimulation, a computational model can be generated to simulate the cardiac artifact's spatial distribution and the magnitude of its voltage deflection. Incorporating the aforementioned assumptions, the computational models predict that for HD-Bifrontal stimulation, anterior recording electrodes would undergo higher voltage amplitude changes during a cardiac pulse, with decreasing voltage deviation with increasingly posterior electrode locations (Fig. 11.7g). These predictions corroborate the notion that tDCS first creates a montage specific distribution of scalp voltages that is then modulated at each pulse by a global change in scalp impedance.

The concerning aspects of the appearance of the cardiac artifact is its stimulation dependent amplitude as well as its time variant scalp distribution. With skin impedance being a dynamic factor, the cardiac artifact could be highly influenced by subjects' physiological and psychological state (Luft and Bhattacharya 2015) during stimulation where anxieties or fears during tDCS can cause a raise in heartbeat and increase sweating, nonlinearly altering acquired data. In electrodes adjacent to stimulation sites, the cardiac artifact can be seen to increase up to approximately

40 μV with 2 mA of current, which is larger than most event-related potentials (ERPs) (Dinteren et al. 2014) and raises concerns with previous concurrent online EEG and stimulation studies that have examined ERPs (Cunillera et al. 2015; Faehling and Plewnia 2016). Detectable changes in the overall voltage offset of the

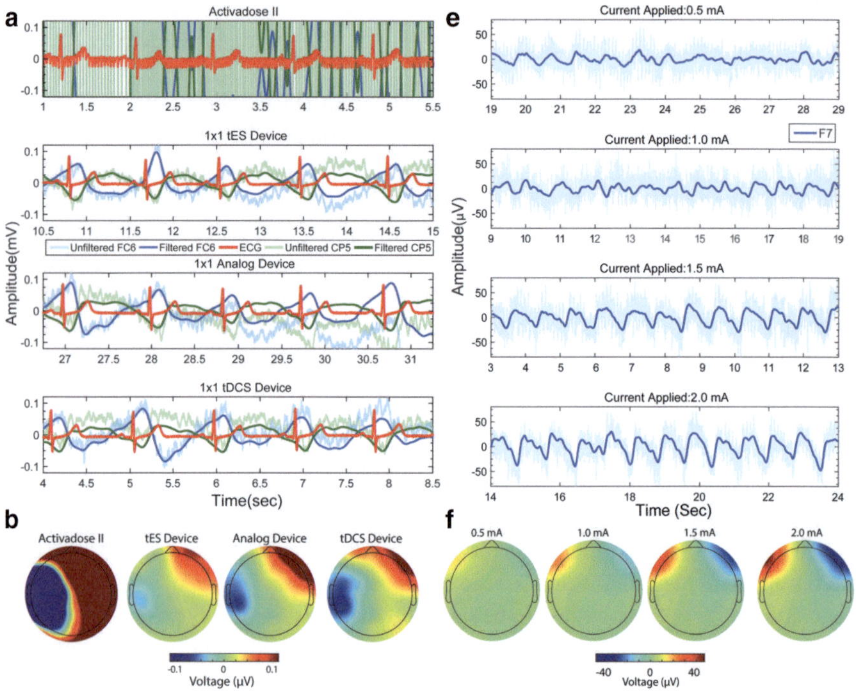

Fig. 11.7 (**a**) The cardiac artifact is reproducible with a range of stimulation devices, with the exception of the Activadose II, which produces large-amplitude, high-frequency broadband noise during stimulation in EEG data as well as in ECG electrodes. The cardiac artifact appears as consistent peaks following the QRS complex but preceding the T-wave of the ECG. Detrended traces for electrodes FC6 and CP5 are also present for comparison. (**b**) Scalp topographies during the peak of the cardiac artifact across stimulation devices show that the artifact is montage specific since the artifacts' spatial distribution is reflective of the stimulation montage. (**c**) A comparison of ECG; and EEG baseline (not powered), during, and post stimulation. A prominent peak at 1–1.2 Hz is present for both the ECG and EEG during stimulation conditions, but not for EEG baseline (not powered) and post stimulation. (**d**) ECG, ECG envelope, and respiration signal over time. During stimulation, the overall ECG signal has a pronounced DC offset. Linear changes in the ECG voltage during the stimulation ramp-up and ramp-down periods are also present. (**e**) The cardiac artifact over time with applied current intensities of 0.5, 1.0, 1.5, and 2.0 mA. (**f**) Mean scalp topographies at the peak of the cardiac artifact during 0.5, 1.0, 1.5, and 2.0 mA of applied current. (**g**) Mean and SEM of cardiac artifact peaks at electrodes F7 and F8 during stimulation for current intensities of 0.5, 1.0, 1.5, and 2.0 mA. (**h**) Computational model prediction of the spatial scalp distribution of the cardiac artifact during HD-Bifrontal stimulation

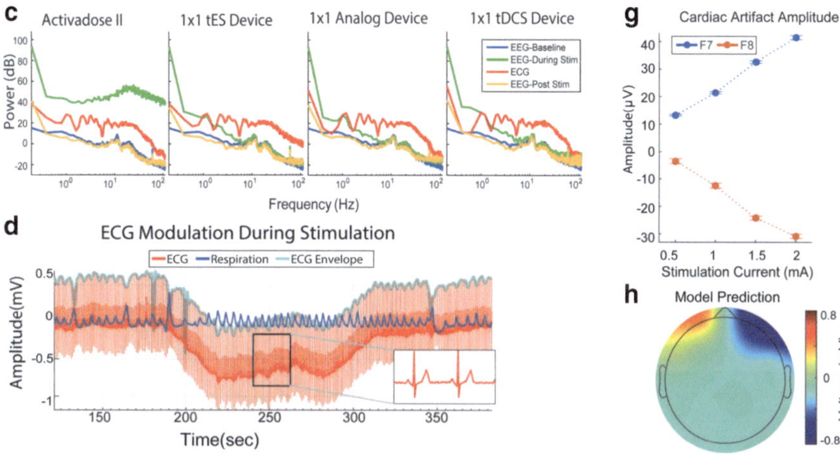

Fig. 11.7 (continued)

ECG signals (~0.5 mV), measured across the chest during stimulation, also raise further questions about how stimulation interacts with autonomic nervous system (Clancy et al. 2014; Schestatsky et al. 2013; Schroeder et al. 2015; Vandermeeren et al. 2010), which could in turn result in changes to the cardiac artifact, as well as heart rate or heart rate variability. In the clinical domain, studies examining the online effects of tDCS are cautioned when it comes to patients who have disorders affecting cardiac function. With the aforementioned studies, concurrent ECG with EEG monitoring is highly recommended. As such, patients with cardiac dysfunctions may introduce further variability to the already time variable cardiac artifacts, which can be misinterpreted as alterations in low frequency Delta activity in acquired EEG data. Reassuringly though, the artifact disappears with the removal of the DC current after both long and short periods of stimulation, attesting to the artifact's dynamics.

Physiological Artifact: Ocular Motor Artifact

During stimulation, strong modulatory effects are observed in relation to ocular motor or blink responses. Amplitudes of these physiologic responses can become highly variable across stimulation current intensities as well as across stimulation montages. The spatial distribution during blink responses become altered during stimulation, in a stimulation montage specific manner.

Depending on the montage used and compared to baseline or no stimulation conditions, the blink artifact amplitude increases, inverts in polarity, or becomes unrecognizably low in amplitude that it appears to be suppressed (see Fig. 11.8a).

These alterations are consistent across DC stimulators (Fig. 11.8b). Interestingly, the latency of the blink propagation between the left and right eye remains unaltered; remaining time-locked under pre, during, and post stimulation conditions. Near the anode, where a positive scalp voltage is present, blink artifacts have large decreases in amplitude opposed to near the cathode, where a negative scalp voltage

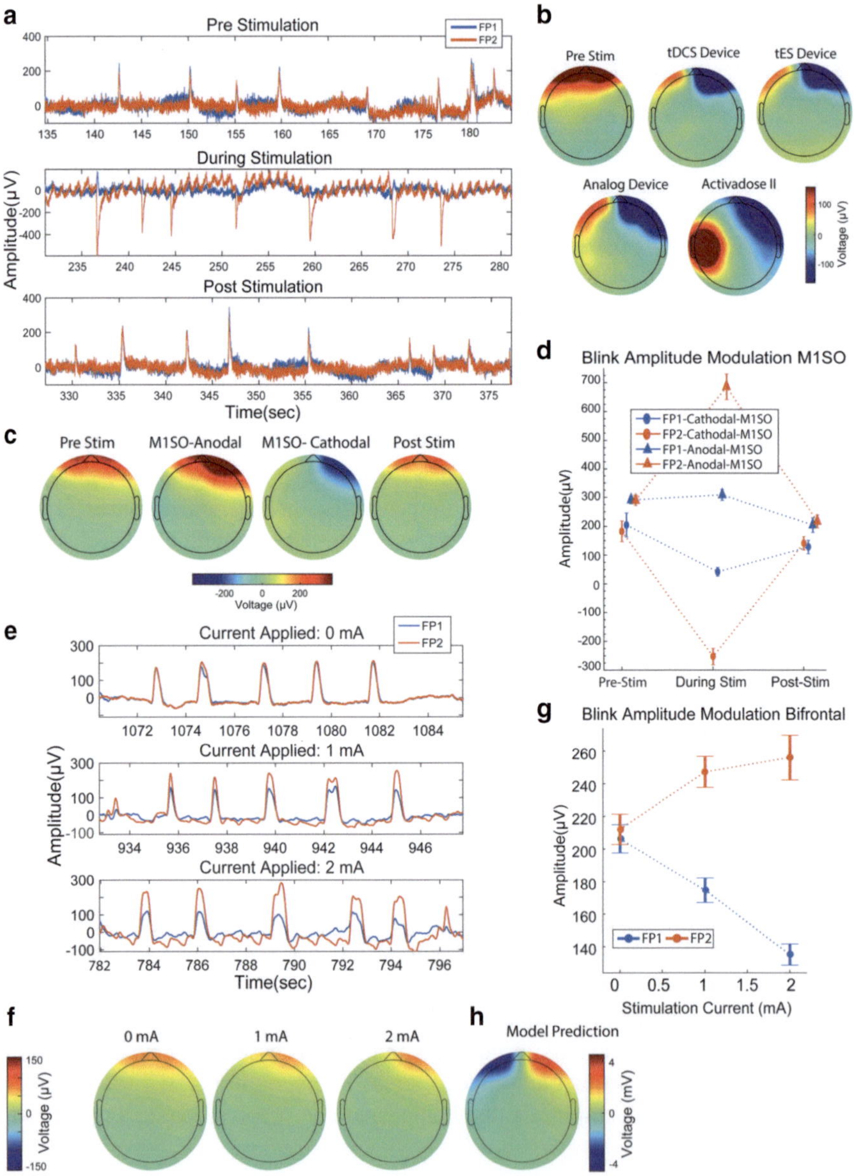

is present, where blink artifacts have large increases in voltage during stimulation (Fig. 11.8c, d). Within stimulation montages the ocular motor amplitude modulation linearly increases or decreases with stimulation intensity (Fig. 11.8e–g). These dramatic changes in amplitude are believed to be a result of eyelid closure with possible smaller contributions from the shifting of the eyes' retinocorneal dipole (Berg and Scherg 1991; Iwasaki et al. 2005). With the eyelids closing during stimulation, they considerably alter the path of the applied current on the scalp and distort the resultant positive amplitude normally seen with Cz referential montages.

These alterations pose problems for automatic artifact rejection algorithms since during stimulation the blink artifact becomes highly distorted in some cases. Previous studies examining tDCS effects on blink responses in healthy subjects using electrooculogram (EOG; Beyer et al. 2017; Cabib et al. 2016; Zuchowski et al. 2014) may also be affected by these artifactual voltage modulations. Similarly, any future studies in the clinical domain using EOG as an online biomarker in tDCS trials with disorders including Parkinson's disease, or multiple sclerosis, would be cautioned. As with other physiologic artifacts the use of traditional control experiments (changing montage) and some signal processing corrections may not suffice. Fortunately though the topographic spatial distribution of scalp voltages during blinks were somewhat predictable based on the overall average topographic scalp distribution during stimulation, which could provide means for development of more dynamic blink artifact rejection methods.

To model the nature of the altered blink responses during concurrent EEG and stimulation computational models can be utilized. In order to model simplistic blink responses, skin over the eye (eyelids) are removed from the computational head

Fig. 11.8 (**a**) During the pre and post-stimulation time periods, both FP1 and FP2 detect positive blink deflections. During the course of cathodal M1SO (referring to cathode:C3, anode:AF8) stimulation the blink responses at FP2 (near the anode) reverse in polarity and show a high amplitude negative deflection, whereas blink responses at FP1 decrease in amplitude and maintain a diminished but positive polarity. (**b**) A comparison of blink responses across stimulating devices compared to pre-stimulation. During stimulation a negative monopole is present in electrodes over the right SO locations (near the anode) and a positive monopole is present in electrodes over the left SO locations, across devices (with the exception of the Activadose II) for the application of 2 mA of cathodal M1SO stimulation, whereas Bifrontal positive dipoles are present over both eyes, pre- stimulation. (**c**) Blink scalp topographies for pre-stimulation, during 1 mA of anodal M1SO stimulation (cathode:AF8, anode:C3), during 1 mA of cathodal M1SO stimulation (cathode:C3, anode:AF8), and post-stimulation conditions. (**d**) Mean and SEM of blink amplitudes at electrodes FP1 and FP2 during 1 mA of M1SO anodal and cathodal stimulation, compared to pre and post-stimulation blink responses. (**e**) Blink responses at FP1 and FP2 over time during 0, 1, and 2 mA of current with a Bifrontal stimulation montage. As the current intensity increases the difference between peak blink amplitude, between FP1 and FP2, increases. (**f**) Blink scalp topographies during 0, 1, and 2 mA of current with a Bifrontal stimulation montage. (**g**) Mean and SEM of blink amplitudes at electrodes FP1 and FP2 for 0 mA, 1 mA, and 2 mA of applied current with a Bifrontal stimulation montage. As the current intensity increases the difference in peak amplitudes between FP1 and FP2 becomes larger. (**h**) Computational model prediction of blink scalp topography during HD-Bifrontal stimulation

models. The difference between model predictions during stimulation with and without eyelids produced an overall scalp topography akin to that seen during EEG. Like topographic voltage distribution seen during EEG, the model prediction demonstrates that with Bifrontal stimulation there is an elevated left SO positive voltage and an elevated right SO negative voltage (Fig. 11.8h). These predictions support the notion that blink responses increase near the cathode whereas they decreased near the anode.

Physiological Artifact: Myogenic Distortions

During stimulation myogenic artifacts, related to facial muscle contraction or jaw clenches, are seen to be montage specific, broadband, and are highly modulated in a current intensity specific manner (Fig. 11.9a–c), similar to the blink and cardiac artifacts. With higher current intensities, the overall broadband activity shifts in amplitude depending on the stimulation montage used. Increasing current intensity, introduces a low frequency drift to the high frequency muscle activity, during muscle contraction. This activity is variable across the scalp and the divergence in amplitude between left and right hemispheric high frequency activity increases with increased bilaterally applied current (HD-Bifrontal; Fig. 11.9a, b). In terms of spatial scalp location, during stimulation and jaw clenching, the DC alters the distribution and polarity of the muscle activity seen on the scalp, compared to muscle activity without stimulation (Fig. 11.9c).

Myogenic interactions during EEG, specifically electromyography (EMG) without stimulation, are the result of contractions of primarily the masseter, temporalis and frontalis muscles (Goncharova et al. 2003; Whitham et al. 2007). These contractions can significantly contaminate acquired data due to its high amplitude, and broadband spectral and anatomical overlap with neurogenic sources (Barlow 1985; Shackman et al. 2009). When combined with stimulation, these myogenic distortions become exacerbated and with their overlap with neurogenic sources, makes it even more difficult for correction algorithms to separate both sources. These myogenic interactions, like the cardiac artifact, can be influenced by subjects' physiological and psychological state (Bradley et al. 2001; Coan and Allen 2003; Tassinary et al. 2007; Waterink and van Boxtel 1994), resulting in variable muscle activation. Even weak facial muscle contractions have been shown to produce low frequency EEG activity that can be mistaken for changes in cognitive related frequency bands like Alpha rhythms (Goncharova et al. 2003; Lee and Buchsbaum 1987; Willis et al. 1993), which can be especially concerning when these artifacts are accentuated by stimulation currents. In the clinical setting, these EMG artifacts may appear in patients with conditions including facial myokymia, hemifacial spasm, or palatal myoclonus (Westmoreland 1996). Caution should be taken in cases like these and other disorders affecting myogenic activity since coupled with stimulation, resultant

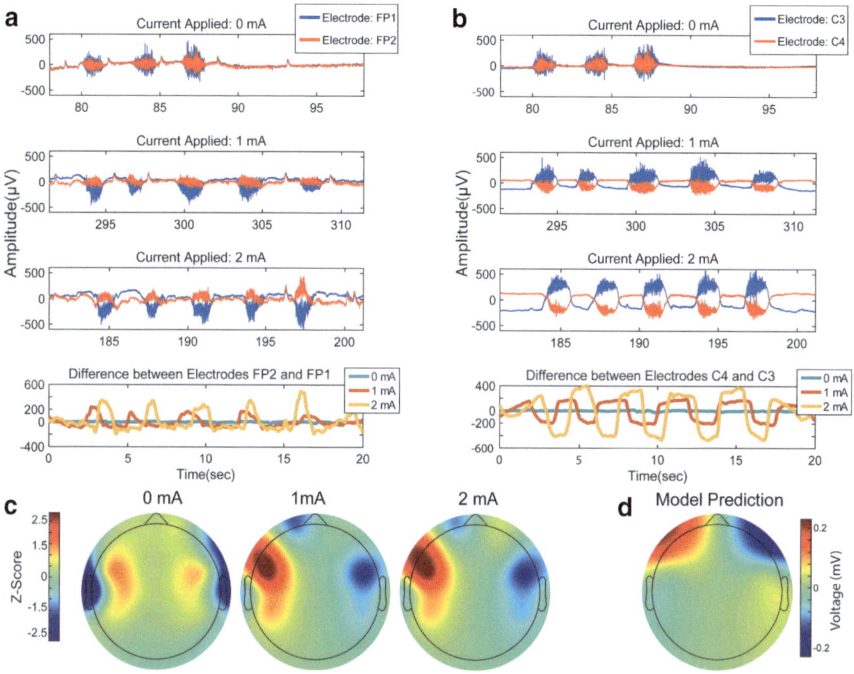

Fig. 11.9 (**a**) Jaw clenches over time detected at bilateral electrodes FP1 and FP2 for applied currents of 0, 1, and 2 mA. Currents were applied in a HD-Bifrontal montage and voltages at FP1 (near the anode) diverged negatively from FP2 with increasing current. (**b**) Jaw clenches over time at bilateral electrodes C3 and C4 for applied currents of 0, 1, and 2 mA. Currents were applied in a HD-Bifrontal montage and voltages at C3 (near the anode) diverged positively from C4 with increasing current. (**c**) Average scalp topographies during jaw clenches plotted as z-scores for comparison. (**d**) Computational model prediction of the spatial scalp distribution of EMG activity resulting from jaw clenches during stimulation

artifacts can be misinterpreted as epileptiform activity or modulations in the frequency domain. These modulations with stimulation however, did not outlast the duration of stimulation and disappeared as the external current was removed.

In order to model EMG activity resulting from jaw clenches during stimulation, the masseter and temporalis muscles are incorporated into MRI-derived computational models. Muscle fibers are represented over the mandible for the masseter muscle and over temporal regions of the skull for the temporalis muscles. The scalp voltages produced by tDCS are then computed with either "relaxed" muscle properties assigned or "active" muscle properties – assuming a 1% muscle conductivity change during to muscle fiber activation. The difference in scalp voltages between the two models gives a prediction of the spatial profile of the myogenic artifact. This muscle activity on the scalp during stimulation, are in accord with the overall DC produced with EEG derived voltages, but do not fully capture the voltage shift during muscle contraction (Fig. 11.9d).

Physiological Artifact: DC Drift

The physiologically related DC drift artifact usually arises from increased perspiration on the scalp (Klass 1995), which consequently alters skin impedance. During EEG this physiologically related DC drift usually takes the form of a low frequency (<0.5 Hz), high amplitude wave (Corby et al. 1974; Picton and Hillyard 1972). During concurrent tDCS and EEG, this non-stationary physiologic artifact can be exacerbated with the introduction of a DC current. With stimulation, this artifact can be high amplitude, low-frequency, narrowbanded, change over the course of the stimulation session, montage specific (normally localized nearest the points of high perspiration, however strongest effect can be seen nearest stimulating electrodes during tDCS), and under some circumstances outlast the duration of stimulation if left unattended. Although not detrimental to data quality since the artifact can be attenuated in post processing, care should be taken to avoid such artifacts in order to acquire the highest quality of EEG data.

Inherent Stimulator Artifacts

With concurrent HD-tDCS and EEG, one source of significant extraphysiologic noise introduction can arise from the stimulators themselves. Stimulators that produce variable current outputs and not a constant direct current can distort and decimate the voltage profile of acquired EEG. These artifacts, referred to as inherent stimulator artifacts, are described as artifacts that are universal to any stimulator/EEG system used, however its severity or impact on data quality is variable. Inherent stimulator artifacts can be divided into three main types of artifactual distortions: broadband noise artifact, "on noise" artifact, and DC-offset artifact.

The broadband noise artifact describes the fact that, under ideal conditions, no simulator can generate an ideal DC without the introduction of power at unintended frequencies. This type of artifact, as its name suggests, produces distortion or non-linear modulations of both signal and noise across several frequencies (hence broadband) including those of physiologic interest with EEG. With this type of artifact, during tDCS the highest modulation can be seen around 0 Hz (the DC frequency) when compared to pre stimulation or no stimulation conditions (device off baseline). The broadband noise artifact can also change over the course of a stimulation session as a result of stimulator reactivity or impedance changes on the scalp. This type of artifact usually does not outlast stimulation and usually disappears after the stimulator is turned off, however residual scalp voltages together with skin impedance changes post stimulation can produce low frequency broadband modulations (see Fig. 11.7c). When it comes to the artifacts spatial variation on the scalp, the broadband noise artifact is seen to be montage and current intensity specific, having maximal distortion in EEG electrodes nearest to the stimulating electrodes in a manner reflective of/tracing the scalp DC voltage.

The “On noise” artifact is the result of leakage or injection of stimulator noise into the recording electrodes while the stimulating device is on yet not stimulating (See time zero onwards in Fig. 11.10a). In some cases large voltage offsets can be seen when the stimulation device is turned on and noise can occur when these devices check impedances before stimulation. This type of artifact has been shown to be broadband, montage specific, additive, and can possibly outlast stimulation if the stimulation device is left connected and on.

The DC-Offset artifact refers to the large voltage offset produced during stimulation (See during stimulation period Fig. 11.2a). This offset, under ideal stimulator and EEG data acquisition conditions, is stable and linear; however, the DC-offset can be somewhat non-stationary and fluctuate over the course of stimulation due to physiologic changes in scalp impedance or subject perspiration. Under non-ideal hardware conditions slow dynamic changes can be seen as the result of the stimulator used, in that the stimulator does not produce a stable DC current; as a result of impedance changes within the stimulator; or as a result of non-linear EEG amplifier performance if voltages reach amplifier limitations.

Non-inherent Artifacts

Artifacts created as a result of non-ideal experimental conditions or set-up can be classified as non-inherent artifacts. These artifacts can easily arise if quality control is not met or strict data monitoring is not performed. Although non-inherent artifacts span a wide range of classifications, here we focus on stimulation and movement distortion, EEG saturation, EEG distortion, and electrode bridging.

Similar to myogenic artifacts, movement disruption during EEG and stimulation can result in robust signal distortion of neural signal. Abrupt or slow head rotation or tilting can introduce broadband noise and in some cases fully distort neural activity during concurrent stimulation and EEG. When examined with concurrent displacement recordings in the X, Y and Z, directions from Cz; spectrograms over time and frequency show that during 2 mA M1SO (anode M1) stimulation, slow neck rolling motions greatly disrupted acquired data. EEG electrodes nearest to the stimulating electrodes (F8) show the largest distortions over time and frequency whereas those further away show lesser distortions (O2; Fig. 11.10b, c). Correlations of EEG electrodes and accelerometer deflections corroborate the notion that the distortions seen in EEG channels during head motion are related to the movement of the head and electrodes, which is most likely exacerbated or amplified by the applied DC. These distortions in most cases are the result of slight movement of the stimulating electrodes as well as the recording EEG electrodes on the scalp. Together with stimulation these distortions are stimulation montage and current intensity dependent, can change over the course of stimulation, and do not outlast the duration of stimulation (depending on the subject). To avoid this, subjects should be comfortably seated and instructed to minimize movement during stimulation and data acquisition. In some cases a headrest can be utilized to keep subjects head in place during experimental procedures.

EEG saturation can occur regardless of stimulation introduction. Saturation occurs when the dynamic range of EEG amplifiers have been reached and EEG signals become "clipped" or do not register voltages above or below a certain range (Light et al. 2010). Amplifier gain settings can, in some cases, influence the dynamic range of the data being acquired and bring the data closer to saturation if gain settings are too high. With concurrent stimulation and EEG this issue can arise very easily and frequently. Since tDCS creates/injects a large voltage offset in EEG recording electrodes, these electrodes become shifted towards their saturation point, designated by the dynamic range of the EEG amplifiers. For example, in Fig. 11.10d current was gradually ramped up during concurrent EEG where the amplifier gain was increased (prior to the commencement of stimulation). Electrodes closest to the anode and cathode (F7 and P8) saturated much sooner than those further away (FP1 and O2), as indicated by the derivative of the EEG voltage (lighter colors) over time (Fig. 11.10d). As the saturation point was reached, the derivative of the EEG voltage over time became zero and voltages beyond the dynamic range of the amplifier were no longer recordable. When the EEG electrodes saturate the data recorded cannot be utilized since any underlying neural data is obliterated. This type of stimulation-related saturated data is usually not broadband, can change during a stimulation session, is highly montage specific, and can sometimes outlast stimulation.

When EEG signals approach the ends of the dynamic range of amplifiers, they can sometimes enter a non-linear amplification range in the EEG amplifiers used. Within this non-linear region EEG signals can sometimes become highly distorted and artifactual. This type of artifact is usually broadband, can change during a stimulation session, is montage specific, and disappears after stimulation ends if it is strictly stimulation related. This type of saturation can be avoided by ensuring that EEG amplifiers that are used have an adequate dynamic range to accommodate large voltage fluctuations.

Electrode bridging in EEG often occurs when too much electrolyte gel is introduced between the scalp electrode interface and the gel merges with neighboring

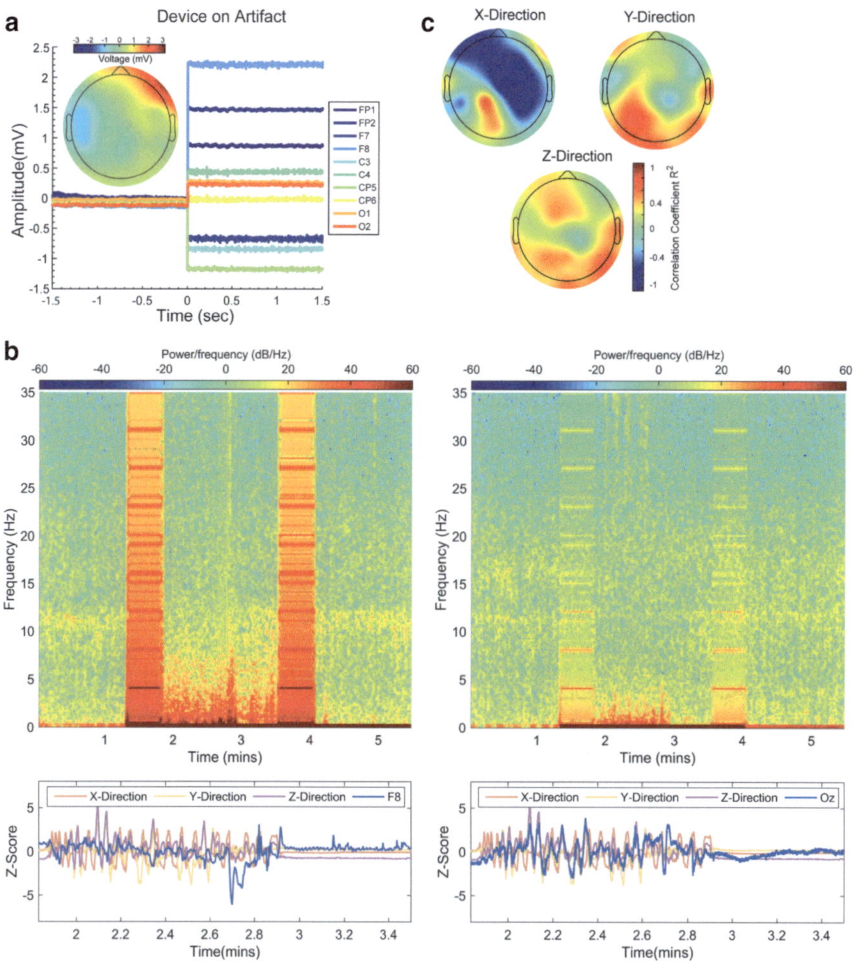

Fig. 11.10 (**a**) Device "On Noise" where time zero onwards indicates the time the stimulation device was switched on but not stimulating. Scalp topography displays the difference in voltage between device on and device off, after zero and before zero respectively. (**b**) Spectrograms at electrodes F8 and O2 over the course of pre, during, and post stimulation with the subject making several head movements during stimulation. EEG electrodes are presented with concurrent time-locked accelerometer recordings, each indicating the direction of displacement. (**c**) Correlation of accelerometer displacement with EEG voltage distortion over time, over the course of stimulation and head movement. (**d**) Electrode saturation over time with increasing current intensity. As current is increased electrodes (F7 and P8) closest to stimulating electrodes saturated earlier in time than those further away (FP1 and O2). Darker colors indicate electrode voltage over time whereas lighter colors indicate the derivative of the voltage over time. When the derivative becomes zero, saturation is reached

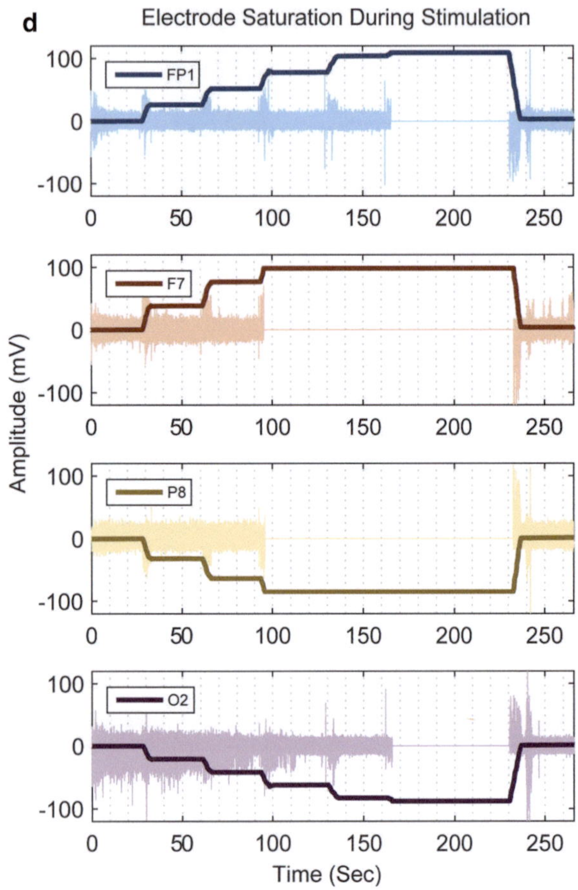

Fig. 11.10 (continued)

recording sites creating low impedance electrical bridges between two or more neighboring electrodes (Alschuler et al. 2014; Greischar et al. 2004; Tenke and Kayser 2001). This issue could be further exacerbated with environmental factors like room temperature that can result in increased scalp perspiration in subjects, which can also act as an electrolyte bridge. In terms of data quality, electrode bridging results in false identical signals being received by multiple electrodes that are bridged. In terms of tDCS though, the effects of electrode bridging of either stimulation electrodes, recording electrodes, or a combination of both; on acquired data can be detrimental. Electrode bridges during stimulation and EEG can result in robust current shunting across the scalp. Not only does the current not reach its proper target but it also gets introduced directly into the EEG recording electrodes distorting any neural data being recorded. Bridging can be avoided by utilizing an appropriate amount of electrolyte gel or saline at recording sites and at stimulation sites. Also ensuring that EEG caps adequately fit (not too tight or too loose), are not moved or do not shift over the course of procedures can help in avoiding bridging.

Artifact Removal

In order to realize the promise of combined EEG-tDCS, it is necessary to develop robust techniques for removing or otherwise mitigating the aforementioned artifacts. Although no straightforward approach exists, due to the robustness of said artifacts, some signal processing techniques exist for cleaning up some aspects of acquired concurrent online EEG- stimulation data. One common feature of all these artifacts is that they possess a seemingly stable spatial topography that is closely related to the tDCS montage. As a result, spatial filtering based techniques that estimate the (spatial) subspace of the artifact may be able to remove a significant proportion of the artifact variance. By regressing the corrupted EEG onto the artifact's subspace and then subtracting the projections (Parra et al. 2005), a large part of the artifact variance should vanish. Unfortunately, even a small amount of residual variability will likely have a confounding effect on any subsequent analysis, as the raw power of the artifacts is very large. It is worth pointing out that this problem is analogous to the one faced when recording EEG in the fMRI environment where artifacts are similarly large (Allen et al. 2000; Niazy et al. 2005). Previous works have employed multistage techniques for removing the residual artifact from the EEG recorded during tACS (Helfrich et al. 2014) and some of these can be adapted for tDCS.

Summary

Integration of tDCS with MRI/MRS, NIRS, and EEG holds great promise for shedding light on the underlying neural mechanisms of stimulation effects. While integration with these methods requires special consideration, a growing body of work provides both evidence of feasibility as well as insight into solutions to common concerns. Integration may not be easily achieved in certain cases, but clearly understand the current limitations of integration is an important first step in designing effective and interpretable studies. In addition, this information provides a clear guide to areas of tDCS integration that require future study and refinement. Regardless of current limitations, recent work in the integration of tDCS with modern neuroscience methods has produced critical insight into tDCS neural mechanisms and provides clear evidence of feasibility. Integration of these methods provide a platform for understanding brain behavior relationships using the inherent strengths of each approaches: tDCS providing a method for directly intervening on brain tissue, EEG providing high degrees of temporal resolution in brain processing, MRI providing a high degree of spatial resolution for structural and functional brain function, MRS providing insight into neurometabolite and neurotransmitter concentrations in brain tissue, and NIRS providing both spatial and temporal resolution of brain activity near the surface of the cortex. This methodological toolbox can be used to answer a wide range of questions about the brain and behavior, as well as underlying neural mechanisms of treatment response and efficacy. In addition, the potential for using this information to better optimize tDCS treatment studies is an exciting frontier in the field. As this field of study grows and our methodological understanding of integration process improves, the range of testable hypotheses about tDCS and the brain will only expand.

References

Aasted, C. M., Yücel, M. A., Cooper, R. J., Dubb, J., Tsuzuki, D., Becerra, L., … Boas, D. A. (2015). Anatomical guidance for functional near-infrared spectroscopy: AtlasViewer tutorial. *Neurophotonics, 2*, 20801.

Abbott, N. J., Rönnbäck, L., & Hansson, E. (2006). Astrocyte–endothelial interactions at the blood–brain barrier. *Nature Reviews. Neuroscience, 7*, 41–53.

Al-Kaysi, A. M., Al-Ani, A., Loo, C. K., Powell, T. Y., Martin, D. M., Breakspear, M., & Boonstra, T. W. (2016). Predicting tDCS treatment outcomes of patients with major depressive disorder using automated EEG classification. *Journal of Affective Disorders, 208*, 597–603.

Allen, P. J., Josephs, O., & Turner, R. (2000). A method for removing imaging artifact from continuous EEG recorded during functional MRI. *NeuroImage, 12*, 230–239.

Alschuler, D. M., Tenke, C. E., Bruder, G. E., & Kayser, J. (2014). Identifying electrode bridging from electrical distance distributions: A survey of publicly-available EEG data using a new method. *Clinical Neurophysiology, 125*, 484–490.

Amadi, U., Ilie, A., Johansen-Berg, H., & Stagg, C. J. (2014). Polarity-specific effects of motor transcranial direct current stimulation on fMRI resting state networks. *NeuroImage, 88*, 155–161.

Antal, A., Bikson, M., Datta, A., Lafon, B., Dechent, P., Parra, L. C., & Paulus, W. (2014). Imaging artifacts induced by electrical stimulation during conventional fMRI of the brain. *NeuroImage, 85*(Pt 3), 1040–1047.

Antal, A., Polania, R., Schmidt-Samoa, C., Dechent, P., & Paulus, W. (2011). Transcranial direct current stimulation over the primary motor cortex during fMRI. *NeuroImage, 55*, 590–596.

Aroniadou, V. A., & Keller, A. (1995). Mechanisms of LTP induction in rat motor cortex in vitro. *Cerebral Cortex, 5*, 353–362.

Attwell, D., Buchan, A. M., Charpak, S., Lauritzen, M., MacVicar, B. A., & Newman, E. A. (2010). Glial and neuronal control of brain blood flow. *Nature, 468*, 232–243.

Bachtiar, V., Near, J., Johansen-Berg, H., & Stagg, C. J. (2015). Modulation of GABA and resting state functional connectivity by transcranial direct current stimulation. *eLife, 4*, e08789.

Barlow, J. S. (1985). A general-purpose automatic multichannel electronic switch for EEG artifact elimination. *Electroencephalography and Clinical Neurophysiology, 60*, 174–176.

Baudewig, J., Nitsche, M. A., Paulus, W., & Frahm, J. (2001a). Regional modulation of BOLD MRI responses to human sensorimotor activation by transcranial direct current stimulation. *Magnetic Resonance in Medicine, 45*, 196–201.

Baudewig, J., Siebner, H. R., Bestmann, S., Tergau, F., Tings, T., Paulus, W., & Frahm, J. (2001b). Functional MRI of cortical activations induced by transcranial magnetic stimulation (TMS). *Neuroreport, 12*, 3543–3548.

Bazargani, N., & Attwell, D. (2016). Astrocyte calcium signaling: The third wave. *Nature Neuroscience, 19*, 182–189.

Beckmann, C. F., Deluca, M., Devlin, J. T., & Smith, S. M. (2005). Investigations into resting-state connectivity using independent component analysis. *Philosophical Transactions of the Royal Society B: Biological Sciences, 360*, 1001–1013.

Berg, P., & Scherg, M. (1991). Dipole models of eye movements and blinks. *Electroencephalography and Clinical Neurophysiology, 79*, 36–44.

Beyer, L., Batsikadze, G., Timmann, D., & Gerwig, M. (2017). Cerebellar tDCS effects on conditioned Eyeblinks using different electrode placements and stimulation protocols. *Frontiers in Human Neuroscience, 11*, 23.

Binkofski, F., Loebig, M., Jauch-Chara, K., Bergmann, S., Melchert, U. H., Scholand-Engler, H. G., ... Oltmanns, K. M. (2011). Brain energy consumption induced by electrical stimulation promotes systemic glucose uptake. *Biological Psychiatry, 70*, 690–695.

Boas, D. A., Culver, J., Stott, J., & Dunn, A. (2002). Three dimensional Monte Carlo code for photon migration through complex heterogeneous media including the adult human head. *Optics Express, 10*, 159–170.

Boggio, P. S., Ferrucci, R., Rigonatti, S. P., Covre, P., Nitsche, M., Pascual-Leone, A., & Fregni, F. (2006). Effects of transcranial direct current stimulation on working memory in patients with Parkinson's disease. *Journal of the Neurological Sciences, 249*, 31–38.

Bonnet, P., Rusch, N. J., & Harder, D. R. (1991). Characterization of an outward K+ current in freshly dispersed cerebral arterial muscle cells. *Pflügers Archiv European Journal of Physiology, 418*, 292–296.

Bottomley, P. A., Edelstein, W. A., Foster, T. H., & Adams, W. A. (1985). In vivo solvent-suppressed localized hydrogen nuclear magnetic resonance spectroscopy: A window to metabolism? *Proceedings of the National Academy of Sciences of the United States of America, 82*, 2148–2152.

Bozzo, L., Puyal, J., & Chatton, J.-Y. (2013). Lactate modulates the activity of primary cortical neurons through a receptor-mediated pathway. *PLoS One, 8*, e71721.

Bradley, M. M., Codispoti, M., Cuthbert, B. N., & Lang, P. J. (2001). Emotion and motivation I: Defensive and appetitive reactions in picture processing. *Emotion, 1*, 276–298.

Brayden, J. E. (1996). Potassium channels in vascular smooth muscle. *Clinical and Experimental Pharmacology & Physiology, 23*, 1069–1076.

Brunoni, A. R., Nitsche, M. A., Bolognini, N., Bikson, M., Wagner, T., Merabet, L., ... Fregni, F. (2012). Clinical research with transcranial direct current stimulation (tDCS): Challenges and future directions. *Brain Stimulation, 5*, 175–195.

Buch, E. R., Santarnecchi, E., Antal, A., Born, J., Celnik, P. A., Classen, J., ... Cohen, L. G. (2017). Effects of tDCS on motor learning and memory formation: A consensus and critical position paper. *Clinical Neurophysiology, 128*, 589–603.

Cabib, C., Cipullo, F., Morales, M., & Valls-Sole, J. (2016). Transcranial direct current stimulation (tDCS) enhances the excitability of Trigemino-facial reflex circuits. *Brain Stimulation, 9*, 218–224.

Cancelli, A., Cottone, C., Tecchio, F., Truong, D. Q., Dmochowski, J., & Bikson, M. (2016). A simple method for EEG guided transcranial electrical stimulation without models. *Journal of Neural Engineering, 13*, 36022.

Castro-Alamancos, M. A., Donoghue, J. P., & Connors, B. W. (1995). Different forms of synaptic plasticity in somatosensory and motor areas of the neocortex. *The Journal of Neuroscience, 15*, 5324–5333.

Charvet, L. E., Kasschau, M., Datta, A., Knotkova, H., Stevens, M. C., Alonzo, A., … Bikson, M. (2015). Remotely-supervised transcranial direct current stimulation (tDCS) for clinical trials: Guidelines for technology and protocols. *Frontiers in Systems Neuroscience, 9*, 26.

Chhabria, K., & Chakravarthy, V. S. (2016). Low-dimensional models of "neuro-Glio-vascular unit" for describing neural dynamics under normal and energy-starved conditions. *Stroke, 7*, 24.

Clancy, J. A., Johnson, R., Raw, R., Deuchars, S. A., & Deuchars, J. (2014). Anodal transcranial direct current stimulation (tDCS) over the motor cortex increases sympathetic nerve activity. *Brain Stimulation, 7*, 97–104.

Clark, V. P., Coffman, B. A., Trumbo, M. C., & Gasparovic, C. (2011). Transcranial direct current stimulation (tDCS) produces localized and specific alterations in neurochemistry: A ^{1}H magnetic resonance spectroscopy study. *Neuroscience Letters, 500*, 67–71.

Coan, J. A., & Allen, J. J. B. (2003). Varieties of emotional experience during voluntary emotional facial expressions. *Annals of the New York Academy of Sciences, 1000*, 375–379.

Cole, D. M., Smith, S. M., & Beckmann, C. F. (2010). Advances and pitfalls in the analysis and interpretation of resting-state FMRI data. *Frontiers in Systems Neuroscience, 4*, 8.

Corby, J. C., Roth, W. T., & Kopell, B. S. (1974). Prevalence and methods of control of the cephalic skin potential EEG artifact. *Psychophysiology, 11*, 350–360.

Cunillera, T., Brignani, D., Cucurell, D., Fuentemilla, L., & Miniussi, C. (2015). The right inferior frontal cortex in response inhibition: A tDCS-ERP co-registration study. *NeuroImage, 140*, 66–75.

Datta, A., Baker, J. M., Bikson, M., & Fridriksson, J. (2011). Individualized model predicts brain current flow during transcranial direct-current stimulation treatment in responsive stroke patient. *Brain Stimulation, 4*, 169–174.

Delpy, D. T., Arridge, S. R., Cope, M., Edwards, D., Reynolds, E. O. R., Richardson, C. E., … van der Zee, P. (1989). *Quantitation of pathlength in optical spectroscopy* (pp. 41–46). Boston, MA: Springer.

Dinteren, R., Arns, M., Jongsma, M. L. A., & Kessels, R. P. C. (2014). P300 development across the lifespan: A systematic review and meta-analysis. *PLoS One, 9*, e87347.

Dutta, A. (2015). Bidirectional interactions between neuronal and hemodynamic responses to transcranial direct current stimulation (tDCS): Challenges for brain-state dependent tDCS. *Frontiers in Systems Neuroscience, 9*, 1–7.

Dutta, A., Jacob, A., Chowdhury, S. R., Das, A., & Nitsche, M. A. (2015). EEG-NIRS based assessment of neurovascular coupling during anodal transcranial direct current stimulation – a stroke case series. *Journal of Medical Systems, 39*, 205.

Edwards, G., & Weston, A. H. (1993). The pharmacology of ATP-sensitive potassium channels. *Annual Review of Pharmacology and Toxicology, 33*, 597–637.

Faehling, F., & Plewnia, C. (2016). Controlling the emotional bias: Performance, late positive potentials, and the effect of anodal transcranial direct current stimulation (tDCS). *Frontiers in Cellular Neuroscience, 10*, 159.

Fang, Q. (2010). Mesh-based Monte Carlo method using fast ray-tracing in Plücker coordinates. *Biomedical Optics Express, 1*, 165–175.

Fantini, S. (2014). Dynamic model for the tissue concentration and oxygen saturation of hemoglobin in relation to blood volume, flow velocity, and oxygen consumption: Implications for functional neuroimaging and coherent hemodynamics spectroscopy (CHS). *NeuroImage, 85*(Pt 1), 202–221.

Faria, P., Fregni, F., Sebastião, F., Dias, A. I., & Leal, A. (2012). Feasibility of focal transcranial DC polarization with simultaneous EEG recording: Preliminary assessment in healthy subjects and human epilepsy. *Epilepsy & Behavior, 25*, 417–425.

Fernández-Corazza, M., Turovets, S., Luu, P., Anderson, E., & Tucker, D. (2016). Transcranial electrical neuromodulation based on the reciprocity principle. *Frontiers in Psychiatry, 7*, 87.
Filippini, N., MacIntosh, B. J., Hough, M. G., Goodwin, G. M., Frisoni, G. B., Smith, S. M., … Mackay, C. E. (2009). Distinct patterns of brain activity in young carriers of the APOE-epsilon4 allele. *Proceedings of the National Academy of Sciences of the United States of America, 106*, 7209–7214.
Fischl, B. (2012). FreeSurfer. *NeuroImage, 62*, 774–781.
Fornito, A., Zalesky, A., & Breakspear, M. (2013). Graph analysis of the human connectome: Promise, progress, and pitfalls. *NeuroImage, 80*, 426–444.
Fox, M. D., & Raichle, M. E. (2007). Spontaneous fluctuations in brain activity observed with functional magnetic resonance imaging. *Nature Reviews. Neuroscience, 8*, 700–711.
Giordano, J., Bikson, M., Kappenman, E. S., Clark, V. P., Coslett, H. B., Hamblin, M. R., … Calabrese, E. (2017). Mechanisms and effects of transcranial direct current stimulation. *Dose Response, 15*, 1559325816685467.
Girouard, H., & Iadecola, C. (2006). Neurovascular coupling in the normal brain and in hypertension, stroke, and Alzheimer disease. *Journal of Applied Physiology, 100*, 328–335.
Goncharova, I. I., McFarland, D. J., Vaughan, T. M., & Wolpaw, J. R. (2003). EMG contamination of EEG: Spectral and topographical characteristics. *Clinical Neurophysiology, 114*, 1580–1593.
Greischar, L. L., Burghy, C. A., Van Reekum, C. M., Jackson, D. C., Pizzagalli, D. A., Mueller, C., & Davidson, R. J. (2004). Effects of electrode density and electrolyte spreading in dense array electroencephalographic recording. *Clinical Neurophysiology, 115*, 710–720.
Guhathakurta, D., & Dutta, A. (2016). Computational pipeline for NIRS-EEG joint imaging of tDCS-evoked cerebral responses-an application in ischemic stroke. *Frontiers in Neuroscience, 10*, 261.
Hahn, C., Rice, J., Macuff, S., Minhas, P., Rahman, A., & Bikson, M. (2013). Methods for extra-low voltage transcranial direct current stimulation: Current and time dependent impedance decreases. *Clinical Neurophysiology, 124*, 551–556.
Hamel, E. (2006). Perivascular nerves and the regulation of cerebrovascular tone. *Journal of Applied Physiology, 100*, 1059–1064.
Helfrich, R. F., Knepper, H., Nolte, G., Strüber, D., Rach, S., Herrmann, C. S., … Engel, A. K. (2014). Selective modulation of interhemispheric functional connectivity by HD-tACS shapes perception. *PLoS Biology, 12*, e1002031.
Hess, G., Aizenman, C. D., & Donoghue, J. P. (1996). Conditions for the induction of long-term potentiation in layer II/III horizontal connections of the rat motor cortex. *Journal of Neurophysiology, 75*, 1765–1778.
Holland, R., Leff, A. P., Josephs, O., Galea, J. M., Desikan, M., Price, C. J., … Crinion, J. (2011). Speech facilitation by left inferior frontal cortex stimulation. *Current Biology, 21*, 1403–1407.
Holmes, C. J., Hoge, R., Collins, L., Woods, R., Toga, A. W., & Evans, A. C. (2015). Enhancement of MR images using registration for signal averaging. *Journal of Computer Assisted Tomography, 22*, 324–333.
Huneau, C., Benali, H., & Chabriat, H. (2015). Investigating human neurovascular coupling using functional neuroimaging: A critical review of dynamic models. *Frontiers in Neuroscience, 9*, 467.
Hunter, M. A., Coffman, B. A., Gasparovic, C., Calhoun, V. D., Trumbo, M. C., & Clark, V. P. (2015). Baseline effects of transcranial direct current stimulation on glutamatergic neurotransmission and large-scale network connectivity. *Brain Research, 1594*, 92–107.
Hunter, M. A., Coffman, B. A., Trumbo, M. C., & Clark, V. P. (2013). Tracking the neuroplastic changes associated with transcranial direct current stimulation: A push for multimodal imaging. *Frontiers in Human Neuroscience, 7*, 495.
Iwasaki, M., Kellinghaus, C., Alexopoulos, A. V., Burgess, R. C., Kumar, A. N., Han, Y. H., … Leigh, R. J. (2005). Effects of eyelid closure, blinks, and eye movements on the electroencephalogram. *Clinical Neurophysiology, 116*, 878–885.

Jasper, H. H. (1958). Report of the committee on methods of clinical examination in electroencephalography. *Electroencephalography and Clinical Neurophysiology. Supplement, 10*, 370–375.

Jenkinson, M., Beckmann, C. F., Behrens, T. E. J., Woolrich, M. W., & Smith, S. M. (2012). FSL. *NeuroImage, 62*, 782–790.

Jindal, U., Sood, M., Dutta, A., & Chowdhury, S. R. (2015). Development of point of care testing device for neurovascular coupling from simultaneous recording of EEG and NIRS during anodal transcranial direct current stimulation. *IEEE Journal of Translational Engineering in Health and Medicine, 3*, 1–12.

Johansen-Berg, H. (2013). Human connectomics – What will the future demand? *NeuroImage, 80*, 541–544.

Jolivet, R., Coggan, J. S., Allaman, I., & Magistretti, P. J. (2015). Multi-timescale modeling of activity-dependent metabolic coupling in the neuron-glia-vasculature ensemble. *PLoS Computational Biology, 11*, e1004036.

Kim, S., Stephenson, M. C., Morris, P. G., & Jackson, S. R. (2014). TDCS-induced alterations in GABA concentration within primary motor cortex predict motor learning and motor memory: A 7T magnetic resonance spectroscopy study. *NeuroImage, 99*, 237–243.

Kirilina, E., Jelzow, A., Heine, A., Niessing, M., Wabnitz, H., Brühl, R., … Tachtsidis, I. (2012). The physiological origin of task-evoked systemic artefacts in functional near infrared spectroscopy. *NeuroImage, 61*, 70–81.

Kitazono, T., Faraci, F. M., Taguchi, H., & Heistad, D. D. (1995). Role of potassium channels in cerebral blood vessels. *Stroke, 26*, 1713–1723.

Klass, D. W. (1995). The continuing challenge of artifacts in the EEG. *The American Journal of EEG Technology, 35*, 239–269.

Komssi, S., Aronen, H. J., Huttunen, J., Kesäniemi, M., Soinne, L., Nikouline, V. V., … Ilmoniemi, R. J. (2002). Ipsi- and contralateral EEG reactions to transcranial magnetic stimulation. *Clinical Neurophysiology, 113*, 175–184.

Kwon, Y. H., Ko, M.-H., Ahn, S. H., Minhas, P., Paulus, W., Kuo, M. F., & Nitsche, M. A. (2008). Primary motor cortex activation by transcranial direct current stimulation in the human brain. *Neuroscience Letters, 435*, 56–59. S0304-3940(08)00180-8 [pii].

Lee, S., & Buchsbaum, M. S. (1987). Topographic mapping of EEG artifacts. *Clinical Electroencephalography, 18*, 61–67.

Lemke, C., Hess, A., Clare, S., Bachtiar, V., Stagg, C., Jezzard, P., & Emir, U. (2015). Two-voxel spectroscopy with dynamic B<inf>0</inf> shimming and flip angle adjustment at 7 T in the human motor cortex. *NMR in Biomedicine, 28*, 852–860.

Leybaert, L., Paemeleire, K., Strahonja, A., & Sanderson, M. J. (1998). Inositol-trisphosphate-dependent intercellular calcium signaling in and between astrocytes and endothelial cells. *Glia, 24*, 398–407.

Light, G. A., Williams, L. E., Minow, F., Sprock, J., Rissling, A., Sharp, R., Swerdlow, N. R., & Braff, D. L. (2010). Electroencephalography (EEG) and event-related potentials (ERPs) with human participants. *Current Protocols in Neuroscience, 52*, 6.25.1–6.25.24.

Lindenberg, R., Nachtigall, L., Meinzer, M., Sieg, M. M., & Flöel, A. (2013). Differential effects of dual and unihemispheric motor cortex stimulation in older adults. *The Journal of Neuroscience, 33*, 9176–9183.

List, J., Lesemann, A., Kübke, J. C., Külzow, N., Schreiber, S. J., & Flöel, A. (2015). Impact of tDCS on cerebral autoregulation in aging and in patients with cerebrovascular diseases. *Neurology, 84*, 626–628.

Logothetis, N. K. (2008). What we can do and what we cannot do with fMRI. *Nature, 453*, 869–878.

Luft, C. D. B., & Bhattacharya, J. (2015). Aroused with heart: Modulation of heartbeat evoked potential by arousal induction and its oscillatory correlates. *Scientific Reports, 5*, 15717.

Mancini, M., Pellicciari, M. C., Brignani, D., Mauri, P., De Marchis, C., Miniussi, C., & Conforto, S. (2015). Automatic artifact suppression in simultaneous tDCS-EEG using adaptive filtering. In: Proceedings of the Annual International Conference of the IEEE Engineering in Medicine and Biology Society, EMBS. pp. 2729–2732

Mangia, A. L., Pirini, M., & Cappello, A. (2014). Transcranial direct current stimulation and power spectral parameters: A tDCS/EEG co-registration study. *Frontiers in Human Neuroscience, 8*, 601.

Mathiisen, T. M., Lehre, K. P., Danbolt, N. C., & Ottersen, O. P. (2010). The perivascular astroglial sheath provides a complete covering of the brain microvessels: An electron microscopic 3D reconstruction. *Glia, 58*, 1094–1103.

Maudsley, A. A., Darkazanli, A., Alger, J. R., Hall, L. O., Schuff, N., Studholme, C., … Zhu, X. (2006). Comprehensive processing, display and analysis for in vivo MR spectroscopic imaging. *NMR in Biomedicine, 19*, 492–503.

Meinzer, M., Lindenberg, R., Sieg, M. M., Nachtigall, L., Ulm, L., & Flöel, A. (2014). Transcranial direct current stimulation of the primary motor cortex improves word-retrieval in older adults. *Frontiers in Aging Neuroscience, 6*, 253.

Minhas, P., Bansal, V., Patel, J., Ho, J. S., Diaz, J., Datta, A., & Bikson, M. (2010). Electrodes for high-definition transcutaneous DC stimulation for applications in drug delivery and electrotherapy, including tDCS. *Journal of Neuroscience Methods, 190*, 188–197.

Mintun, M. A., Vlassenko, A. G., Rundle, M. M., & Raichle, M. E. (2004). Increased lactate/pyruvate ratio augments blood flow in physiologically activated human brain. *Proceedings of the National Academy of Sciences of the United States of America, 101*, 659–664.

Monai, H., Ohkura, M., Tanaka, M., Oe, Y., Konno, A., Hirai, H., … Hirase, H. (2016). Calcium imaging reveals glial involvement in transcranial direct current stimulation-induced plasticity in mouse brain. *Nature Communications, 7*, 11100.

Mulligan, S. J., & MacVicar, B. A. (2004). Calcium transients in astrocyte endfeet cause cerebrovascular constrictions. *Nature, 431*, 195–199.

Muthalib, M., Besson, P., Rothwell, J., Ward, T., & Perrey, S. (2016). Effects of anodal high-definition transcranial direct current stimulation on bilateral sensorimotor cortex activation during sequential finger movements: An fnirs study. *Advances in Experimental Medicine and Biology, 876*, 351–359.

Muthalib, M., Ferrari, M., Quaresima, V., Kerr, G., & Perrey, S. (2017). Functional near-infrared spectroscopy to probe sensorimotor region activation during electrical stimulation-evoked movement. *Clinical Physiology and Functional Imaging.*

Nelson, M. T., Patlak, J. B., Worley, J. F., & Standen, N. B. (1990). Calcium channels, potassium channels, and voltage dependence of arterial smooth muscle tone. *The American Journal of Physiology, 259*, C3–C18.

Niazy, R. K., Beckmann, C. F., Iannetti, G. D., Brady, J. M., & Smith, S. M. (2005). Removal of FMRI environment artifacts from EEG data using optimal basis sets. *NeuroImage, 28*, 720–737.

Nitsche, M. A., & Paulus, W. (2000). Excitability changes induced in the human motor cortex by weak transcranial direct current stimulation. *The Journal of Physiology, 527*(Pt 3), 633–639.

Nitsche, M. A., Schauenburg, A., Lang, N., Liebetanz, D., Exner, C., Paulus, W., & Tergau, F. (2003). Facilitation of implicit motor learning by weak transcranial direct current stimulation of the primary motor cortex in the human. *Journal of Cognitive Neuroscience, 15*, 619–626.

Noetscher, G. M., Yanamadala, J., Makarov, S. N., & Pascual-Leone, A. (2014). Comparison of cephalic and extracephalic montages for transcranial direct current stimulation – A numerical study. *IEEE Transactions on Biomedical Engineering, 61*, 2488–2498.

Noury, N., Hipp, J. F., & Siegel, M. (2016). Physiological processes non-linearly affect electrophysiological recordings during transcranial electric stimulation. *NeuroImage, 140*, 99–109.

Obrig, H. (2014). NIRS in clinical neurology – A "promising" tool? *NeuroImage, 85*, 535–546.

Okamoto, M., Dan, H., Sakamoto, K., Takeo, K., Shimizu, K., Kohno, S., … Dan, I. (2004). Three-dimensional probabilistic anatomical cranio-cerebral correlation via the international 10-20 system oriented for transcranial functional brain mapping. *NeuroImage, 21*, 99–111.

Oomagari, K., Buisson, B., Dumuis, A., Bockaert, J., & Pin, J. P. (1991). Effect of glutamate and lonomycin on the release of arachidonic acid, prostaglandins and HETEs from cultured neurons and astrocytes. *The European Journal of Neuroscience, 3*, 928–939.

Parra, L. C., Spence, C. D., Gerson, A. D., & Sajda, P. (2005). Recipes for the linear analysis of EEG. *Neuroimage, 28*, 326–341

Paulson, O. B., & Newman, E. A. (1987). Does the release of potassium from astrocyte endfeet regulate cerebral blood flow? *Science, 237*, 896–898.

Picton, T. W., & Hillyard, S. A. (1972). Cephalic skin potentials in electroencephalography. *Electroencephalography and Clinical Neurophysiology, 33*, 419–424.

Pievani, M., de Haan, W., Wu, T., Seeley, W. W., & Frisoni, G. B. (2011). Functional network disruption in the degenerative dementias. *Lancet Neurology, 10*, 829–843.

Pievani, M., Filippini, N., Van Den Heuvel, M. P., Cappa, S. F., & Frisoni, G. B. (2014). Brain connectivity in neurodegenerative diseases – From phenotype to proteinopathy. *Nature Reviews. Neurology, 10*, 620–633.

Polanía, R., Nitsche, M. A., Korman, C., Batsikadze, G., & Paulus, W. (2012). The importance of timing in segregated theta phase-coupling for cognitive performance. *Current Biology, 22*, 1314–1318.

Polanía, R., Nitsche, M. A., & Paulus, W. (2011a). Modulating functional connectivity patterns and topological functional organization of the human brain with transcranial direct current stimulation. *Human Brain Mapping, 32*, 1236–1249.

Polanía, R., Paulus, W., Antal, A., & Nitsche, M. A. (2011b). Introducing graph theory to track for neuroplastic alterations in the resting human brain: A transcranial direct current stimulation study. *NeuroImage, 54*, 2287–2296.

Pulgar, V. M. (2015). Direct electric stimulation to increase cerebrovascular function. *Frontiers in Systems Neuroscience, 9*, 54.

Raichle, M. E., MacLeod, A. M., Snyder, A. Z., Powers, W. J., Gusnard, D. A., & Shulman, G. L. (2001). A default mode of brain function. *Proceedings of the National Academy of Sciences of the United States of America, 98*, 676–682.

Reis, J., Schambra, H. M., Cohen, L. G., Buch, E. R., Fritsch, B., Zarahn, E., … Krakauer, J. W. (2009). Noninvasive cortical stimulation enhances motor skill acquisition over multiple days through an effect on consolidation. *Proceedings of the National Academy of Sciences of the United States of America, 106*, 1590–1595.

Roy, A., Baxter, B., & He, B. (2014). High-definition transcranial direct current stimulation induces both acute and persistent changes in broadband cortical synchronization: A simultaneous tDCS-EEG study. *IEEE Transactions on Biomedical Engineering, 61*, 1967–1978.

Roy, C. S., & Sherrington, C. S. (1890). On the regulation of the blood-supply of the brain. *The Journal of Physiology, 11*, 85–158.17.

Rubin, D., & Daube, J. (2016). Adult EEG: Artifacts and the EEG. *Clinical Neurophysiology.* Oxford University Press.

Schestatsky, P., Simis, M., Freeman, R., Pascual-Leone, A., & Fregni, F. (2013). Non-invasive brain stimulation and the autonomic nervous system. *Clinical Neurophysiology, 124*, 1716–1728.

Schmitt, S. (2017). Artifacts resembling seizures. In *Continuous EEG monitoring* (pp. 153–171). Cham, Switzerland: Springer International Publishing.

Scholkmann, F., Kleiser, S., Metz, A. J., Zimmermann, R., Mata Pavia, J., Wolf, U., & Wolf, M. (2014). A review on continuous wave functional near-infrared spectroscopy and imaging instrumentation and methodology. *NeuroImage, 85*, 6–27.

Schroeder, P. A., Ehlis, A. C., Wolkenstein, L., Fallgatter, A. J., & Plewnia, C. (2015). Emotional distraction and bodily reaction: Modulation of autonomous responses by anodal tDCS to the prefrontal cortex. *Frontiers in Cellular Neuroscience, 9*, 482.

Sehm, B., Kipping, J., Schäfer, A., Villringer, A., & Ragert, P. (2013). A comparison between Uni- and bilateral tDCS effects on functional connectivity of the human motor cortex. *Frontiers in Human Neuroscience, 7*, 183.

Sehm, B., Schäfer, A., Kipping, J., Margulies, D., Conde, V., Taubert, M., … Ragert, P. (2012). Dynamic modulation of intrinsic functional connectivity by transcranial direct current stimulation. *Journal of Neurophysiology, 108*, 3253–3263.

Shackman, A. J., McMenamin, B. W., Slagter, H. A., Maxwell, J. S., Greischar, L. L., & Davidson, R. J. (2009). Electromyogenic artifacts and electroencephalographic inferences. *Brain Topography, 22*, 7–12.

Smith, S. M., Fox, P. T., Miller, K. L., Glahn, D. C., Fox, P. M., Mackay, C. E., … Beckmann, C. F. (2009). Correspondence of the brain's functional architecture during activation and rest. *Proceedings of the National Academy of Sciences, 106*, 13040–13045.

Snyder, A. Z., & Raichle, M. E. (2012). A brief history of the resting state: The Washington University perspective. *NeuroImage, 62*, 902–910.

Sood, M., Besson, P., Muthalib, M., Jindal, U., Perrey, S., Dutta, A., & Hayashibe, M. (2016). NIRS-EEG joint imaging during transcranial direct current stimulation: Online parameter estimation with an autoregressive model. *Journal of Neuroscience Methods, 274*, 71–80.

Sood, M., Jindal, U., Chowdhury, S. R., Das, A., Kondziella, D., & Dutta, A. (2015). Anterior temporal artery tap to identify systemic interference using short-separation NIRS measurements: A NIRS/EEG-tDCS study. Conf proc. *Annual International Conference of the IEEE Engineering in Medicine and Biology Society. IEEE Engineering in Medicine and Biology Society. Annual Conference, 2015*, 1239–1242.

Stagg, C. J., Bachtiar, V., & Johansen-Berg, H. (2011a). The role of GABA in human motor learning. *Current Biology, 21*, 480–484.

Stagg, C. J., Best, J. G., Stephenson, M. C., O'Shea, J., Wylezinska, M., Kincses, Z. T., … Johansen-Berg, H. (2009a). Polarity-sensitive modulation of cortical neurotransmitters by transcranial stimulation. *The Journal of Neuroscience, 29*, 5202–5206.

Stagg, C. J., Jayaram, G., Pastor, D., Kincses, Z. T., Matthews, P. M., & Johansen-Berg, H. (2011b). Polarity and timing-dependent effects of transcranial direct current stimulation in explicit motor learning. *Neuropsychologia, 49*, 800–804.

Stagg, C. J., Lin, R. L., Mezue, M., Segerdahl, A., Kong, Y., Xie, J., & Tracey, I. (2013). Widespread modulation of cerebral perfusion induced during and after transcranial direct current stimulation applied to the left dorsolateral prefrontal cortex. *The Journal of Neuroscience, 33*, 11425–11431.

Stagg, C. J., & Nitsche, M. A. (2011). Physiological basis of transcranial direct current stimulation. *The Neuroscientist, 17*, 37–53.

Stagg, C. J., O'Shea, J., Kincses, Z. T., Woolrich, M., Matthews, P. M., & Johansen-Berg, H. (2009b). Modulation of movement-associated cortical activation by transcranial direct current stimulation. *The European Journal of Neuroscience, 30*, 1412–1423.

Stagg, C. J., Wylezinska, M., Matthews, P. M., Johansen-Berg, H., Jezzard, P., Rothwell, J. C., & Bestmann, S. (2009c). Neurochemical effects of Theta burst stimulation as assessed by magnetic resonance spectroscopy. *Journal of Neurophysiology, 101*, 2872–2877.

Strangman, G. E., Li, Z., & Zhang, Q. (2013). Depth sensitivity and source-detector separations for near infrared spectroscopy based on the Colin27 brain template. *PLoS One, 8*, e66319.

Stucht, D., Danishad, K. A., Schulze, P., Godenschweger, F., Zaitsev, M., & Speck, O. (2015). Highest resolution in vivo human brain MRI using prospective motion correction. *PLoS One, 10*, e0133921.

Tachtsidis, I., & Scholkmann, F. (2016). False positives and false negatives in functional near-infrared spectroscopy: Issues, challenges, and the way forward. *Neurophotonics, 3*, 31405.

Takai, H., Tsubaki, A., Sugawara, K., Miyaguchi, S., Oyanagi, K., Matsumoto, T., … Yamamoto, N. (2016). Effect of transcranial direct current stimulation over the primary motor cortex on cerebral blood flow: A time course study using near-infrared spectroscopy. *Advances in Experimental Medicine and Biology, 876*, 335–341.

Tassinary, L. G., Cacioppo, J. T., & Vanman, E. J. (2007). The skeletomotor system. In G. Berntson, J. T. Cacioppo, & L. G. Tassinary (Eds.), *Handbook of psychophysiology* (pp. 267–300). Cambridge: Cambridge University Press.

Tenke, C. E., & Kayser, J. (2001). A convenient method for detecting electrolyte bridges in multichannel electroencephalogram and event-related potential recordings. *Clinical Neurophysiology, 112*, 545–550.

Torricelli, A., Contini, D., Pifferi, A., Caffini, M., Re, R., Zucchelli, L., & Spinelli, L. (2014). Time domain functional NIRS imaging for human brain mapping. *NeuroImage, 85*, 28–50.

Trepel, C., & Racine, R. J. (1998). Long-term potentiation in the neocortex of the adult, freely moving rat. *Cerebral Cortex, 8*, 719–729.

Trepel, C., & Racine, R. J. (2000). GABAergic modulation of neocortical long-term potentiation in the freely moving rat. *Synapse, 35*, 120–128.

Tsytsarev, V., Hu, S., Yao, J., Maslov, K., Barbour, D. L., & Wang, L. V. (2011). Photoacoustic microscopy of microvascular responses to cortical electrical stimulation. *Journal of Biomedical Optics, 16*, 76002.

Tzourio-Mazoyer, N., Landeau, B., Papathanassiou, D., Crivello, F., Etard, O., Delcroix, N., … Joliot, M. (2002). Automated anatomical labeling of activations in SPM using a macroscopic anatomical parcellation of the MNI MRI single-subject brain. *NeuroImage, 15*, 273–289.

Vaishnavi, S. N., Vlassenko, A. G., Rundle, M. M., Snyder, A. Z., Mintun, M. A., & Raichle, M. E. (2010). Regional aerobic glycolysis in the human brain. *Proceedings of the National Academy of Sciences, 107*, 17757–17762.

Vandermeeren, Y., Jamart, J., & Ossemann, M. (2010). Effect of tDCS with an extracephalic reference electrode on cardio-respiratory and autonomic functions. *BMC Neuroscience, 11*, 38.

Vernieri, F., Assenza, G., Maggio, P., Tibuzzi, F., Zappasodi, F., Altamura, C., … Rossini, P. M. (2010). Cortical neuromodulation modifies cerebral vasomotor reactivity. *Stroke, 41*, 2087–2090.

Villamar, M. F., Volz, M. S., Bikson, M., Datta, A., Dasilva, A. F., & Fregni, F. (2013). Technique and considerations in the use of 4x1 ring high-definition transcranial direct current stimulation (HD-tDCS). *Journal of Visualized Experiments*, e50309.

Wachter, D., Wrede, A., Schulz-Schaeffer, W., Taghizadeh-Waghefi, A., Nitsche, M. A., Kutschenko, A., … Liebetanz, D. (2011). Transcranial direct current stimulation induces polarity-specific changes of cortical blood perfusion in the rat. *Experimental Neurology, 227*, 322–327.

Wagner, S., Lucka, F., Vorwerk, J., Herrmann, C. S., Nolte, G., Burger, M., & Wolters, C. H. (2016). Using reciprocity for relating the simulation of transcranial current stimulation to the EEG forward problem. *NeuroImage, 140*, 163–173.

Waterink, W., & van Boxtel, A. (1994). Facial and jaw-elevator EMG activity in relation to changes in performance level during a sustained information processing task. *Biological Psychology, 37*, 183–198.

Westmoreland, B. F. (1996). Periodic patterns in the EEG. *American Journal of Electroneurodiagnostic Technology, 36*, 1–17.

Whitham, E. M., Pope, K. J., Fitzgibbon, S. P., Lewis, T., Clark, C. R., Loveless, S., … Willoughby, J. O. (2007). Scalp electrical recording during paralysis: Quantitative evidence that EEG frequencies above 20 Hz are contaminated by EMG. *Clinical Neurophysiology, 118*, 1877–1888.

Willis, J., Nelson, A., Rice, J., & Black, F. W. (1993). The topography of muscle activity in quantitative EEG. *Clinical Electroencephalography, 24*, 123–126.

Windhoff, M., Opitz, A., & Thielscher, A. (2013). Electric field calculations in brain stimulation based on finite elements: An optimized processing pipeline for the generation and usage of accurate individual head models. *Human Brain Mapping, 34*, 923–935.

Woods, A. J., Antal, A., Bikson, M., Boggio, P. S., Brunoni, A. R., Celnik, P., … Nitsche, M. A. (2016). A technical guide to tDCS, and related non-invasive brain stimulation tools. *Clinical Neurophysiology, 127*, 1031–1048.

Woods, A. J., Hamilton, R. H., Kranjec, A., Minhaus, P., Bikson, M., Yu, J., & Chatterjee, A. (2014). Space, time, and causality in the human brain. *NeuroImage, 92*, 285–297.

Yang, J., Ruchti, E., Petit, J.-M., Jourdain, P., Grenningloh, G., Allaman, I., & Magistretti, P. J. (2014). Lactate promotes plasticity gene expression by potentiating NMDA signaling in neurons. *Proceedings of the National Academy of Sciences of the United States of America, 111*, 12228–12233.

Zheng, X., Alsop, D. C., & Schlaug, G. (2011). Effects of transcranial direct current stimulation (tDCS) on human regional cerebral blood flow. *NeuroImage, 58*, 26–33.

Zuchowski, M. L., Timmann, D., & Gerwig, M. (2014). Acquisition of conditioned eyeblink responses is modulated by cerebellar tDCS. *Brain Stimulation, 7*, 525–531.

Chapter 12
Methodological Considerations for Transcranial Direct Current Stimulation in Clinical Trials

Roy H. Hamilton, Sudha K. Kessler, Laura Castillo-Saavedra, Felipe Fregni, Donel Martin, Colleen Loo, Helena Knotkova, and Adam J. Woods

R. H. Hamilton (✉)
Department of Neurology, University of Pennsylvania, Philadelphia, PA, USA

Department of Physical Medicine and Rehabilitation, University of Pennsylvania, Philadelphia, PA, USA

Goddard Laboratories, Room 518, University of Pennsylvania, Philadelphia, PA, USA
e-mail: Roy.Hamilton@uphs.upenn.edu

S. K. Kessler
Departments of Neurology and Pediatrics, Perelman School of Medicine at the University of Pennsylvania, Philadelphia, PA, USA

Children's Hospital of Philadelphia, Philadelphia, PA, USA

L. Castillo-Saavedra · F. Fregni
Spaulding Neuromodulation Center, Department of Physical Medicine and Rehabilitation, Spaulding Rehabilitation Hospital, Harvard Medical School, Boston, MA, USA

D. Martin
Black Dog Institute, The University of New South Wales, Sydney, NSW, Australia

C. Loo
School of Psychiatry, Black Dog Institute, The University of New South Wales, Sydney, NSW, Australia

H. Knotkova
MJHS Institute for Innovation in Palliative Care, New York, NY, USA

Department of Family and Social Medicine, Albert Einstein College of Medicine, Bronx, NY, USA

A. J. Woods
Center for Cognitive Aging and Memory (CAM), McKnight Brain Institute, Department of Clinical and Health Psychology, College of Public Health and Health Professions, University of Florida, Gainesville, FL, USA

H. Knotkova et al. (eds.), *Practical Guide to Transcranial Direct Current Stimulation*, https://doi.org/10.1007/978-3-319-95948-1_12

Introduction

In recent years, transcranial direct current stimulation (tDCS) has been explored as a treatment for a variety of disorders in psychiatry, neurology, rehabilitation, and pain medicine. This technology has a number of features that make it appealing as a potential clinical application, including a favorable safety profile, low cost, and ease of use. However, despite its advantages, tDCS currently has no FDA-approved indications. Further development of tDCS as an approved therapy requires that investigators pursue clinical trials that are of sufficient size and methodological rigor to convincingly establish the efficacy of tDCS for treating specific disorders. In turn, implementation of these well-designed trials requires consideration of a number of important factors, including study design, patient selection, use of appropriate control conditions, and the selection of optimal stimulation parameters. While many of these issues are similar to those facing the development of other novel treatments such as pharmacologic agents or other medical devices, the fact that tDCS is designed to leverage and enhance brain plasticity can add further complexity to these concerns. This chapter will address a range of methodological considerations in the design and execution of clinical trials involving tDCS.

Overview of tDCS Study Designs

Clinical trial design methodology has largely been driven by the study of pharmaceuticals, and this accumulated knowledge and experience informs the design of clinical trials of all types. However, clinical trial methods must be adapted to specific issues that arise in device trials in general, and noninvasive brain stimulation (NIBS) and tDCS studies specifically. The progression of a pharmaceutical compound to a clinically available medication includes pre-clinical studies in animal models; phase 1 trials (whose primary role is initial safety assessments and/or dose finding, and may be performed in healthy adults or a disease population); phase 2 trials (whose role is evaluating safety and tolerability, and gaining preliminary evidence of efficacy in a limited sample of patients with the disorder of interest); phase 3 studies (pivotal trials of efficacy in a large sample of patients which are needed for regulatory body approval for commercial marketing); and phase 4 post-marketing studies which conduct surveillance of the therapy after it is in widespread commercial use.

In contrast to the development of pharmaceutical treatments, in tDCS and other NIBS trials the initial evidence of potential efficacy does not typically come from animal studies, but rather from small, open label (non-randomized) case series or comparative observational studies that provide "proof-of-concept" of a treatment goal. Though this is an important step for determining whether to move forward with further studies, and for beginning to work out the best stimulation parameters, the gold standard for showing efficacy is to conduct randomized controlled studies, which will be the focus of this discussion. In device trials in general, the progression to proof of efficacy is often simpler: *pilot studies* (smaller studies showing safety, tolerability, and preliminary evidence of efficacy), and *pivotal studies* (larger studies aiming to establish clinically meaningful efficacy), particularly for implantable devices whose safety cannot be studied in healthy people because of the permanence and risk of implantation. Non-invasive brain stimulation falls somewhere in between these two poles – with some similarities to drugs, and other similarities to implantable devices. Thus, clinical trial methodology needs to be tailored to the specific issues of tDCS, and of course to the specific disease processes being targeted for treatment.

It is important to note the reasons why open label and non-randomized studies are inadequate to prove efficacy. A comparator group is essential to testing the efficacy of a treatment because there may be random fluctuations in disease severity that lead to a false appearance of effect. Moreover, the act of enrolling patients in a trial may in itself result in them receiving additional attention that may positively influence their function or outcome. Randomization is critical for efficacy trials in order to balance these and other measured and unmeasured confounders between the treatment groups, so that differences in outcome can be attributed to the treatment without bias. An example of balancing measurable confounders is the case in which enrolled patients are on CNS active medications either for the disorder being studied or for a comorbid condition. For instance, if by chance a higher proportion of patients on an SSRI are treated with verum (real) stimulation compared to sham (placebo) tDCS, the result may be inadvertently biased toward showing an effect of tDCS. While it might be possible to account for a measurable confounder like this (by accounting for that factor in the statistical analyses), unmeasured confounders cannot be dealt with in ways outside of randomization. Unmeasurable confounders include intrinsic biological factors, such as capacity for neural plasticity, that are not easily assessed. Randomization and adequate study sample sizes are critical for balancing factors like these, which are otherwise difficult to control explicitly.

There are several ways of structuring a clinical trial. Study design choices salient for tDCS trials include: parallel (between subjects) versus cross-over (within subjects), and single interventions versus factorial (more than one intervention tested simultaneously). The classic trial design is a 2-arm parallel enrollment study of treatment (A) versus placebo/sham or other treatment, including a different dose of active tDCS (B). In this design, patients are randomized to A or B, outcomes are measured at a specified time point, and comparisons are made between the two independent groups. The advantages of this design include shorter duration of participation for an individual patient and thus shorter overall study duration. In addition, this design is more conducive to evaluating long term outcomes. The disadvantages of a parallel design study include the requirement for larger numbers of patients than cross-over studies, and the potential for recruitment difficulty if patients dislike the idea of being randomized to sham treatment.

The alternative to a parallel study is the cross-over study, in which patients are randomized to one treatment arm first (treatment A, for example), followed by assessment of outcome at a specified time point, followed by entry into the other treatment arm (treatment B) with assessment of outcome at a specified time point (Fig. 12.1). The advantages of this design are that smaller numbers of patients are required to populate each treatment arm, every patient is exposed to the experimental treatment, and there is less heterogeneity between the two treatment arms because they are not

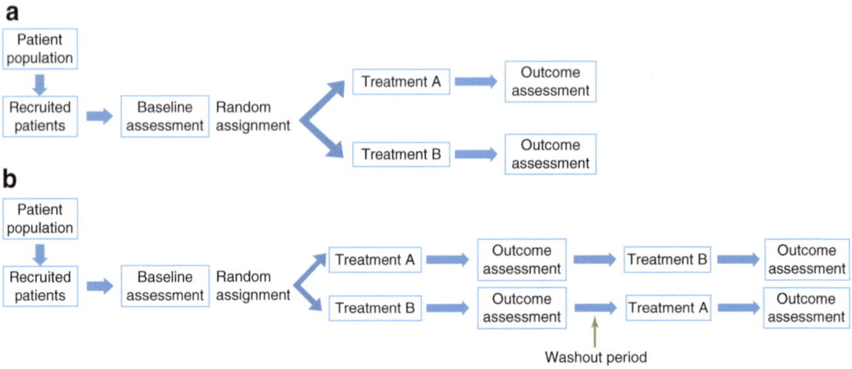

Fig. 12.1 (**a**) Two-arm parallel and (**b**) two-arm crossover trial designs

independent of each other. The major disadvantage of this design is the "wash out period" – that is, the amount of time necessary after a treatment for the effects of that treatment to dissipate. This design has been popular in NIBS studies because many studies have offered short term treatment exposure (even a single session sometimes) and have measured short term outcomes. However, in studies in which tDCS and other NIBS methods are being investigated for possible long term, or even permanent, effects, this design may eventually prove adequate. Furthermore, in clinical trials of tDCS for cognitive rehabilitation or augmentation, practice effects that occur when subjects undergo the same cognitive test multiple times must also be accounted for. Cross-over studies can also be challenging to implement and interpret in studies of neurodegenerative disease, wherein neurologic performance declines over time irrespective of clinical intervention. Another limitation to this design is that the sensory experience of sham tDCS may not be completely indistinguishable from verum stimulation, in which care it may be more difficult to achieve a true sham effect if patients are exposed to verum treatment prior to sham stimulation (Kessler et al. 2012).

A related trial design is the partial cross-over study, in which patients are randomized to either verum or sham treatment, and after the first outcome assessment, patients in the sham arm are crossed over to the verum arm. This method reduces or eliminates the concern about a wash out period for verum treatment, but there are statistical considerations that must be addressed in assessing the effect when the comparison groups are only partially independent.

Finally, another related trial design is the placebo run-in study – this is a relatively newer method that is gaining popularity in fields where there are historically high degrees of placebo effect, such as depression and headache. In the placebo run-in design, all subjects are started on placebo first, and subjects who are robust placebo responders are then removed from the study prior to randomization of the remaining subjects to placebo or active treatment. In this way, the randomization population is enriched for subjects who are not placebo responders, and thus the difference (effect size) between the two arms may be bigger, and the study would require fewer subjects to have the power to detect a true difference. This issue may be particularly relevant for tDCS trials because the treatment requires equipment and is more time and labor intensive for the investigative team than an oral pharmaceutical that can be dispensed to be taken at home. However, some investigators in fields using this design have raised concerns about whether it artificially elevates the absolute effect size and have called for it not to be used, particularly in phase 3 pivotal trials (Lee et al. 2004; Rosenkranz 2016).

In the study designs discussed so far, one treatment is compared to another or to placebo. In a factorial design, a combination of treatment can be compared to individual treatment and to placebo. In the classic 2 × 2 factorial study design, patients are randomized to treatment A, treatment B, treatment A and B together, or no treatment (sham). All patients undergo outcome assessment at a specified time point after enrollment. This study design may be particularly useful in tDCS studies when tDCS is believed to be augmentative, not independently effective. For example, this design may be useful in evaluating whether tDCS is more effective than standard rehabilitation techniques in a stroke population, or whether tDCS plus rehabilitation is more effective than either single treatment alone. The major disadvantage of this design is the requirement for a larger sample size than a simple 2 arm parallel group design, and the logistical challenges that attends combining two therapies (particularly if neither is a pharmaceutical that can be taken independently at home).

One of the most critical elements of clinical trials is the choice of control subjects and conditions. Clearly, the choice of study design is critical in determining who the control group is, as discussed above. In prior commentaries on tDCS treatment for neurologic or psychiatric disorders, and indeed in the broader medical literature, some investigators have raised concerns about the ethical issues of comparing treatment to placebo. However, this issue is nuanced. Randomization of patients to different treatment arms, including placebo, is ethical when there is clinical equipoise – genuine uncertainty about which treatment is safer and more beneficial, or whether treatment is safe and beneficial at all compared to placebo. Investigators who have invested time and effort into developing a new treatment which is inherently exciting to them may be inclined to believe that not providing the therapy is unethical – however, it is important for investigators to remember that strong preclinical evidence, or evidence from uncontrolled studies in humans, or in humans outside of the target population is rarely if ever robust enough to remove clinical equipoise. A strong argument can be made that it is, in fact, unethical to offer treatment with a weak evidence base (without randomized controls trials). Special cases arise in disorders that are rapidly life threatening, but under most circumstances the importance of properly conducted comparative trials when possible is hard to over-emphasize.

Recent advances in the science of clinical trial design have focused on adaptive trial designs, modifications to classical clinical trial methods which address key barriers to study completion such as expense, achieving adequate sample size, lengthy duration of studies, and the need for sequential studies to identify optimal treatments (Chow and Chang 2008). Adaptive designs allow for modifications to the trial procedures or statistical analyses after trial initiation without undermining its validity or integrity. The general goal is to achieve adequate statistical power with smaller sample sizes. Examples of adaptive designs include adaptive randomization, in which the probability of randomization to one treatment arm changes based on prior treatment assignments, in order to increase the likelihood of success; group sequential design, which allows for stopping a trial early for safety reasons or efficacy reasons during interim analyses; pick the winner design, which is employed when multiple treatments are being compared simultaneously, and allows for the least efficacious treatment arms to be dropped during interim analyses to allow subsequent patients to be assigned to treatments with higher likelihood of effect; and adaptive dose finding, which is used in early phase trials to find the minimum effective dose or maximally tolerated dose to determine the best dose range for the next phase trial.

Adaptive trial designs employ Bayesian statistical methods to determine the likelihood that study findings are true or false. This approach is based on the notion of updating the probability for a hypothesis as more evidence or information becomes available. A major advantage of adaptive trial designs for patients is that they may increase the likelihood of a patient being allocated to treatment that is beneficial to that patient while minimizing the risk of being exposed to potential harms – therefore enhancing the risk benefit balance. In this way, adaptive designs may also address some of the concerns raised in the discussion above about the ethics of enrolling patients in sham controlled studies. Studies involving tDCS may be especially well-suited for adaptive designs. Because there are many parameters that can affect outcome with tDCS, an adaptive design might employ Bayesian statistical methods to first find which electrode montage has the greatest effect, followed by which dose is most efficacious with the least discomfort. Of note, these approaches work best when short-term outcomes are being assessed.

Time Course and Natural History of Disease on tDCS Trials

Understanding the clinical characteristics and natural history of the disease being studied is essential to the decision-making process that takes place when designing a treatment trial. This is especially true for treatments like tDCS that involve long-term modulation of cortical activity. One of the critical functional properties of the central nervous system is its ability to form dynamic neuronal connections that can adjust and accommodate to new stimuli and situations. This capacity for neuroplasticity is considered the foundation of many behavioral and cognitive processes, and is also the basis for recovery after brain injury. Aberrant neuroplastic changes are also a critical component of several neurologic and psychiatric conditions. Modifying the dynamic processes that leads to plastic changes in the nervous system is the main goal of noninvasive neuromodulation approaches like tDCS. Importantly, patterns of altered cortical excitability and the ability of the brain to adapt vary according to the time course of injury (i.e. acute, subacute, or chronic) and the natural history (i.e. improving, static, or declining) of specific diseases.

Therefore, these factors must be taken into account when considering the appropriate design of clinical trials involving tDCS.

In the next two sections of this chapter we will use stroke as an example of a neurologic condition in which the timing of tDCS intervention and the time course of the disease have a tremendous impact on study design. Stroke is one of the best-studied neurologic conditions with respect to response to tDCS treatment, in that there is a large body of evidence that supports the use of tDCS for the treatment of both motor and cognitive post-stroke deficits (Elsner et al. 2013; Flöel 2014; Kang et al. 2015). Although the mechanisms through which tDCS exerts its beneficial effects are somewhat understood, there is no clear consensus as to what stage of stroke recovery will benefit most from NBIS techniques. We will discuss some of the benefits and disadvantages of selecting patients in the acute/subacute versus chronic stages of post-stroke recovery for clinical trials, and how the natural evolution of the disease through each specific stage affects trial design.

Acute and Subacute Conditions

Post-stroke recovery is often classified into acute, subacute, and chronic, although the time lapses that define such stages tend to vary in the literature. In general, the first 7 days after the injury are referred to as acute, 1 week–3 months are known as the subacute stage, and the time period after 3 months is the chronic stage (Duncan et al. 2003; Ng et al. 2008; Werner et al. 2002). It is important to point out that the acute and subacute phases stages of stroke recovery are widely considered to be critical periods in disease rehabilitation, when most synaptic reorganization normally occurs. Correspondingly, several studies (Cramer 2008; Hankey et al. 2007; Jørgensen et al. 1995, 1999) have shown that the most significant proportion of functional recovery in patients who have suffered a stroke will occur between months 3 and 6 after an injury, with a very small proportion of patients accomplishing some degree of recovery after 18 months (Hankey et al. 2007). In general, neural recovery usually precedes motor recovery by approximately 2 weeks, and the severity of the initial lesion will predict the rate of recovery, with those suffering from more severe injuries taking longer to experience improvement in the motor area (Jørgensen et al. 1995, 1999).

Based on what is known about the natural progression of recovery, it would seem logical that stroke patients would benefit most from therapeutic interventions started very early during their convalescent period. In support of this, some studies have shown that starting rehabilitation with physical (PT) and occupational therapy (OT) early in the hospital stay of patients admitted with stroke improves outcomes (Horn et al. 2005). However, the use of tDCS for stroke rehabilitation has, to date, mainly been reserved for the subacute and chronic periods of recovery. Given the physiologic changes that take place in the recovering post-stroke brain, one may think that introducing tDCS as early in the recovery process as possible would add a significant advantage to neural recovery, by enhancing beneficial neuroplasticity taking place in the damaged area, and by decreasing the maladaptive plastic changes in compensatory areas. However, there are a number of drawbacks that complicate the design of rigorous and interpretable clinical trials using tDCS in the acute stage of post-stroke recovery.

One of the most important challenges to designing tDCS trials in the early phases of stroke recovery is disambiguating natural recovery from treatment effects. As previously noted, the natural history of stroke is for most recovery to occur early after injury. This is of great importance for designing any study assessing the efficacy of a stroke rehabilitation intervention, in that it makes it more difficult for researchers to prove that improvements in either motor or cognitive function are a direct result of the introduced treatment, and not a normal consequence of the spontaneous recovery process. In addition, one could theorize that if there is a significant amount of plasticity that normally takes place very early on after neural injury, further increasing excitability in critical networks with tDCS may offer little added advantage. Moreover, it is important to consider that the degree to which tDCS and other neuromodulation therapies may benefit patients in the acute and subacute phases after stroke may vary from individual to individual. It has therefore been argued that it may be critical to correctly select subjects that would be responsive to early tDCS intervention, though the means for selecting such patients have not yet been determined.

The fact that the functional capacities of post-stroke patients can improve dramatically over a short period of time in the acute and subacute phases of recovery makes it difficult, if not impossible, to gather stable baseline behavioral assessments at different timepoints in the course of a prolonged clinical study. Because of these "period effects," crossover designs that use patients as their own controls must always carefully consider the impact of disease stage on the validity and interpretability of data, especially when subjects are being tested in the early phases of recovery. Unfortunately, while using a between-subject approach allows for treatment assumptions that are more robust and less complex, this study design approach also requires a larger number of subjects and measurements to achieve statistical power, as well as careful selection of patient characteristics in order to reduce variability related to baseline differences between patient groups.

We conducted a search on PubMed for clinical trials analyzing the effects of tDCS on patients in the early post-stroke stage, either acute or subacute. Only two of the retrieved studies included a sample of acute post-stroke subjects (Di Lazzaro et al. 2014; Sattler et al. 2015). Both trials were conducted within 4 weeks of injury and had a 2-group parallel design, and one was completed in an in-hospital setting. Although results from these two studies were inconsistent, they both addressed the possibility of spontaneous motor recovery as a possible limitation. Similarly, all subacute stage studies had a 2-group parallel design. However, most trials sampling subjects in the subacute stage did not include this aspect as a possible limitation for analysis of results (Bang and Bong 2015; Chang et al. 2015; Fusco et al. 2014; Hesse et al. 2007; Khedr et al. 2013; Kim et al. 2010; You et al. 2011). Only one of the retrieved studies mentioned the possibility of spontaneous recovery as a possible confounding factor in their trial (You et al. 2011).

Chronic Conditions

Conducting clinical studies with tDCS in the chronic phase of recovery of stroke introduces a different set of benefits and concerns with respect to trial design. It is generally accepted that late in the course of convalescence most subjects have reached a steady state of performance, which allows researchers to test their hypotheses regarding the efficacy of interventions against stable baseline performance. Nonetheless, a well-designed control condition is typically necessary in these investigations in order to assess other effects related to improvement, such as motivation and the Hawthorne effect, which is alteration of behavior by the subjects of a study due to their awareness of being observed.

After approximately 6 months following stroke, recovery becomes more stable and fewer changes in cognitive and motor function are seen. This makes baseline measurements of performance more stable and amenable to being compared in a crossover design. Between-subject comparisons remain more robust, but require a larger number of subjects. Large sample size requirements can become burdensome in studies with chronic patients; because patients in this stage of recovery are often at home and not hospitalized or in special care centers, access to them may be more limited, making recruitment more challenging. Patients who are coming in from home to participate in studies also have higher rates of attrition than patients studied in the inpatient environment. Most subjects after a moderate to severe stroke require some type of assistance in daily living activities, including transportation. Therefore, being part of a long clinical trial can become especially taxing to them and their caregivers, undermining their motivation to continue participating in studies. The different challenges facing within- and between-subject tDCS involving patients with chronic stroke are reflected in the existing literature. Of the 11 current studies that use a sample of chronic post-stroke patients, four included a crossover design (Celnik et al. 2009; Lefebvre et al. 2013, 2014; Zimerman et al. 2012), which allowed them to have relatively smaller sample sizes because of their decreased baseline heterogeneity and variance.

Management of Pre-existing Therapies in Chronic Conditions

In addition to conditions like stroke, where there is a single initiating event followed by a period of acute, subacute, and chronic recovery, tDCS has also been explored in clinical trials aimed at treating disorders in which the underlying disease process may be chronic, fluctuating or recurrent. For many such conditions, there are already pre-existing treatments that are believed to have some degree of efficacy (e.g. SSRIs for depression). Therefore, a key consideration in the design of clinical trials for this category of disorders is whether tDCS should be given in addition to existing treatments or whether current clinical treatments are withdrawn before tDCS is given. In this section, we will consider this dilemma in detail using depression as our main clinical example.

Many regulatory authorities require that a new experimental intervention (here tDCS) should be tested in the absence of other interventions, so that one can gauge the "pure" effect of the intervention without interference or interaction with other treatments. At face value this may seem reasonable, but in reality it poses several problems. The process of withdrawing a patient who has been stably established on drug treatments for several months, for the purpose of initiating tDCS in a clinical trial, is complex. First, withdrawal of existing treatments may lead to worsening of the clinical state of the patient. For example, in depression, one may see, paradoxically, an initial brief improvement, then followed by a decline in mental state. This means a complex and difficult-to-predict time course of mood changes, around the time that one is then introducing tDCS as an intervention. In clinical trials where participants have been withdrawn from prior treatments, for depression this has often involved a 2-week "wash out" period. However, the above effects may not have resolved by 2 weeks and a longer period may be necessary from the point of view of scientific purity. However a longer period is often not feasible within a clinic trial design.

Withdrawal of a participant from concurrent treatments also poses clinical risks and thus ethical questions. For example, someone who has partially responded to antidepressant treatment but still meets the entry criteria for a trial in terms of severity, may decline to a substantially worse mental state if current treatments are withdrawn, then become too unwell to enter the research trial and possibly even require urgent treatment due to suicide risk. This may happen in a not insignificant proportion of patients (personal observations). Thus, the participant is then denied trial entry and has gone from being stable though only partially responsive to treatment, to unstable and at acute risk. This not uncommon scenario arises because treatments to which the patient has failed to fully respond may still be partially effective (in this example with antidepressant effects) or may be providing specific beneficial effects e.g. antidepressants may improve anxiety and sleep without improving mood per se.

Withdrawal of concurrent medications also raises the challenging question of which medications should be withdrawn, since many medications have more than one effect. For example, in the case of a depression trial, one may specify that antidepressant medications should be withdrawn. However, the patient may also be on antipsychotic medications, some of which have independent antidepressant effects (e.g. quetiapine) or which may augment the effect of antidepressant treatments (e.g. aripiprazole). Further, depressed patients may often be on benzodiazepines to assist with sleep and anxiety. Patients with bipolar disorder (who may also be treated in depression trials) may be on mood stabilisers. If these are withdrawn, the participant is likely to be at increased risk of a manic upswing in mood i.e. a serious adverse event.

Withdrawal of concurrent treatments also means that it is difficult to know how the outcomes of the clinical trial then apply to a general clinical population, in whom concurrent treatments would not be withdrawn unless required for safety reasons. Thus, though the clinical trial may have been a useful "proof of concept" study testing the effects of tDCS in isolation, the results may not actually be generalizable to clinical practice. Translation into clinical practice is the ultimate aim of clinical trials of new interventions.

Given the above concerns, depending on the disorder being treated, the best compromise may be to require participants to be on stable doses of those medications which have effects on the specific outcomes being tested, and that these doses remain stable for a substantial period of time prior to the trial entry. This period should be informed by the disorder being treated and the time course for anticipated treatment effects to emerge with changes in dose. For example, for depression trials, this should be at least 6 weeks of a stable dose for new medications, or 4 weeks without change of dose for an established medication.

Later in this chapter, we will discuss specific interactions between tDCS and psychopharmacologic and nonpharmacologic interventions and further underscore the importance of considering the role of concurrent medication use on study design.

Impact of Disease Symptoms, Functional Impairments, and Medical Co-morbidities on tDCS Studies

In addition to the natural history and time course of the diseases being studied, disease-related symptoms, co-morbidities, and overall limitations of functional status associated with disease can substantially impact an overall feasibility and outcomes of any clinical trial, including trials employing tDCS. These factors often influence enrollment, retention, procedure compliance and data collection, and therefore require careful considerations in the planning stage of a study. Here we discuss three specific ways in which patient-related clinical factors can impact clinical trials involving tDCS: the ability of patients to provide informed consent, the ability of patients to travel to a research facility to participate in trials, and the ability of investigators to collect reliable data.

Informed Consent

The adverse cognitive effects of many neuropsychiatric diseases—and in some cases, the treatments for these diseases—may compromise patients' ability to fully consider risks and benefits of the study and to make informed decisions about study participation. While the nuances of determining whether a patient is in full command of the faculties required to provide consent are beyond the scope of this chapter, patients can be categorized broadly into individuals who are cognitively intact, those with cognitive deficits who possess decisional capacity, and those lacking decisional capacity.

Enrollment of study participants who are cognitively intact follows the usual consenting procedures delineated by regulatory authorities, such as the Institutional

Review Boards employed in the U.S. Adjustments to the consenting process are required if cognitively intact subjects suffer from sensory deficits (e.g. blind subjects); in such cases, regulatory bodies can provide specific guidance as to how to obtain the informed consent. The presence of patient's legal representative and/or an additional witness is often required.

Inclusion of subjects who present with cognitive difficulties but maintain decisional capacity, is more challenging (Galeotti et al. 2012; Giampieri 2012; Iacono and Carling-Jenkins 2012). These individuals have the legal capacity to provide informed consent for the study, but it is the responsibility of the investigator to ascertain (and sufficiently document) that these subjects understand the risks and benefits of the study as well as the study procedures and rights and responsibilities pertaining to study participation (Palmer et al. 2013). A suitable and frequently used approach to this issue is to include a brief quiz as a part of the informed consent (e.g. Knotkova et al. 2014; Nikulina et al. 2016; Rosedale et al. 2012). The quiz, approved by the regulatory authorities prior to the study together with the consent, usually includes a set of True/False statements, such as "If I participate in this study, I will be asked to come to the research facility for three visits"; "If I participate in the study I may not receive the real tDCS treatment"; "If I decide to participate in the study, I may withdraw from the study any time." A quiz such as this should cover all important aspects of study participation and procedures. If a patient answers incorrectly, the study personnel review the consent form with the patient again and provide clarification. A written note signed or initialized by both the investigator and the patient should be made to document that clarification was provided and that the patient verbalized understanding.

Regarding participants who lack decisional capacity, at least in the U.S. there are clear regulations on how to proceed with research consent (e.g. "Electronic Code of Federal Regulations 2016"; "New England Institutional Review Board 2016"). Consent is provided by the patient's legally authorized representative, and the study protocol often includes co-participation of a consented assistant or representative. It is expected that an authorized representative and/or the co-participating assistant will act in best interest of a patient, carefully weighing the anticipated risks and benefits of the trial, as well as an overall burden for the patient. Clinical trials involving participants lacking decisional capacity are extremely challenging in all aspects, but can yield valuable data on the potential utility of tDCS to treat serious medical conditions. To illustrate, a tDCS study by Angelakis et al. (2014) applied tDCS to subjects lacking decisional capacity due to disorders of consciousness (a persistent vegetative and minimally conscious states), and determined that tDCS may have the potential for clinical benefit in a field where effective treatments are sorely needed.

Limitations in Mobility and Travel

Because repeated administrations of tDCS are typically required to achieve long-lasting clinically meaningful changes in functional outcomes (Boggio et al. 2006; Cruciani et al. 2009; Fregni et al. 2006; Knotkova et al. 2009, 2012; Mori et al. 2010; Palm et al. 2012; Park et al. 2014; Sandrini et al. 2014; Valle et al. 2009; and others), participation in tDCS clinical trials often requires frequent travels to a research facility. This may be a substantial burden or barrier for some patient populations, such as patients with motor impairments or other symptoms that confer a high level of disability and/or low overall performance status. Until recently, participation in tDCS studies for such patients was either very limited or impossible. However, at-home systems for tDCS delivery have become available (Cha et al. 2016; Charvet et al. 2015; Kasschau et al. 2016; Knotkova et al. 2016). At-home tDCS requires that patients or individuals assisting them undergo comprehensive training in tDCS administration. This approach also requires a way to collect and transmit data that accounts for patient-specific limitations, systems that enable compliance and safety monitoring, and the ability to regulate critical stimulation parameters, such as stimulation intensity and duration. Experience indicates that the at-home tDCS approach, which is discussed in detail in Chap. 14, overcomes a number of barriers to participation in tDCS trials and enables inclusion of subjects with wide range of physical disabilities.

Another possible way to include subjects with decreased mobility or low performance status is an in-patient study. This approach has been successfully used in tDCS to accommodate the needs of patients with acute conditions in postoperative settings (Borckardt et al. 2013; Glaser et al. 2016), but can be extended also to tDCS trials in elderly patients or in persons with advanced illness who are in skilled-nursing facilities, nursing homes or hospice settings.

Limitations in Data Collection

Patient-related constrains pertaining to data collection arise from several issues that are often intertwined: sensory, motor and cognitive deficits, or overall low stamina. While an adjustment of data collection procedures for a specific deficit is usually straightforward, making adjustments for patients with overall low performance status, such as in patients with advanced illness or in elderly, is problematic because the volume of collected data has to be kept at minimum in order to maintain feasibility and to prevent excessive patient attrition. These constrains on data collection can be substantial and require careful selection of assessment tools and careful consideration of the duration of testing, the properties and demands of the assessments, and the anticipated value of the information to be gained. The issue of limited data collection in participants with low overall performance status can be at least partially mitigated by data collection assisted by patients' medical or informal caregivers, or supplementary data collection from a collateral source (Kutner et al. 2015). This approach has been successfully used in tDCS applications in patients with low performance status due to advanced life-threatening illness (Knotkova et al. 2016).

Balancing Inclusion and Exclusion of Patient Characteristics

The features of the population to be enrolled in any clinical trial are reflected in the inclusion and exclusion criteria employed to screen patients into and out of the investigation. The specifics of these criteria dramatically impact the heterogeneity or uniformity of study cohorts and the degree to which they are likely to be impaired by the disease being studied or by other comorbid conditions. The breadth or narrowness of these criteria must be largely informed by the purpose of the planned study.

If the purpose of the proposed trial is to determine the efficacy of tDCS (i.e. answering a research question "Does tDCS work for specific disease, symptom or population?"), the study sample should be well selected, and many potentially confounding conditions should be set as exclusion criteria at screening. This reflects the accepted notion that efficacy trials should be conducted with the study population that has the best likelihood of detecting effects (Friedman et al. 2014; Gartlehner et al. 2006). For that reason, many tDCS efficacy trials plan for exclusion of concomitant medication, either via wash-out prior the enrollment or by including medication-naive participants. However, it is also important to keep in mind that an excessive stringency in patient enrollment can paradoxically undermine a clinical trial. Study inclusion and exclusion criteria must be clinically relevant, and allow for generalization of the findings. For instance, it is important that the cluster of "core" symptoms typical for a disease of interest not be excluded, because that would render interpretation of the trial results in the broader clinical context problematic. From a practical standpoint, excessive exclusion can also jeopardize enrollment. For example, fatigue is a common symptom in many diseases, such as fibromyalgia, cancer, multiple sclerosis. Thus, excluding subjects with fatigue in clinical trials involving these patient populations would substantially affect both the generalizability of the study results and the feasibility of enrollment.

In contrast to efficacy trials, if the purpose of a proposed trial is to determine effectiveness, (answering the question "Does tDCS work in real life settings?"), inclusion of relatively broad study population is more appropriate. In such trials, patients' clinical characteristics, including co-morbidities and medication regimen should be built into the study protocol. This requires thorough considerations about strengths and weaknesses of different study designs because not all types of design are suitable for patients saddled with complex symptoms, multiple co-morbidities, polypharmacy or low stamina.

In summary, the inclusion of patient populations with complex symptoms, functional impairments, and medical co-morbidities is a complicated challenge, but one that promises to yield positive advances for tDCS as a potential therapeutic intervention. Taking complex patient factors into account further facilitates the development of approaches and protocols that target multiple symptoms and enhances exploration of tDCS paired with conventional non-tDCS treatments (Mendonca et al. 2016; Oliveira et al. 2015; and others). Hopefully, more comprehensive engagement with the various characteristics and co-morbities of patients' diseases will ultimately allow investigators to uncover the potential of tDCS to treat larger numbers of patients with currently unmet needs.

The Influence of Concurrent Treatments on tDCS Effects

Earlier in this chapter, we discussed concurrent treatments as a complicating factor in the design of tDCS studies in areas such as depression and chronic pain. One important reason to consider concurrent treatments very carefully when designing tDCS studies is that other clinical interventions—both pharmacologic agents and behavioral therapies—may influence the effects of tDCS in additive, synergistic, or in some cases, unexpected ways. Here we will review some of these issues.

Interactions with Pharmacologic Agents

In some cases, tDCS can be combined with other treatments to intentionally increase efficacy by eliciting additive and/or synergistic effects. Perhaps the best know example of this is the addition of SSRI antidepressant medications to tDCS in the treatment of depression. First, an initial proof of concept study in healthy volunteers showed that tDCS given concurrently with citalopram (an SSRI medication) led to enhanced and prolonged effects of anodal tDCS (Nitsche et al. 2009). Brunoni et al. (2013) then applied this principle in a two-factor clinical trial, showing that tDCS was superior to sham stimulation in treating depression, but that the combination of an SSRI (sertraline) and tDCS had superior effects to tDCS alone. Brunoni et al. (2012) also showed in a retrospective analysis of data from other clinical trials that a similar enhancement of antidepressant effects may also occur with antidepressants from another class. An early, open label pilot trial of tDCS in unipolar and bipolar depression suggested that effects of tDCS in bipolar depression may be superior, i.e. more prolonged, than in unipolar depression. The authors speculated that this lasting effect may have been due to the 14 bipolar patients involved being treated with concurrent mood stabilizer medications.

Combining tDCS with other concurrent treatments may also have complex, unintended and difficult to predict effects. For example, Nitsche et al. (2004) found that giving tDCS concurrently with a benzodiazepine (lorazepam) delayed the effects of anodal tDCS, though effects were later facilitated. However, an analysis by Brunoni et al. (2012) found that in depressed participants, receiving tDCS in the presence of a benzodiazepine may reduce the efficacy of tDCS. Similarly, Nitsche's group found that carbamazapine negated the cortical excitability- enhancing effects of anodal tDCS (Nitsche et al. 2003a). However, the analysis by Brunoni et al. (2012) in depressed participants did not find any effect of non-benzodiazepine anticonvulsant medications on stimulation efficacy. It is perhaps not surprising that experiments based on a single session of tDCS in the motor cortex of healthy volunteers, in a highly controlled, proof of concept setting do not translate into clinical findings when tDCS is given repeatedly in a clinical population of heterogeneous phenomenology, in combination with a variety of medications, even though they may belong to the same class. Apart from the examples discussed above, there are also multiple other pharmacological agents and receptor systems which may be involved, e.g. glutamate/NMDA, dopamine etc. (for review see Stagg and Nitsche 2011).

Other important considerations are whether the concurrent treatment is commenced with tDCS or whether it is a preexisting treatment. It is important that clinical treatment trials clearly demarcate between these two scenarios. Further, even if the concurrent treatment is initiated with tDCS, the brain's prior exposure to this particular medication, or medications from this class may also be important in determining stimulation outcomes, due to receptor changes which outlast the actual period of medication administration.

Interaction with Behavioral Tasks and Therapies

As with pharmacologic agents, there is evidence that tDCS has additive or synergistic effects when combined with behavioral tasks and interventions. Such effects have been observed with tDCS combined with motor and language rehabilitation following stroke (Meinzer et al. 2016), cognitive behavioral therapy for the treatment of depression (D'Urso et al. 2013), cognitive training for cognitive enhancement (Martin et al. 2013), and specialized skill learning for military application (Clark et al. 2010). Given the many possible interactions between tDCS physiological and behavioral effects, attempts should be made to both standardize patient behavior during an intervention and monitor both intentional and potential unintentional effects. This is important for understanding treatment effects, ensuring patient safety, and maintaining adequate blinding.

Evidence indicates that the physiological effects of tDCS are different when subjects perform a task during stimulation. Measurement of motor evoked potentials (MEPs) using single pulse TMS has been the most commonly used model to investigate tDCS physiological effects following stimulation. Antal et al. (2007) investigated the effects on post-stimulation MEPs after subjects performed two different tasks during anodal tDCS administered to the primary motor cortex, a cognitive task (general knowledge questions) and a motor task (pushing a ball with the right hand), compared to subjects sitting at rest during active tDCS. The type of behavioral task performed during tDCS was found to significantly affect the magnitude of MEPs post-stimulation. Task intensity has also been found to affect outcomes. Performance of fast thumb movements during anodal tDCS administered to the primary motor cortex reduced post stimulation MEPs, whilst slow thumb movements increased MEPs compared to sham (Bortoletto et al. 2015).

Functional neuroimaging studies further support the notion that behavioral tasks influence the effect of concurrent tDCS administration. Using fMRI, Antal et al. (2011) showed that concurrent finger tapping during anodal tDCS administered to the primary motor cortex decreased the BOLD response in the supplementary motor area compared to finger tapping with sham tDCS. In contrast, increased BOLD response in the primary sensorimotor cortex occurred with grasp hand movements during anodal tDCS administered to the primary motor cortex compared to the same movements during sham tDCS (Kwon and Jang 2011). In patients with mild cognitive impairment, Meinzer et al. (2015) found reduced BOLD responses in bifrontal task-relevant regions during performance on a verbal fluency task with active anodal tDCS administered to the left ventral inferior frontal gyrus compared to during sham tDCS. Using EEG, picture naming during concurrent tDCS caused differences in event related potentials (ERPs) during active compared to during sham tDCS, as well as reduced delta power immediately following active stimulation (Wirth et al. 2011). While the aforementioned neuroimaging studies are important in demonstrating different physiological effects of tDCS during performance of behavioral tasks, it is important to note that these studies did not examine the effects of active tDCS alone, so potential additive or synergistic physiological effects are unclear.

There is substantial evidence that tDCS has cognitive effects both during and following stimulation. These effects should be considered when designing a clinical trial. What patients do cognitively whilst receiving tDCS may influence treatment outcomes due to potential interactions between stimulation and task performance. For example, Segrave et al. (2014) found that antidepressant effects were improved when depressed participants performed cognitive tasks during tDCS compared to tDCS alone. Performing a task during concurrent tDCS over repeated sessions has also been found to both improve task performance and learning. For example, on a difficult motor learning task, anodal tDCS administered to the primary motor cortex improved performance during concurrent training over 5 consecutive days, with an increase in between-session compared to training during sham tDCS (Reis et al. 2009). In a subsequent study using the same task, this learning effect was found to be dependent on the duration of time between repeated sessions, with a period of at least 3 h following tDCS and training identified as necessary for consolidation effects (Reis et al. 2015). Concurrent anodal tDCS administered to the left dorsolateral prefrontal cortex (LDLPFC) also improved performance on a cognitive training task compared to sham tDCS over 10 daily sessions, though no effect was found for learning (Martin et al. 2013; Richmond et al. 2014). Task performance during concurrent tDCS over repeated sessions therefore may improve both performance on the task and learning between sessions. These effects though likely depend on the task in question, regions of stimulation, and interval between sessions. They also depend on the timing of the task relative to stimulation.

There is also the potential for unintended behavioral effects when patients perform tasks during tDCS. Such unintended effects first came to attention in a study which involved concurrent tDCS and task performance over repeated sessions. Iuculano and Kadosh (2013) administered numerical tasks during concurrent anodal tDCS administered either to the posterior parietal cortex or LDLPFC. While parietal tDCS improved learning on the trained task, performance on the second task was impaired compared to during sham tDCS. Interestingly, the opposite effect was observed in the LDLPFC condition, thus showing a double dissociation with task and stimulation effects. Given the limited evidence for adverse effects such as these, careful monitoring of potential unintended effects is recommended for protocols involving tDCS in combination with task performance, particularly in those involving repeated treatments. This can be achieved through incorporating comprehensive standardized assessments.

Choosing tDCS Parameters for Clinical Trials

Determining the appropriate approach for delivery of tDCS and the optimal parameters of stimulation is a critical consideration for the use of tDCS in clinical trials. As discussed in prior chapters, tDCS parameters include the size, number, and location of electrodes, the duration and intensity of stimulation, and the number of stimulation sessions. In this final section of Chap. 12, we will review practical considerations for the selection of stimulation parameters in clinical trials and highlight current challenges to appropriate parameter selection.

Electrode Properties: Size, Number, and Location

Because electrodes are the point of delivery of current generated by a tDCS stimulator, their properties—size, location and number—are important variables to consider in any stimulation study. The size of electrodes dictates the spatial distribution of current across the scalp at the point of contact with the head (Nitsche and Paulus, 2000; Woods et al. 2016). This feature can alter the distribution of current flow through brain tissue (Datta et al. 2009). Larger electrodes tend to result in distribution of current across a larger area of tissue, but also result in lower levels of stimulation intensity within stimulated tissue (Bikson et al. 2010; Datta et al. 2009). Thus, if the goal of a clinical trial was to deliver stimulation to a larger overall area of tissue with a lower stimulation intensity at any given region, larger anode and cathode electrodes would be appropriate (Bikson et al. 2010). However, if the goal of a trial was to deliver more intense stimulation to smaller area of the brain, smaller electrodes would be more appropriate. It is critical to note that a two-electrode tDCS approach (also referred to as 1×1 tDCS or conventional tDCS) using electrodes that are several centimeters in size (e.g., 5.0×5.0 cm) generally delivers stimulation

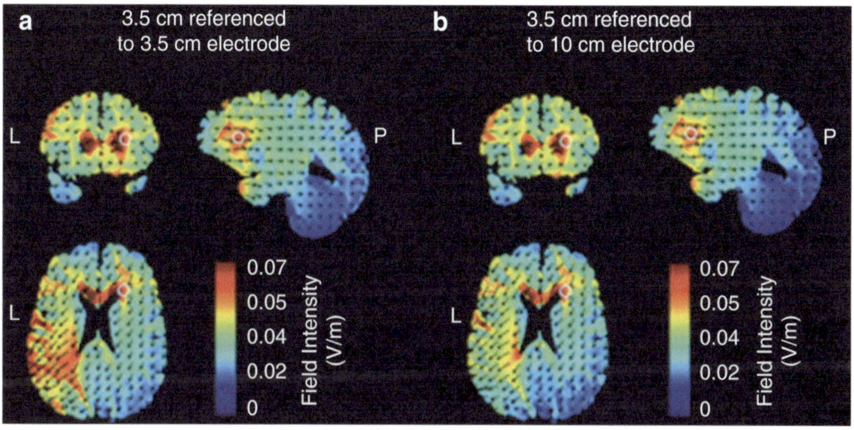

Fig. 12.2 (**a**) 3.5 cm^2 electrode over the right supraorbital (SO) area referenced to a 3.5 cm^2 electrode over CP3 (10–20 nomenclature) on the contralateral left hemisphere. (**b**) 3.5 cm^2 electrode over the right supraorbital (SO) area referenced to a 10 cm^2 electrode over CP3 on the contralateral left hemisphere. L left, P posterior, V/m = volts per meter, white circle = center of current model sampling location. Note the difference in current intensity between A and B

that has a low spatial resolution compared to other neuromodulation technologies like transcranial magnetic stimulation (TMS), so the notion of administering tDCS with either more or less focality is relative. Nonetheless, the size of the electrode directly impacts the overall distribution of current and the intensity of current flow at a given unit of tissue. For example, a trial might aim to distribute current more broadly with less overall intensity under one electrode (e.g., cathode) to potentially minimize the impact of current flowing from or to that electrode. In this case, a trial should use of a large electrode (e.g., 10 cm^2) paired with a smaller electrode (e.g., 3.5 cm^2; see Fig. 12.2). One caveat regarding this approach is that it is predicated on an assumption from the early tDCS literature that stimulation with different electrode polarities has opposite effects on brain activity (i.e. neuronal excitation under the anode and inhibition under the cathode), and that the delivery of more intense stimulation to a site is associated with more robust physiologic and behavioral effects. While this appears to be the case for certain combinations of parameters, this assumption is not universal and does not apply to all parameters used in tDCS (Nitsche and Paulus 2000, 2001; Stagg et al. 2013). It is also noteworthy that at least some recent data suggest that the relationship between electrode size and tDCS-induced changes cortical excitability may not be as predictable as had previously been presumed (Ho et al. 2016). Thus, it is not entirely clear whether it is always the case that a large electrode referenced to a small electrode serves to minimize effects under the larger electrode.

Most studies and trials using tDCS have employed a conventional two-electrode (1 anode and 1 cathode) approach. However, more recently, a number of studies have experimented with multi-electrode arrays in an attempt to alter the focality of current delivery to brain tissue (Borckardt et al. 2012; Edwards et al. 2013; Kuo et al. 2013; Nikolin et al. 2015; Villamar et al. 2013). For example, so-called High-Definition

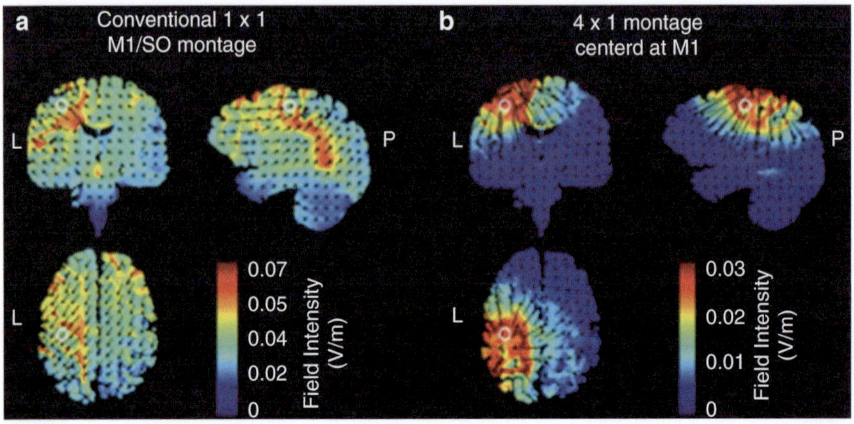

Fig. 12.3 (**a**) 3.5 cm² electrode over the right supraorbital (SO) area referenced to a 3.5 cm² electrode over M1 on the contralateral left hemisphere. (**b**) 4 × 1 montage centered at M1 using 1 cm diameter electrodes. L left, P posterior, V/m = volts per meter, white circle = center of current model sampling location. Note the difference in the stimulation intensity range in V/m between models indicates less stimulation intensity with the 4 × 1 montage

(HD) tDCS employs a 4 × 1 array of small electrodes, typically 1 cm² silver-silver chloride electrodes. This method places either a single anode or cathode electrode in the center of an array of four surrounding electrodes (Edwards et al. 2013; Woods et al. 2016). Modeling data demonstrates that the 4 × 1 high definition approach delivers current to a region of cortical tissue within the area defined by these electrodes, with little stimulation of deeper brain structures (Fig. 12.3) (Datta et al. 2009; Kessler et al. 2013; Minhas et al. 2012). Thus, if a trial seeks to stimulate only brain tissue near the cortical surface in a focal area, HD-tDCS could provide the necessary focality of stimulation for such a trial. Unlike the broad pattern of stimulation described with larger electrodes, the combination of small electrode size, higher electrode number, and careful placement of electrodes on the scalp interact to provide a level of spatial resolution that is not achievable with conventional tDCS (Woods et al. 2016).

It is possible to exceed five electrodes when administering tDCS. Some stimulators provide the option of using up to 20 or more electrodes with custom control of intensity of current delivery at each electrode (Park et al. 2011). While modeling software exists that can allow one to estimate the potential impact of "dense array" tDCS, the potential impact of this approach is almost entirely unexplored. Thus, it is not currently advisable to pursue dense array tDCS in clinical trials until further research on mechanism and impact are performed, or in the presence of clear pilot data supporting the effectiveness of the approach. Moreover, while traditional two- and five-electrode approaches are more common in the literature and have received significantly more investigation, the impact of varying parameters in these relatively well-established approaches are not well known. Thus, in the absence of pilot data that supports the use of a novel stimulation approach, radical modification or combination of parameters should be viewed with caution when planning a trial.

Electrode location is one of the most important properties for consideration when selecting stimulation parameters for a clinical trial (Bikson et al. 2010; DaSilva et al. 2011; Woods et al. 2015, 2016, since electrode placement dictates where in the brain stimulation is delivered, as well as the areas of greatest current density within brain tissue (Bikson et al. 2010; Dasilva et al. 2011; Woods et al. 2015, 2016). As noted above, conventional two-electrode (or 1 × 1) tDCS delivers a relatively broad pattern of current across large areas of brain tissue (Datta et al. 2009). However, while it is generally important for investigators to avoid the misconception that conventional tDCS has a high degree of spatial resolution for targeting brain structures (Woods et al. 2016), careful selection of electrode locations can help to make 1 × 1 tDCS more focal than simply stimulating the entire brain (Bikson et al. 2010; DaSilva et al. 2011; Woods et al. 2015, 2016). For example, placing conventional electrodes at F3 and F4 appears to produce stimulation that alters current density throughout the frontal cortices (Woods et al. 2014), whereas placing electrodes at CP3 and CP4 stimulates the entire parietal cortex, as well as posterior frontal, occipital, and superior temporal regions (Woods et al. 2014). While there is some overlap in areas of stimulation, the current flow patterns of these two electrode montages are sufficiently different to allow for experimental comparison of frontal vs. parietal effects of tDCS (Woods et al. 2015). Thus, careful electrode placement is critical to reassure investigators that regions that are meant to be stimulated are receiving a relatively high current, while areas that ought to be avoided are not. Various available modeling software packages—both free and for purchase—can be used to generate estimated current flow and density maps from model brains. However, caution should be exercised in interpreting these models, as they largely reflect the physical properties of the brain (e.g. tissue conductances), but not its physiological properties (e.g. patterns of brain activity at the time of stimulation). Moreover, these models do not typically account for the unique variations in individual brain anatomy. Currently, generating individualized models is a process that requires significant computing resources and personnel hours (López-Alonso 2014; Parazzini et al.2015). However, as modeling technology improves, it is likely that an individually optimized approach will provide improved guidance in electrode placement for clinical trials.

Number of Sessions, Stimulation Intensity, and Stimulation Duration

Other critical choices in the design of tDCS clinical trial include the number of stimulation sessions and the spacing of these sessions. While mechanistic, proof-of principle, and brain-behavior relationship oriented experiments typically involve designs where participants undergo a single session of active stimulation compared to a single session of sham stimulation in a within-subject design, or a single session of either tDCS or sham in a between subject design, a single-session approach is generally not useful for trials exploring tDCS as a clinical intervention (Gill et al. 2014; Woods et al. 2014). Because the effects achieved from a single session of tDCS are typically quite small, repeated stimulation sessions over multiple days are generally required to elicit larger, sustained, clinically meaningful impact (Faber et al. 2012; Ferrucci et al. 2014; Martin et al. 2014; Mattioli et al. 2015; Rushmore et al. 2013; Triccas et al. 2016; Villamar et al. 2013). Many studies have thus employed either a 1 week (e.g., five consecutive days) or 2 week (e.g., 10 days out of 14 possible days) repeated session design. Of note, the common use of these specific time periods is largely driven by feasibility rather than by any demonstrated difference in efficacy between specific periods of stimulation. Unfortunately, there is little information regarding the optimal number of sessions required to achieve maximal clinical effectiveness in any domain currently under study. Furthermore, it is also unclear whether multiple stimulation sessions within a single day could have more clinical benefit that single daily session approaches. While the ideal duration of multiday and multisession tDCS studies is yet to be determined, at literature currently strongly suggests that tDCS clinical trials are best suited to multiday repeated session approaches.

Stimulation intensity is another important but complex tDCS parameter that must be selected carefully in clinical trials. A very common assumption in the field is that stimulation under the anode electrode equates to excitation of underlying cortical structures, stimulation under the cathode equates to inhibition. However, this oversimplified account of the effects of tDCS derives in part from early neurophysiology studies of tDCS that examined the effect of 1 mA on TMS-elicited motor evoked potentials (MEPs) (Antal et al. 2004; Nitsche and Paulus, 2000; Nitsche et al. 2003b). These classic studies demonstrated that when the anode electrode was placed over the primary motor cortex (M1) and the cathode electrode was placed over the contralateral supraorbital region of the head (SO, i.e., above the eye), TMS-induced MEPs increased, consistent with increased motor excitability. The opposite pattern was found, smaller MEPs, when the cathode electrode was placed over M1, with the anode over SO. This finding has been replicated many times across numerous labs. However, more recent work has shown that when stimulation intensity is increased to 2 mA, MEPs increase when either the anode or cathode are placed over M1, with the opposing polarity electrode over SO (Batsikadze et al. 2013). This finding contradicts the assumption that brain areas under the anode and cathode are always excited and inhibited, respectively, and also indicates that the relationship between stimulation intensity and the physiologic effects of stimulation is not linear. Moreover, it remains unclear whether simple assumptions regarding electrode polarity and stimulation effects extend to regions in the brain outside the motor cortex. Further still, the effect of higher levels of stimulation (>2 mA) on tissue response is almost completely unknown. Thus, it is currently not recommended for clinical trials to exceed 2 mA of stimulation intensity in the absence of clear pilot data supporting the potential benefit of such a change.

Just as with stimulation intensity, stimulation duration is another tDCS parameter for which the assumption that “more is better” has been shown to be both oversimplified and potentially misleading. In most tDCS studies, the duration of stimulation ranges between 10 and 20 min. The effects of stimulation in this duration range are estimated to last from minutes to hours, or perhaps days in the case of multi-day repeated stimulation sessions (Nitsche et al. 2008; Woods et al. 2016). However, recent research demonstrates that stimulation lasting 20 min or more may alter the direction of tDCS-based effects on brain tissue (Batsikadze et al. 2013). Specifically, when 2 mA of stimulation was administered with the cathode over the primary motor cortex for 20 min, there was an increase in motor excitability, as reflected by increased motor evoked potentials elicited by TMS. This shift in direction of effect could have unintended negative consequences in the context of trials seeking to alter the excitability of brain tissue in specific ways. Of note, these effects were observed in healthy individuals; the effects of prolonged stimulation duration are likely to be even more unpredictable in patients. Thus, in the absence of clear pilot data demonstrating the efficacy of prolonged stimulation, investigators are advised to use caution in designing tDCS trials that employ stimulation durations that exceed 20 min.

Passive Versus Task-Associated Application of tDCS

In clinical trials tDCS has been explored as either a in a passive manner (i.e. no associated activity) or paired with a concurrent cognitive or behavioral task or activity. For example, in the case of depression, tinnitus, or pain, tDCS is often delivered while participants wait passively (Brunoni et al. 2011, 2013; Faber et al. 2012; Fagerlund et al. 2015). By contrast, in clinical trials attempting to treat cognitive symptoms of aging, stroke, traumatic brain injury, or other conditions, tDCS is often paired with a behavioral intervention, with the goal of strengthening the set of behaviors or mental operations elicited during stimulation (Jones et al. 2015; Martin et al. 2013, 2014; Mattioli et al. 2015). Recent research suggests that tDCS effects on cognition are state-dependent, meaning that stimulation appears to be most effective when people are stimulated when engaged in tasks that induce cognitive states of interest (Gill et al. 2014; Martin et al. 2014). In studies comparing "online" vs. "offline" applications of tDCS and cognitive training, online (i.e. concurrent) stimulation and training has shown the greatest effect on cognitive function (Martin et al. 2014). Further still, recent research suggests that tDCS effects occur when cognitive demands on the participant are relatively high in the domain of interest (Gill et al. 2014). For example, Gill et al. (2014) demonstrated that persons undergoing stimulation during a challenging working memory task showed effects of tDCS on neurocognitive measures of working memory function, whereas persons stimulated during a less challenging working memory task failed to evidence significant effects. Thus, while tDCS as a passive intervention is appropriate for certain clinical trials (e.g., depression, tinnitus, pain), trials that employ tDCS to treat disorders of cognition may be best suited to pair the application of stimulation with relevant tasks.

In summary, current knowledge of the optimal stimulation parameters tDCS in clinical trials remains fairly rudimentary. At present the parameter space of tDCS is very often oversimplified. Even in this brief section, we have outlined several misconceptions that permeate the field of tDCS. In this section of the chapter, we provided initial guidelines for consideration when designing the parameter space of a clinical trial. However, additional foundational studies are needed to more fully explore key variables such as electrode size, number, and location, stimulation intensity, duration, and frequency, and the role of concurrent behavioral tasks. In the meantime, clinicians and researchers designing clinical trials are best advised to work within common parameter space or based on specific pilot data when venturing outside common parameter space.

Conclusions

Designing robust and informative clinical trials for any intervention can prove to be formidable challenge. Investigators must select a study design that best fits the characteristics of the patient population, including the chronicity, clinical features, functional impairments, and co-morbidities of the disease being studied. In addition, there are a number of concerns that must be addressed in trials that employ tDCS, including but not limited to the interactions that arise between stimulation and other pharmacologic and behavioral interventions. Finally, a number of considerations relate specifically to the parameters of tDCS administration, such as the location, intensity, duration, and frequency of stimulation. In light of this extensive list of potential concerns, it is important for the field to look for ways to promote the consistency and quality of clinical trials involving tDCS.

One important way to achieve this goal is to use commonly agreed upon standards of practice in the design and reporting of tDCS clinical trial data. One such set of standards is spelled out in the Consolidated Standards of Reporting Trials (CONSORT) statement ("The CONSORT Statement 2016"), an evidence-based, minimum set of recommendations for reporting randomized trials. This statement has been endorsed by prominent peer-reviewed journals and editorial organizations, and a modified set of these standards has been supported by a growing number of investigators pursuing clinical trials employing tDCS (e.g. Brunoni and Fregni 2011). In addition, clinical trials involving tDCS should be registered at ClinicalTrials.gov ("ClinicalTrials.gov 2016"), an NIH-run registry and results database of publicly and privately supported clinical studies involving human participants. Registration at this site is now widespread practice in clinical research, and some journals now decline to publish trials that are not registered.

In summary, although it has yet to be approved by the FDA for any clinical indication, tDCS has a number of features that make it attractive as a potential intervention, and is actively being explored for treatment of a wide variety of disorders.

Careful consideration of the many issues that accompany the design and implementation of tDCS studies and the adoption of common standards for reporting clinical trial data will permit investigators to greatly accelerate the pace of discovery of successful tDCS treatments.

References

Angelakis, E., Liouta, E., Andreadis, N., Korfias, S., Ktonas, P., Stranjalis, G., & Sakas, D. E. (2014). Transcranial direct current stimulation effects in disorders of consciousness. *Archives of Physical Medicine and Rehabiliattion, 95*(2), 283–289.

Antal, A., Kincses, T. Z., Nitsche, M. A., Bartfai, O., & Paulus, W. (2004). Excitability changes induced in the human primary visual cortex by transcranial direct current stimulation: Direct electrophysiological evidence. *Investigative Opthalmology & Visual Science, 45*, 702–707.

Antal, A., Polania, R., Schmidt-Samoa, C., Dechent, P., & Paulus, W. (2011). Transcranial direct current stimulation over the primary motor cortex during fMRI. *NeuroImage, 55*(2), 590–596.

Antal, A., Terney, D., Poreisz, C., & Paulus, W. (2007). Towards unravelling task-related modulations of neuroplastic changes induced in the human motor cortex. *European Journal of Neuroscience, 26*(9), 2687–2691.

Bang, D., & Bong, S. (2015). Effect of combination of transcranial direct current stimulation and feedback training on visuospatial neglect in patients with subacute stroke: A pilot randomized controlled trial. *Journal of Physical Therapy Science, 27*(9), 2759–2761.

Batsikadze, G., Moliadze, V., Paulus, W., Kuo, M.-F., & Nitsche, M. A. (2013). Partially non-linear stimulation intensity-dependent effects of direct current stimulation on motor cortex excitability in humans. *Journal of Physiology, 591*, 1987–2000.

Bikson, M., Datta, A., Rahman, A., & Scaturro, J. (2010). Electrode montages for tDCS and weak transcranial electrical stimulation: Role of " return" electrode's position and size. *Clinical Neurophysiology, 121*, 1976–1978.

Boggio, P. S., Ferrucci, R., Rigonatti, S. P., Covre, P., Nitsche, M., Pascual-Leone, A., & Fregni, F. (2006). Effects of transcranial direct current stimulation on working memory in patients with Parkinson's disease. *Journal of the Neurological Sciences, 249*(1), 31–38.

Borckardt, J. J., Bikson, M., Frohman, H., Reeves, S. T., Datta, A., Bansal, V., … George, M. S. (2012). A pilot study of the tolerability and effects of high-definition transcranial direct current stimulation (HD-tDCS) on pain perception. *Journal of Pain, 13*, 112–120.

Borckardt, J. J., Reeves, S. T., Robinson, S. M., May, J. T., Epperson, T. I., Gunselman, R. J., … George, M. S. (2013). Transcranial direct current stimulation (tDCS) reduces postsurgical opioid consumption in total knee arthroplasty (TKA). *The Clinical Journal of Pain, 29*(11), 925–928.

Bortoletto, M., Pellicciari, M. C., Rodella, C., & Miniussi, C. (2015). The interaction with task-induced activity is more important than polarization: A tDCS study. *Brain Stimulation, 8*(2), 269–276.

Brunoni, A. R., Ferrucci, R., Bortolomasi, M., Scelzo, E., Boggio, P. S., Fregni, F., … Priori, A. (2012). Interactions between transcranial direct current stimulation (tDCS) and pharmacological interventions in the major depressive episode: Findings from a naturalistic study. *European Psychiatry, 28*(6), 356–361.

Brunoni, A. R., Ferrucci, R., Bortolomasi, M., Vergari, M., Tadini, L., Boggio, P. S., … Priori, A. (2011). Transcranial direct current stimulation (tDCS) in unipolar vs. bipolar depressive disorder. *Progress in Neuro-Psychopharmacology & Biological Psychiatry, 35*, 96–101.

Brunoni, A. R., & Fregni, F. (2011). Clinical trial design in non-invasive brain stimulation psychiatric research. *International Journal of Methods in Psychiatric Research, 20*(2), E19–E30.

Brunoni, A. R., Valiengo, L., Baccaro, A., Zanão, T. A., Oliveira, J. F., Goulart, A., … Fregni, F. (2013). The sertraline vs electrical current therapy for treating depression clinical study: Results from a factorial, randomized, controlled trial. *JAMA Psychiatry, 70*(4), 383–391.

Celnik, P., Paik, N., Vandermeeren, Y., Dimyan, M., & Cohen, L. G. (2009). Effects of combined peripheral nerve stimulation and brain polarization on performance of a motor sequence task after chronic stroke. *Stroke, 40*(5), 1764–1771.

Cha, Y., Urbano, D., & Pariseau, N. (2016). Randomized single blind sham controlled trial of adjunctive home-based tDCS after rTMS for Mal De Debarquement syndrome: Safety, efficacy, and participant satisfaction assessment. *Brain Stimulation, 9*(4), 537–544.

Chang, M. C., Kim, D. Y., & Park, D. H. (2015). Enhancement of cortical excitability and lower limb motor function in patients with stroke by transcranial direct current stimulation. *Brain Stimulation, 8*(3), 561–566.

Charvet, L. E., Kasschau, M., Datta, A., Knotkova, H., Stevens, M. C., Alonzo, A., … Bikson, M. (2015). Remotely-supervised transcranial direct current stimulation (tDCS) for clinical trials: Guidelines for technology and protocols. *Frontiers in Systems Neuroscience, 9*.

Chow, S.-C., & Chang, M. (2008). Adaptive design methods in clinical trials – A review. *Orphanet Journal of Rare Diseases, 3*, 11.

Clark, V. P., Coffman, B. A., Mayer, A. R., Weisend, M. P., Lane, T. D., Calhoun, V. D., … Wassermann, E. M. (2010). TDCS guided using fMRI significantly accelerates learning to identify concealed objects. *NeuroImage, 59*(1), 117–128.

ClinicalTrials.gov. (2016). Retrieved July 14, 2016, from http://clinicaltrials.gov/

Cramer, S. C. (2008). Repairing the human brain after stroke: I. Mechanisms of spontaneous recovery. *Annals of Neurology, 63*(3), 272–287.

Cruciani, R. A., Esteban, S., Sibirceva, U., & Knotkova, H. (2009). Non-invasive brain stimulation therapy for the management of complex regional pain syndrome (CRPS). *Journal of Pain Management, Special issue on "Brain stimulation for treatment of pain", 2*(3), 277–285.

D'Urso, G., Mantovani, A., Micillo, M., Priori, A., & Muscettola, G. (2013). Transcranial direct current stimulation and cognitive-behavioral therapy: Evidence of a synergistic effect in treatment-resistant depression. *Brain Stimulation, 6*(3), 465–467.

Dasilva, A. F., Volz, M. S., Bikson, M., & Fregni, F. (2011). Electrode positioning and montage in transcranial direct current stimulation. *Journal of Visualized Experiments, 54*.

Datta, A., Bansal, V., Diaz, J., Patel, J., Reato, D., & Bikson, M. (2009). Gyri-precise head model of transcranial direct current stimulation: Improved spatial focality using a ring electrode versus conventional rectangular pad. *Brain Stimulation, 2*(4), 201–207.e1.

Di Lazzaro, V., Dileone, M., Capone, F., Pellegrino, G., Ranieri, F., Musumeci, G., … Fregni, F. (2014). Immediate and late modulation of interhemipheric imbalance with bilateral transcranial direct current stimulation in acute stroke. *Brain Stimulation, 7*(6), 841–848.

Duncan, P., Studenski, S., Richards, L., Gollub, S., Lai, S. M., Reker, D., … Johnson, D. (2003). Randomized clinical trial of therapeutic exercise in subacute stroke. *Stroke, 34*(9), 2173–2180.

Edwards, D., Cortes, M., Datta, A., Minhas, P., Wassermann, E. M., & Bikson, M. (2013). Physiological and modeling evidence for focal transcranial electrical brain stimulation in humans: A basis for high-definition tDCS. *NeuroImage, 74*, 266–275.

Electronic Code of Federal Regulations. (2016). Retrieved July 15, 2016, from http://www.ecfr.gov/

Elsner, B., Kugler, J., Pohl, M., & Mehrholz, J. (2013). Transcranial direct current stimulation (tDCS) for improving function and activities of daily living in patients after stroke. *Cochrane Database of Systematic Reviews, 11*.

Faber, M., Vanneste, S., Fregni, F., & Ridder, D. D. (2012). Top down prefrontal affective modulation of tinnitus with multiple sessions of tDCS of dorsolateral prefrontal cortex. *Brain Stimulation, 5*(4), 492–498.

Fagerlund, A. J., Hansen, O. A., & Aslaksen, P. M. (2015). Transcranial direct current stimulation as a treatment for patients with fibromyalgia. *Pain, 156*(1), 62–71.

Ferrucci, R., Vergari, M., Cogiamanian, F., Bocci, T., Ciocca, M., Tomasini, E., … Priori, A. (2014). Transcranial direct current stimulation (tDCS) for fatigue in multiple sclerosis. *NeuroRehabilitation, 34*, 121–127.

Flöel, A. (2014). TDCS-enhanced motor and cognitive function in neurological diseases. *NeuroImage, 85*(3), 934–947.

Fregni, F., Boggio, P. S., Nitsche, M. A., Rigonatti, S. P., & Pascual-Leone, A. (2006). Cognitive effects of repeated sessions of transcranial direct current stimulation in patients with depression. *Depression and Anxiety, 23*(8), 482–484.

Friedman, L. M., Furberg, C. D., & DeMets, D. L. (2014). *Fundamentals of clinical trials* (3rd ed.). Cham, Switzerland: Springer.

Fusco, A., Assenza, F., Iosa, M., Izzo, S., Altavilla, R., Paolucci, S., & Vernieri, F. (2014). The ineffective role of cathodal tDCS in enhancing the functional motor outcomes in early phase of stroke rehabilitation: An experimental trial. *BioMed Research International, 2014*, 1–9.

Galeotti, F., Vanacore, N., Gainotti, S., Izzicupo, F., Menniti-Ippolito, F., Petrini, C., … Raschetti, R. (2012). How legislation on decisional capacity can negatively affect the feasibility of clinical trials in patients with dementia. *Drugs Aging Drugs & Aging, 29*(8), 607–614.

Gartlehner, G., Hansen, R. A., & Nissman, D. (2006). Criteria for distinguishing effectiveness from efficacy trials in systematic reviews. *Agency for Healthcare Research and Quality, 12*, 1–17.

Giampieri, M. (2012). Communication and informed consent in elderly people. *Minerva Anestesiologica, 78*(2), 236–242.

Gill, J., Shah-Basak, P. P., & Hamilton, R. (2014). It's the thought that counts: Examining the task-dependent effects of transcranial direct current stimulation on executive function. *Brain Stimulation, 8*, 253–259.

Glaser, J., Reeves, S. T., Stoll, W. D., Epperson, T. I., Hilbert, M., Madan, A., … Borckardt, J. J. (2016). Motor/prefrontal transcranial direct current stimulation (tDCS) following lumbar surgery reduces postoperative analgesia use. *Spine, 41*(10), 835–839.

Hankey, G. J., Spiesser, J., Hakimi, Z., Bego, G., Carita, P., & Gabriel, S. (2007). Rate, degree, and predictors of recovery from disability following ischemic stroke. *Neurology, 68*(19), 1583–1587.

Hesse, S., Werner, C., Schonhardt, E. M., Bardeleben, A., Jenrich, W., & Kirker, S. B. (2007). Combined transcranial direct current stimulation and robot-assisted arm training in subacute stroke patients: A pilot study. *Restorative Neurology & Neuroscience, 25*(1), 9–15.

Ho, K., Taylor, J. L., Chew, T., Gálvez, V., Alonzo, A., Bai, S., … Loo, C. K. (2016). The effect of transcranial direct current stimulation (tDCS) electrode size and current intensity on motor cortical excitability: Evidence from single and repeated sessions. *Brain Stimulation, 9*(1), 1–7.

Horn, S. D., Dejong, G., Smout, R. J., Gassaway, J., James, R., & Conroy, B. (2005). Stroke rehabilitation patients, practice, and outcomes: Is earlier and more aggressive therapy better? *Archives of Physical Medicine and Rehabilitation, 86*(12), 101–114.

Iacono, T., & Carling-Jenkins, R. (2012). The human rights context for ethical requirements for involving people with intellectual disability in medical research. *Journal of Intellectual Disability Research, 56*(11), 1122–1132.

Iuculano, T., & Kadosh, R. C. (2013). The mental cost of cognitive enhancement. *Journal of Neuroscience, 33*(10), 4482–4486.

Jones, K. T., Stephens, J. A., Alam, M., Bikson, M., & Berryhill, M. E. (2015). Longitudinal neurostimulation in older adults improves working memory. *PLoS One, 10*(4), e0121904.

Jørgensen, H. S., Nakayama, H., Raaschou, H. O., & Olsen, T. S. (1999). Stroke: Neurologic and functional recovery. The Copenhagen stroke study. *Physical Medicine and Rehabilitation Clinics of North America, 10*(4), 887–906.

Jørgensen, H. S., Nakayama, H., Raaschou, H. O., Vive-Larsen, J., Støier, M., & Olsen, T. S. (1995). Outcome and time course of recovery in stroke. Part II: Time course of recovery. The Copenhagen stroke study. *Archives of Physical Medicine and Rehabilitation, 76*(5), 406–412.

Kang, N., Summers, J. J., & Cauraugh, J. H. (2015). Transcranial direct current stimulation facilitates motor learning post-stroke: A systematic review and meta-analysis. *Journal of Neurology, Neurosurgery & Psychiatry, 87*(4), 345–355.

Kasschau, M., Reisner, J., Sherman, K., Bikson, M., Datta, A., & Charvet, L. E. (2016). Transcranial direct current stimulation is feasible for remotely supervised home delivery in multiple sclerosis. *Neuromodulation: Technology at the Neural Interface, 19*, 824–831.

Kessler, S. K., Minhas, P., Woods, A. J., Rosen, A., Gorman, C., & Bikson, M. (2013). Dosage considerations for transcranial direct current stimulation in children: A computational modeling study. *PLoS One, 8*(9), e76112.

Kessler, S. K., Turkeltaub, P. E., Benson, J. G., & Hamilton, R. H. (2012). Differences in the experience of active and sham transcranial direct current stimulation. *Brain Stimulation, 5*(2), 155–162.

Khedr, E. M., Shawky, O. A., El-Hammady, D. H., Rothwell, J. C., Darwish, E. S., Mostafa, O. M., & Tohamy, A. M. (2013, September 22). Effect of anodal versus cathodal transcranial direct current stimulation on stroke rehabilitation: A pilot randomized controlled trial. *Neurorehabilitation and Neural Repair, 27*(7), 592–601.

Kim, D., Lim, J., Kang, E. K., You, D. S., Oh, M., Oh, B., & Paik, N. (2010). Effect of transcranial direct current stimulation on motor recovery in patients with subacute stroke. *American Journal of Physical Medicine & Rehabilitation, 89*(11), 879–886.

Knotkova, H., Homel, P., & Cruciani, R. A. (2009). Cathodal tDCS over the somatosensory cortex relieved chronic neuropathic pain in a patient with complex regional pain syndrome (CRPS/RSD). *Journal of Pain Management, Special issue on "Brain stimulation for treatment of pain", 2*(3), 365–368.

Knotkova, H., Malamud, S. C., & Cruciani, R. A. (2014). Transcranial direct current stimulation (TDCS) improved cognitive outcomes in a cancer survivor with chemotherapy-induced cognitive difficulties. *Brain Stimulation, 7*(5), 767–768.

Knotkova, H., Riggs, A., Patel, V., Troung, D., Arce, D., Datta, A., & Bikson, M. (2016). *Adjustment of headgear for easy use by chronically ill patients performing non-invasive neurostimulation at home. Poster*. New York, NY: Metropolitan Jewish Health System Research Day.

Knotkova, H., Rosedale, M., Strauss, S. M., Horne, J., Soto, E., Cruciani, R. A., … Malamud, D. (2012). Using transcranial direct current stimulation to treat depression in HIV-infected persons: The outcomes of a feasibility study. *Frontiers in Psychiatry, 3*.

Kuo, H., Bikson, M., Datta, A., Minhas, P., Paulus, W., Kuo, M., & Nitsche, M. A. (2013). Comparing cortical plasticity induced by conventional and high-definition 4 × 1 ring tDCS: A neurophysiological study. *Brain Stimulation, 6*(4), 644–648.

Kutner, J. S., Blatchford, P. J., Taylor, D. H., Ritchie, C. S., Bull, J. H., Fairclough, D. L., … Abernethy, A. P. (2015). Safety and benefit of discontinuing statin therapy in the setting of advanced, life-limiting illness. *JAMA Internal Medicine, 175*(5), 691–700.

Kwon, Y. H., & Jang, S. H. (2011). The enhanced cortical activation induced by transcranial direct current stimulation during hand movements. *Neuroscience Letters, 492*(2), 105–108.

Lee, S., Walker, J. R., Jakul, L., & Sexton, K. (2004). Does elimination of placebo responders in a placebo run-in increase the treatment effect in randomized clinical trials? A meta-analytic evaluation. *Depression and Anxiety, 19*(1), 10–19.

Lefebvre, S., Dricot, L., Laloux, P., Gradkowski, W., Desfontaines, P., Evrard, F., … Vandermeeren, Y. (2014). Neural substrates underlying stimulation-enhanced motor skill learning after stroke. *Brain, 138*(1), 149–163.

Lefebvre, S., Laloux, P., Peeters, A., Desfontaines, P., Jamart, J., & Vandermeeren, Y. (2013). Dual-tDCS enhances online motor skill learning and long-term retention in chronic stroke patients. *Frontiers in Human Neuroscience, 6*.

López-Alonso, V., Cheeran, B., Río-Rodríguez, D., & Fernández-Del-Olmo, M. (2014). Inter-individual variability in response to non-invasive brain stimulation paradigms. *Brain Stimulation, 7*(3), 372–380.

Martin, D. M., Liu, R., Alonzo, A., Green, M., & Loo, C. K. (2014). Use of transcranial direct current stimulation (tDCS) to enhance cognitive training: Effect of timing of stimulation. *Experimental Brain Research, 232*(10), 3345–3351.

Martin, D. M., Liu, R., Alonzo, A., Green, M., Player, M. J., Sachdev, P., & Loo, C. K. (2013). Can transcranial direct current stimulation enhance outcomes from cognitive training? A randomized controlled trial in healthy participants. *The International Journal of Neuropsychopharmacology, 16*(9), 1927–1936.

Mattioli, F., Bellomi, F., Stampatori, C., Capra, R., & Miniussi, C. (2015, May 26). Neuroenhancement through cognitive training and anodal tDCS in multiple sclerosis. *Multiple Sclerosis Journal, 22*(2), 222–230.

Meinzer, M., Darkow, R., Lindenberg, R., & Floel, A. (2016). Electrical stimulation of the motor cortex enhances treatment outcome in post-stroke aphasia. *Brain, 139*(4), 1152–1163.

Meinzer, M., Lindenberg, R., Phan, M. T., Ulm, L., Volk, C., & Floel, A. (2015). Transcranial direct current stimulation in mild cognitive impairment: Behavioral effects and neural mechanisms. *Alzheimer's & Dementia, 11*(9), 1032–1040.

Mendonca, M. E., Simis, M., Grecco, L. C., Battistella, L. R., Baptista, A. F., & Fregni, F. (2016). Transcranial direct current stimulation combined with aerobic exercise to optimize analgesic responses in fibromyalgia: A randomized placebo-controlled clinical trial. *Frontiers in Human Neuroscience*, 10.

Minhas, P., Bikson, M., Woods, A. J., Rosen, A. R., & Kessler, S. K. (2012). Transcranial direct current stimulation in pediatric brain: A computational modeling study. *2012 Annual International Conference of the IEEE Engineering in Medicine and Biology Society*.

Mori, F., Codecà, C., Kusayanagi, H., Monteleone, F., Buttari, F., Fiore, S., ... Centonze, D. (2010). Effects of anodal transcranial direct current stimulation on chronic neuropathic pain in patients with multiple sclerosis. *The Journal of Pain, 11*(5), 436–442.

New England Institutional Review Board. (2016). Retrieved August 15, 2016, from http://www.neirb.com/

Ng, M. F., Tong, R. K., & Li, L. S. (2008). A pilot study of randomized clinical controlled trial of gait training in subacute stroke patients with partial body-weight support electromechanical gait trainer and functional electrical stimulation: Six-month follow-up. *Stroke, 39*(1), 154–160.

Nikolin, S., Loo, C. K., Bai, S., Dokos, S., & Martin, D. M. (2015). Focalised stimulation using high definition transcranial direct current stimulation (HD-tDCS) to investigate declarative verbal learning and memory functioning. *NeuroImage, 117*, 11–19.

Nikulina, V., Guarino, H., Acosta, M. C., Marsch, L. A., Syckes, C., Moore, S. K., ... Rosenblum, A. (2016). Patient vs provider reports of aberrant medication-taking behavior among opioid-treated patients with chronic pain who report misusing opioid medication. *Pain, 157*(8), 1791–1798.

Nitsche, M. A., Cohen, L. G., Wassermann, E. M., Priori, A., Lang, N., Antal, A., ... Pascual-Leone, A. (2008). Transcranial direct current stimulation: State of the art 2008. *Brain Stimulation, 1*(3), 206–223.

Nitsche, M. A., Fricke, K., Henschke, U., Schlitterlau, A., Liebetanz, D., Lang, N., ... Paulus, W. (2003a). Pharmacological modulation of cortical excitability shifts induced by transcranial direct current stimulation in humans. *Journal of Physiology, 553*(1), 293–301.

Nitsche, M. A., Kuo, M. F., Karrasch, R., Wachter, B., Liebetanz, D., & Paulus, W. (2009). Serotonin affects transcranial direct current-induced neuroplasticity in humans. *Biological Psychiatry, 66*(5), 503–508.

Nitsche, M. A., Liebetanz, D., Schlitterlau, A., Henschke, U., Fricke, K., Frommann, K., ... Tergau, F. (2004). GABAergic modulation of DC stimulation-induced motor cortex excitability shifts in humans. *European Journal of Neuroscience, 19*(10), 2720–2726.

Nitsche, M. A., Nitsche, M. S., Klein, C. C., Tergau, F., Rothwell, J. C., & Paulus, W. (2003). Level of action of cathodal DC polarisation induced inhibition of the human motor cortex. *Clinical Neurophysiology, 114*(4), 600–604.

Nitsche, M. A., & Paulus, W. (2000). Excitability changes induced in the human motor cortex by weak transcranial direct current stimulation. *The Journal of Physiology, 527*(3), 633–639.

Nitsche, M. A., & Paulus, W. (2001). Sustained excitability elevations induced by transcranial DC motor cortex stimulation in humans. *Neurology, 57*(10), 1899–1901.

Oliveira, L. B., Lopes, T. S., Soares, C., Maluf, R., Goes, B. T., Sá, K. N., & Baptista, A. F. (2015, April 20). Transcranial direct current stimulation and exercises for treatment of chronic temporomandibular disorders: A blind randomised-controlled trial. *Journal of Oral Rehabilitation, 42*(10), 723–732.

Palm, U., Schiller, C., Fintescu, Z., Obermeier, M., Keeser, D., Reisinger, E., … Padberg, F. (2012). Transcranial direct current stimulation in treatment resistant depression: A randomized double-blind, placebo-controlled study. *Brain Stimulation, 5*(3), 242–251.

Palmer, B. W., Savla, G. N., Roesch, S. C., & Jeste, D. V. (2013, June 09). Changes in capacity to consent over time in patients involved in psychiatric research. *The British Journal of Psychiatry, 202*(6), 454–458.

Parazzini, M., Fiocchi, S., Liorni, I., & Ravazzani, P. (2015). Effect of the interindividual variability on computational modeling of transcranial direct current stimulation. *Computational Intelligence and Neuroscience, 2015*, 1–9.

Park, J., Hong, S. B., Kim, D., Suh, M., & Im, C. (2011). A novel array-type transcranial direct current stimulation (tDCS) system for accurate focusing on targeted brain areas. *IEEE Transactions on Magnetics, 47*(5), 882–885.

Park, S., Seo, J., Kim, Y., & Ko, M. (2014). Long-term effects of transcranial direct current stimulation combined with computer-assisted cognitive training in healthy older adults. *Neuroreport, 25*(2), 122–126.

Reis, J., Fischer, J. T., Prichard, G., Weiller, C., Cohen, L. G., & Fritsch, B. (2015). Time- but not sleep-dependent consolidation of tDCS-enhanced visuomotor skills. *Cerebral Cortex, 25*(1), 109–117.

Reis, J., Schambra, H. M., Cohen, L. G., Buch, E. R., Fritsch, B., Zarahn, E., … Krakauer, J. W. (2009). Noninvasive cortical stimulation enhances motor skill acquisition over multiple days through an effect on consolidation. *Proceedings of the National Academy of Sciences of the United States, 106*(5), 1590–1595.

Richmond, L. L., Wolk, D., Chein, J., & Olson, I. R. (2014). Transcranial direct current stimulation enhances verbal working memory training performance over time and near transfer outcomes. *Journal of Cognitive Neuroscience, 26*(11), 2443–2454.

Rosedale, M., Malaspina, D., Malamud, D., Strauss, S. M., Horne, J. D., Abouzied, S., … Knotkova, H. (2012). Developing patient-centered treatment protocols in brain stimulation: A rationale for combining quantitative and qualitative approaches in persons with HIV. *Journal of the American Psychiatric Nurses Association, 18*(3), 166–174.

Rosenkranz, G. K. (2016). Remarks on designs enriching for placebo non-responders. *Clinical Trials, 13*(3), 338–343.

Rushmore, R. J., Desimone, C., & Valero-Cabré, A. (2013). Multiple sessions of transcranial direct current stimulation to the intact hemisphere improves visual function after unilateral ablation of visual cortex. *European Journal of Neuroscience, 12*, 3799–3807.

Sandrini, M., Brambilla, M., Manenti, R., Rosini, S., Cohen, L. G., & Cotelli, M. (2014). Noninvasive stimulation of prefrontal cortex strengthens existing episodic memories and reduces forgetting in the elderly. *Frontiers in Aging Neuroscience, 6*.

Sattler, V., Acket, B., Raposo, N., Albucher, J., Thalamas, C., Loubinoux, I., … Simonetta-Moreau, M. (2015). Anodal tDCS combined with radial nerve stimulation promotes hand motor recovery in the acute phase after ischemic stroke. *Neurorehabilitation and Neural Repair, 29*(8), 743–754.

Segrave, R. A., Arnold, S., Hoy, K., & Fitzgerald, P. B. (2014). Concurrent cognitive control training augments the antidepressant efficacy of tDCS: A pilot study. *Brain Stimulation, 7*(2), 325–331.

Stagg, C. J., Lin, R. L., Mezue, M., Segerdahl, A., Kong, Y., Xie, J., & Tracey, I. (2013). Widespread modulation of cerebral perfusion induced during and after transcranial direct current stimulation applied to the left dorsolateral prefrontal cortex. *Journal of Neuroscience, 33*(28), 11425–11431.

Stagg, C. J., & Nitsche, M. A. (2011). Physiological basis of transcranial direct current stimulation. *The Neuroscientist, 17*(1), 37–53.

The CONSORT Statement. (2016). Retrieved July 7, 2016, from http://www.consort-statement.org/

Triccas, L. T., Burridge, J., Hughes, A., Pickering, R., Desikan, M., Rothwell, J., & Verheyden, G. (2016). Multiple sessions of transcranial direct current stimulation and upper extremity rehabilitation in stroke: A review and meta-analysis. *Clinical Neurophysiology, 127*(1), 946–955.

Valle, A., Roizenblatt, S., Botte, S., Zaghi, S., Riberto, M., Tufik, S., … Fregni, F. (2009). Efficacy of anodal transcranial direct current stimulation (tDCS) for the treatment of fibromyalgia: Results of a randomized, sham-controlled longitudinal clinical trial. *Journal of Pain Management, 2*(3), 353–362.

Villamar, M. F., Wivatvongvana, P., Patumanond, J., Bikson, M., Truong, D. Q., Datta, A., & Fregni, F. (2013). Focal modulation of the primary motor cortex in fibromyalgia using 4×1-ring high-definition transcranial direct current stimulation (HD-tDCS): Immediate and delayed analgesic effects of cathodal and anodal stimulation. *The Journal of Pain, 14*(4), 371–383.

Werner, C., Frankenberg, S. V., Treig, T., Konrad, M., & Hesse, S. (2002). Treadmill training with partial body weight support and an electromechanical gait trainer for restoration of gait in subacute stroke patients: A randomized crossover study. *Stroke, 33*(12), 2895–2901.

Wirth, M., Rahman, R. A., Kuenecke, J., Koenig, T., Horn, H., Sommer, W., & Dierks, T. (2011). Effects of transcranial direct current stimulation (tDCS) on behaviour and electrophysiology of language production. *Neuropsychologia, 49*(14), 3989–3998.

Woods, A., Antal, A., Bikson, M., Boggio, P., Brunoni, A., Celnik, P., … Nitsche, M. (2016). A technical guide to tDCS, and related non-invasive brain stimulation tools. *Clinical Neurophysiology, 127*(2), 1031–1048.

Woods, A. J., Bryant, V., Sacchetti, D., Gervits, F., & Hamilton, R. (2015). Effects of electrode drift in transcranial direct current stimulation. *Brain Stimulation, 8*(2), 320–321.

Woods, A. J., Hamilton, R. H., Kranjec, A., Minhaus, P., Bikson, M., Yu, J., & Chatterjee, A. (2014). Space, time, and causality in the human brain. *NeuroImage, 92*, 285–297.

You, D. S., Kim, D., Chun, M. H., Jung, S. E., & Park, S. J. (2011). Cathodal transcranial direct current stimulation of the right Wernicke's area improves comprehension in subacute stroke patients. *Brain and Language, 119*(1), 1–5.

Zimerman, M., Heise, K. F., Hoppe, J., Cohen, L. G., Gerloff, C., & Hummel, F. C. (2012). Modulation of training by single-session transcranial direct current stimulation to the intact motor cortex enhances motor skill acquisition of the paretic hand. *Stroke, 43*(8), 2185–2191.

Chapter 13
Home-Based Patient-Delivered Remotely Supervised Transcranial Direct Current Stimulation

Helena Knotkova, Ashley Clayton, Michael Stevens, Alexa Riggs, Leigh E. Charvet, and Marom Bikson

Introduction

The attractive idea of tDCS application in home settings has been propelled by encouraging findings on tDCS neurophysiological and behavioral effects, as well as by a notion that tDCS effects are cumulative and a single application is not enough to elicit longer lasting effects.

The trend toward tDCS applications at home resonates with different groups of users, addressing variety of unmet needs (Knotkova et al. 2013, 2015; Rosedale et al. 2012; Woods et al. 2016). In research, tDCS application at home may improve retention of study subjects, decrease costs for subject's travel to the research facility and costs associated with the personnel time needed for the applications. It also opens new possibilities for participation in tDCS studies to seriously ill patients, and patients with specific disabilities that make travel to research facility excessively burdensome or impossible. The idea of tDCS applied at home

H. Knotkova (✉)
MJHS Institute for Innovation in Palliative Care, New York, NY, USA

Department of Family and Social Medicine, Albert Einstein College of Medicine, Bronx, NY, USA
e-mail: HKnotkov@mjhs.org

A. Clayton · L. E. Charvet
Department of Neurology, New York University Langone Medical Center, New York, NY, USA

M. Stevens
Department of Psychiatry, Yale University School of Medicine, New Haven, CT, USA

A. Riggs
MJHS Institute for Innovation in Palliative Care, New York, NY, USA

M. Bikson
Department of Biomedical Engineering, The City College of New York, New York, NY, USA

H. Knotkova et al. (eds.), *Practical Guide to Transcranial Direct Current Stimulation*, https://doi.org/10.1007/978-3-319-95948-1_13

may also be attractive from the scope of clinical/therapeutic settings, yielded by the vision of a medical professional sending selected patients home with a tDCS stimulator instead of a bottle of pills. And, of course, the at-home tDCS concept has been attractive to specific segments of the general healthy public, especially in recent years, as the evidence on tDCS effects is growing and medical and public attention to possibilities of functional enhancement in healthy subjects intensifies.

As with any other innovative idea, the use of tDCS in home settings has enormous potential - to enhance the tDCS practice-at-large, and to facilitate the overall development of the neurostimulation field - if used responsibly; on the other hand, careless/reckless tDCS use without provisions for safety, proper training, or access to assistance or resources can be counterproductive and lead to undesired outcomes for involved individuals or the field.

Therefore, it is of interest of all involved to facilitate the environment for tDCS applications in home settings in a safe and effective way.

Potential Benefits of At-Home tDCS

While there is warranted opposition against using "do-it-yourself" (DIY) devices of unknown origin or devices that do not have safety certifications, there are many potential benefits to conducting tDCS at-home as opposed to in a clinic setting. tDCS is a convenient and low cost method of treatment. The size and weight of the device is minimal and it is usually battery-powered making the ability for administration extremely user-friendly. Because of the device configuration and portability, tDCS has the most potential for use outside of a clinic setting (Alonzo and Charvet 2016; Knotkova et al. 2017a).

Another aspect in favor of an at-home approach is that the burden on the patient as well as the institution or clinic is reduced. tDCS sessions often take place at least one time daily, 5 days a week. Daily travel to a treatment facility is often not feasible for most individuals. Work and family schedules and often limited transportation capabilities contribute to the impracticality of daily in-clinic sessions (Kasschau et al. 2016). For those patients living in remote areas without the means of traveling to large cities where academic institutions are located, and are often the ones offering such services, the ability to conduct sessions at home is a tremendous benefit.

Further, remote tDCS is cost effective. The cost associated with trips to the clinic is lessened considerably when sessions are conducted in the home setting. For institutions, at-home tDCS is also financially beneficial. By minimizing the number of in-clinic visits, the cost of dedicated space and allotted staff time at the treatment facility is reduced.

Research has shown that cumulative sessions of tDCS may be more beneficial than a single treatment session (Monte-Silva et al. 2013). The availability of a tDCS treatment option that does not consist of a need for recurring, in-person visits, may lead to a higher retention rate in research protocols.

At-home tDCS is also more accessible than other similar non-invasive brain stimulation techniques such as transcranial magnetic stimulation or TMS. Unlike tDCS, TMS involves strong magnetic field induction and cannot be performed outside of the clinic setting.

Still, another benefit to at-home tDCS use stems from the physical limitations often seen in patients with a number of various medical conditions. Many neurologic conditions, for example, can result in an inability to ambulate easily from place to place, making trips to clinic both challenging and frustrating for the patient. For example, multiple sclerosis, or MS, patients may benefit from tDCS in regards to a number of related symptoms, but these patients often have ongoing problems with ambulation. Recent survey results indicate that the majority of the MS population face mobility challenges on a daily basis (Larocca 2011). Such limitation can prevent patients from independently attending clinic visits, thus, requiring the need for caregiver assistance, and further increasing the existing patient burden. By limiting the need for such in-clinic visits, a potential larger number of subjects are able to complete protocols through to the final session.

Approaches to At-Home tDCS

There is still an underlying concern of safety and clinical guidance regarding at-home use and tDCS in general. Non-invasive brain stimulation, especially the use of tDCS, will eventually be available on a much greater scale. Therefore, it's important to look at the current approaches in at-home use, along with the pros and cons of these methods, in order to carefully inform those looking towards expanding this implementation.

The variety of approaches to at-home tDCS arises from differences in several elements:

- Specificity in selection of good candidates for at-home application
- Quality/intensity of training of the prospective user (and assurance of competence to perform tDCS safely and in accordance with good practices)
- Degree of adjustment of the tDCS procedure with regards to efficacious and safe use (e.g. adjustments allowing for precise electrode positioning at home)
- Quality and technological advancement of the device (e.g. including or not including functionalities allowing for dose control)
- Degree of rigor pertaining to monitoring for safety (adverse events) and compliance with the protocol
- Degree of rigor pertaining to outcome assessment and data collection
- Degree of support and remote assistance provided to the tDCS user

On the continuum of variability in these elements, the top tier is represented by approaches implementing the highest level of control/rigor, aiming for replicability and thus, suitable for conditions with high rigor requirement, such as clinical controlled trials, and we discuss them in detail below (Charvet et al. 2015; Knotkova et al. 2017a, b; Riggs et al. 2017a, b).

The low end of the continuum includes DIY tDCS application by untrained individuals on their own, using devices that often do not meet the good manufacturing practices (CGMP) for quality assurance and internationally accepted standards, such as those codified by ISO 13485. Currently, there are several DIY websites and blogs that are making it as convenient as possible for the average lay person to obtain and/or construct their own DIY tDCS device. Many of these sites promote simply purchasing a 9-volt battery, wires, and sponges in order to meet the "requirements" of at-home brain stimulation. There are also devices currently being marketed for online purchase such as foc.us and The Brain Stimulator (Alonzo and Charvet 2016). While the cost of these products varies, they are still readily available to the average consumer. Purchase of devices such as these or creation of DIY tDCS kits should not be encouraged. There is no prescription needed to purchase these devices. With that, comes no supervision, safety standards, or the ability to control dosing over repeated sessions.

The ability to control dose administration incorporates correct electrode preparation, montage, and waveform. Although it can be argued that no formal oversight is required for a private use of publicly available tDCS devices (even those of questionable quality), it is important to understand that the potential adverse effects due to careless/uninformed tDCS application can negatively impact the entire tDCS field.

Besides the two approaches defining the top and lowest tier, there are other approaches of tDCS applications in home settings, utilizing various degree of compliance control, support or training. One approach in research involving tDCS in home settings has been to provide patient participants with devices and instruction for self-administration (Andre et al. 2016; Hagenacker et al. 2014; Hyvarinen et al. 2016). Another approach has been to combine tDCS with an extension of in-clinic treatments such as TMS (Cha et al. 2016). The advantage of this approach is that it most closely approximates real-world use, simulating a potential model of prescription use. However, in addition to any potential safety concerns, there are limitations to these studies in terms of understanding the exact doses administered and, especially, reproducibility of the findings. Further, participants may have some difficulty with self-administration if they have cognitive or motor disabilities, and may require ongoing guidance for use. Some clinicians are utilizing tDCS home-use to sustain clinical benefit (Andrade 2013; Narayanaswamy et al. 2014). This tailored individual approach can be helpful to the patient, but does not serve to answer overall research questions and is completed without parameters or guidance.

Home-Based Patient-Delivered Remotely-Supervised tDCS

The idea of remotely-supervised versus non-supervised at-home tDCS is one of the largest distinctions between the current approaches. The implementation of a remotely-supervised method is overall favored, as it adheres to the necessary safety and standardized procedures previously mentioned. Further, in terms of the most important aspect of an at-home approach to tDCS is safety. A currently used remotely supervised (RS) tDCS protocol implements a number of safety features to minimize risk, maximize benefit that other at-home devices disregard. Sessions are conducted under direct supervision of a tDCS trained technician. The training the technician receives goes beyond the real-time supervision during sessions. Prior to any interaction with patients, technicians are trained on the proper technique of tDCS, how to correctly place the headset, the ability to identify unexpected adverse events, and how to overall screen for potential eligible subjects. With safety being one of the primary concerns surrounding remote tDCS sessions, a structured protocol inclusive of real-time monitoring helps to alleviate such unease (Charvet et al. 2015; Knotkova et al. 2017a, b).

In summary, the increased interest surrounding tDCS has been overall well-received in the scientific and medical communities. While it is clear that tDCS will ultimately be used at home, either directly by the consumer or through a prescription, research is needed to answer critical questions of safety and tolerability of extended treatments and dosing optimization. If an individual self-administers tDCS for treatment, there are currently no known parameters for how many sessions, and of what duration and strength, are safe and effective. In addition, they would not have objective measurements at baseline in which to measure any progress or response to treatment. Therefore, directed and monitored home use in a research context is essential for the guidance of the future of tDCS as a therapy.

Protocols, Technologies and Consumers

It has been recognized that even within the most rigorous remotely-supervised tDCS application in home settings, the treatment protocol and technology (functionality of the tDCS device) must reflect specific needs and limitations of the user. Below, we discuss three examples of specific patient-tailored adjustments of the remotely-supervised tDCS application in home settings to various patient populations – those with the Attention-Deficit/Hyperactivity Disorder (ADHD), Multiple Sclerosis (MS) and seriously ill polymorbid, polysymptomatic patients who are candidates for- or receiving specialist-level community-based palliative care.

Attention-Deficit/Hyperactivity Disorder

ADHD is a behaviorally-defined disorder affecting 5–7% of children and adolescents (Barkley et al. 2002; Kessler et al. 2006). DSM 5-defined ADHD (American Psychiatric Association 2013) is marked by excessive impulsivity/hyperactivity and inattention as well as frequent and diverse cognitive impairments (Frazier et al. 2004; Willcutt et al. 2012) that cause significant, academic, employment, legal or psychosocial problems (Barkley et al. 2006; Breslau et al. 2009, 2011; Hinshaw 1992a, b; Polderman et al. 2010; Raggi and Chronis 2006) despite the best-supported treatments (Jensen et al. 2007; Molina et al. 2009; The MTA Cooperative Group 1999), and is linked to increased risk for other psychopathology and substance disorder (Breslau et al. 2011; Levin et al. 1998; Wilens 2004). These symptoms and the problems that are associated with ADHD represent a substantial burden to patients and typically require treatment to improve functioning. First- and second-line recommended treatment for ADHD is pharmacotherapy with psychostimulants that increase extracellular levels of dopamine or with atomoxetine that blocks reuptake of norepinephrine (Kooij et al. 2010; Pliszka and Issues AWGoQ 2007). Although the majority of ADHD patients show some degree of clinical improvement when using these medications, the parents of a surprisingly high number of ADHD-diagnosed children and adolescents seek alternative treatments to manage the behavioral and cognitive problems associated with the disorder. The reasons why medications are so unpopular with many parents are varied (Dosreis et al. 2003; McLeod et al. 2004), but often involve parent attitudes towards medications, such as misunderstanding of safety or concerns about the long-term effects of medication use (DosReis et al. 2009), as well as perceived social stigma or other concerns. Moreover, ADHD medications have meager effects on academic performance (Langberg and Becker 2012; Prasad et al. 2013), inconsistent effects on adult psychosocial outcome (Advokat 2009; Barkley and Cunningham 1978; Carlson and Bunner 1993; Cunningham and Barkley 1978; Gadow 1983; Loe and Feldman 2007; Swanson et al. 1991), and carry a high substance abuse potential (Bright 2008; Faraone and Upadhyaya 2007; Harpur et al. 2008; Johnston et al. 2008).

Among numerous non-pharmacological treatments that have been examined in ADHD (typically behavioral interventions or cognitive training) (Evans et al. 2014; Hodgson et al. 2014; Rabipour and Raz 2012; Rutledge et al. 2012; Sonuga-Barke et al. 2013; Toplak et al. 2008) tDCS has recently garnered interest based on theoretical arguments that it could have a potential clinical benefit (Demirtas-Tatlidede, et al. 2013; Rubio et al. 2016). Despite the interest, the available empirical evidence that tDCS has a meaningful positive effect on ADHD still remains limited at present. Laboratory studies conducted so far have typically examined whether single-session tDCS has an immediate facilitative effect on cognitive abilities found to be abnormal in ADHD. Most published evidence is supportive. For instance, anodal tDCS over the left dorsolateral prefrontal cortex improves attention and behavioral inhibition (Bandeira et al. 2016) or response accuracy (Soltaninejad et al. 2015). However, contrary evidence also exists; e.g., a similar study in ADHD adults found no improvement in inhibitory control after 1 mA anodal stimulation (Cosmo et al. 2015a, b). However, it remains unclear whether the differences compared to other studies are due to the age of the patients or other experimental factors. In addition, other applications of tDCS have been shown to influence ADHD-related cognitive deficits and suggest alternative uses for tDCS to treat ADHD that might engage different mechanisms of action. In one study,

ADHD-diagnosed children exposed to 0.75 Hz oscillating tDCS increased EEG-recorded slow wave oscillation during sleep, and improved subsequent memory recall the next day (Prehn-Kristensen et al. 2014), while in another study ADHD-diagnosed boys undergoing a similar treatment had less variable motor performance and generally slower reaction time during Go/NoGo task the next day (Munz et al. 2015). Also, cathodal tDCS was found to improve ADHD behavioral inhibition in one study (Soltaninejad et al. 2015). The basis of these potentially beneficial tDCS effects on neural function is not yet well understood, but so far appears consistent with known models of ADHD pathophysiology. A study using a spontaneously hyperactive rat model of ADHD not only found repeated tDCS administration over 8 days improved animal analogues of ADHD-related behavioral abnormalities, but also that dopamine levels in the striatum – a brain region linked to ADHD pathophysiology by several lines of research (Del Campo et al. 2011) – were higher after tDCS treatment (Leffa et al. 2016). In another study, anodal tDCS applied over the left prefrontal cortex altered ADHD brain dysfunction not only under the target area, but also in brain regions known to be interconnected within neural networks (Cosmo et al. 2015a, b). This indicates tDCS effects can propagate among brain regions within extended neural systems that numerous studies have implicated as dysfunctional in ADHD (Cao et al. 2014; Cortese et al. 2012; Rubia et al. 2014; Weyandt et al. 2013).

This emerging evidence that tDCS acutely improves neurocognitive task performance known to often be abnormal in ADHD along with the well-documented safety, general tolerability, and established long-term effects of tDCS on both cognitive performance (Ditye et al. 2012) and brain function (Miniussi and Ruzzoli 2013; Sale et al. 2015) suggest tDCS might be an option for an unmet ADHD treatment need that arises from patient and parent concerns about medication use, tolerability, or inadequate response. However, before tDCS can be used clinically, it must be validated by properly-designed clinical trials to test its clinical efficacy. To date, no study has looked at the effects of repeated tDCS administration in ADHD to determine if it has cumulative benefits on cognitive function. More importantly, there has not yet been a study to determine whether tDCS might reduce ADHD symptoms or associated social, academic, related functional impairments. The practical difficulties of such studies are considerable. For instance, a prototypical treatment protocol would require ADHD patients and their families to attend near-daily clinic visits over 2–4 weeks. This duration and frequency are needed not only to ensure adequate "dose" of neurostimulation, but also because such a timeframe is needed to evaluate meaningful change in clinical function. Typical families contend with the schedules of two working parents, school demands and extra-curricular activities, and often have to manage more than one child's needs. Therefore, any clinic-based tDCS trial for ADHD not only would miss potential recruitment opportunities because of family refusal, but would also likely be plagued by poor compliance and high dropout. Probably only the most motivated of families and subjects would complete treatment, complicating generalizability and efficacy inferences. Remotely-supervised tDCS represents a means to accelerate the pace and feasibility of such clinical trials by opening interventions to a wider potential ADHD participant pool than would otherwise be possible.

There are two primary considerations for population-specific recommendations for tDCS performed at home for ADHD. The first is the patient or research participant age. Unlike many other clinical groups for which tDCS is being considered as a potential treatment, ADHD is a disorder usually diagnosed in childhood when problem behavior becomes severe enough to bring the patient to clinical attention. Administering tDCS at home for ADHD children and adolescents should require a family member to participate to help ensure proper protocol adherence. While some adolescents might have the maturity to set up and administer tDCS without direct parental assistance using remote supervision, it is an impractical idea for most children. Furthermore, most institutional review boards are unlikely to approve research trial protocols where youth are asked to set up and administer tDCS themselves. This suggests effective clinical trial design must overcome additional issues arising from parent training, parent-child interactions, and joint tDCS procedure troubleshooting in order to ensure that tDCS is administered properly each and every treatment session. Second, unlike other clinical populations who benefit from tDCS (e.g., stroke or multiple sclerosis) whose patients often require assistance in tDCS set up due to fine motor impairment, ADHD does not have frank motor disabilities to overcome. ADHD cognitive deficits not only are varied and not found in all ADHD patients (Willcutt et al. 2005), they also typically are not particularly severe – most often merely relative weaknesses. Thus, there are no specific disabilities in ADHD that require careful planning for the population as a whole to overcome. However, the problems with distractibility, inattention to detail, and persistence are hallmark problem behaviors in ADHD. ADHD neurobiological theory also implicates motivational brain systems in the disorder (Sonuga-Barke 2005), which could represent a similar hindrance to remaining engaged throughout a clinical trial of tDCS without proper oversight. Therefore, ADHD-specific recommendations for remotely-supervised tDCS fall primarily into the category of efforts tailored to the population to help ensure treatment protocol adherence, patient motivation, and continuity of optimal tDCS administration by capitalizing on parental engagement. As such, most recommendations would apply equally to either research-based clinical trials or to clinical services that eventually might be offered to ADHD patients if research evidence for tDCS efficacy ultimately is found.

Fortunately, considerable effort already has been made to understand what specific factors influence ADHD patients' compliance with treatment. This body of published research focuses on ADHD medication adherence, for which non-compliance or discontinuation rates vary from 13 to 81% across studies (Adler and Nierenberg 2010; Ferrin et al. 2012). Medication adherence can be operationalized in different ways. Typically, it is taken to mean the patient's and family's engagement in and consistency using a medication regimen that both the medical provider and family believe could be beneficial (Gearing et al. 2011). Although some reasons why ADHD patients choose to discontinue pharmacological treatment are highly specific to medication use (e.g., drug side-effect intolerance), many of its lessons can be directly translated to non-pharmacological interventions. As might be expected, there are age-specific predictors of ADHD treatment adherence that track the developmental maturity of patients. For instance, younger children are more likely to adhere to treatment recommendations if they have more troublesome ADHD symptoms or associated problems (Charach and Gajaria 2008; Coletti et al. 2012), except for when those problems cause such severe levels of family discord they interfere with treatment (Coletti et al. 2012; Gau et al. 2006). ADHD-diagnosed adolescents often take increasing responsibility for managing their treatment as they develop insight into the functional aspect of medication in their lives (Brinkman et al. 2012). Adolescent treatment adherence is higher when academic benefits are perceived, side-effects are low, and any social stigma is controlled (Bussing et al. 2012). Adult ADHD medication non-compliance rates are similar to that found in youth, e.g., between 11–64% (Christensen et al. 2010; Olfson et al. 2007). For adults with ADHD, treatment adherence is lower when patients have more severe symptoms or engage in illicit substance use (Semerci et al. 2016). Factors that predict medication adherence for all ages of ADHD patients include beliefs that ADHD is a biological disorder (Charach and Gajaria 2008; Coletti et al. 2012), understanding the treatment safety profile (Bussing et al. 2012), and efforts to reduce the practical burden of treatment (Gau et al. 2006). It is also clear that familial and medical support are highly important. Not only does higher socioeconomic status and two-parent households predict treatment compliance (Charach and Gajaria 2008), studies that find patients and their families have active, supportive relationships with treatment providers are more likely to adhere to treatment as well (Coletti et al. 2012).

Taken together, these factors suggest several practical suggestions for ADHD tDCS treatment protocols performed at home. These suggestions emphasize establishing an effective treatment relationship between the clinicians or researchers overseeing the treatment and the ADHD patients and their families, educating parents and children about what to expect with tDCS treatment, and devising ways to plan, structure and otherwise facilitate interactions between parents and their children. All recommendations should be tailored to the developmental age of the patient. Nearly all should be considered for protocols involving ADHD-diagnosed adults.

Establish an Effective Treatment/Research Relationship Because research shows that ADHD treatment compliance is supported by a well-established relationship between patients and caregivers, tDCS protocol adherence likely will be facilitated if effort is made to explain the ways in which patients or their families can seek support during the treatment protocol. Although the protocols of clinical trials will differ from study to study, it is recommended that all protocols include a) a clinic visit for consent, clinical assessment, and training with particular attention paid to educating families that treatment must be a "whole family" cooperative effort, b) a home visit prior to treatment so that research staff can assess and advise tDCS equipment set up and other technical issues, and c) a schedule of contacts for when the medical/research team will contact the family to check in about the protocol. Contact information for ways to reach a member of the treatment team should be provided not only for emergencies or reporting any adverse events believed to be related to the treatment, but also for routine questions. Having a direct and responsive avenue of contact is useful to avoid frustration that can lead to treatment non-compliance.

Provide tDCS Psychoeducation Because ADHD treatment adherence is greater when patients and the their parents understand ADHD is a neurobiological disorder, tDCS clinical trials or clinical treatment performed at home should include a standardized discussion that educates both the patient and family member who will be assisting the trial about (a) how tDCS is believed to work neurobiologically and its purported therapeutic effect on specific aspects of ADHD neural dysfunction, (b) tDCS risk profile, in particular age-specific caveats to existing safety/tolerability research for children where less information is known than for tDCS in adults (Brunoni et al. 2011a, b), (c) expectations for therapeutic effects that emphasize that treatment in clinical trials might not show an effect at all, or that effects might be small and not emerge until the end of treatment or long after. The latter should also include that current models of ADHD believe it likely is caused by multiple different etiologies (Sonuga-Barke, 2005), which may or may not be responsive to tDCS.

Describe Outcome Evaluation Process Perceived lack of benefit is a key reason for ADHD treatment discontinuation. For ADHD tDCS treatment protocols, it is recommended to explain that tests of attention, response inhibition, or other cognitive abilities are surrogate outcome measures that may or may not predict actual behavioral change. Evaluation of ADHD symptoms and associated problems is best done over a longer timeframe. For research protocols, this means explaining the use of standardized ADHD behavioral outcome measures (e.g., parent- or teacher-report ADHD symptom severity checklists) so parents can understand how the study plans to gauge the impact of the treatment over time. For clinical treatment, this might include goals for outcome evaluation that are patient-specific (e.g., sibling arguments, homework compliance, etc.) and devising ways to for parents and patients to measure gains towards those goals.

Parent Preparedness/Training When the patient is a child or adolescent, parental involvement should be required or at least strongly recommended. However, the interpersonal nature of the parent-child relationship should be discussed as a factor that can facilitate or hinder treatment adherence. A potentially effective approach is for each to articulate their hopes and goals for the treatment, i.e., to make clear what is motivating them. The role of the parent as a “coach” instead of “drill sergeant” should be emphasized. Youth with greater developmental maturity can take more responsibility for the practical issues, relegating parental involvement to oversight and documentation. Because interpersonal factors that might influence both tDCS protocol adherence and outcome in ADHD are unknown, it is advised that formal assessments of parent-child dyadic interactions or familial relationship styles be conducted at treatment baseline of research studies. Such metrics can be examined as potential outcome moderators in the statistical analysis of outcome data. Finally, it should be emphasized that the trial should be a "whole family" effort. A pre-treatment training session should discuss family schedules such as extra-curricular activities for both the patient and other children in the family to identify in advance potential hurdles. Practical issues such as establishing a regular tDCS time, ensuring lack of interruption by siblings, etc. should be emphasized.

tDCS Equipment Training A trial using remotely-supervised tDCS is unlikely to succeed if patients or their families are unable to access the technology required. As described elsewhere in this chapter, training should cover both proper use of the tDCS equipment, but also the communication medium used for the study. Ideally, a videoconferencing system will be employed so that staff can confirm the proper positioning of tDCS electrodes. If concurrent cognitive stimulation (e.g., a "cognitive training" framework) is included as part of a tDCS experimental protocol, training on how to start those exercises must be provided. As intimated above, the roles of parents versus ADHD-diagnosed children or adolescents might optimally fall into one of two categories: a) one in which parents perform all set up, communication with caregiver staff, and documentation, or b) one in which parents supervise, but older youth might take responsibility for much of the practical set up.

Contingency Management The goal of tDCS treatment adherence ultimately is to complete a prescribed number and duration of stimulation sessions within a particular timeframe. As such, some ADHD patients might benefit from contingency management approaches (Kaiser et al. 2008). A system of small incentives might be established that rewards increasing levels of compliance throughout any lengthy treatment protocol. For example, a small reward can be provided after each daily tDCS session is successfully completed, followed by a choice of a larger reward on the weekend if all sessions that week were done. The benefit of such a system likely will depend on the age of the patients and developmental appropriateness of the rewards, but likely should be considered standard for the youngest patients. Moreover, if a contingency management approach is included in any treatment protocol, parents should be trained how to properly present contingencies in order to avoid a punitive or coercive approach. Protocol-specific guidelines on how and when to provide positive reinforcements should be made explicit, and their use should be quantified by trial staff weekly.

Multiple Sclerosis

For individuals living with multiple sclerosis (MS), tDCS has shown early promise in ameliorating many frequent and often disabling symptoms including cognitive impairment, fatigue, pain, and motor problems (Ayache et al. 2016; Cuypers et al. 2013; Ferrucci et al. 2014; Mattioli et al. 2016; Meesen et al. 2014; Palm et al. 2014). However, at-home use is critical for providing adequate access for patients for both treatment and participation in clinical study. Many of those living with MS are not able to travel to a clinic to receive treatment, especially if sessions span weeks or even months of daily stimulation. As MS often occurs in younger adults, typically with both work and family responsibilities, time for treatment, especially involving in-clinic appointments, is a major obstacle. In addition, for those that are more advanced in disability, traveling to a clinic appointment can be a tremendous burden, in terms of time and the need to make specific transportation arrangements, for both the patient and caregiver as well. To provide remote treatment for both clinical and research purposes in MS, there are several considerations for optimal use.

First, there is consideration for cognitive capacity to understand and participate in the tDCS procedures. While cognitive impairment is frequent (occurring in up to 70% of all individuals), deficits are typically marked by cognitive slowing and difficulty with new learning, but are not at the severity seen in dementias. A brief cognitive screening procedure can ensure that the potential tDCS candidate will be successful in executing the procedures. This can include checking for understanding during the screening process and completion of brief measures such as reading recognition (as a proxy for premorbid intellectual functioning) and information processing speed (e.g., Symbol Digit Modalities Test [SDMT]).

A second concern is sufficient fine motor functioning for headset placement. MS is frequently associated with fine motor impairment and slowed motor functioning. Therefore, devices must be designed as simplistically as possible. This includes easily-held devices with large buttons and press points for operation. In addition, headsets must be designed for simple placement (Fig. 13.1).

Headsets in a current MS protocol have been re-configured to include an adjustable headpiece so electrode placement is optimal for varying head sizes (Kasschau et al. 2015). The wires attached to the headset are color coded black and red for simple connection to the device. The anode and cathode are labeled red and black, respectively to also assist in proper, simplistic placement. In general, a cap-like design that can be easily grasped, lifted, and placed is important. Electrodes and sponges must also be easy to manipulate and place. This latter concern has been especially challenging, but pre-moistened sponges (that do not require the use of a saline syringe), provided in perforated single use packaging, have been most helpful. In addition, a snap connection placement for sponges to join the headset is preferred over a button connection.

In some cases, the individual with MS may meet screening requirements for cognitive ability, but might have too severe motor involvement to adequately place the headset and operate the device. In these cases, a caregiver proxy may be enlisted

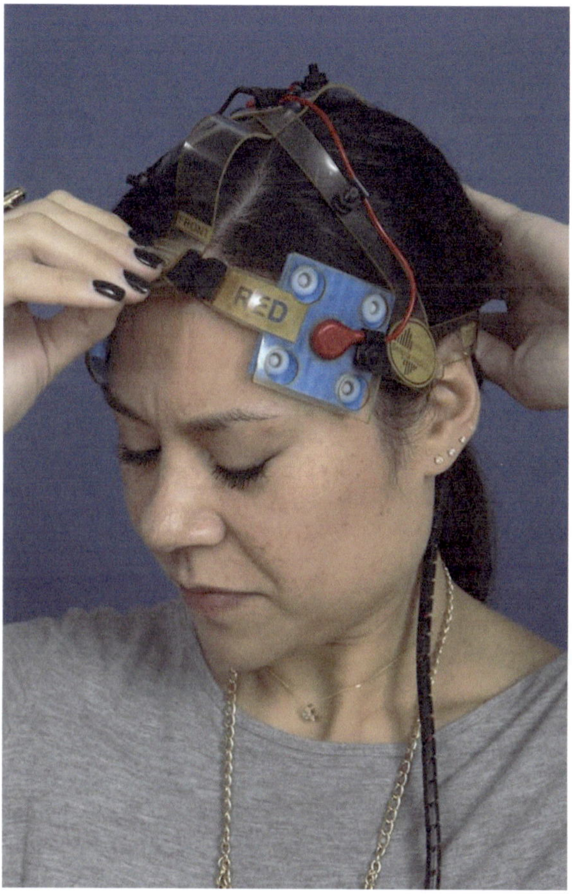

Fig. 13.1 4 × 4 tDCS headgear. Custom-made headgear has been modified with the goal of simplifying placement and minimizing dependence on manual dexterity. Electrodes will be securely attached to specific markings on the headset with the use of pre-moistened sponges. The sponges are provided in single-use packets, and once opened, can be readily attached in the correct placement to the headgear. A marker guides accurate user placement of the headgear. (The figure is courtesy of L. Charvet)

depending on institution requirements. In these cases, the proxy must be screened and trained during the baseline visit in all procedures.

During the training period, tolerability can be tested as well as capacity. Once cleared, the MS participant (with or without a caregiver proxy) can be required to demonstrate successful headset placement and device operation. In addition, while in-clinic, the targeted dose should be tested on the participant, for at least 1 min, in order to ensure that the individual can tolerate the treatment. If the subject does not pass the initial tolerability test, they are terminated from further protocol participation. If the tolerability test is successful, it is then recommended to complete the first full session under the supervision of a study technician to stimulate the individual's daily experience from home, and provide an extra measure of clearance. Only once cleared, they can be provided an "at-home" tDCS kit for remote sessions. Once again, the tDCS technician reviews with the subject and/or proxy each part of the tDCS kit (headset, device, laptop, and sponges) prior to departure so that at-home sessions are confidently and safely administered.

At-home devices must be designed for safety, reliability of stimulation delivery, and optimal remotely supervised operation. For instance, one device that has been studied, the Soterix Mini-CT, is dependent on a code to "unlock" delivery of only one "dose" for stimulation (or sham) to be administered. Once connected, the technician can coach the participant and/or proxy on correct placement and ensure all safety criteria are met. An impedance meter is included in the device which prevents access until the placement is adequate. The previously mentioned code is not provided until the device displays a "good" connection. Through the videoconferencing platform, visual confirmation of correct placement can also be made. Then, the session is monitored in real-time to ensure consistent stimulation and no unexpected adverse events including poor tolerance.

In addition, parameters to assess such adverse events and participant experiences must minimize user burden. For example, the study technician should adhere to brief, visual analog scales to assess pain and fatigue, with a standardized, verbal interview of any side effects experienced.

The currently used MS protocol includes extensive training procedures as well as highly detailed "stop" criteria that provide the technician with specific steps and guidelines to initiate and oversee each session. In cases of violations, including failure to observe safety features or report of any pain over a moderate level, the use code is not provided and/or the remote use is discontinued.

This protocol was initially demonstrated to be feasible in a sample of adults with MS (Kasschau et al. 2016). Twenty participants (n = 26), ages 30–69 years with a range of neurologic disability form mild to severe (using a proxy) and subtype including both relapsing remitting and progressive forms, were enrolled to test the feasibility of the methods. Protocol adherence exceeded what has been observed in studies with clinic-based treatment delivery, with all but one participant (95%) completing at least eight of the ten sessions. Across a total of 192 supervised treatment sessions, no session required discontinuation and no adverse events were reported. The most common side effects were itching/tingling at the electrode site with no side effect exceeding an intensity of moderate. The study was met with strong patient interest and highly positive feedback.

In a second and ongoing study, n = 32 MS participants have been randomized to either active or sham 2.0 mA tDCS for 20 sessions. Those in the sham condition are offered an additional 10 open-label active sessions at study end. A third trial has expanded this protocol to patients with Parkinson's disease (n = 12) for an initial 10 open-label sessions for feasibility. We continue to see very high protocol adherence with both the expanded session number (20 sessions) and sham conditions, as well as when applying the procedures to those with Parkinson's disease. In over 800 remotely-supervised sessions to date, only one session has been discontinued during stimulation (due to headache). There have been no serious adverse events, and tolerability remains consistent with what is published in the extensive literature of in-clinic application (Bikson et al. 2016). In sum, remote supervision offers a platform to provide in-home treatment to those living with MS and potentially many other neurologic conditions.

Chronically Ill Patients with Multiple Symptoms

With aging of the worldwide population, the prevalence of chronic illness is rising (Centers for Medicare and Medicaid Services 2012; Hasselman 2013; Ortman et al. 2014). In the U.S., approximately 50% of adults have one or more chronic illness. Symptom management is challenging in those with multiple chronic conditions, particularly when age-related risk from drug therapy compounds the risks associated with disease-related organ dysfunction. Distress associated with poorly controlled symptoms such as pain, fatigue, depressed mood or cognitive difficulties, is highly prevalent in the chronically ill, and it can substantially affect patient's functional independence, as well as drive health-care costs (Dhingra et al. 2017; Hasselman 2013; Ortman et al. 2014).

Most chronically ill patients live at home and seek care that aims to mitigate illness burden and maintain a good quality of life. Therefore, adjunct non-pharmacological strategies for symptom control in home settings are highly relevant for this patient population. Although tDCS has shown promising potential for symptom control, the burden of repeated visits to receive tDCS in medical- or research facilities has been among the major obstacles that made an access to tDCS difficult for many chronically ill patients. Therefore, the development of tDCS protocols suitable for the patient's use in home settings represents a great opportunity specifically for those with multiple illnesses, complex symptoms and lower functional status. However, designing an at-home tDCS protocol for this potentially vulnerable patient population requires specific considerations, such as the following:

Involvement of Family Caregiver Seriously ill patients frequently rely on assistance of family caregivers. Therefore, it is likely that home-based tDCS applications in some patients may need to be assisted by an informal caregiver rather than self-applied by the patient. However, patients with higher functional status may find it important to be directly involved in tDCS application. Thus, both options should be included in the tDCS protocol and offered to the patient and the family.

Minimal Burden Both the patient and the informal caregiver bear the enormous burden of the illness and the level of their overall distress may be high. Therefore, study procedures pertaining to the tDCS administration and data collection must be user friendly, easy and not time-demanding. While data collection in healthy populations or patients with higher performance status may include extensive questionnaire sets and testing, data collection in frail, seriously ill patients must be carefully selected and include only a brief set of assessment tools.

Time Flexibility It is difficult for the patient and their informal caregiver to accommodate multiple day-to-day chores in daily life affected by the illness. Adding another element, such as participation in an at-home tDCS study only adds to an already full schedule. Therefore, time planning of tDCS procedures should leave reasonable margins acceptable for both the patient-caregiver dyad and the study personnel, for example when scheduling the real-time video monitoring of the procedure.

Maintaining the Medication Regimen Medical care and symptom management in seriously ill patients relies largely on pharmacological treatments, often including multiple medications. Due to ethic as well as regulatory reasons (seriously ill patients are considered potentially vulnerable subjects), medication wash-out prior to participation in a tDCS study is not feasible. This may represent a substantial methodological hurdle, because certain agents (such as NMDA antagonists) may alter tDCS effects. It requires careful consideration when planning the tDCS protocol and the study inclusion and exclusion criteria.

Other Considerations It has to be taken into account that the tDCS stimulation session usually takes 20–30 min during which the patient should remain seated or in a bed, without walking around. Therefore, subjects who are restless or are not comfortably able to comply with that requirement are not good candidates for the tDCS procedure.

Overall, the feasibility of home-delivered remotely-monitored tDCS in seriously ill patients is multifaceted, including (but not limited to) the following elements: (a) Patient's and family caregiver's understanding of the procedure, their willingness and ability to participate in tDCS applications; (b) Patient's or caregiver's ability to perform tDCS specific procedures after training; (c) Patient's acceptability and tolerability of the procedure, including being able to remain seated or in bed for the 20-min stimulation; (d) Patient's ability to provide a brief feedback or numerical rating when asked; (e) Home environment, including sufficient arrangements to accommodate tDCS administration; and tDCS acceptability in the frame of spiritual/religious beliefs and overall settings of the household (Riggs et al. 2017b).

A schema of a tDCS patient-tailored protocol suitable for polysymptomatic seriously ill patients aiming for symptom control in home settings (Knotkova et al. 2017a) is depicted in Fig. 13.2.

The protocol allows for an optional inclusion of assisting informal caregiver. There is 1 home visit for consenting, screening and familiarization with the tDCS device, followed by in-person initiation of training that will then continue in remote.

To facilitate familiarization with tDCS at the home visit, the tDCS technician demonstrates the equipment and function of the device, and the patient has an opportunity to experience the sensory sensation associated with tDCS procedure: the patient undergoes 1 min of tDCS first on their arm and then on their head, at the default intensity of 1.5 mA. As the protocol is tailored to the patient's needs,

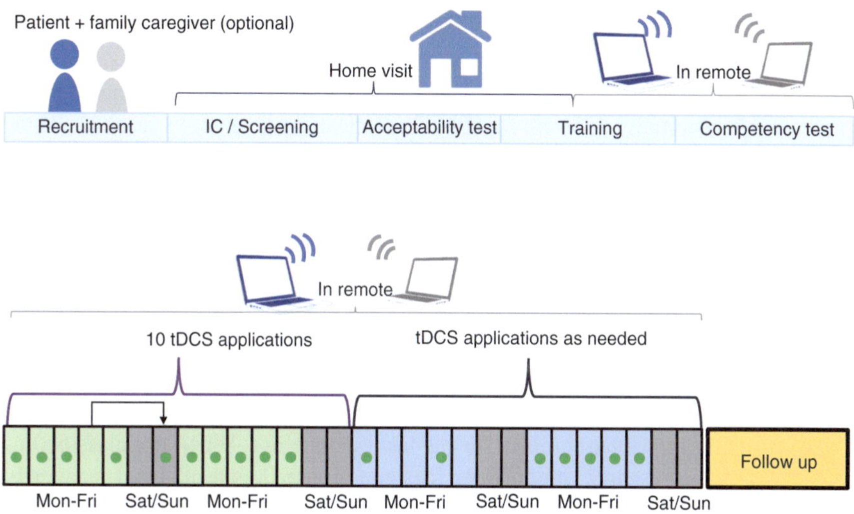

Fig. 13.2 Schema of tDCS protocol suitable for home-bound seriously ill patients with multiple symptoms. The protocol includes 1 at-home visit and has specific patient-tailored elements, such as an optional inclusion of an assisting informal caregiver, as well as elements that enhance compliance and safety, including remote visual contact with the patient via telehealth tablet. (The figure is courtesy of H. Knotkova and A. Riggs)

those who find the sensation not acceptable, may repeat the acceptability test at lower intensity of 1.0 mA, which - if accepted - then become the patient-specific stimulation intensity through the protocol. Patients who do not find the lower intensity acceptable are not suitable candidates for tDCS. Although tDCS is in general well accepted even at higher intensities, such as 2 mA, some patients may have increased skin sensitivity due to clinical condition, medications or other factors. After familiarization with the device and sensory sensation, the tDCS technician initiates patient's or informal caregiver's training in tDCS application. The training continues in remote for about 1 week with an assistance from the tDCS technician via videoconference as needed. tDCS skill-building is extremely important for tDCS applications in home settings and for that reason the training is concluded with a competency test, to assure that the designated individual (the patient or the caregiver) is able to perform tDCS in accordance with good practice.

After conclusion of the competency test, patients are encouraged to apply one tDCS session per day on multiple consecutive days. In the second phase, patients are allowed to apply tDCS as needed, ranging from none to two applications per day, and the applications are remotely supervised. The level of remote supervision is patient-tailored and varies upon the patient's/caregiver's tDCS skills and compliance with good practices for tDCS applications.

The initial feasibility and face validity of this protocol has been determined in an IRB-approved study (Riggs et al. 2017b).

Regulatory and Ethical Aspects Pertaining to At-Home tDCS

The regulatory framework that applies to tDCS in general, including at-home applications, is substantially different for tDCS in clinical/medical use vs research. Thus, regulations that apply to use of off-label devices in medical practice vs research differ, and the distinction between the two is guided by the respective definitions: The goal of medical practice is to "provide diagnosis, preventative treatment or therapy", while research is "designed to test a hypothesis, permit conclusions to be drawn, and thereby to develop or contribute to generalizable knowledge." (Riley and Basilius 2007; Wittich et al. 2012). The FDA (and comparable organizations that regulate device manufacturers) does not regulate the practice of medicine, which instead is subject to the direction of state and federal professional and licensing boards. Thus, the federal Food, Drug, and Cosmetic Act of 1938 does not play a role in creating physician liability for off-label device use. When not classified as tools involved in research, medical devices can be used in an off-label manner in medical practice without FDA regulatory oversight. Currently, the general legality and value of off-label use is integral for medical practice, and under the U.S. law, physicians may prescribe drugs and devices for off-label use (Wittich et al. 2012). A limitation to this rule is that physicians may only prescribe off-label devices if the physicians are not employed by the medical or pharmaceutical companies in question. (Wilkes and Johns 2008).

Entirely different regulatory framework, however, applies to tDCS medical devices in clinical research outside of or contrary to FDA approval, and the following requirements must be met: (i) Approval by an institutional review board (IRB); and additionally, if the study involves a significant risk device (defined as one that presents a potential for serious risk to the health, safety, or welfare of a subject), approval of an investigational device exemption (IDE) by FDA; (ii) Informed consent from research participants; (iii) Labeling of the device for investigational use only; (iv) Monitoring of the study; and (v) Compliance with required records and reports.

In summary, there is duality in the regulatory framework that applies to tDCS use in research settings vs off-label clinical use, and this duality applies not only to a general tDCS use, but encompasses also at-home applications.

Challenges, Open Questions and Future Trends in At-Home tDCS

Any new approach faces hurdles to its widespread use and acceptance. The ability to conduct tDCS treatment or research outside of a clinic setting does not simply require technological advances to make it possible, but also must be able to surmount valid concerns about feasibility, safety, and proper oversight. As described above, many of the safety concerns can be addressed using technical design features that prevent harm through uncontrolled stimulation. Oversight concerns are largely addressed both through focused training and by the ability to provide videoconferencing-based interaction to ensure proper tDCS use – either as periodic check-in assessments or at every tDCS treatment session if deemed necessary or useful. At this stage of remotely-supervised tDCS, feasibility issues are largely addressed. It currently is possible to conduct tDCS clinical trials in a wide range of clinical populations in home settings. However, a concise, thoughtful, and effective series of guidelines and recommendations is needed to navigate the development of protocols for these trials. We have endeavored to provide a generalized set of expectations for such protocols in this chapter and in our previous reports (Charvet et al. 2015).

- Although some remotely-supervised tDCS studies are underway (Kasschau et al. 2015, 2016; Knotkova et al. 2016), additional clinical trials conducted in a variety of patient populations are needed to ultimately demonstrate the feasibility of generalized use. Not only will more trials identify other possible practical barriers that might need to be overcome, continued demonstration that patients can effectively and reliably administer tDCS at home with remote supervision will promote general acceptance of the method as viable and informative. It is hoped that with increasing empirical support for tDCS as an effective treatment, there will be increased demand to streamline equipment for remotely-supervised use. One can envision that as technology progresses, so will construction of new devices that more seamlessly integrate tDCS delivery, videoconferencing-based telecommunications using built-in cellular capability, optional cognitive stimulation, and features to automatically upload clinical trial-relevant data via internet to a central monitoring site into a single unit such as a handheld PDA or tablet device. Such integrated systems would go even further to offer remotely-supervised tDCS to a greater number of households, including households without computers. However, smartphones are commonplace now, suggesting that families without extensive computer experience are likely to be able to use such devices with less familiarization and training.
- Perhaps the most significant near-term challenge for remotely-supervised tDCS is to facilitate the process of empirical research needed to validate the treatment approach in various disorders. Currently, tDCS shows the strongest empirical support for potential efficacy in Major Depressive Disorder, stroke and selected chronic pain conditions. However, complexity arises as there are a variety of ways to deliver tDCS in potentially therapeutic ways. The combination of these different tDCS approaches and different patient groups offers numerous options for exploratory treatment trial agendas. As with any new set of options to explore, potential delays and risks to scientific progress arise from the difficulty comparing the results across several small trials when they use disparate methodology. So in addition to a set of recommendations for optimal remotely-supervised tDCS protocol construction, a likely next step to facilitate tDCS research might be the construction of a tDCS-specific clinical trials informatics platform for researchers. Two things might specifically help. First, reporting standards should be developed

that detail the minimal information that should be collected about remotely-supervised tDCS in all future clinical trials. Such a system should not only follow, but expand upon CONSORT 2010 guidelines (Schulz et al. 2010) for clinical trial reporting with tDCS-specific information about tDCS equipment configuration, ratings of the quality of each session set up, the number and duration of tDCS treatment sessions, which tDCS equipment was used, and what methods were employed to remotely-supervise patients, etc. Second, a repository should be established so that patient-based data across different studies could be integrated. Such resources typically are feasible only when they are voluntary, but that clear expectations are made by the researchers who lead the field that investigator reporting compliance is in the field's best scientific interest. Moreover, there is an increasing trend for federally-funded research to require researchers to contribute data to such repositories. Therefore, it is possible that if such a system is made available, the reporting of tDCS-specific administration information might eventually be mandated for any tDCS research funded by the National Institutes of Health. However, the potential payoff for this effort is considerable. By fostering large-scale remotely-supervised tDCS clinical trial reporting, such standards would not merely facilitate accurate and rigorous reporting of tDCS trial results, they would guide the aggregation of a database that can be continually mined to assess the quality of remotely-supervised tDCS methodology as more research is done. If participant demographic data, basic clinical characteristics, and outcome data were included in this repository, it also could facilitate future meta-analytic studies. Such information could be integrated at the meta-analytic level to characterize factors that moderate tDCS protocol adherence or even outcome, determine whether those factors are disorder- or population-specific or generalized, etc. The availability of such a standardized reporting framework/repository likely would prompt other useful additions. For instance, researchers might develop a brief, standardized questionnaire to assess patient attitudes about tDCS and reasons for seeking tDCS treatment or participating in tDCS research trials.

- This sort of recommendation is feasible because the number of tDCS researchers currently is limited, and is unlikely to grow to unmanageable proportions unless tDCS becomes fully validated as a treatment for specific disorders and people begin arguments about whether tDCS should be offered to specific patient groups as standard care options. Looking forward, it is possible to envision future challenges involving how remotely-supervised tDCS is best delivered clinically. Although the technical demands are not prohibitive, it is unlikely that at home tDCS will ever become "over the counter" or practically fit into the scope of general medical practice. More reasonably it will be used by specialty medical clinics, whose staff are fully trained to manage the technical, education, and oversight responsibilities necessary for at-home tDCS to be administered validly. This raises questions about how those staff members should best be trained. The guidelines we offer here are geared to the state of the field today, which is far more dominated by research-related concerns than issues of clinical delivery. However, they provide a blueprint of many issues that will also be relevant when considering the development of clinical care protocols. For instance, at

minimum, future training standards for tDCS clinical services should be developed that are specific to remotely-supervised procedures. This includes training and possible accreditation of technical staff. Here, the remotely-supervised tDCS can learn from standards applied in telehealth centers where medical staff remotely monitors biomedical information from at-home patients. In fact, the remotely supervised tDCS would fit well into the scope of practice of specialized telehealth centers or units, and the adoption would not require excessive additional resources.
- It is possible that the availability of at-home tDCS with remote supervision may trigger interest in physicians prescribing tDCS application at home for therapeutic purposes. In the U.S., different regulations apply to research vs medical practice.

Conclusions

In conclusion, tDCS applied in home settings can have multiple benefits to all involved. However, existing approaches in at-home tDCS vary in many elements, such as degree of rigor pertaining to patients' training, data collection, compliance with stimulation protocol, and level of supervision or necessary assistance in administration. The top tier is represented by approaches implementing highest level of control/rigor, aiming for replicability and enhanced safety. An approach utilizing remote supervision and enhanced compliance monitoring and safety monitoring, with high requirement for replicability, is suitable for tDCS clinical trials in various populations; population-specific adjustments of protocol and technology, as illustrated on examples in this chapter, document wide usefulness of this approach. The future trends in the field of tDCS applied in home settings include further development of the tDCS technology paired with technical solutions for remote monitoring/supervision; broad data sharing via data repositories; and rigorous results-reporting that may facilitate replication studies.

References

Adler, L. D., & Nierenberg, A. A. (2010). Review of medication adherence in children and adults with ADHD. *Postgraduate Medicine, 122*(1), 184–191.

Advokat, C. (2009). What exactly are the benefits of stimulants for ADHD? *Journal of Attention Disorders, 12*(6), 495–498.

Alonzo, A., & Charvet, L. (2016). Home-based tDCS: Design, feasibility, and safety considerations. In *Transcranial direct current stimulation in neuropsychiatric disorders* (pp. 351–361). Springer.

American Psychiatric Association. (2013). *Diagnostic and statistical manual of mental disorders (DSM-5®)* (5th ed.). Arlington, TX: American Psychiatric Pub.

Andrade, C. (2013). Once- to twice-daily, 3-year domiciliary maintenance transcranial direct current stimulation for severe, disabling, clozapine-refractory continuous auditory hallucinations in schizophrenia. *The Journal of ECT, 29*(3), 239–242.

Andre, S., Heinrich, S., Kayser, F., Menzler, K., Kesselring, J., Khader, P. H., … Mylius, V. (2016). At-home tDCS of the left dorsolateral prefrontal cortex improves visual short-term memory in mild vascular dementia. *Journal of the Neurological Sciences, 369*, 185–190.
Ayache, S. S., Palm, U., Chalah, M. A., Al-Ani, T., Brignol, A., Abdellaoui, M., … Lefaucheur, J. P. (2016). Prefrontal tDCS decreases pain in patients with multiple sclerosis. *Frontiers in Neuroscience, 10*, 147.
Bandeira, I. D., Guimaraes, R. S., Jagersbacher, J. G., Barretto, T. L., de Jesus-Silva, J. R., Santos, S. N., … Lucena, R. (2016). Transcranial direct current stimulation in children and adolescents with attention-deficit/hyperactivity disorder (ADHD) a pilot study. *Journal of Child Neurology, 31*(7), 918–924.
Barkley, R. A., & Cunningham, C. E. (1978). Do stimulant drugs improve the academic performance of hyperkinetic children? A review of outcome studies. *La Clinica Pediatrica, 17*(1), 85–92.
Barkley, R. A., Fischer, M., Smallish, L., & Fletcher, K. (2002). The persistence of attention-deficit/hyperactivity disorder into young adulthood as a function of reporting source and definition of disorder. *Journal of Abnormal Psychology, 111*(2), 279–289.
Barkley, R. A., Fischer, M., Smallish, L., & Fletcher, K. (2006). Young adult outcome of hyperactive children: Adaptive functioning in major life activities. *Journal of the American Academy of Child and Adolescent Psychiatry, 45*(2), 192–202.
Bikson, M., Grossman, P., Thomas, C., Zannou, A. L., Jiang, J., Adnan, T., … Woods, A. J. (2016). Safety of transcranial direct current stimulation: Evidence based update 2016. *Brain Stimulation, 9*(5), 641–661.
Breslau, J., Miller, E., Breslau, N., Bohnert, K., Lucia, V., & Schweitzer, J. (2009). The impact of early behavior disturbances on academic achievement in high school. *Pediatrics, 123*(6), 1472–1476.
Breslau, J., Miller, E., Joanie Chung, W. J., & Schweitzer, J. B. (2011). Childhood and adolescent onset psychiatric disorders, substance use, and failure to graduate high school on time. *Journal of Psychiatric Research, 45*(3), 295–301.
Bright, G. M. (2008). Abuse of medications employed for the treatment of ADHD: Results from a large-scale community survey. *Medscape Journal of Medicine, 10*(5), 111.
Brinkman, W. B., Sherman, S. N., Zmitrovich, A. R., Visscher, M. O., Crosby, L. E., Phelan, K. J., & Donovan, E. F. (2012). In their own words: Adolescent views on ADHD and their evolving role managing medication. *Academic Pediatrics, 12*(1), 53–61.
Brunoni, A. R., Amadera, J., Berbel, B., Volz, M. S., Rizzerio, B. G., & Fregni, F. (2011a). A systematic review on reporting and assessment of adverse effects associated with transcranial direct current stimulation. *The International Journal of Neuropsychopharmacology, 14*(8), 1133–1145.
Brunoni, A. R., Fregni, F., & Pagano, R. L. (2011b). Translational research in transcranial direct current stimulation (tDCS): A systematic review of studies in animals. *Reviews in the Neurosciences, 22*(4), 471–481.
Bussing, R., Koro-Ljungberg, M., Noguchi, K., Mason, D., Mayerson, G., & Garvan, C. W. (2012). Willingness to use ADHD treatments: A mixed methods study of perceptions by adolescents, parents, health professionals and teachers. *Social Science & Medicine, 74*(1), 92–100.
Cao, M., Shu, N., Cao, Q., Wang, Y., & He, Y. (2014). Imaging functional and structural brain connectomics in attention-deficit/hyperactivity disorder. *Molecular Neurobiology, 50*(3), 1111–1123.
Carlson, C. L., & Bunner, M. R. (1993). Effects of methylphenidate on the academicperformance of children with attention deficit hyperactive disorder and learning disabilities. *School Psychology Review, 22*, 184–198.
Centers for Medicare and Medicaid Services. (2012). *Chronic conditions among medicare beneficiaries*. Baltimore, MD: Chartbook.
Cha, Y. H., Urbano, D., & Pariseau, N. (2016). Randomized single blind sham controlled trial of adjunctive home-based tDCS after rTMS for mal de debarquement syndrome: Safety, efficacy, and participant satisfaction assessment. *Brain Stimulation, 9*(4), 537–544.

Charach, A., & Gajaria, A. (2008). Improving psychostimulant adherence in children with ADHD. *Expert Review of Neurotherapeutics, 8*(10), 1563–1571.

Charvet, L. E., Kasschau, M., Datta, A., Knotkova, H., Stevens, M. C., Alonzo, A., … Bikson, M. (2015). Remotely-supervised transcranial direct current stimulation (tDCS) for clinical trials: Guidelines for technology and protocols. *Frontiers in Systems Neuroscience, 9*, 26.

Christensen, L., Sasane, R., Hodgkins, P., Harley, C., & Tetali, S. (2010). Pharmacological treatment patterns among patients with attention-deficit/hyperactivity disorder: Retrospective claims-based analysis of a managed care population. *Current Medical Research and Opinion, 26*(4), 977–989.

Coletti, D. J., Pappadopulos, E., Katsiotas, N. J., Berest, A., Jensen, P. S., & Kafantaris, V. (2012). Parent perspectives on the decision to initiate medication treatment of attention-deficit/hyperactivity disorder. *Journal of Child and Adolescent Psychopharmacology, 22*(3), 226–237.

Cortese, S., Kelly, C., Chabernaud, C., Proal, E., Di Martino, A., Milham, M. P., & Castellanos, F. X. (2012). Toward systems neuroscience of ADHD: A meta-analysis of 55 fMRI studies. *The American Journal of Psychiatry, 169*(10), 1038–1055.

Cosmo, C., Baptista, A. F., de Araujo, A. N., do Rosario, R. S., Miranda, J. G., Montoya, P., & de Sena, E. P. (2015a). A randomized, double-blind, sham-controlled trial of transcranial direct current stimulation in attention-deficit/hyperactivity disorder. *PLoS One, 10*(8), e0135371.

Cosmo, C., Ferreira, C., Miranda, J. G., do Rosario, R. S., Baptista, A. F., Montoya, P., & de Sena, E. P. (2015b). Spreading effect of tDCS in individuals with attention-deficit/hyperactivity disorder as shown by functional cortical networks: A randomized, double-blind, sham-controlled trial. *Frontiers in Psychiatry*.

Cunningham, C. E., & Barkley, R. A. (1978). The role of academic failure in hyperactive behavior. *Journal of Learning Disabilities, 11*(5), 274–280.

Cuypers, K., Leenus, D. J., Van Wijmeersch, B., Thijs, H., Levin, O., Swinnen, S. P., & Meesen, R. L. (2013). Anodal tDCS increases corticospinal output and projection strength in multiple sclerosis. *Neuroscience Letters, 554*, 151–155.

Del Campo, N., Chamberlain, S. R., Sahakian, B. J., & Robbins, T. W. (2011). The roles of dopamine and noradrenaline in the pathophysiology and treatment of attention-deficit/hyperactivity disorder. *Biological Psychiatry, 69*(12), 145–157.

Demirtas-Tatlidede, A., Vahabzadeh-Hagh, A. M., & Pascual-Leone, A. (2013). Can noninvasive brain stimulation enhance cognition in neuropsychiatric disorders? *Neuropharmacology, 64*, 566–578.

Dhingra, L., Barrett, M., Knotkova, H., Chen, J., Riggs, A., Lee, B., … Portenoy, R. (2017). Symptom sistress among diverse patients referred for community-based palliative care: Sociodemographic and medical correlates. *Journal of Pain and Symptom Management, 55*, 290–296.

Ditye, T., Jacobson, L., Walsh, V., & Lavidor, M. (2012). Modulating behavioral inhibition by tDCS combined with cognitive training. *Experimental Brain Research, 219*(3), 363–368.

DosReis, S., Mychailyszyn, M. P., Evans-Lacko, S. E., Beltran, A., Riley, A. W., & Myers, M. A. (2009). The meaning of attention-deficit/hyperactivity disorder medication and parents' initiation and continuity of treatment for their child. *Journal of Child and Adolescent Psychopharmacology, 19*(4), 377–383.

Dosreis, S., Zito, J. M., Safer, D. J., Soeken, K. L., Mitchell, J. W., Jr., & Ellwood, L. C. (2003). Parental perceptions and satisfaction with stimulant medication for attention-deficit hyperactivity disorder. *Journal of Developmental and Behavioral Pediatrics, 24*, 155–162.

Evans, S. W., Owens, J. S., & Bunford, N. (2014). Evidence-based psychosocial treatments for children and adolescents with attention-deficit/hyperactivity disorder. *Journal of Child & Adolescent Psychopharmacology, 43*(4), 527–551.

Faraone, S. V., & Upadhyaya, H. P. (2007). The effect of stimulant treatment for ADHD on later substance abuse and the potential for medication misuse, abuse, and diversion. *The Journal of Clinical Psychiatry, 68*(11), 15–22.

Ferrin, M., Ruiz-Veguilla, M., Blanc-Betes, M., Abd, S. E., Lax-Pericall, T., Sinclair, M., & Taylor, E. (2012). Evaluation of attitudes towards treatment in adolescents with attention deficit hyperactivity disorder (ADHD). *European Child & Adolescent Psychiatry, 21*(7), 387–401.

Ferrucci, R., Vergari, M., Cogiamanian, F., Bocci, T., Ciocca, M., Tomasini, E., … Priori, A. (2014). Transcranial direct current stimulation (tDCS) for fatigue in multiple sclerosis. *NeuroRehabilitation, 34*(1), 121–127.

Frazier, T. W., Demaree, H. A., & Youngstrom, E. A. (2004). Meta-analysis of intellectual and neuropsychological test performance in attention-deficit/hyperactivity disorder. *Neuropsychology, 18*(3), 543–555.

Gadow, K. D. (1983). Effects of stimulant drugs on academic performance in hyperactive and learning disabled children. *Journal of Learning Disabilities, 16*(5), 290–299.

Gau, S. S., Shen, H. Y., Chou, M. C., Tang, C. S., Chiu, Y. N., & Gau, C. S. (2006). Determinants of adherence to methylphenidate and the impact of poor adherence on maternal and family measures. *Journal of Child & Adolescent Psychopharmacology, 16*(3), 286–297.

Gearing, R. E., Townsend, L., MacKenzie, M., & Charach, A. (2011). Reconceptualizing medication adherence: Six phases of dynamic adherence. *Harvard Review of Psychiatry, 19*(4), 177–189.

Hagenacker, T., Bude, V., Naegel, S., Holle, D., Katsarava, Z., Diener, H. C., & Obermann, M. (2014). Patient-conducted anodal transcranial direct current stimulation of the motor cortex alleviates pain in trigeminal neuralgia. *The Journal of Headache and Pain.*

Harpur, R. A., Thompson, M., Daley, D., Abikoff, H., & Sonuga-Barke, E. J. (2008). The attention-deficit/hyperactivity disorder medication-related attitudes of patients and their parents. *Journal of Child and Adolescent Psychopharmacology, 18*(5), 461–473.

Hasselman, D. (2013). *Super-utilizer summit: Common themes from innovation complex care management programs* (pp. 1–32). Center for Health Care Strategies Available via https://www.chcs.org/resource/super-utilizer-summit-common-themes-from-innovative-complex-care-management-programs/ Accessed 10 Oct 2017

Hinshaw, S. P. (1992a). Academic underachievement, attention deficits, and aggression: Comorbidity and implications for intervention. *Journal of Consulting and Clinical Psychology, 60*(6), 893–903.

Hinshaw, S. P. (1992b). Externalizing behavior problems and academic underachievement in childhood and adolescence: Causal relationships and underlying mechanisms. *Psychological Bulletin, 111*(1), 127–155.

Hodgson, K., Hutchinson, A. D., & Denson, L. (2014). Nonpharmacological treatments for ADHD: A meta-analytic review. *Journal of Attention Disorders, 18*(4), 275–282.

Hyvarinen, P., Makitie, A., & Aarnisalo, A. A. (2016). Self-administered domiciliary tDCS treatment for tinnitus: A double-blind sham-controlled study. *PLoS One, 11*(4), e0154286.

Jensen, P. S., Arnold, L. E., Swanson, J. M., Vitiello, B., Abikoff, H. B., Greenhill, L. L., … Hur, K. (2007). 3-year follow-up of the NIMH MTA study. *Journal of the American Academy of Child and Adolescent Psychiatry, 46*(8), 989–1002.

Johnston, C., Hommersen, P., & Seipp, C. (2008). Acceptability of behavioral and pharmacological treatments for attention-deficit/hyperactivity disorder: Relations to child and parent characteristics. *Behavior Therapy, 39*(1), 22–32.

Kaiser, N. M., Hoza, B., & Hurt, E. A. (2008). Multimodal treatment for childhood attention-deficit/hyperactivity disorder. *Expert Review of Neurotherapeutics, 8*(10), 1573–1583.

Kasschau, M., Reisner, J., Sherman, K., Bikson, M., Datta, A., & Charvet, L. E. (2016). Transcranial direct current stimulation is feasible for remotely supervised home delivery in multiple sclerosis. *Neuromodulation, 19*(8), 824–831.

Kasschau, M., Sherman, K., Haider, L., Frontario, A., Shaw, M., Datta, A., … Charvet, L. (2015). A protocol for the use of remotely-supervised transcranial direct current stimulation (tDCS) in multiple sclerosis (MS). *Journal of Visualized Experiments, 106*, e53542.

Kessler, R. C., Adler, L., Barkley, R., Biederman, J., Conners, C. K., Demler, O., … Zaslavsky, A. M. (2006). The prevalence and correlates of adult ADHD in the United States: Results from the National Comorbidity Survey Replication. *The American Journal of Psychiatry, 163*(4), 716–723.

Knotkova, H., Greenberg, A., Leuschner, Z., Soto, E., & Cruciani, R. A. (2013). Evaluation of outcomes from transcranial direct current stimulation (tDCS) for the treatment of chronic pain. *Clinical Neurophysiology, 124*(10), 125–126.

Knotkova, H., Riggs, A., Patel, V., Harounian, J., Heshmati, P., Arce, D., … Bikson, M. (2016). Advances in transcranial direct current stimulation (tDCS): Adjustment of technology, protocol and training for home-based, self-delivered remotely supervised tDCS for community-dwelling patients with advanced chronic illness. *Neuromodulation, 19*, e10.

Knotkova, H., Riggs, A., Patel, V., Truong, D., Arce, D., Bernstein, H., … Bikson, M. (2017a). A novel approach to determining M1 tDCS montage without neuronavigational measurements, suitable for patients in home settings. *Brain Stimulation, 10*(4), 78–80.

Knotkova, H., Riggs, A., & Portenoy, R. K. (2017b). A patient-tailored protocol of tDCS stimulation paired with telehealth support for at-home symptom management in seriously ill patients with multiple chronic symptoms. *Brain Stimulation, 10*(4), 77–78.

Knotkova, H., Woods, A., & Bikson, M. (2015). Transcranial direct current stimulation (tDCS): What pain practitioners need to know. *Practical Pain Management, 15*(3), 58–65.

Kooij, S. J., Bejerot, S., Blackwell, A., Caci, H., Casas-Brugue, M., Carpentier, P. J., … Asherson, P. (2010). European consensus statement on diagnosis and treatment of adult ADHD: The European network adult ADHD. *BMC Psychiatry, 10*, 67.

Langberg, J. M., & Becker, S. P. (2012). Does long-term medication use improve the academic outcomes of youth with attention-deficit/hyperactivity disorder? *Clinical Child and Family Psychology Review, 15*(3), 215–233.

Larocca, N. G. (2011). Impact of walking impairment in multiple sclerosis: Perspectives of patients and care partners. *Patient, 4*(3), 189–201.

Leffa, D. T., de Souza, A., Scarabelot, V. L., Medeiros, L. F., de Oliveira, C., Grevet, E. H., … ILS, T. (2016). Transcranial direct current stimulation improves short-term memory in an animal model of attention-deficit/hyperactivity disorder. *European Neuropsychopharmacology, 26*(2), 368–377.

Levin, F. R., Evans, S. M., & Kleber, H. D. (1998). Prevalence of adult attention-deficit hyperactivity disorder among cocaine abusers seeking treatment. *Drug and Alcohol Dependence, 52*(1), 15–25.

Loe, I. M., & Feldman, H. M. (2007). Academic and educational outcomes of children with ADHD. *Ambulatory Pediatrics, 7*(1), 82–90.

Mattioli, F., Bellomi, F., Stampatori, C., Capra, R., & Miniussi, C. (2016). Neuroenhancement through cognitive training and anodal tDCS in multiple sclerosis. *Multiple Sclerosis, 22*(2), 222–230.

McLeod, J. D., Pescosolido, B. A., Takeuchi, D. T., & White, T. F. (2004). Public attitudes toward the use of psychiatric medications for children. *Journal of Health and Social Behavior, 45*(1), 53–67.

Meesen, R. L., Thijs, H., Leenus, D. J., & Cuypers, K. (2014). A single session of 1 mA anodal tDCS-supported motor training does not improve motor performance in patients with multiple sclerosis. *Restorative Neurology and Neuroscience, 32*(2), 293–300.

Miniussi, C., & Ruzzoli, M. (2013). Transcranial stimulation and cognition. *Handbook of Clinical Neurology, 116*, 739–750.

Molina, B. S., Hinshaw, S. P., Swanson, J. M., Arnold, L. E., Vitiello, B., Jensen, P. S., … MTA Cooperative Group. (2009). The MTA at 8 years: Prospective follow-up of children treated for combined-type ADHD in a multisite study. *Journal of the American Academy of Child and Adolescent Psychiatry, 48*(5), 484–500.

Monte-Silva, K., Kuo, M. F., Hessenthaler, S., Fresnoza, S., Liebetanz, D., Paulus, W., & Nitsche, M. A. (2013). Induction of late LTP-like plasticity in the human motor cortex by repeated non-invasive brain stimulation. *Brain Stimulation, 6*(3), 424–432.

Munz, M. T., Prehn-Kristensen, A., Thielking, F., Molle, M., Goder, R., & Baving, L. (2015). Slow oscillating transcranial direct current stimulation during non-rapid eye movement sleep improves behavioral inhibition in attention-deficit/hyperactivity disorder. *Frontiers in cellular neuroscience, 9*, 307:1–8.

Narayanaswamy, J. C., Shivakumar, V., Bose, A., Agarwal, S. M., Venkatasubramanian, G., & Gangadhar, B. N. (2014). Sustained improvement of negative symptoms in schizophrenia with add-on tDCS: A case report. *Clinical Schizophrenia & Related Psychoses, 8*(3), 135–136.

Olfson, M., Marcus, S. C., Zhang, H. F., & Wan, G. J. (2007). Continuity in methylphenidate treatment of adults with attention-deficit/hyperactivity disorder. *Journal of Managed Care Pharmacy, 13*(7), 570–577.

Ortman, J. M., Velkoff, V. A., & Hogan, H. (2014). *An aging nation: The older population in the United States, current population reports*. Washington, DC: U.S. Census Bureau.

Palm, U., Ayache, S. S., Padberg, F., & Lefaucheur, J. P. (2014). Non-invasive brain stimulation therapy in multiple sclerosis: A review of tDCS, rTMS and ECT results. *Brain Stimulation, 7*(6), 849–854.

Pliszka, S., & Issues AWGoQ. (2007). Practice parameter for the assessment and treatment of children and adolescents with attention-deficit/hyperactivity disorder. *Journal of the American Academy of Child and Adolescent Psychiatry, 46*(7), 894–921.

Polderman, T. J., Boomsma, D. I., Bartels, M., Verhulst, F. C., & Huizink, A. C. (2010). A systematic review of prospective studies on attention problems and academic achievement. *Acta Psychiatrica Scandinavica, 122*(4), 271–284.

Prasad, V., Brogan, E., Mulvaney, C., Grainge, M., Stanton, W., & Sayal, K. (2013). How effective are drug treatments for children with ADHD at improving on-task behaviour and academic achievement in the school classroom? A systematic review and meta-analysis. *European Child & Adolescent Psychiatry, 22*(4), 203–216.

Prehn-Kristensen, A., Munz, M., Goder, R., Wilhelm, I., Korr, K., Vahl, W., … Baving, L. (2014). Transcranial oscillatory direct current stimulation during sleep improves declarative memory consolidation in children with attention-deficit/hyperactivity disorder to a level comparable to healthy controls. *Brain Stimulation, 7*(6), 793–799.

Rabipour, S., & Raz, A. (2012). Training the brain: Fact and fad in cognitive and behavioral remediation. *Brain and Cognition, 79*(2), 159–179.

Raggi, V. L., & Chronis, A. M. (2006). Interventions to address the academic impairment of children and adolescents with ADHD. *Clinical Child and Family Psychology Review, 9*(2), 85–111.

Riggs, A., Patel, V., Charvet, L., Kassachau, M., Harounian, J., & Knotkova, H. (2017a). Developing patient and caregiver instructional materials and training for at-home, remotely-supervised, transcranial direct current stimulation (tDCS) in seriously ill patients with multiple symptoms. *Brain Stimulation, 10*(4), 44.

Riggs, A., Patel, V., Harounian, J., Bikson, M., Paneri, B., et al. (2017b). A novel telehealth-neurostimulation intervention for at-home symptom management in chronically ill patients with multiple symptoms. *Neuromodulation, 20*(7), 232.

Riley, J. B., & Basilius, J. P. A. (2007). Physicians' liability for off-label prescriptions. *Hematology & Oncology News & Issues, 6*(5), 24–37.

Rosedale, M., Malaspina, D., Malamud, D., Strauss, S. M., Horne, J. D., Abouzied, S., … Knotkova, H. (2012). Developing patient-centered treatment protocols in brain stimulation: A rationale for combining quantitative and qualitative approaches in persons with HIV. *Journal of the American Psychiatric Nurses Association, 18*(3), 166–174.

Rubia, K., Alegria, A., & Brinson, H. (2014). Imaging the ADHD brain: Disorder-specificity, medication effects and clinical translation. *Expert Review of Neurotherapeutics, 14*(5), 519–538.

Rubio, B., Boes, A. D., Laganiere, S., Rotenberg, A., Jeurissen, D., & Pascual-Leone, A. (2016). Noninvasive brain stimulation in pediatric attention-deficit hyperactivity disorder (ADHD): A review. *Journal of Child Neurology, 31*(6), 784–796.

Rutledge, K. J., van den Bos, W., McClure, S. M., & Schweitzer, J. B. (2012). Training cognition in ADHD: Current findings, borrowed concepts, and future directions. *Neurotherapeutics, 9*(3), 542–558.

Sale, M. V., Mattingley, J. B., Zalesky, A., & Cocchi, L. (2015). Imaging human brain networks to improve the clinical efficacy of non-invasive brain stimulation. *Neuroscience and Biobehavioral Reviews, 57*, 187–198.

Schulz, K. F., Altman, D. G., Moher, D., & Group C. (2010). CONSORT 2010 statement: Updated guidelines for reporting parallel group randomised trials. *BMJ, 340*, c332.

Semerci, B., Taskiran, S., Tufan, E., & Sanli, I. (2016). Factors predicting treatment adherence in patients with adult attention-deficit/hyperactivity disorder: A preliminary study. *ADHD Attention Deficit and Hyperactivity Disorders, 8*(3), 139–147.

Soltaninejad, Z., Nejati, V., & Ekhtiari, H. (2015). Effect of anodal and cathodal transcranial direct current stimulation on DLPFC on modulation of inhibitory control in ADHD. *Journal of Attention Disorders*.

Sonuga-Barke, E. J. (2005). Causal models of attention-deficit/hyperactivity disorder: From common simple deficits to multiple developmental pathways. *Biological Psychiatry, 57*(11), 1231–1238.

Sonuga-Barke, E. J., Brandeis, D., Cortese, S., Daley, D., Ferrin, M., Holtmann, M., … European ADHD Guidelines Group. (2013). Nonpharmacological interventions for ADHD: Systematic review and meta-analyses of randomized controlled trials of dietary and psychological treatments. *The American Journal of Psychiatry, 170*(3), 275–289.

Swanson, J. M., Cantwell, D., Lerner, M., McBurnett, K., & Hanna, G. (1991). Effects of stimulant medication on learning in children with ADHD. *Journal of Learning Disabilities, 24*(4), 219–230.

The MTA Cooperative Group. (1999). A14-month randomized clinical trial of treatment strategies for attention-deficit/hyperactivity disorder. Multimodal treatment study of children with ADHD. *Archives of General Psychiatry, 56*(12), 1073–1086.

Toplak, M. E., Connors, L., Shuster, J., Knezevic, B., & Parks, S. (2008). Review of cognitive, cognitive-behavioral, and neural-based interventions for attention-deficit/hyperactivity disorder ADHD. *Clinical Psychology Review, 28*(5), 801–823.

Weyandt, L., Swentosky, A., & Gudmundsdottir, B. G. (2013). Neuroimaging and ADHD: fMRI, PET, DTI findings, and methodological limitations. *Developmental Neuropsychology, 38*(4), 211–225.

Wilens, T. E. (2004). Attention-deficit/hyperactivity disorder and the substance use disorders: The nature of the relationship, subtypes at risk, and treatment issues. *The Psychiatric Clinics of North America, 27*(2), 283–301.

Wilkes, M., & Johns, M. (2008). Informed consent and shared decision-making: A requirement to disclose to patients off-label prescription. *PLoS Medicine, 5*(11), 1553–1556.

Willcutt, E. G., Doyle, A. E., Nigg, J. T., Faraone, S. V., & Pennington, B. F. (2005). Validity of the executive function theory of attention-deficit/hyperactivity disorder: A meta-analytic review. *Biological Psychiatry, 57*(11), 1336–1346.

Willcutt, E. G., Nigg, J. T., Pennington, B. F., Solanto, M. V., Rohde, L. A., Tannock, R., … Lahey, B. B. (2012). Validity of DSM-IV attention deficit/hyperactivity disorder symptom dimensions and subtypes. *Journal of Abnormal Psychology, 121*(4), 991–1010.

Wittich, C. M., Burkle, C. M., & Lanier, W. L. (2012). Ten common questions (and their answers) about off-label drug use. *Mayo Clinic Proceedings, 87*(10), 982–990.

Woods, A. J., Antal, A., Bikson, M., Boggio, P. S., Brunoni, A. R., Celnik, P., … Nitsche, M. A. (2016). A technical guide to tDCS, and related non-invasive brain stimulation tools. *Clinical Neurophysiology, 127*(2), 1031–1048.

Chapter 14
Transcranial Direct Current Stimulation Ethics and Professional Conduct

Andrea Antal, Adam J. Woods, and Helena Knotkova

Introduction

Low intensity transcranial direct current stimulation (tDCS) is increasingly used in research and clinical practices around the world including a wide range of neurological and psychiatric conditions, where patients have no or few alternative treatment options. In parallel, the regulatory, safety and ethical considerations (Maslen et al. 2014, 2015; Maslen et al. 2013, 2014; Wexler 2016) and related problems using this methodology started to grow rapidly. Nevertheless, important ethical concerns with regard to different kind of electrical stimulation methods emerged already more than 200 years ago, since electrophysiology was born, mainly through incidental findings. E.g. Aldini travelled through Europa promoting his belief that electrical stimulation could reanimate the dead (Parent 2004). In early clinical applications the risk-benefit ratio was frequently ignored: a well-known example is a case study in 1874, when Dr. Bartholow applied electrical current to the exposed dura in a female patient. After the induction of muscular twitches, he increased the applied current intensity until distress, convulsion and finally coma were reported (Harris and Almerigi 2009). About 100 years later in the twentieth century, one of

A. Antal (✉)
Department of Clinical Neurophysiology, University Medical Center, Georg-August University Göttingen, Göttingen, Germany
e-mail: aantal@gwdg.de

A. J. Woods
Center for Cognitive Aging and Memory (CAM), McKnight Brain Institute, Department of Clinical and Health Psychology, College of Public Health and Health Professions, University of Florida, Gainesville, FL, USA

H. Knotkova
MJHS Institute for Innovation in Palliative Care, New York, NY, USA

Department of Family and Social Medicine, Albert Einstein College of Medicine, Bronx, NY, USA

H. Knotkova et al. (eds.), *Practical Guide to Transcranial Direct Current Stimulation*, https://doi.org/10.1007/978-3-319-95948-1_14

the most shocking and ethically unacceptable incident raised relevant public attention. Two physicians at the Tulane University aimed to treat a patient because of his homosexuality. Combining electrical stimulation applied over the septum with sexual interactions provided by a female prostitute, they reported a 10-month suppression of the homosexual behavior (Moan and Heath 1972). However, by evaluating these events in the past, we have to consider that the ethical awareness was/is always linked to the social definitions and moral, both in health and disease. Nowadays a very careful assessment of the Institutional Review Boards and Ethical Committees of a given clinic or university is required before a study is initiated. Nevertheless, the main responsibility with regard to the appropriate conduct and keeping a rigorous ethical framework remains always by the investigators. In this chapter we provide an overview of the present ethical issues associated with the scientific and therapeutic application of tDCS, including recommendations, in which ways these issues should be addressed.

Regulatory Framework and System of Regulations

As research involving human subjects must comply with ethical principles and standards. Although the regulatory framework differs among countries, the leading principles revolve around topics of protection and safety of participating subjects, and professional conduct. This in general involves multiple aspects addressed by a complex system of regulations, recommendations and principles, for example Good Practices in Clinical Research, Code of Federal Regulations (CFR) or Food and Drug Administration (FDA) in the USA, the Medical Devices Directive (MDD) and European health authorities in the EU. CFR is accessible to public online and regulations pertaining to protection of human subjects appear in CRF Titles 21 and 45. At present, tDCS is not approved in the United States by the FDA as a medical treatment for any indication. Devices from two companies, Soterix or Neuroconn, whose have an ‘investigational device exemption’ from the FDA, can be obtained by researchers and by medical personnel for investigational use.

Generally, non-invasive brain stimulation medical devices (NIBS), like transcranial magnetic stimulator (TMS), are classified as class IIa devices according to the Council Directive 93/42/CEE for medical devices and should conform to standards and directives. The MDD distinguishes two main cases for medical devices made available to the user, with and without CE marking. Devices without CE marking are either custom-made devices or devices intended for clinical evaluation. All other devices necessitate CE marking. Devices intended for clinical evaluation should be evaluated by the manufacturer with regard to the possibility of undesirable side effects during use. All medical devices must fulfill the Essential Requirements for safety and performance described in Annex I of the MDD, which state that a device used for its intended purpose shall not compromise the safety of any person (patients and professional users, who are applying the stimulation. The manufacturer should trace each device on the market in order to perform post-market surveillance by implementing a systematic procedure (with regard to malfunction of the stimulators, appearance and frequency of side and adverse effects, etc). Medical practitioners are required to report all incidents, related to the use of stimulator.

In 2016 the European Parliament and Council reached an agreement for better surveillance and traceability of medical devices, the Commission published a communication concerning the position of the Council on the adoption of the regulation on 9 March, 2017. The medical devices regulation will enter into force 3 years after publication, on 26 May 2020 (http://www.europarl.europa.eu/legislative-train/theme-environment-public-health-and-food-safety/file-regulation-on-medical-devices).

Ethical Considerations Pertaining to tDCS Personnel

It is the responsibility of the clinician and researcher to obtain appropriate training to insure optimal safety of patients and participants receiving tDCS. In the absence of such training, the patients or participants are exposed to an unnecessary increased risk of burn or other adverse event (AE) that would be otherwise avoidable. Suitable training should involve formal knowledge acquisition including lectures, hands-on training, and supervised administration. At a minimum, training should include: (1) knowledge of relevant background (2) knowledge of information relevant to common safety concerns, (3) knowledge of necessary precautions for reduction of AEs and serious AEs (SAEs), and the correct documentation of these, if they occur, (4) hands on training with the preparation and application of tDCS electrodes, (5) hands on training with tDCS stimulator operation, (6) supervised preparation and application of tDCS electrodes, (7) supervised operation of the tDCS stimulator, and (8) demonstration of mastery of the above training components.

1. Knowledge of relevant background. This element of training should include information regarding the physiological mechanisms underlying tDCS, with specific focus on the impact of tDCS on tissue properties including all of the neuronal elements, neurotransmitters, and possible interaction with common medications and medical conditions.
2. Knowledge of information relevant to common safety concerns. Training should also include information on how variations on contact medium, electrode properties, electrode preparation, equipment sanitization, and other tDCS parameters and their interactions that could impact the overall efficacy and safety of tDCS application.
3. Knowledge of necessary precautions for reduction of AEs and SAEs. In addition, training should involve information for optimizing safety of tDCS electrode preparation and application, medical conditions that may increase the likelihood of adverse events or serious adverse events (e.g., existing skin lesions, history of epilepsy, etc.), and special considerations for potentially vulnerable populations (e.g., children, persons with skull defects) and the correct documentation and process in case of these occur.

4. Hands on training with the preparation and application of tDCS electrodes. Training should include demonstration and hands on practice with the preparation and application of electrodes. This should include appropriate localization of electrodes (e.g., 10–20 International Electrode Measurement System, by using neuronavigation or TMS), application of contact medium to electrodes, placement of electrodes on the head, safe removal of electrodes, and equipment sanitization procedures.
5. Hands on training with tDCS stimulator operation. This element of training should involve demonstration and hands on experience with the tDCS stimulator and all of the possible settings on the device. This should include, at least, methods for powering on and off the device, knowledge of the unit power supply, how to check impedance or contact quality metrics, blinding procedures, ramp-up and down, stimulation intensity and duration settings, and emergency procedures for stopping stimulation in the middle of a session.
6. Supervised preparation and application of tDCS electrodes. This component of training must take place before a person is allowed to independently stimulate a patient or participant. This should involve supervision of the trainee in the full preparation and application of electrodes to a patient or participant, with guided feedback when necessary. A single observation is not sufficient, at least two, but preferably three or more, sessions should be supervised.
7. Supervised operation of the tDCS stimulator. Similar to the preceding component, trainees should be supervised in operation of the tDCS stimulator with guided feedback on at least two occasions, but preferably three or more.
8. Demonstration of mastery of the above training components. Following completion of components 1–7, trainees should be required to demonstrate independent mastery of each component through demonstration of necessary knowledge and skills. This demonstration of mastery should ideally involve a formal test of relevant knowledge and observation of expertise through independent application of electrodes and stimulator operation. Only after this demonstration of mastery should the trainee be allowed to work independently.

Until recently, relatively few formal courses were available for tDCS training. Several courses have become available that meet the above criteria. These courses provide the best opportunity for optimal training of clinicians and researchers new to tDCS. In the absence of a formal course work, materials with the relevant information for items 1–3 can be obtained from the literature (e.g., Antal et al. 2004; Batsikadze et al. 2013; Bikson et al. 2010; Boggio et al. 2007; Datta et al. 2009; Kessler et al. 2013; Minhas et al. 2012; Monte-Silva et al. 2010; Nitsche et al. 2000, 2003a, b, 2004a, b, 2005, 2007, 2008; Palm et al. 2008; Stagg and Nitsche 2011; Stagg et al. 2009, 2013; Woods et al. 2015, 2016) or in textbooks like this one. However, hands-on training and supervision must be acquired from either a formal course or in the lab of someone with extensive expertise in tDCS application. To reiterate, it is never advised for persons without training to apply tDCS to another person. Whether it is in a research, clinical or at-home settings, the administrator of tDCS has an ethical responsibility to protect the person receiving tDCS from AEs to the best of their ability, even when that person is administrator stimulation to him or herself.

Any research team carrying out a tDCS study has to be arranged for several specific functions and roles, some pertaining to general research activities and some specific to the tDCS use. Although one individual may assume more than one role and responsibilities associated with the role, the duties have to be clearly described, assigned, accepted and documented. Key roles within the research team and a typical scope of responsibilities include:

Principal investigator (PI) bears the overall responsibility for the whole research project. An important aspect from the regulatory and ethical point of view is that PI can delegate specific responsibilities and duties to others, such as co-investigators, but *the PI's accountability pertaining to the project is not transferable*. Therefore, it is in the best interest of PI to have the process of duty delegation well-defined and documented, so that an effective oversight of the personnel and quality checks can be made. Co- investigators substantially contribute to the scientific component of the project (such as contributing to design of the study) and/or to day-to-day study procedures (such as participant's screening). Co-investigators as all study personnel must comply with mandatory regulatory requirements clearly stated in the ethic proposals and report to the PI.

Study coordinator is mainly responsible for day-to-day study activities, such as contact with study participants, deployment of equipment, carrying out study procedures, and maintaining study documentation including participants individual study files, mandatory regulatory files, and study database. An important consequence pertaining to study coordinator's responsibilities is that the study coordinator is the core person dealing with regulatory files and associated documents and processes, such as mandatory time-frames pertaining to reporting or standard operating procedures to be followed. Thus, misconduct, negligence or insufficient training will likely have direct effects on the regulatory compliance of the study. Therefore, assigning duties to study coordinator for a specific study should emphasize this aspect and should be discussed in detail before the duty is assigned, and through training pertaining to regulatory agenda should be issued and documented. In many research teams the day-to-day study procedures are carried out by post-graduate trainees (such as post-doctoral students), it is important to keep in mind that still all duties that typically belong to the study coordinator have to be covered. They can either be assigned in full to the trainee, or can be split with a co-investigator or other senior member of the team, so that the trainee carries out the day-to-day study procedures and the senior member is responsible for maintaining the mandatory regulatory files.

Assisting personnel supports day-to-day study operations. Ethical and regulatory issues pertaining to assisting personnel encompass mostly two broad areas: (i) the supporting personnel have to have sufficient knowledge of the study so that they input is in compliance with the study protocol and regulatory requirements, and (ii) responsibilities on a specific study have to be really clearly defined. Although it seems to be trivial, substantial difficulties may arise if the responsibilities of supporting personnel are in the "gray zone", not clearly clarified. For example: Is assisting personnel allowed to contact study participants? If yes, for all which purpose? A phone call for scheduling purpose has an entirely different regulatory framework than a call to follow-up on a serious adverse event. In real life, the issue of responsibility of assisting personnel gets more complicated due to possible multitude of studies that the assisting personnel support. Thus, a clear check list of activities/support provided and not provided for each study helps keep track and ease the compliance oversight for the assisting personnel, and an at-a-glance duty delegation log provides an overview of specific responsibilities of each individual contributing to the study.

It is a frequently discussed issue whether researchers have a responsibility to laypersons who appropriate their research, or not. Many scientists agree that research results should be made freely available in order to better inform e.g. those engaging in do-ot yourself (DIY) practices. Indeed, a lay summary in scientific publications might help to avoid misinterpretation and misuse of the methodology by individuals who may lack the scientific background to understand the details. Nevertheless, there is no clear agreement with regard to these points.

Ethical Considerations Concerning Recipients, Including Research Participants and Patients

As the research and clinical value of tDCS grows, questions concerning treatment guidelines and the continuous updating of these guidelines must be considered. First, have to contemplate what criteria should we adopt before recommending tDCS, and not another treatment as a possible option. Furthermore, the scientific actuality about what tDCS can and cannot do must be explicitly stated, and every effort to balance a patient's hopes and expectations should be fairly done. Informed consent and any kind of communication with potential participants must be clear, and the objectives transparent. Risk – benefit determinations, (including an evaluation of the possible and probable risks the type, magnitude, and duration of benefit; the level of uncertainty, patients' tolerance for risk and perception of benefit) should always part of the informed consent. Moreover, participants should fully understand that they have the option to choose another alternative treatment options. Here, the basic ethical and legal requirements for inclusion of human subjects to tDCS are summarized.

Informed Consent

In the USA and in the EU the federal regulations for the protection of human subjects require investigators to obtain legally effective informed consent (IC) from individuals participating in research. IC is considered legally effective if (a) all federally required elements of IC (discussed below) as set forth in the Code of Federal Regulations, section 45 CFR 46.116 (USA) are contained in the consent form document, *and* (b) the consent of the participant is obtained prior to conducting any study-related procedure or intervention, *and* (c) the person signing the consent form is the participant or the participant's legally authorized representative. Although there are exceptions to this requirement, such as a waiver of consent, these exceptions are limited and must be approved by the IRB or Ethical Committee before the commencement of the study. Importantly, IC is not a single event or form to be signed, but an educational process that takes place between the authorized study personnel and the prospective participant. The process should include providing information in several sessions or phone calls, providing written information and allowing enough time, so that the information can be reviewed by the prospective participant. Further, sufficient time has to be allowed for questions and answers before the consent is obtained. The following are the required conditions and elements of IC:

1. Consent must be sought under circumstances that provide the participant or the legally authorized representative sufficient opportunity to consider whether or not to participate, and to minimize the possibility of coercion or undue influence.
2. Consent may not include any exculpatory language (a) through which the participant or the legally authorized representative is made to waive or appear to waive any of the participant's legal rights, or (b) which releases, or appears to release, the investigator, the Sponsor, or its agents from liability for negligence.
3. The consent must include the following elements:

   – Explicit statement that the subject is consenting to research (including prominent use of the term "research").
   – The purposes of the research, including the name of the study and who is conducting the study.
   – The description of the procedures to be followed/what will happen to the participant and the methods will be used. The ethics application must specify what other measures or stimulation methods (if any) will be employed in conjunction with tDCS. It must indicate the expected duration of the participant's involvement, including the time commitment for each component of the study and the total expected time to complete the study. If there are experimental procedures as part of the research, these must be identified.
   – Description of any reasonably foreseeable risks, AEs, SAEs, or discomforts to the participant.
   – Description of any benefits to the participant or others, which may be reasonably expected from the research.
   – Disclosure of appropriate alternative procedures or courses of treatment/therapy, if any, that might be advantageous to the participant.
   – Description of the manner and extent to which the confidentiality of records identifying the participant will be maintained.
   – Statement as to what audio or visual recording devices will be used, if any, and what will be done with such recordings upon completion of the study. The

consent form should include a separate signature line for the participant to agree to be video- or audio-taped or photographed.
- Explanation as to whether and what compensation is provided and schedule of payments.
- When appropriate, contact information and emergency contact information for the participant in the event of a research-related injury to the participant.
- When appropriate, information about the insurance during the experiments, available medical treatments for research-related injuries, payments for these treatments, and contact information for additional information about these issues.
- Name and contact information of the PI and contact persons for answers to pertinent questions by the participant about the research and his or her rights as a participant, at any time before or during the research.
- Statement that participation is voluntary, that refusal to participate will not involve any penalty or loss of benefits to which the participant is otherwise entitled, and that the participant may discontinue participation at any time without penalty or loss of benefits to which the participant is otherwise entitled.
- IRB and Ethic Committee contact information and statement that the participant may contact the IRB and Ethic Committee at any time with any questions or complaints.
- Statement that the participant will be given a copy of the consent form.

In the USA and in Europa the IRB or Ethical Committee has the final authority as to the content of the consent form presented to the prospective study participants and may require adding additional elements to the consent, for example if the research involves potentially vulnerable population, such as chronically ill patients, children, pregnant women and prisoners; or subjects with sensory disabilities, language barrier, or if inclusion of subjects without decisional capacity is planned. Further, the IRB and Ethical Committee have the authority to determine the way how IC will be obtained and documented. For example, they may approve obtaining verbal IC or an abbreviated written IC, but in most studies IC is obtained in written using a full length consent form.

The process of the consent must be documented in the participant's study files. As the study files are confidential and do not bear the participant's name (only an individual study participation code), the signed consent has to be kept in a separate location from the individual study files in order to maintain confidentiality.

It is mandated that no study procedures take place until the IC is obtained. Thus, screening for the full Inclusion/Exclusion criteria is carried out after obtaining the IC and those who do not fully meet the Inclusion/Exclusion criteria are noted in the study files as screen failures and discharged from the study. It is important to note that any study participant may withdraw from study at any time. In addition, participants may be removed from the study by study personnel for specified reasons. A clear criteria for removal of a participant from the study by the study personnel have to be in place, noted in written in the study protocol as well as in the text of the informed consent. Criteria for removal from the study vary among studies, but often include the following events:

- Not following the study protocol or instructions from study personnel.
- If a SAEs or repeated AEs related or potentially related to the study procedure occurs.
- For administrative reasons, such as if the study closes.

Screening of Subjects

It is of the utmost importance that subjects or patients be carefully screened using the Inclusion/Exclusion criteria that maximize their safety during tDCS in a research or clinical protocol, as discussed above. For a study investigating the role of a brain regions in a given behavior in healthy adults would include common items, including but not limited to: absence of head injury or neurological disease, no personal or family history of seizures, a minimum age or a specific age-range for participants, no metal implanted in the head (e.g., stent, plate, metal shavings in the eye, hearing aids, etc.) or body (e.g., pacemaker, insulin pump, etc.) that could be affected or the function altered by current flow, no pregnancy, drug and alcohol abuse, no glutamatergic or GABA-ergic medications that could alter tDCS effects, no major psychiatric illness (depression, schizophrenia, etc.). However, some of these criteria will differ based on the intended application or treatment use of tDCS. For example, a depression trial would specifically target persons with a clinical diagnosis of depression, but might maintain all other criteria.

Appropriate screening methods of the population of study or treatment must use appropriate methods. For research studies in otherwise healthy populations, a detailed self-reported medical history is the typical method for acquiring this information. When using this method, it is important to stress in the consenting process or phone interview prior to consent, the importance and relevance of the screening criteria and how they can impact the person, is critical. For example, relaying how metal in the head could interact with the electrical current flow to cause damage helps to fully inform the participant of risks, should they misreport information on the self-reported medical screening. In addition, and when possible, permission to review of the person's medical records can help the researcher to cross-validate self-reported information and further enhance study/participant safety. However, the availability of medical records is not universal when working with healthy populations.

In contrast, when working in patient populations, self-report can be used, but should also be verified using medical records and/or in collaboration with the person's physician. These materials should be reviewed by a study physician and the subject should optimally be interviewed by the study physician before study entry and after they have had the opportunity to review the medical records. In clinical treatment studies, the availability of medical records will provide much of the needed information for study screening. However, medical records are often incomplete, especially when patients use different health care systems for treatment across the lifespan (extremely common). Thus, it is also important to cross validate this information with self-reported information to identify discrepancies that deserve further investigation.

In the case of patients or participants with compromised cognitive abilities, self-report information should be obtained from the caregiver and cross-validated with medical records. Nonetheless, it is not always easy to identify compromised cognitive function, thus matching medical records to self-report from the patient/participant and the caregiver provides optimal insight into premorbid conditions or other factors that may prevent a participant from participating in a study or treatment.

Ethical Issues Related to Choosing Subject Population

Choosing a sample size For prospective research applications of tDCS, sample size calculations should be performed prior to initiation of a study using either pilot data or best available data in the literature to estimate the necessary minimum sample size for appropriate tDCS effect estimation. If a study is underpowered with no potential for appropriate effect estimation, subjects are exposed to study risks, even if minimal, without any potential for scientific benefit. However, in the absence of appropriate data, a pilot study in a small sample of subject may be used to acquire the data needed for appropriate estimation. Again, the minimum number of subjects necessary for initial effect size estimation should be used in pilot studies, minimizing any exposure to risk for the participants. Furthermore, appropriate sample size estimation is critical for avoiding an oversampling of the population and, in effect, the unethical process of "chasing a statistical p-value." As is the case with parametric statistics, a significant effect can be "found", if a study collected enough subjects. This issue highlights the importance of not only reporting test-statistics, but also measures of effect size. Simply put, if a test statistic is significant, but the effect size estimate is small (e.g., Cohen's d less than 0.2), this is an indication of a small and perhaps negligible effect of stimulation even in the presence of statistical significance. Nevertheless, the scientific aim should always be considered, e.g. with regard to clinical studies including a small number of patients for the global test comparing primary and secondary endpoints of the study among treatment groups a p value less than 0.2 indicates a possible treatment effect and warrants further studies (Kianifard and Islam 2011),

Another point of consideration is the use of appropriate statistical procedures to investigate tDCS effects. If a sample size does not allow for assumptions necessary for parametric statistics (and a normal distribution of the data is a necessary condition related to the study aim) non-parametric statistics should be used. Furthermore, general or generalized linear modeling approaches accounting for covariates of interest and non-interest are important for understanding the meaning and potential impact of data. The use of t-tests as primary test statistics for data analyses is generally not the best choice, unless used as a planned contrast following prior appropriate statistical procedures (e.g., ANOVA, ANCOVA, multiple linear regression).

Choosing appropriate inclusion/exclusion criteria Identifying the appropriate population and selecting inclusion/exclusion criteria to minimize subject risk is an important part of the overall study design and ethical execution of a study or clinical treatment using tDCS. Inclusion/exclusion criteria will vary significantly depending on the population of interest and the applied experimental procedures. For example, while personal or family history of epilepsy would be major exclusion criteria for a study using tDCS to enhance cognitive function in older adults, it would be an inclusion criteria for a study seeking to enhance cognitive function in patients with epilepsy. Very few inclusion/exclusion criteria are universal, except for exclusion of persons with metal implanted or lodged in the head, neck or face. In the case of metal piercings or studs that cannot be removed, these persons should also be excluded from tDCS. Stimulation of persons with face tattoos that may use inks containing metals should be avoided as well. Another exclusion criteria important to consider is the exclusion of persons with implanted devices in the body that control autonomic function or perform a function that, if altered by introduction of current, could endanger the patient (e.g. pacemaker, implanted medication pump, etc). In the absence of technical and medical specialist that can verify the continued functionality of such devices during and after tDCS, these persons should be excluded from research or clinical applications of tDCS.

Other criteria important for consideration to minimize risk and maximize possible benefit include significant medical histories that may predispose a person to seizure activity. While no cases of seizure have been reported to date from tDCS, introduction of electrical current to the brain, no matter how small, requires careful consideration and minimization of risk when considering of the study outweigh the possible increased risk profile of including someone with a personal history or family history of epilepsy. Conditions related to vascular, traumatic, tumoral, infectious or metabolic lesions of the brain, even without history of seizure, administration of drugs that potentially lower seizure threshold, sleep deprivation, alcoholism should always carefully evaluated. As in the example above, it is possible that seizure history can be an inclusion criteria in a clinical study, but for most applications it is a common exclusion criteria.

Medications that can alter the impact of tDCS on brain function are yet another criteria important for consideration. For example, prior research shows that 1 mA stimulation while a person is on an selective serotonin reuptake inhibitor (SSRI) changes the typical inhibitory effects related to cathodal stimulation in the motor system to a net excitatory effect and enhances and prolongs the efficacy of anodal stimulation (Nitsche et al. 2009). Depending on the study goals (e.g., adjunctive depression treatment), this may be a desirable effect. However, in other applications where selective inhibition and excitation under different electrodes is desired (e.g., some inhibitory control paradigms), use of concurrent SSRI could have unintended consequences and change the potential benefit/risk profile for specific subjects. Another careful consideration is exclusion of persons on drugs that either block NMDA receptors or GABA agonists, as these have been shown to undermine the overall neuroplastic effect of tDCS (Nitsche et al. 2004a, b). This would mean that a person may have limited to no potential benefit from tDCS in the presence of such drugs, and this would alter the benefit/risk ratio for the participant or patient, too. As dose-response relationships are relatively poorly understood in many applications of tDCS, careful consideration and caution are required to maximize safety of participants and patients.

Ethically, it is also important not to use biased inclusion/exclusion criteria, providing equitable access to tDCS studies or treatments. For example, exclusion based on gender or ethnic background must be clearly justified by the scientific aims of a study. For example, a study examining ethnic differences between analgesic tDCS response for two ethnic groups with differing pain profiles could be justified in a series of ethnicity based inclusion/exclusion criteria. In contrast, ethnic or gender-based inclusion/inclusion criteria are never acceptable for consideration of clinical treatment options of tDCS. Age of participant is another factor that must be carefully considered regarding potential for benefit vs. risk. Several studies suggest (Kessler et al. 2013; Minhas et al. 2012) that application of 'adult' tDCS protocols to children does not result in the same effects that were observed in adults. For example, application of 2 mA tDCS can produce current density much higher in the brain of an 8 year old a child versus an adult. Aside from parameter considerations, inclusion/exclusion of children should be considered very carefully relative to potential benefit vs. risk. It is entirely unknown what long-term effects of repeated applications of tDCS in a developing brain might have on the plastic development of neuronal tissue. While no negative data have been produced, no data exist to support or refute possible long-term effects. Thus, inclusion of participants that are still in a phase of neural development must be strongly justified by potential benefit to the participant. The human brain is reported to continue development in frontal regions into the mid-twenties. However, most work in tDCS has been applied to college age students participating in research studies. While the effects on a "mostly" developed brain may be negligible or even positive, there is yet again an absence of data supporting either notion. Nevertheless, here a distinction should be made between repeated stimulation sessions and a single application that does not induce a long lasting physiological change.

Ethical Considerations Related to the tDCS Implications of Involuntary or Coercive Use

As tDCS becomes more commonly applied in clinical settings, the potential for coercive use of tDCS as a treatment becomes a realistic possibility that deserves careful consideration. tDCS has been shown effective in treating a number of symptoms and disease states that have potential for impact on this issue. For example, some studies have shown efficacy in treating symptoms of schizophrenia. As such, it is possible that a psychiatrist could order treatment within a mental health facility, as is the case with electroconvulsive therapy (ECT) or pharmaceutical treatment. It is within the purview of informed and trained clinicians to make medically relevant decisions regarding treatment of their patients when that treatment has a potential for alleviating the medical condition afflicting the patient. There is also the potential for clinicians or researchers to apply tDCS to children at the request of their parents. Prior to the age of consent within a given country, this is within the legal rights of the parents, as they are deemed best qualified to dictate the treatment of their child in collaboration with a trained and certified clinician. This is not disputed here. However, a strong word of caution is needed regarding such applications – as the long-term consequences of tDCS for developing tissue is yet undetermined. In cases where the clinician and parents deem the potential benefit to the child to outweigh unknown risks to the developmental process, these applications may be warranted. However, the quantification of unknown risk is difficult at best, similarly to many other interventions in children.

Furthermore, as tDCS is a technology that can be acquired by the community at large with little effort, yet using devices that have inferior or no device qualifications (discussed further in a following section below), there is also the possibility of tDCS being applied without consent to children by their parents, without consultation of a clinician. This is both ill-advised and unethical, as the technology's consequences are not at a stage where this process could be considered safe – due to unknown optimal dosing parameters, unknown long-term effects and risks, and increased potential for harm when using uncertified devices available to the public. At a future date where these factors are better understood, this application may become possible within an ethical space, but this is currently not the case.

Ethical Aspects of Reimbursement (and Methods How to Mitigate Coercive Effect)

It has been widely accepted that participants in research may be reimbursed for their time or discomfort, but ethical considerations are needed to mitigate coercive effect of the reimbursement. It is recommended (and in some studies required) to derive the level of reimbursement from the characteristics of each involved study procedure, such as time-demand, burden for the participant, or need for frequent travel to the research facility. It is recommended to dispense the reimbursement at time points along the study protocol (e.g. at each study visit), avoiding all-in-once payment at the beginning or end of a study, in order to avoid potential bias of "buying participants to the study" or potential coercive effect as some participants may tend to under-report AEs in order to be eligible for the reimbursement at the end of study. Importantly, the process of reimbursement must be planned and codified in the approved study protocol, and each reimbursement transaction must be documented and kept on files.

Ethics Pertaining to tDCS Procedures

Independently from the type of the study, stimulation parameters and schedules must always be chosen with clear clinical goals and safety considerations in mind and these parameters and protocols must be accepted by the IRB and Ethical Committee before initiation of a study. However, it could happen that during a given study the approved research protocol cannot be or was not followed, i.e. due to a change in a research activity. If an unanticipated or unintentional divergence from the approved protocol happens (e.g. higher intensity, longer stimulation duration was applied) it must be reported to the IRB/ Ethical Committee (usually within 7 days of their discovery). Generally, the only ethically acceptable intentional protocol deviation is when urgent action is required to eliminate an immediate hazard to a subject.

Other single occurrence deviations could occur e.g. in inclusion/exclusion criteria that are often planned exceptions in clinical studies. They should receive IRB or Ethical Committee approval before being implemented.

Like in every research and clinical application, the potential benefit of the tDCS must be found by an independent assessment to outweigh the risk. In any case, the decision on the risk-benefit ratio of a given study needs to be made by each PI and the local IRB or Ethical Committee. The requirement of equal distribution of the burdens and benefits of research can be violated when tDCS is conducted on seriously ill patients or patients made vulnerable by physical or social or conditions, bearing only its burdens. Nevertheless, in these patients alternative therapies also have significant risks (e.g. neurosurgical procedures). It is not only sufficient that the subject be willing to accept the risk involved and it is advised that the likelihood of clinical benefit must always outweigh the potential risks.

tDCS studies in patients with primary therapeutic objective, including the development of new protocols that have been not yet tested for safety, e.g. cumulative daily or weekly applications of tDCS for therapeutic purposes, has a potential resulting in direct individual clinical benefit, nevertheless with potential risk(s). Studies with indirect benefit and related moderate risk might involve patients where the potential clinical benefit is speculative or where no clinical benefit is anticipated, but the study might result in a better understanding of pathophysiological mechanisms of different disorders. Here the exposure to AEs (when clinical benefit is uncertain) for patients and many times healthy controls subjects should carefully be evaluated by the PI and the IRB or Ethical Committee.

Appropriate safety measures related to a given study must permanently be introduced. It is important to assess the subject/patient's acute condition prior to each tDCS application. Thus, participants would answer a series of questions regarding their experience with various symptoms prior to the first stimulation session, to establish a baseline. Furthermore, subjects must be continuously monitored during and after the stimulation sessions. It is advised that following each session participants should complete an Adverse Effects Questionnaire, (http://www.neurologie.uni-goettingen.de/downloads.html) which requires participants to rate of any

AEs such as local pain, tingling, burning, headaches, perception, or cognitive effects before, during and after stimulation. At the next session, they would report on these questions regarding the interval between the last stimulation to immediately before the day's stimulation session. After stimulation, they would again report on the experience during and immediately after stimulation. This approach provides the researcher or clinician to assess for AEs or changes that could warrant concern for study continuation. These questionnaires typically query participants using either a visual analog scale or a basic Likert scale that can be quickly evaluated by the researcher or clinician and quantified for further analyses. These data might also provide information important for validating effectiveness of sham versus real tDCS stimulation in both clinical and research settings.

Participants should remain in the laboratory for min. fifteen minutes after stimulation has ended. If they feel unwell, they should be seen by a medical doctor. With respect to the skin contact, there is a possibility of electrochemical production of toxins and electrode dissolution products at the electrode tissue interface that occurs very rarely, probably due to using non-suitable electrode material. Repeated applications of tDCS over several days might cause skin irritation under the electrodes in some individuals. Participants should therefore be interviewed for the existence of skin diseases and the condition of the skin under the electrodes should be inspected before and after stimulation. In the case of notable skin irritation caused in sensitive individuals it should be decided at case by case basis whether to proceed with the experiment.

Long-term negative cognitive and neuropsychological changes of single tDCS applications seem negligible. However, at least one study has suggested that using tDCS to "enhance" certain functions may impair others (Iuculano and Kadosh 2013). Therefore, neuropsychological monitoring is strongly recommended when repeated daily sessions of tDCS are administered for therapeutic purposes, or when new parameters of stimulation (e.g. higher intensities) are investigated (even in healthy subjects). Many laboratories apply physiological monitoring (TMS, EEG) of every subject undergoing new tDCS protocols. It is responsibility of the PI to decide the most appropriate tests to be applied. These additional procedures should also be approved by the IRB.

Open Questions and Gray Areas in the tDCS Ethics

There is much discussion about the difference between treatment and neuroenhancement. Where does tDCS treatment versus neuroenhancement differ? Does it matter? On the one hand, tDCS has been shown efficacious in addressing a variety of clinical issues in patient populations: depression, pain, post-stroke cognitive or motor deficits, etc. When the case of tDCS as a neuroenhancer is discussed, it is more often the situation that this refers to the use of tDCS by otherwise healthy adults or young adults in an attempt to enhance their abilities beyond their normal aptitude. In contrast, others are currently using the technique to address cognitive decline associated with the normal aging process. Thus, otherwise healthy older adults that experience a natural decline in cognitive abilities are treated with tDCS, typically in conjunction with another therapy, such as cognitive training, to help alleviate symptoms of cognitive aging. While this case falls under the category of neuroenhancement, in many ways it also fits with examples of tDCS use that treat symptoms associated with a given disorder. To researchers who are investigating the process of aging, it is a disorder that affects all systems in the body and its preclusion may prevent the development of debilitating diseases, like Alzheimer's.

Where is the fine line between neuroenhancement and treatment? This most likely exists in the overall "intent" of the tDCS application by the user. From a simple perspective, an application to recover function (e.g., aging, stroke) is a treatment approach, whereas, an attempt to enhance function beyond baseline levels fits within the category of neuroenhancement. Does this distinction between treatment and neuroenhancement matter? In and of itself, perhaps not. However, there are caveats based on our current knowledge in the field that must be considered. From one perspective, adults attend higher education to enhance their fluid abilities beyond their current stage. This is not unethical. We take caffeine to enhance our current state of arousal to optimize performance. Thus, the simple act of neuroenhancement itself is not unethical, as it represents a fundamental component of human life and development. However, the current lack of understanding of long term consequences of tDCS and poor understanding of its effect on developing brain tissue suggests that application of this technique as a neuroenhancer may or may not have the intended consequences. Thus, while neuroenhancement in and of itself is likely not unethical by definition, its application at the current state of our understanding of tDCS deserves extreme caution. Thus, application as a neuroenhancer prior to necessary understanding of the technologies long-term consequences could be viewed as ethically questionable outside of research applications exploring impact. As the longitudinal consequences of this technology become more clearly defined, both treatment and neuroenhancement approaches will become viable avenues of use.

Ethical Aspects of Using Neuromodulation Devices Outside of Therapeutic Use

Should the ability to facilitate brain function be reserved for clinical treatment and research applications or should it be available to the community at large? There are different perspectives that are important to consider.

1. *Should we self-stimulate because we can stimulate?* There is a long human history of performing techniques or consuming substances to enhance function/performance. The use of caffeine serves as an example of self-stimulating behavior common across the world. Indeed, many people take supplements to potentially enhance health. Furthermore, nonsteroidal anti-inflammatory drugs (NSAIDs) are commonly taken without a prescription for treatment of pain.

Thus, if tDCS can provide some form of health benefit, alleviate pain, or enhance cognition, one perspective would argue that it should be available to all persons that might benefit. However, while tDCS can affect the domains from these examples, the long-term consequences remain relatively unknown. Further still, optimal dosing parameters require further study to evaluate what long-term effects tDCS might have on the brain. In fact, few studies have stimulated participants outside of a 2-week window of stimulation for 10 out of 14 days (Loo et al. 2012). E.g. Loo et al. in one study investigated 3 weeks of treatment (15 days over 3 weeks). This means that there is little to no evidence of stimulation consequences for extended long-term use. Until these data become available, a level of regulation is necessary. Thus, the absence of knowledge for long-term consequences suggests that tDCS as a self-administered neuroenhancer or treatment requires regulation for the time being.

2. *Is it safe for everyone to stimulate?* The safety profile for "enhancers" like caffeine, NSAIDs, or other supplements are quite different from tDCS. When tDCS is performed incorrectly, e.g. if the scalp is broken in any way, skin lesions and deep burns can occur. The full safety profile and contraindications for tDCS are not well explored. Any metal in the head could lead to damage to brain tissue or death, if for example a metal stent was inside the head of a person. Thus, if readily available over the counter for self-use, there is a significant potential for unintended irreversible damage to person. Counter to this, one could also argue that overuse of any of the counter example products could also lead to damage of the liver, stomach, etc. However, the quantities required for irreparable damage would be high, whereas, a single session of tDCS in a person with a metal stint could cause irreparable harm. Further still, there is a possibility for parents of children to apply tDCS to enhance classroom performance, to attempt to treat some aspect of neurodevelopmental disability or to enhance the normal developmental process. As discussed above, the consequences of tDCS for developing brain tissue in children is currently unknown (Kessler et al. 2013; Minhas et al. 2012; Woods et al. 2016). Thus, ready access for self-dosing of children by parents is ill advised and should be avoided. As the application of tDCS to a human can lead to harm in a single session (e.g. using to long stimulation duration or higher intensities) and could be misused with potential for harm in those untrained or uninformed, over the counter use/off the shelf availability of tDCS outside of research or clinical settings is not advised from safety and potential for harm perspectives.
3. *Are all tDCS devices the same?* Compared to other forms of transcranial neuromodulation, tDCS relies on devices that are relatively easy to build and therefore cheaper (e.g compared to TMS). Due to this fact, a movement arose starting in 2010–2011, in which lay persons started modifying iontophoresis devices or building tDCS devices for use on themselves, with the main aims of cognitive enhancement or self-treatment. This movement, which is known as do-it-yourself (DIY) tDCS, comprises people, who are mainly communicating online, largely using the most dedicated forum called Reddit.com. Therefore, it is not surprising that in this rapidly expanding DIY culture and based on the perceived simplicity

of the engineering principles behind creating a device capable of delivering current through two or more wires to two or more electrodes, the world market is quickly becoming flooded with individuals or companies offering tDCS devices for home-stimulation or plans for construction of such devices. Furthermore, since many direct-to-consumer brain stimulation companies, mainly in the USA and Asia do not make medical claims, they are marketing their products for enhancement and/or "wellness," and they can sell them even cheaper. However, these devices often meet none of the certified device criteria discussed in Chap. 7. Thus, these devices often fail to have mechanisms for ramping current, methods for maintaining a controlled and constant current at a safe level of intensity (e.g., preventing surges/spikes in electrical current that could increase chance of burns or other harmful effects), or other features that maximize the safety of the person receiving tDCS or the DIY user (Woods et al. 2016). Through a simple internet search, one can find 9-volt batteries soldered to wires ending in bare wires or gator clips, intended to be clamped or inserted into the top of kitchen sponges or some other porous material. This should not be considered a tDCS device, as it fails to meet even the most basic safety criteria or necessary precision required for current delivery in tDCS. While such a device has limited risk of current spikes, there are in fact numerous aspects of such a device that can drastically increase the opportunity for burns by such a device (e.g., metal to skin contact, inconsistent electrode material, no ability to deliver a controlled and constant current with ramping safety features, etc.). Ethically, these devices do little to nothing to minimize the safety risks of the person being stimulated and should be avoided. Again, based on the perspective of safety, as well as the necessary engineering principles required to maintain safety, there is at least a minimum level of regulation necessary for devices made available to the public.

Conclusions

The aim of this chapter was to provide an overview of the present ethical issues associated with the scientific and therapeutic use of tDCS. Overall, the perspectives of knowledge and safety suggest that tDCS is ethically ready for supervised research and clinical applications but not for mass availability for DIY application/self/home administration. From an engineering perspective, once the devices are available, there is a minimum level of features and criteria necessary for device safety, meaning that at least a minimum level of regulation is suggested. The former argument is likely a matter of scientific and clinical research over time, while the latter is already well explored. Once the science of tDCS and our understanding of dosing and long-term consequences equal our understanding of the engineering principles behind tDCS, this is a technology that may well be suited to ready availability across the world market. Nevertheless, until this point several critical ethical issues should also be clarified, including e.g. the possible interaction with behavior by tDCS, such as impulsivity, risk taking behaviour (Cheng and Lee 2016; Fecteau et al. 2013).

Indeed, many commonly used psychiatric drugs could theoretically be understood as "personality" modifiers, nevertheless, the regulation of medical treatments using drugs have a long history and generally, the intake of these medications is relatively good regulated. Other important point is whether tDCS-induced enhancement can or should be accepted for educational purposes or not. At present, we have not reached this stage, and it is ethically questionable to make such technologies available to the public before the risks associated with their long-term use or application in vulnerable populations is understood.

References

Antal, A., Nitsche, M. A., Kruse, W., Kincses, T. Z., Hoffmann, K.-P., & Paulus, W. (2004). Direct current stimulation over V5 enhances visuomotor coordination by improving motion perception in humans. *Journal of Cognitive Neuroscience, 16*, 521–527.

Batsikadze, G., Moliadze, V., Paulus, W., Kuo, M.-F., & Nitsche, M. A. (2013). Partially non-linear stimulation intensity-dependent effects of direct current stimulation on motor cortex excitability in humans. *The Journal of Physiology, 591*, 1987–2000.

Bikson, M., Datta, A., Rahman, A., & Scaturro, J. (2010). Electrode montages for tDCS and weak transcranial electrical stimulation: Role of " return" electrode's position and size. *Clinical Neurophysiology, 121*, 1976–1978.

Boggio, P. S., Nunes, A., Rigonatti, S. P., Nitsche, M. A., Pascual-Leone, A., & Fregni, F. (2007). Repeated sessions of noninvasive brain DC stimulation is associated with motor function improvement in stroke patients. *Restorative Neurology and Neuroscience, 25*, 123–129.

Cheng, G. L., & Lee, T. M. (2016). Altering risky decision-making: Influence of impulsivity on the neuromodulation of prefrontal cortex. *Social Neuroscience, 11*(4), 353–356.

Datta, A., Bansal, V., Diaz, J., Patel, J., Reato, D., & Bikson, M. (2009). Gyri-precise head model of transcranial direct current stimulation: Improved spatial focality using a ring electrode versus conventional rectangular pad. *Brain Stimulation, 2*, 201–207.e1.

Fecteau, S., Boggio, P., Fregni, F., & Pascual-Leone, A. (2013). Modulation of untruthful responses with non-invasive brain stimulation. *Front Psychiatry, 3*, 97.

Harris, L. J., & Almerigi, J. B. (2009). Probing the human brain with stimulating electrodes: The story of Roberts Bartholow's (1874) experiment on Mary Rafferty. *Brain and Cognition, 70*, 92–115.

Kianifard, F., & Islam, M. Z. (2011). A guide to the design and analysis of small clinical studies. *Pharmaceutical Statistics, 10*(4), 363–368.

Kessler, S. K., Minhas, P., Woods, A. J., Rosen, A., Gorman, C., & Bikson, M. (2013). Dosage considerations for transcranial direct current stimulation in children: A computational modeling study. *PLoS One, 8*, e76112.

Iuculano, T., & Cohen Kadosh, R. J. (2013). The mental cost of cognitive enhancement. *Neuroscience, 33*, 4482–4486.

Loo, C. K., Alonzo, A., Martin, D., Mitchell, P. B., Galvez, V., & Sachdev, P. (2012). Transcranial direct current stimulation for depression: 3-week, randomised, sham-controlled trial. *The British Journal of Psychiatry, 200*, 52–59.

Maslen, H., Douglas, T., Cohen Kadosh, R., Levy, N., & Savulescu, J. (2014a). The regulation of cognitive enhancement devices: Extending the medical model. *Journal of Law and the Biosciences, 1*, 68–93.

Maslen, H., Douglas, T., Cohen Kadosh, R., Levy, N., & Savulescu, J. (2015). Do-it-yourself brain stimulation: A regulatory model. *Journal of Medical Ethics, 41*, 413–414.

Maslen, H., Earp, B. D., Cohen Kadosh, R., & Savulescu, J. (2014b). Brain stimulation for treatment and enhancement in children: An ethical analysis. *Frontiers in Human Neuroscience, 8*, 953.

Maslen, H., Savulescu, J., Douglas, T., Levy, N., & Cohen Kadosh, R. (2013). Regulation of devices for cognitive enhancement. *Lancet, 382*, 938–939.

Minhas, P., Bikson, M., Woods, A. J., Rosen, A. R., & Kessler, S. K. (2012). Transcranial direct current stimulation in pediatric brain: A computational modeling study. *Conference Proceedings: Annual International Conference of the IEEE Engineering in Medicine and Biology Society, 2012*, 859–862.

Moan, C. E., & Heath, R. G. (1972). Septal stimulation for initiation of heterosexual behavior in a homosexual male. *Journal of Behavior Therapy and Experimental Psychiatry, 3*, 23–30.

Monte-Silva, K., Kuo, M.-F., Liebetanz, D., Paulus, W., & Nitsche, M. A. (2010). Shaping the optimal repetition interval for cathodal transcranial direct current stimulation (tDCS). *Journal of Neurophysiology, 103*, 1735–1740.

Nitsche, M. A., Cohen, L. G., Wassermann, E. M., Priori, A., Lang, N., Antal, A., … Pascual-Leone, A. (2008). Transcranial direct current stimulation: State of the art 2008. *Brain Stimulation, 1*, 206–223.

Nitsche, M. A., Doemkes, S., Karaköse, T., Antal, A., Liebetanz, D., Lang, N., … Paulus, W. (2007). Shaping the effects of transcranial direct current stimulation of the human motor cortex. *Journal of Neurophysiology, 97*, 3109–3117.

Nitsche, M. A., Jaussi, W., Liebetanz, D., Lang, N., Tergau, F., & Paulus, W. (2004a). Consolidation of human motor cortical neuroplasticity by D-cycloserine. *Neuropsychopharmacology, 29*, 1573–1578.

Nitsche, M. A., Kuo, M. F., Karrasch, R., Wachter, B., Liebetanz, D., & Paulus, W. (2009). Serotonin affects transcranial direct current-induced neuroplasticity in humans. *Biological Psychiatry, 66*, 503–508.

Nitsche, M. A., Liebetanz, D., Lang, N., Antal, A., Tergau, F., & Paulus, W. (2003a). Safety criteria for transcranial direct current stimulation (tDCS) in humans. *Clinical Neurophysiology, 114*, 2220–2222. author reply 2222–2223.

Nitsche, M. A., Liebetanz, D., Schlitterlau, A., Henschke, U., Fricke, K., Frommann, K., … Tergau, F. (2004b). GABAergic modulation of DC stimulation-induced motor cortex excitability shifts in humans. *The European Journal of Neuroscience, 19*, 2720–2726.

Nitsche, M. A., Nitsche, M. A., Paulus, W., & Paulus, W. (2000). Excitability changes induced in the human motor cortex by weak transcranial direct current stimulation. *The Journal of Physiology, 527*(Pt 3), 633–639.

Nitsche, M. A., Nitsche, M. S., Klein, C. C., Tergau, F., Rothwell, J. C., & Paulus, W. (2003b). Level of action of cathodal DC polarisation induced inhibition of the human motor cortex. *Clinical Neurophysiology, 114*, 600–604.

Nitsche, M. A., Seeber, A., Frommann, K., Klein, C. C., Rochford, C., Nitsche, M. S., … Tergau, F. (2005). Modulating parameters of excitability during and after transcranial direct current stimulation of the human motor cortex. *The Journal of Physiology, 568*, 291–303.

Palm, U., Keeser, D., Schiller, C., Fintescu, Z., Reisinger, E., Padberg, F., & Nitsche, M. (2008). Skin lesions after treatment with transcranial direct current stimulation (tDCS). *Brain Stimulation, 1*, 386–387.

Parent, A. (2004). Giovanni Aldini: From animal electricity to human brain stimulation. *The Canadian Journal of Neurological Sciences Le journal canadien des sciences neurologiques, 31*, 576–584.

Stagg, C. J., Best, J. G., Stephenson, M. C., O'Shea, J., Wylezinska, M., Kincses, Z. T., … Johansen-Berg, H. (2009). Polarity-sensitive modulation of cortical neurotransmitters by transcranial stimulation. *The Journal of Neuroscience, 29*, 5202–5206.

Stagg, C. J., Lin, R. L., Mezue, M., Segerdahl, A., Kong, Y., Xie, J., & Tracey, I. (2013). Widespread modulation of cerebral perfusion induced during and after transcranial direct current stimulation applied to the left dorsolateral prefrontal cortex. *The Journal of Neuroscience, 33*, 11425–11431.

Stagg, C. J., & Nitsche, M. A. (2011). Physiological basis of transcranial direct current stimulation. *The Neuroscientist, 17*, 37–53.

Wexler, A. (2016). The practices of do-it-yourself brain stimulation: Implications for ethical considerations and regulatory proposals. *Journal of Medical Ethics, 42*, 211–215.

Woods, A. J., Antal, A., Bikson, M., Boggio, P. S., Brunoni, A. R., Celnik, P., … Nitsche, M. A. (2016). A technical guide to tDCS, and related non-invasive brain stimulation tools. *Clinical Neurophysiology, 127*, 1031–1048.

Woods, A. J., Bryant, V., Sacchetti, D., Gervits, F., & Hamilton, R. (2015). Effects of electrode drift in transcranial direct current stimulation. *Brain Stimulation, 8*, 515–519.

Part III
Clinical Potential and Applications

Chapter 15
Transcranial Direct Current Stimulation in Psychiatry: Mood Disorders, Schizophrenia and Other Psychiatric Diseases

Andre Russowsky Brunoni and Ulrich Palm

Introduction

Mental and substance abuse disorders are an important cause of morbidity and mortality worldwide. According to data from the Global Burden of Disease (GBD), Injuries and Risk factors study, in 2010 these disorders accounted for up to 184 million disability-adjusted life years (DALYs) in the world, which is 7.4% of all DALYs, also considering non-psychiatric diseases. This study also revealed that mental and substance abuse disorders are the leading cause of years lived with disability (YLD) worldwide. Of them, affective disorders (depressive disorder and bipolar disorder) account for almost 50% of the YLD, followed by substance abuse (almost 20%), anxiety disorders (14.6%) and schizophrenia (7.4%). This burden increased by 37.6% between 1990 and 2010, mainly due to population growth and ageing (Whiteford et al. 2013). As these factors are still present and important, it is expected that the burden of mental disorders continues to increase in the upcoming years.

The treatment of mental disorders is challenging because these conditions are usually chronic, prevalent and present a multifactorial etiology. The therapeutic success of pharmacological therapies usually ranges between 40–70%, which translates into 30–60% of patients with mental conditions being treatment-resistant to phar-

Andre Russowsky Brunoni and Ulrich Palm contributed equally with all other contributors.

A. R. Brunoni (✉)
Service of Interdisciplinary Neuromodulation, Laboratory of Neurosciences (LIM-27), Department and Institute of Psychiatry, University of São Paulo, São Paulo, Brazil

Department of Psychiatry and Psychotherapy, Ludwig-Maximilian University Munich, Munich, Germany
e-mail: brunoni@usp.br

U. Palm
Department of Psychiatry and Psychotherapy,
Ludwig-Maximilian University Munich, Munich, Germany

H. Knotkova et al. (eds.), *Practical Guide to Transcranial Direct Current Stimulation*, https://doi.org/10.1007/978-3-319-95948-1_15

macotherapy. Although different forms of psychotherapy are useful in the treatment of some mental disorders, they are not always accessible and their success depends on patient's adherence and commitment. Thus, there is an urgent need for the development of novel strategies for treating these disorders.

In fact, the past decade has seen a rapid increase in the application of neuromodulatory non-pharmacological techniques for the treatment of mental disorders. Non-invasive brain stimulation (NIBS) encompasses several techniques (such as repetitive transcranial magnetic stimulation, rTMS; electroconvulsive therapy, ECT and transcranial direct current stimulation, tDCS) that use electric and/or magnetic fields to induce changes in cortical excitability and/or activity. The most effective technique is ECT, an already established therapy for treatment of acute cases of affective disorders and schizophrenia, which is nonetheless continuously studied for parameter optimization and improvement of tolerability and adverse effects profile (Allan and Ebmeier 2011). RTMS is a relatively novel technique that is effective in the treatment of major depression and possibly effective for other conditions such as negative and positive symptoms of schizophrenia, post-traumatic stress disorder and nicotine dependence (Lefaucheur et al. 2014).

In this context, tDCS is a more recent technique; although, in fact, there are reports of its clinical use since the 1960s and 1970s on mood and alertness in healthy volunteers and psychiatric samples, such as depression and psychoses. During this period, in most of the reports this method was termed "brain polarization". At least two randomized clinical trials and four open-label trials were performed during this time period for the treatment of depression, achieving initially positive but overall mixed results (for a review, see Nitsche et al. 2009a). Due to these mixed results, the development of psychopharmacotherapy and the stigma of ECT as prototype of electrical brain stimulation, among other factors, tDCS was largely forgotten between 1970 and 2000 (Nitsche et al. 2009a). The reappraisal of brain polarization only took place after the seminal studies of Priori et al. (1998) and Nitsche and Paulus (2000), discussed elsewhere in this book. A few years later, different research groups started to evaluate the efficacy of tDCS in psychiatric disorders using open-label designs and randomized clinical trials (RCTs).

Probing tDCS efficacy in psychiatric disorders is under intensive investigation because, comparatively to other treatment modalities, tDCS might present some relevant advantages. For instance, tDCS is cheaper and easier to use than rTMS (Priori et al. 2009). Also, rTMS is a non-portable device that can be handled only by trained staff, whereas tDCS is a handheld device – in fact, patients can be trained to use tDCS at home (Charvet et al. 2015). As compared to pharmacotherapy, taking a pill is indeed easier than using tDCS, even considering handheld devices. However, tDCS could be still a useful alternative to drug treatment in selected groups, such as pregnancy, depression associated with clinical comorbidities (where pharmacological interactions with antidepressants are an issue) and patients intolerant to drug adverse effects. TDCS is a more targeted intervention (i.e., more localized) compared to antidepressant drugs. Also, tDCS can be combined with antidepressant drugs, as the combination might induce increased and faster effects than each treatment alone (Brunoni et al. 2013a, d).

Another important advantage of tDCS is its acceptability, i.e., dropout rate (unpublished data). In a recent systematic review and meta-analysis of 64 clinical tDCS trials (n = 2262 subjects) enrolling psychiatric and neurologic disorders in adults, it was found that the dropout rate in the active group was 6%, similar to the dropout rate in the sham group (7.2%) (Fig. 15.1). In a sub-analysis of studies describing the dropout reasons, only 4.1% and 3.7% of patients in the active and sham groups, respectively, abandoned the trial due to adverse events (other reasons were protocol violation, inefficacy of treatment or not reported). Taken together, this findings suggest that even though adverse events such as tingling, itching and discomfort are commonly reported in tDCS trials, they are not important order to lead to treatment discontinuation, given that dropout rates between active and sham groups were similar.

In this present chapter we discuss the results of recent studies that evaluated tDCS efficacy in several psychiatric disorders, including mood disorders, schizophrenia, obsessive-compulsive disorder (OCD), addiction and others.

Major Depressive Disorder

Major Depressive Disorder is an incapacitating condition associated with significant personal, social and economic impairment. Its main symptoms include persistent low mood, anhedonia, anxiety, negative thoughts, impairment in sleep, psychomotor retardation and weight changes. Moreover, depression is a chronic, recurrent disorder, as nearly 80% of patients relapse after the treatment of an episode (Anderson et al. 2008); moreover, about one third of patients have treatment-resistant depression (TRD) – i.e., the failure to achieve adequate response of symptoms after adequate antidepressant treatment trials (Berlim and Turecki 2007; Nemeroff 2007). Due to its chronicity, modest rates of treatment and high prevalence (8–12% lifetime prevalence), major depressive disorder is projected to be the second most disabling condition by 2020 (Murray and Lopez 1997), reinforcing the need for the development of novel treatment modalities.

Current Treatments for Major Depressive Disorder

Antidepressant drug treatment for depression includes first-generation antidepressants (tricyclic antidepressants and monoamine oxidase inhibitors), SSRIs (serotonin selective reuptake inhibitors, such as sertraline and fluoxetine), SNRIs (such as venlafaxine and duloxetine) and others (e.g., bupropion and mirtazapine). It was suggested that escitalopram and sertraline are the antidepressants that best combine

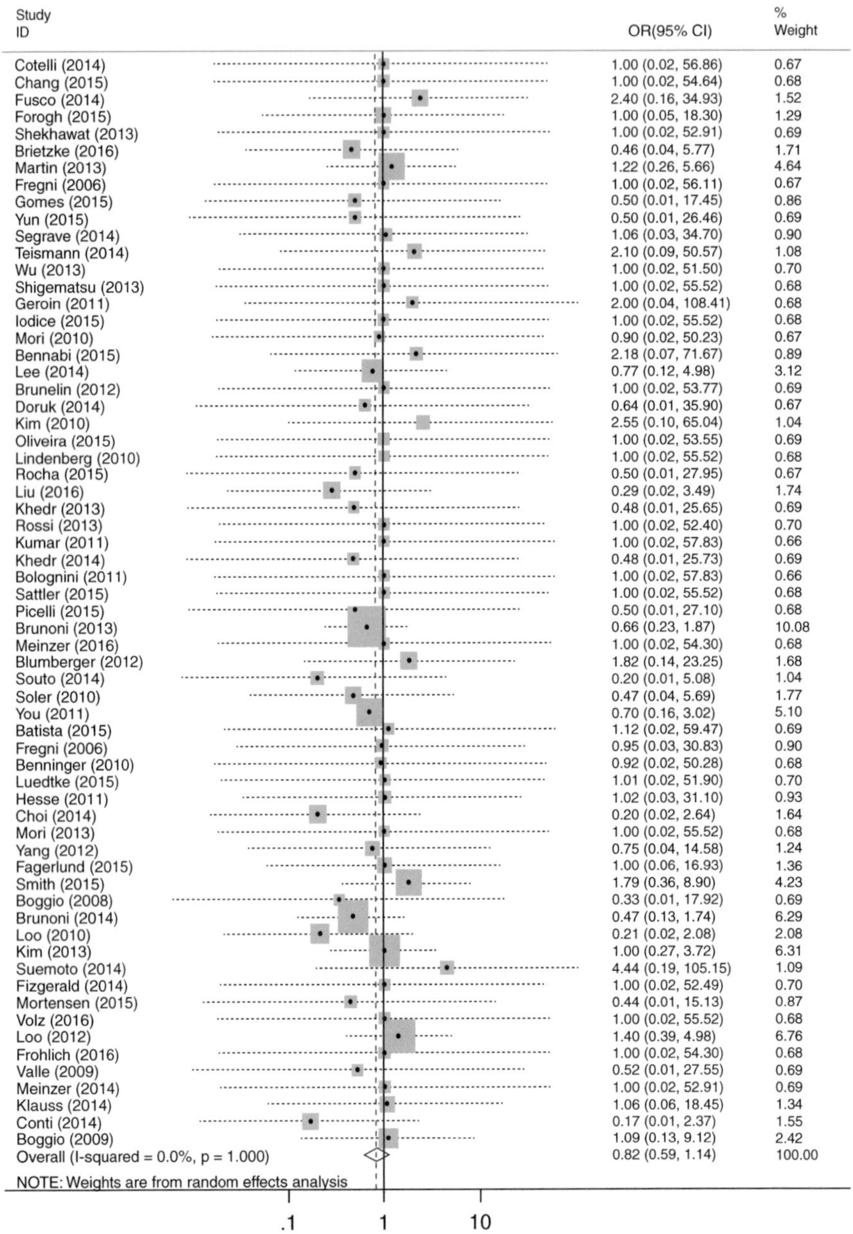

Fig. 15.1 Meta-analysis of tDCS dropout rate (a proxy for acceptability) of 64 clinical trials. The odds ratio was 0.82 (0.59–1.14) showing no significant differences in acceptability between active and sham groups in all neurologic and psychiatric tDCS trials published to date. (Unpublished data)

effectiveness with tolerability and therefore should be the choice for treatment (Cipriani et al. 2010). The STAR*-D (Sequenced Treatment Alternatives to Relieve Depression), a NIMH-sponsored trial, enrolled almost 3000 patients to evaluate the efficacy of several antidepressant treatments (Rush et al. 2006). Its main results were that, indeed, 30% of patients do not remit after 4 consecutive treatment trials and that there is no substantial difference, in terms of efficacy, among the different antidepressants tested.

Regarding non-pharmacological therapies, ECT is a very effective treatment for major depressive disorder (Group, 2003). Compared to sham ECT, active ECT is significantly more effective. A pooled analysis of ECT comparisons against amitriptyline, imipramine, phenelzine, or other pharmacotherapies also favored ECT. However, ECT is also associated with important cognitive deficits, especially in subgroups of patients and in specific protocols (Nobler and Sackeim 2008).

Finally, at the present time, rTMS for the treatment of major depressive disorder is an approved therapy worldwide. A recent review of the efficacy of rTMS in neurology and psychiatry disorders classified rTMS for major depressive disorder treatment as a level "A" of evidence (Lefaucheur et al. 2014). RTMS is well tolerated, it is associated only with few adverse effects and a low risk of treatment-emergent mania (Xia et al. 2008). Its efficacy rates seem to be similar compared to pharmacotherapy (Brunelin et al. 2012, 2014, 2015).

Mechanisms of Action

Although its antidepressant mechanisms of action are still elusive, it is supposed that tDCS acts by inhibiting or enhancing activity of pathways involved in the pathophysiology of major depressive disorder. The dorsolateral prefrontal cortex (DLPFC) is an important site of dysfunction in depression mainly due to left hypo-function and right hyper-function (Mayberg et al. 2000). Neuroimaging studies also show structural alterations in fronto-cingulo-striatal (FCS) circuits (Bora et al. 2012). The imbalance between cortical and subcortical brain activities might also be involved in major depressive disorder pathophysiology. Response to fluoxetine was associated with a marked reduction in local cerebral blood flow as well as changes in downstream limbic and cortical sites as measured with positron emission tomography (Mayberg et al. 2000). Other brain areas, such as the amygdala and the hippocampus, have a lower volume in depressed patients when compared to controls (Campbell and Macqueen 2004; Hamilton et al. 2008b). In addition, functional studies suggest a high level of activity in the ventro-medial prefrontal cortex (vmPFC) and a low level of activity in the DLPFC. In addition, patients with major depression display lower excitability in the left motor cortex (Maeda et al. 2000), in the left hemisphere (Bajwa et al. 2008) and a higher brain activity in the right cortex (Janocha et al. 2009).

Putatively, tDCS acts by increasing cortical excitability and neuroplasticity of the DLPFC, thus restoring this brain area to normal activity. For example, tDCS has been shown to improve affective and cognitive processing in depressed patients

(Moreno et al. 2015; Wolkenstein and Plewnia 2013; Zanao et al. 2014) – since the DLPFC is involved in such processing in depression, these findings suggest that tDCS modulates DLPFC activity.

The neurotrophin hypothesis of depression states that the depressive state is associated with decreased expression of several neurotrophins associated with neuroplasticity, such as the blood-derived neurotrophic factor (BDNF) (Brunoni et al. 2008). BDNF is a neurotrophin related to neuronal survival, synaptic signaling and synaptic consolidation (Allen and Dawbarn 2006); it is also associated with late phase of Long Term Potentiation (LTP), the property of neurons to persistently increase synaptic strength (Gartner and Staiger 2002). It was shown, for instance, that the amygdala of patients with major depressive disorder present volume loss that increases after antidepressant treatment (Hamilton et al. 2008a). Hence, the neurotrophin hypothesis of depression also states that the amelioration of depressive symptoms is accompanied by an increase in neuroplasticity. For instance, peripheral levels of BDNF increase after successful treatment (Brunoni et al.). Thus, another mechanism of action of tDCS in depression might be enhancing LTP-like plasticity. For example, Fritsch et al. (2010) showed that direct current stimulation promoted BDNF-dependent synaptic plasticity in mice and Antal et al. (2010) showed that BDNF gene polymorphisms influence tDCS-induced plasticity. However, the findings in depressed patients were mixed. Although one study found that depressed patients presented increased motor cortex neuroplasticity after receiving tDCS (Player et al. 2014), two studies showed that blood levels of BDNF in depressed patients did not increase after tDCS treatment (Brunoni et al. 2014c; Palm et al. 2012, 2013, 2016).

The 5-HT system might also be involved in tDCS antidepressant effects. One study found that the serotonin transporter genetic polymorphism (SLC6A4), which codifies the pre-synaptic serotonin reuptake transporter (SERT), predicts antidepressant tDCS efficacy. This polymorphism is characterized by a functional 44-bp insertion/deletion polymorphism (5HTTLPR) in its promoter region (Collier et al. 1996). The short allele (s) is related to a lower disposal and function in SERT in comparison to its long (l) form. Subjects with allele *s* display a worse clinical response to serotonergic antidepressants, since they act on the SERT, and thus will be less efficient in case of a hypo-functional transporter (Serretti et al. 2007). In our study, using the depression sample of SELECT-TDCS, we found that long/long homozygotes displayed a larger improvement comparing active vs. sham tDCS, but not short-allele carriers (i.e., the same patter of response usually identified in serotonergic antidepressants) (Brunoni et al. 2013c). In fact, antidepressant effects of tDCS seem to involve the serotonergic system, as shown in pharmacological studies of Nitsche et al. (2009a, b, c), and Kuo et al. (2015), which found that the excitability-enhancing effects of anodal tDCS were boosted with citalopram whereas the excitability-decreasing cathodal effects were reversed – leading to, in fact, excitability-enhancing effects. A proof of concept was subsequently demonstrated in the SELECT clinical trial, which showed the antidepressant effects of tDCS were enhanced by sertraline (Brunoni et al. 2011b, 2013d).

Dopamine might also be relevant for the antidepressant mechanisms of tDCS, considering that the use of dopamine agonists and antagonists modify tDCS-induced cortical excitability (Monte-Silva et al. 2009; Nitsche et al. 2009b). Moreover, it was shown that genetic polymorphisms of the catechol-*o*-methyltransferase (COMT, an enzyme that degrade catecholamines such as dopamine) influence tDCS effects on executive functions and response inhibition in healthy volunteers (Nieratschker et al. 2015; Plewnia et al. 2013). However, COMT polymorphisms have not been evaluated in depressed patients receiving tDCS.

Conversely, there is no evidence to date that tDCS induces any specific changes in peripheral biomarkers that have been associated to major depressive disorder pathophysiology. For instance, decreased heart rate variability (HRV) is observed in depression, which reflects autonomic dysfunction (decreased vagal tone) (Kemp et al. 2010), although HRV levels do not change after tDCS treatment (Brunoni et al. 2013b). Moreover, decreased brain-derived neurotrophic factor (BDNF) levels have been found in depression, suggesting that depression is associated with decreased neuroplasticity (the "neurotrophin hypothesis of depression"), and BDNF levels increase after treatment with pharmacotherapy (Brunoni et al.), but not after tDCS – this was also observed for non-BDNF neurotrophins (Brunoni et al. 2014b, c). One possibility for these negative findings is that the effects of tDCS are restricted to the brain, exerting no or minimal influence on peripheral activity. Nonetheless, to date no peripheral biomarker associated with tDCS efficacy in major depressive disorder is available.

Clinical Evidence

To date, at least 8 open-label trials and 11 RCTs using tDCS for major depressive disorder have been published. Treatment protocols vary between studies: the current dose applied ranged from 1 to 2 mA; the number of sessions from 5 to 15; the interval between sessions from every other day to twice a day; the cathode positioning between the right DLPFC, supra-orbital area, and extracephalic positions. Nonetheless, left DLPFC was the site of anode positioning in virtually all studies, reflecting the rationale of applying an excitability-enhancing electrode (the anode) over a hypoactive area.

Some open-label studies provided important findings that were further explored in RCTs, including the finding that tDCS and SSRI could have the same efficacy (Rigonatti et al. 2008), and that tDCS effects might be enhanced with antidepressant drugs and decreased with benzodiazepines (Brunoni et al.2011a, 2013a).

Fregni et al. (2006a), in the first modern, sham-controlled, randomized clinical trial, found a significant decrease in depression scales after 5 days of active stimulation, with a mean reduction in depression scores of 60–70% for the active tDCS group relative to baseline. In contrast, improvement in the placebo group was only 10–30%. Similar results were demonstrated in a further study in antidepressant-free patients with recurrent major depressive episodes after 5 days of active tDCS (Fregni et al. 2006b) with 18 patients. Boggio et al. (2008) recruited 40 patients with moderate to severe depression, evaluating depression improvement immediately after 10 consecutive weekdays of stimulation and 30 days later. Only prefrontal, but not occipital or sham tDCS reduced depressive symptoms significantly, with effects sustained at 30-day follow up.

After these initial positive results, other studies reported negative findings. Loo et al. (2010, 2012) recruited 40 patients to receive active vs. sham tDCS and did not find significant differences between these groups. Palm et al. (2012, 2013, 2016) recruited 22 patients with depression and randomized them to receive 1 mA stimulation, 2 mA stimulation or sham tDCS in a cross-over design. Active and placebo tDCS was applied for 2 weeks, but no differences in depression improvement were found. Finally, Blumberger et al. (2012) did not find significant differences between active vs. sham tDCS in a sample of 24 highly refractory patients.

After that, larger trials found that tDCS was an effective treatment for depression. Loo et al. (2010, 2012) randomized 64 patients to receive active or sham tDCS (2 mA, 15 sessions over 3 weeks), followed by a 3-week open-label active treatment phase. Mood and neuropsychological effects were assessed. There was a significantly greater improvement in mood after active than sham treatment. This study also showed that attention and working memory improved after a single session of active but not sham tDCS. There was no decline in neuropsychological functioning after 3–6 weeks of active stimulation. Brunoni et al. (2011b, 2013d) enrolled 120 antidepressant-free patients with moderate and severe depression who were randomized in four arms (2 × 2 design): sham tDCS and placebo pill, sham tDCS and sertraline, active tDCS and placebo pill and active tDCS and sertraline (the study name was Sertraline vs. Electric Current Therapy to Treat Depression Clinical Trial – SELECT-TDCS; its design is described in (Valiengo et al. 2013)). The tDCS parameters were 2 mA per 30 min/day, for 2 weeks and 2 extra tDCS sessions every other week until week 6 (study endpoint); the dose of sertraline was fixed (50 mg/day). The main findings, shown in Fig. 15.2, were that: (1) combined tDCS / sertraline was significantly more effective than the other treatment groups in reducing depressive symptoms; (2) tDCS and sertraline efficacy did not differ; (3) active tDCS as a monotherapy was also more effective than the placebo group.

In 2014, two randomized, sham-controlled trials evaluated the efficacy of tDCS combined with cognitive control therapy (CCT), an intervention that aims to increase prefrontal cortical activity through working memory tasks (in both cases, an adapted version of the Paced Serial Addition Task, PASAT). Segrave et al. (2013) enrolled 27 patients to receive tDCS and CCT, sham tDCS and CCT, and sham CCT and tDCS (2 mA, 5 sessions). All treatments led to a reduction in depression severity after 5 tDCS sessions, but only the combined tDCS / CCT treatment resulted in sustained antidepressant response at week 4. In contrast, Brunoni et al. (2014a) randomized 37 participants to receive sham tDCS and CCT or active tDCS and CCT (2 mA, 10 sessions) and found similar antidepressant improvement in both groups. However, further analysis showed that in older patients, those with greater improve-

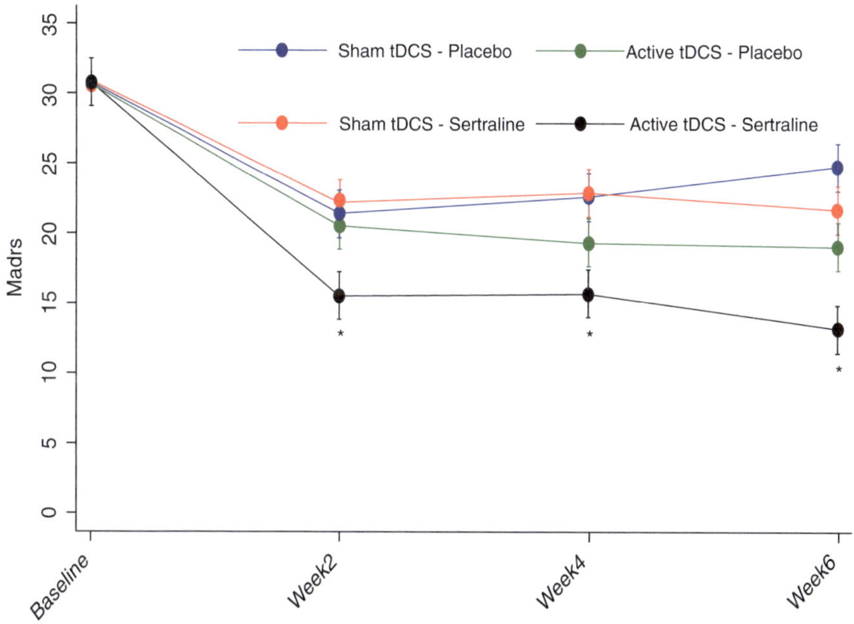

Fig. 15.2 Results from SELECT-TDCS trial. The figure shows the main results of SELECT-TDCS trial Brunoni et al. 2011b, 2013d). Combined treatment (tDCS and sertraline) presented a larger, faster response. At endpoint, tDCS and sertraline efficacy were similar, although tDCS, but not sertraline, was superior to placebo

ment in CCT task performance also had greater antidepressant improvement with active tDCS.

The last RCT published hitherto was a phase-II trial in which 24 escitalopram-resistant depressed patients were randomized to receive two daily sessions, with a time interval between sessions of 2 h, of tDCS for 5 days (2 mA, 10 sessions over 1 week). In this study, tDCS did not induce clinically relevant antidepressant effects in active and sham stimulation groups at endpoint (Bennabi et al. 2015).

A recent meta-analysis (Meron et al. 2015) enrolling 393 patients and 10 studies observed that tDCS was more effective than sham stimulation when considering continuous outcomes but not categorical ones (i.e., response and remission), suggesting that larger studies are still needed to evaluate tDCS efficacy. Also, an individual patient data meta-analysis (Brunoni et al.) was recently performed in order to further assess efficacy and to identify predictors of response, pooling data from six randomized sham-controlled trials, enrolling 289 patients. Active tDCS was significantly superior to sham in all outcomes. Treatment-resistant depression (Fig. 15.3a) and higher tDCS "doses" (Fig. 15.3b) were respectively negatively and positively associated with tDCS efficacy.

Adverse Effects

The rate and intensity of adverse effects observed in the abovementioned studies were similar to those reported when using tDCS in other contexts; however, the issue of treatment-emergent hypomania/mania (TEM) should be discussed. There are four stand-alone case reports in literature (Arul-Anandam et al. 2010;

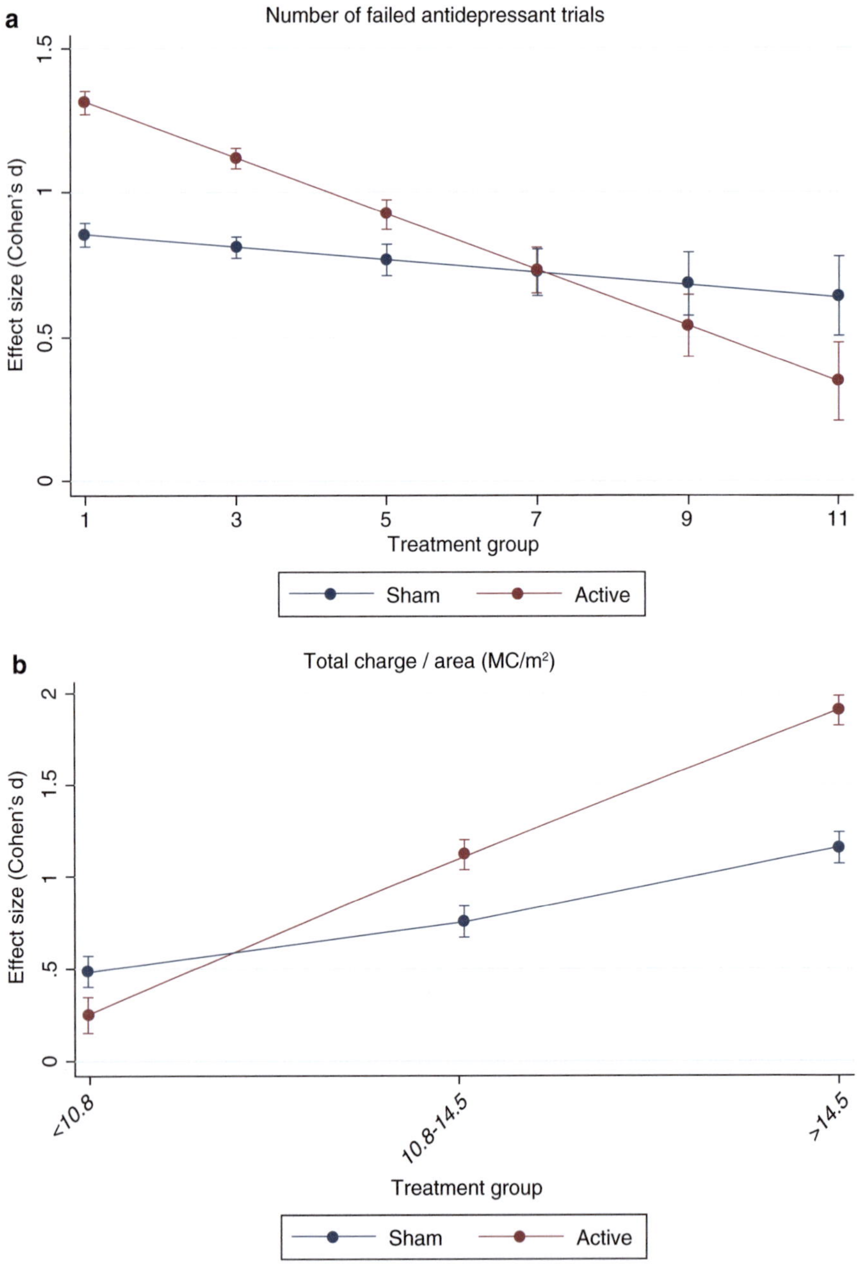

Baccaro et al. 2010; Brunoni et al. 2011b, 2013d; Galvez et al. 2011) and some reports of TEM in RCTs. Most of these episodes resolved spontaneously, with tDCS withheld for a few days, or with small dose adjustments / introduction of a new pharmacotherapy, although one of them was a full-blown episode of mania with psychotic features (Brunoni et al. 2011b, 2013d). It is difficult to estimate the precise frequency of this adverse effect or, even, if it is directly caused by tDCS or if the case reports represent a casual event that occurred coincidently with the repeated tDCS sessions. Therefore, the same recommendations of care for depressed patients are also valid when using tDCS as an antidepressant treatment – i.e., careful observation of the patients' clinical outcomes while on a clinical treatment. Further, patients should be carefully assessed for history of bipolar disorder and history of switching into mania with past antidepressant treatments, as these factors may indicate a higher risk of manic switch with tDCS. In these patients, concurrent treatment with mood stabilizer medication during tDCS treatment course should be considered. Nonetheless, it should be underscored that mood stabilizers that are sodium and/or calcium channel blockers (such as some anticonvulsant drugs) might abolish at least some physiological tDCS effects, as it was shown that blocking voltage-gated sodium and calcium channels decreases the excitability-enhancing effect of anodal tDCS (Liebetanz et al. 2002; Nitsche et al.) over the motor cortex. In addition, it was found that antipsychotics (also commonly used in the treatment of bipolar disorder) of high dopaminergic D2-receptor affinity decreased, compared to antipsychotics of low D2-receptor affinity, the efficacy of tDCS in the treatment of schizophrenia symptoms (Agarwal et al. 2016). These data reinforce the need of trials investigating the safety and efficacy of tDCS in patients with bipolar depression.

Schizophrenia

About 1–2% of the population is suffering from schizophrenia, a disabling disorder with a variety of impairments in cognition, mood, impetus, interaction and social functioning. Syndromal diversity of schizophrenia and related disorders includes

Fig. 15.3 (**a**) Results from an individual patient data meta-analysis showing the influence of treatment-resistant depression on tDCS efficacy. (**b**) Results from an individual patient data meta-analysis showing the influence of treatment-resistant depression on tDCS efficacy. This figure shows results from analyses done in the study of Brunoni et al. that pooled individual patient data from 289 patients from six randomized, sham-controlled studies. The y-axis represents treatment efficacy in terms of Cohen's d: the higher the number, the larger the efficacy. In (**a**), the x-axis represents number of previous antidepressant failed trials, a measure directly associated with treatment refractoriness. As it can be seen, active tDCS efficacy decreases in more refractory patients. In (**b**), three tDCS "doses" were estimated: "low" (<36 C or < 10285C/m^2), "medium" (36C or 10,286-14500C/m^2) and "high" (43.2 C or > 14500C/m^2). Therefore, "dose" is a composite measure of current density, session duration and number of sessions. As it can be seen, higher doses were associated to larger active-sham difference

highly heterogeneous symptoms that have been classified into five dimensions that are represented in the most common clinical rating scale, the Positive and Negative Symptom Scale (PANSS) (Kay et al. 1987) and reflecting typical clinical symptoms, e.g. delusions and hallucinations (positive symptoms), avolition and emotional withdrawal (negative symptoms), cognitive impairment and disorganization (cognition), depressed mood and fear (depression/anxiety), and impairment of social interaction (excitement/hostility). Although psychopharmacologic treatment of schizophrenia has advanced in recent years, even adequate drug regimen does not exert full remission in up to 30% of patients (Murphy et al. 2006; Shergill et al. 1998). Especially auditory hallucinations and negative symptoms can be refractory to treatment (Hasan et al. 2012). Finally treatment-resistant symptoms impair global functioning, recovery, occupational rehabilitation, and social integration.

Current Treatments for Schizophrenia

Standard treatment of schizophrenia includes a combined psychopharmacologic, psychoeducational, psychosocial, and rehabilitation treatment.

Current guidelines suggest second-generation antipsychotics to treat psychotic episodes; however first generation antipsychotics are still used for otherwise treatment-resistant cases (Hasan et al. 2012). Electroconvulsive therapy is a treatment option to improve persistent positive symptoms and catatonia. rTMS has shown some efficacy in the treatment of auditory hallucinations and negative symptoms, however results are inconsistent regarding negative symptoms (Wobrock et al. 2015) and cognitive symptoms (Hasan et al. 2012, 2015).

Mechanisms of Action

The rationale of tDCS application in schizophrenia is based on neuroimaging findings and results of clinical rTMS studies. Neuroimaging suggests a dysfunction of cortical areas with temporoparietal hyperactivation during auditory hallucinations (Jardri et al. 2011), frontal hypoactivation in negative symptoms and cognitive dysfunction (Sanfilipo et al. 2000), and a fronto-temporal dysconnectivity (Lawrie et al. 2002; Schmitt et al. 2011). Thus, tDCS can be used for neuromodulation of dysfunctional areas, i.e. to decrease activity in temporo-parietal regions to reduce auditory hallucinations or to increase activity in frontal regions to enhance mood, impetus, and cognition. For this purpose, a mono-hemisperic electrode montage with the cathode over the left temporo-parietal junction and the anode over the left DLPFC has been successfully used to treat auditory hallucinations (Brunelin et al. 2012; Mondino et al. 2015), however a bihemispheric montage with the anode over the left DLPFC and the cathode contralaterally has also been applied to improve negative symptoms with a focus of current distribution on frontal brain areas (Gomes et al. 2015) (Table 15.1).

Clinical Evidence

More than twenty single case reports and several open label studies and RCTs are available addressing various symptoms of schizophrenia, predominantly auditory hallucinations. Negative symptoms and improvement of cognition were investigated in either single case reports or some small open label studies and RCTs. To provide only clinical evidence from RCTs and open label studies, single case reports are not discussed here, however can be found in a respective review article (Mondino et al. 2015) (Table 15.2).

The first randomized placebo-controlled clinical trial which reported an improvement of *auditory hallucinations* by tDCS was published in 2012 by Brunelin et al. (2012). Thirty patients with medication-resistant auditory hallucinations were randomized to either receive twice-daily 20 min of 2 mA tDCS over 5 days with the anode over the left DLPFC and the cathode over the left temporo-parietal junction or sham tDCS. The active group showed a significant reduction of auditory hallucinations by 31% up to 3 months after stimulation. (Fig. 15.4).

In contrast, Fitzgerald et al. (2014) found no superiority of active tDCS over sham in an RCT with monohemisperic (F3-Tp3) and bihemisperic electrode montage (F3-Tp3, F4-Tp4, 2 tDCS devices) in 24 patients with treatment-resistant auditory hallucinations, although this study used an adequate total dosage (2 mA, 20 min, 15 sessions). Furthermore there was no difference between monohemisperic and bihemispheric active stimulation.

Mondino et al. (2015) used a partially overlapping sample and the same procedure as Brunelin et al. (2012) and found a significant reduction of 28% in auditory hallucinations after active tDCS compared to 10% after sham tDCS. Analysis of resting state functional magnetic resonance imaging (rsfMRI) revealed a reduction of connectivity between temporo-parietal regions and the left inferior frontal cortex after active tDCS, whereas connectivity between temporo-parietal regions and the left DLPFC increased. A second study in 2015 by Mondino et al. (2015) also used a partially overlapping sample to Brunelin et al. (2012) and found a decrease in source-monitoring confusions between covert and overt speech after active compared to sham tDCS and a reduction of auditory hallucinations by 46% in the active group compared to an increase by 7.5% in the sham group.

Fröhlich et al. (2016) included 26 patients with auditory hallucinations in a randomized placebo controlled trial with the anode over the left DLPFC (2 mA, 20 min, 5 sessions) and the cathode over the left temporo-parietal junction and found a significant decrease of auditory verbal hallucinations in both active and sham groups with a pronounced reduction of hallucinations by 34% in the sham group. Furthermore symptom changes measured by PANSS did not differ between groups.

Overall, tDCS has shown some efficacy in the treatment of auditory hallucinations; however there are two studies reporting no benefit. Studies with positive results usually performed two stimulations per day whereas studies with negative results applied one stimulation per day. It may be hypothesized that two stimulations per

Table 15.1 Summary of controlled tDCS trials in major depression

Author	Sample (n)	Anode	Cathode	Current (mA)/ electrode size (cm^2)	Intensity (A/m^2)	Number of sessions	Results
Fregni et al. (2006a)	10	F3	R SO	1 / 35	0.28	5 (every other day)	Positive
Fregni et al. (2006b)	18	F3	R SO	1 /35	0.28	5 (every other day)	Positive
Boggio et al. (2008)	40	F3	F4	1 / 35	0.28	10 (1×/ day)	Positive
Loo et al. (2010)	40	F3	R SO	1 /35	0.28	5 (every other day)	Negative
Palm et al. (2012)	22	F3	R SO	1 or 2 / 35	0.28/0.57	10 (1×/ day)	Negative
Blumberger et al. (2012)	24	F3	F4	2 /35	0.57	15 (1×/ day)	Negative
Loo et al. (2012)	64	F3	R SO	2 /35	0.57	15 (1×/ day)	Positive
Brunoni et al. (2013d)	120	F3	F4	2/ 25	0.8	10 (1×/ day)	Positive
Segrave et al. (2014)	27	F3	RSO	2/35	0.57	5 (1×/ day)	Mixed
Brunoni et al. (2014a)	37	F3	F4	2/25	0.8	10 (1×/ day)	Mixed
Bennabi et al. (2015)	23	F3	R SO	2/35	0.57	10 (2×/ day)	Negative

R SO right supraorbital area, *F4* right dorsolateral prefrontal cortex

day induce prolonged neuroplasticity after-effects and that a higher cumulative tDCS dosage leads to sustained treatment efficacy. Furthermore, negative studies included patients with higher treatment resistance and symptom heterogeneity. Future tDCS have to take into account syndromal diversity and duration of illness to control for potentially symptom specific effects of tDCS.

Gomes et al. (2015) investigated the effects of bifrontal tDCS (anode: left DLPFC, cathode: right DLPFC) in 15 patients with negative symptoms and reported a significant reduction of negative and general subscales after active tDCS, however depression ratings (Calgary Depression Scale in Schizophrenia, CDSS) did not change after active tDCS compared to sham tDCS.

Kurimori et al. (2015) conducted an open label study with 9 patients with *negative symptoms* and found a significant reduction of the negative subscale of the PANSS but not in the other subscales after 5× anodal tDCS over the left DLPFC with the cathode over the right deltoid muscle. A RCT by Palm et al. with 20 patients

Table 15.2 Summary of controlled tDCS trials in schizophrenia

Author	Sample (n)	Anode	Cathode	Current (mA)/ electrode size (cm^2)	Number of sessions	Results
Brunelin et al. (2012)	30	F3	Tp3	2/35	10	Positive
Fitzgerald et al. (2014)	24	F3 (F4)	Tp3 (Tp4)	2/35	15	Negative
Mondino et al. (2015)	23[a]	F3	Tp3	2/35	10	Positive
Gomes et al. (2015)	15	F3	F4	2/25	10	Positive
Mondino et al. (2015)	28[a]	F3	Tp3	2/35	10	Positive
Frohlich et al. (2016)	26	F3	Tp3	2/35	5	Negative
Nienow et al. (2016)	10	F3	R SO	1/35	28	Positive
Reinhart et al. (2015)	19	FCz	R cheek	1.5/19.25 and 52	1	Positive
Vercammen et al. (2011)	20	F3	Fp2	2/35	1	Mixed
Hoy et al. (2014)	18	F3	Fp2	1 and 2/35	1	Positive
Göder et al. (2013)	14	F3	F4	0–0.03 at 0.75 Hz/4 × 0.05	5	Positive
Smith et al. (2015)	37	F3	Fp2	2/5.08	5	Mixed
Rassovsky et al. (2015)	36	F1/F2	R UA	2 × 1/35	1	Negative
Palm et al. (2016)	20	F3	Fp2	2/35	10	Positive

R SO right supraorbital, *FCz* medial-frontal cortex, *R cheek* right cheek between cheilion and condylion, *Fp2* right fronto-polar, *R UA* right upper arm

[a]15 patients of this sample are overlapping with the study of Brunelin et al. (2012), temporoparietal junction (midway between T3 and P3)

receiving either active or sham tDCS over the left DLPFC reported a significant reduction of negative symptoms in the Scale for the Assessment of Negative Symptoms (SANS) and PANSS after 10 sessions of active tDCS compared to sham stimulation. To date, two RCT and one open label study suggest an efficacy of left prefrontal tDCS on the improvement of negative symptoms (Fig. 15.5); however sample sizes are small and larger studies are needed to corroborate these preliminary findings.

There are several studies without clinical improvement as primary outcome criterion although reporting on clinical efficacy as well. These studies primarily refer to an improvement of cognition, neurophysiological parameters, or cigarette craving in schizophrenia patients by tDCS. *Cognition* was investigated in a trial by Nienow et al. (2016). The authors found a significant improvement of cognitive functions in a word and picture 2-back test and the MATRICS Consensus Cognitive Battery (MCCB) after anodal compared to sham tDCS in 10 patients. Vercammen et al. (2011) conducted a randomized placebo-controlled study in 20 schizophrenia patients who were treated with a single-session of active and sham tDCS with the anode over the left DLPFC (F3) and the cathode contralateral supraorbital (Fp2) before undergoing a probabilistic learning test (cue and outcome reaction). They found no tDCS effect in the whole sample, however patients with adequate performance at baseline showed a significant

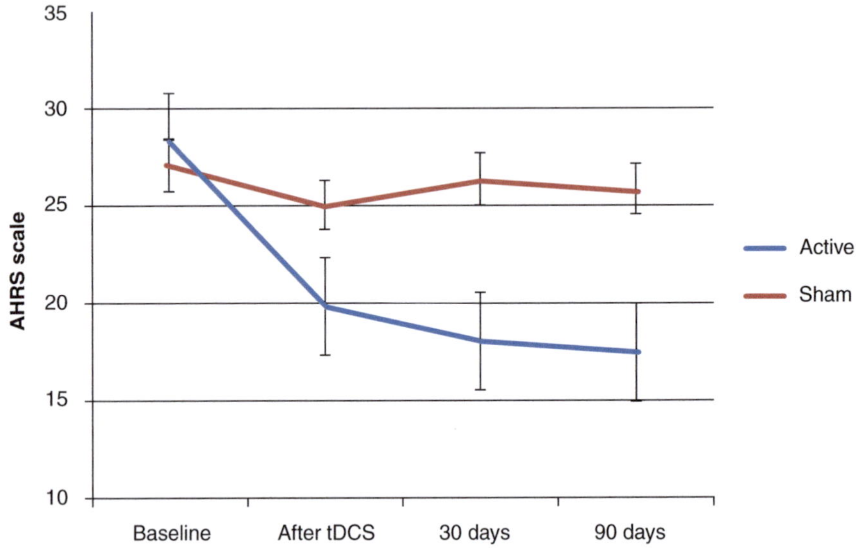

Fig. 15.4 Results from Brunelin et al. study. The figure shows superiority of active tDCS over sham tDCS in decreasing symptoms in the Auditory Hallucination Rating Scale (AHRS) after 5 days of stimulation twice a day. These effects persisted for up to 3 months after stimulation. Bars represent standard error (SE). (Adapted from Brunelin et al. 2012)

improvement of performance in the following tests. Hoy et al. (2014) assessed changes of working memory after tDCS in a crossover trial in 18 schizophrenia patients. Prefrontal tDCS (anode F3, cathode Fp2) was delivered in two active (1 and 2 mA) and sham condition and led to improvement of working memory in the n-back task up to 40 min after 2 mA active tDCS compared to sham and 1 mA tDCS. Ribolsi et al. (2013) investigated the effect of left and right hemisphere tDCS on spatial pseudoneglect in a sample of 15 schizophrenia patients and found that anodal stimulation of the right parietal cortex (P4) normalized pseudoneglect bias in the line bisection task. Göder et al. (2013) applied slow-oscillating tDCS (so-tDCS, 0.75 Hz, anodes F3/F4, cathodes mastoids) during sleep stage 2 in 14 schizophrenia patients and found a significant improvement of the Rey Auditory–Verbal Learning Test after active stimulation compared to sham. Rassowsky et al. (2015) randomized 36 schizophrenia patients to either receive anodal, cathodal or sham tDCS over both prefrontal cortices (F1/F2) with the reference at the right upper arm. They found no superiority of any condition after a single session of tDCS in four different cognitive tests except for an intra-group effect in facial recognition in the active tDCS group. Bose et al. (2015) reported a reduction of auditory hallucinations by 32% and an increase in insight by 156% in an open label study with 21 patients after 10 × 2 mA tDCS with the anode over left frontal areas and the cathode over the left temporo-parietal junction.

The impact of tDCS on *neurophysiological* changes in schizophrenia patients was assessed by Reinhardt et al. (2015) with an investigation into the impact of tDCS on EEG-related error-related mismatch negativity (ERN) over frontal brain

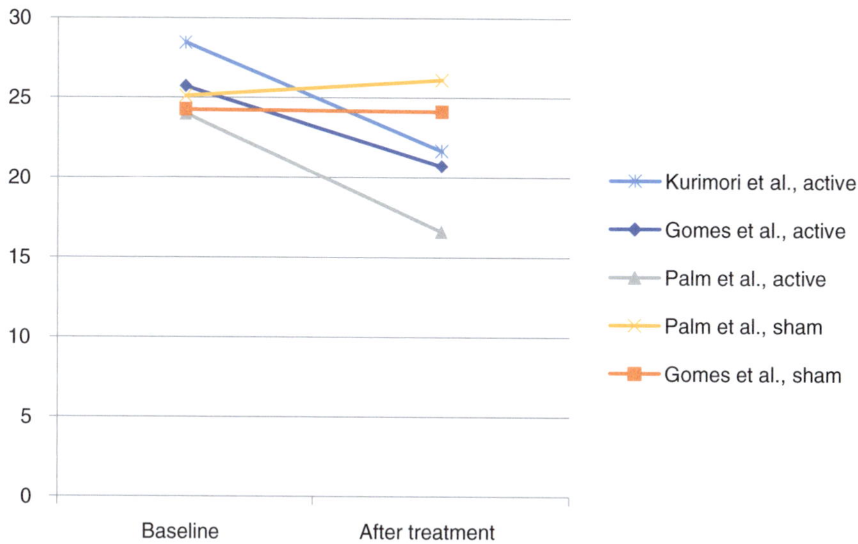

Fig. 15.5 Changes in mean PANSS negative dimension score (y-axis) in 3 studies addressing schizophrenia with predominant negative symptoms

regions in a visual learning task as a predictor of error signaling in the brain of 19 schizophrenia patients and 18 healthy controls. They found a reduced ERN in patients compared to healthy controls indicating impaired prediction error calculation in patients and slower response and less accuracy in patients compared to healthy controls. Anodal tDCS over the medio-frontal cortex (FCz) boosted ERN amplitude in both, schizophrenia patients and healthy controls, compared to sham stimulation. In schizophrenia patients, velocity and accuracy of the visual learning task after active stimulation was similar to the sham stimulation results of the healthy controls. Subramaniam et al. (2015) conducted an open-label study in 13 patients with schizophrenia, treated with 10 sessions of 2 mA tDCS with the anode over F3 and the cathode over Tp3. They reported a significant reduction in antisaccade error percentage (eye-tracking antisaccade task) and severity of auditory verbal hallucinations.

Cigarette craving, cognition and clinical symptoms were assessed in a randomized placebo controlled trial by Smith et al. (2015) with 37 schizophrenia patients. They investigated the effects of prefrontal tDCS on psychiatric symptoms (PANSS), hallucinations (PSYRATS), cigarette craving, and cognitive tasks (MCCB). Only cognitive improvement could be detected after five sessions of 2 mA prefrontal tDCS (anode F3, cathode, Fp2) whereas psychiatric symptoms and cigarette craving did not change in the active group compared to sham.

Furthermore, two studies investigated the effects of *pharmacological interaction* and tDCS in schizophrenia patients. The impact of antipsychotic medication on the effects of tDCS was investigated by Agarwal et al. (2016) in an open label study in 36 patients individually treated with various antipsychotics. After 10 sessions of

2 mA tDCS, they found less improvement of auditory hallucinations in female patients treated with high D2-receptor affinity antipsychotics compared to low D2 receptor-affinity antipsychotics.

The impact of tobacco smoking on tDCS effects on auditory hallucinations was investigated by Brunelin et al. (2015) in an open label study. They found a lower effect of tDCS on the improvement of auditory hallucinations in smokers than in non-smokers.

Adverse Events

No specific treatment-emergent adverse effects of tDCS in schizophrenia trials have been reported so far.

Obsessive-Compulsive Disorder

Obsessive-compulsive disorder (OCD) is disabling neuropsychiatric disorder with an estimated lifetime prevalence of 2% (Ruscio et al. 2010). OCD is characterized by the presence of obsessive, recurrent, intrusive thoughts and/or compulsions, which are usually rituals performed by the patient in an attempt to control the obsessive thinking. Patients with OCD also usually present excessive worry, rumination, and an increased perception of threat. Common obsessive thoughts are dedicated to contamination, losing control, harm, perfectionism, unwanted sexual thoughts, scrupulosity, whereas common compulsions are washing/cleaning, checking, repeating, and mental compulsions. Other conditions of the OCD spectrum include body dysmorphic disorders, hypochondriasis, tic disorders and trichotillomania.

Current Treatments for OCD

Conventional interventions for OCD patients involve medication, usually SSRIs and/or cognitive behavior therapy (Foa et al. 2005). Although the majority of people with OCD benefit from these therapies, some patients (about one third) are resistant to conventional treatments. Among non-pharmacological therapies, rTMS has been intensively investigated. It has been hypothesized that the inhibitory effects of low-frequency rTMS may be useful in treating some OCD symptoms. Nevertheless, the results regarding rTMS efficacy in OCD are mixed (Berlim et al. 2013). Deep brain stimulation (DBS) might be an interesting alternative for OCD-resistant patients (Alonso et al. 2015); however, the invasive nature of this treatment makes it a last resource option only for refractory cases.

Mechanisms of Action

Neuroimaging studies suggest that alterations at the cortico-striato-thalamo-cortical (CSTC) loop are implicated in the pathophysiology of OCD (Maia et al. 2008). Particularly, OCD involves failures in two main inhibitory loops, frontostriatal and the orbitofrontal loops responsible for behavioral and cognitive inhibition, respectively (Goncalves et al. 2011). This model inspired the neurosurgical approaches to OCD, which turned out to be effective treatments, as evidenced by the FDA humanitarian use approval for high frequency deep brain stimulation (DBS) in treatment-resistant cases (Shah et al. 2008). DLPFC is a crucial area for cognitive and emotional control as well as the most frequently targeted region in psychiatric applications of non-invasive brain stimulation (NIBS) techniques. In addition, based upon the neuroimaging evidence of hyperactivity in the orbito-frontal cortex (OFC) of OCD patients, other studies targeted this region using low-frequency rTMS (Berlim et al. 2013).

Another suitable area of tDCS application in OCD is the pre-SMA, which has been found to be hyperactive in OCD patients during performance of cognitive tasks related to attentional aspects of action control (de Wit et al. 2012; Yucel et al. 2007). In fact, evidence derived from the clinical efficacy of inhibitory rTMS on this area (Mantovani, et al. 2010) and from neurophysiological measures of altered motor cortex excitability in OCD (Greenberg et al. 2000), that normalized after 1-Hz rTMS to the pre-SMA (Mantovani et al. 2010, 2013), suggests that the pre-motor/motor system is abnormally hyperactive in OCD, and that there is a pathophysiological link between such hyperexcitability and OCD symptoms.

Clinical Evidence

4 original case-reports investigated the clinical effect of tDCS in patients with OCD. In one case study, 10 daily sessions of tDCS with the cathode placed over the left DLPFC and the anode over the neck (2 mA for 20 min) improved both depression and anxiety scores, but had no effects on OC symptoms in an adult with OCD (Volpato et al. 2013). Another study showed that 20 sessions of tDCS with the anode placed over the left pre-SMA and the cathode to the right supraorbital area (2 mA for 20 min) in an adult with OCD lead to significant reduction of OC symptoms (Narayanaswamy et al. 2015). Another case report found a significant reduction on OC symptoms after 10 sessions (2 sessions per day during 5 days) of tDCS with the anode placed over the right cerebello-occipital region and the cathode over the left OFC (2 mA for 20 min) (Mondino et al. 2015). Finally, D'Urso et al. (2016) describe a patient with treatment-resistant OCD who received 20 daily consecutive 2 mA/20 min tDCS sessions with the active electrode placed on the pre-SMA. The first 10 sessions were anodal, while the last 10 were cathodal. In the end of anodal stimulation, OCD symptoms had worsened. Subsequent cathodal stimulation

induced a dramatic clinical improvement, which led to an overall 30% reduction in baseline symptoms severity.

At the present time, there is only one open-label, pilot study available using tDCS for OCD (Bation et al. 2016). Eight patients with treatment-resistant OCD received 10 sessions (twice a day) of 2 mA tDCS applied with the cathode over the left OFC and the anode over the right cerebellum. These patients presented a significant (26.4%) improvement of symptoms, which lasted during the 3 month follow-up.

Adverse Events

No specific treatment-emergent adverse effects of tDCS in OCD studies have been reported so far.

Addiction

Addiction disorders are among the most frequent psychiatric disorders and present an important socioeconomic burden. Word Health Organization data suggest that alcohol abuse causes 3.3 million deaths per year and 15.3 million persons have a drug use disorder (WHO 2016). Especially the beginning of drug abuse during adolescence substantially increases the burden of disease and worsens the outcome (Degenhardt et al. 2016). For instance, alcohol and illicit substance use are responsible for 14% of the total health burden in young men aged 20–24 years, with predominant alcohol abuse in Eastern Europe, and illicit drug abuse in the USA, Canada, Australia, New Zealand, and Western Europe (Degenhardt et al. 2016).

Current Treatments for Addiction

The treatment outcome of addiction disorders is based on an effective reduction of craving and maintenance of abstinence. Abstinence is influenced by lifestyle and psychosocial factors and can be enhanced by psychotherapeutic interventions, usually cognitive behavioral therapy (Dutra et al. 2008; Magill and Ray 2009), however the average effect size of cognitive behavioral therapy is only moderate for addiction disorders - although contingency management, a form of behavioral therapy, seems to be a promising intervention in addiction disorders (Prendergast et al. 2006; Stitzer and Petry 2006). Pharmacological treatments are used to reduce craving or to support abstinence, e.g. disulfiram, nalmefene, naltrexone, or acamprosate in alcohol dependency. Since several years, varenicline and bupropion are used to reduce craving in tobacco dependency.

Mechanisms of Action

Although drugs modulate neuronal pathways in different ways, e.g. by increasing dopaminergic (cocaine), serotonergic or noradrenergic (amphetamines) transmission or by GABAergic disinhibition (opiates, alcohol), they mostly have a common final pathway with impact on the reward circuitry in the ventral striatum-ventral tegmental area (VTA) pathway (Nestler 2005) and a concomitant hypofunction of the dorsal anterior cingulate cortex (dACC) and insula (Dunlop et al. 2016). The association between restoration of dACC activation and improvement in abstinence control point to a causal role of the dACC in addiction disorders (Moeller et al. 2012). Furthermore, activity in the ventral striatum, ventromedial prefrontal cortex and orbitofrontal cortex seems to be associated with cue reactivity and craving (Kilts et al. 2004; Li et al. 2012; Risinger et al. 2005). Non-invasive brain stimulation techniques, including tDCS, are able to modulate activity in superficial and more remote brain areas by modulation of networks that can be measured by functional connectivity magnet resonance imaging (fcMRI) (Dunlop et al. 2016; Keeser et al. 2011).

Clinical Evidence

The first study using tDCS in *tobacco dependency* was published in 2008 (Fregni et al. 2008). In this randomized placebo-controlled clinical trial, 24 smokers received anodal or sham stimulation over the left respectively right DLPFC (electrode size 35 cm^2) with the reference electrode (100 cm^2) placed contralateral. Craving with and without cue exposition was significantly reduced in the active compared to the sham group. A replication study by Boggio et al. (2009) with 27 smokers showed reduced craving for cigarettes after anodal stimulation of the left DLPFC with the reference electrode over the right DLPFC compared to no changes in craving after sham stimulation. The number of smoked cigarettes was slightly reduced in the active group. Another study by Fecteau et al. (2014) showed a significant reduction of cigarette consumption after anodal tDCS of the right DLPFC with the cathode over the left DLPFC (bilateral stimulation) compared to sham stimulation. Additionally, participants of the active group showed more frequent refusal of cigarettes, but not money, in the Ultimatum Game.

Xu et al. (2013) conducted a cross-over study in 24 smokers staying abstinent overnight and showed that the negative affect in the Profile of Mood States (POMS) was improved by anodal tDCS of the left DLPFC with the cathode contralateral (bilateral stimulation); however craving did not differ after anodal and sham tDCS. An alternative electrode placement was investigated by Meng et al. (2014) in a sham-controlled cross-over study to test whether right hemispheric cathodal stimulation and left hemispheric anodal stimulation alone was responsible for reducing nicotine consumption or if a bihemispheric cathodal stimulation with the reference electrodes over both occipital regions is superior. Therefore, in the single cathodal stimulation, they placed the cathode over the right fronto-parieto-temporal area and the anode over the respective area on the left side, and for the double cathodal stimulation, they placed two cathodal electrodes over both right and left fronto-parieto-temporal areas and two anodes over the both occipital lobes. Active bihemispheric cathodal stimulation turned out to be superior to the other conditions in terms of reduction of cigarette consumption.

Pripfl et al. (2013) conducted a randomized placebo controlled study in 17 participants with tobacco dependence in a cross over design with anodal left, cathodal right, and sham stimulation. Three small cup electrodes were positioned over F1, F3, and AF1 respectively over F2, F4, and AF2 to increase focality of anodal stimulation. The standard size reference electrode (35 cm^2) was placed contralateral and was assumed to be ineffective. Anodal tDCS over the right DLPFC was able to reduce negative affect, however did not modulate craving. Anodal left stimulation did not induce any effects.

Finally, Smith et al. (2015) reported on a first RCT investigating the effects of tDCS in schizophrenia patients with comorbid tobacco dependency. Thirty-three schizophrenia patients underwent five sessions of 2 mA tDCS with the anode over the left DLPFC and the cathode over the contralateral orbit. There was a significant improvement of cognitive functions in the active group; however cigarette consumption and craving were unchanged after active tDCS compared to sham.

Treatment of *alcohol dependency* with tDCS was first investigated in 2008 by Boggio et al. (2008b) in a double-blind randomized controlled trial with anodal versus cathodal versus sham stimulation of the left DLPFC with the reference electrode contralateral (bilateral stimulation). There was a significant superiority of both active conditions compared to sham stimulation in craving with and without cue exposition. Nakamura-Palacios et al. (2012) conducted a RCT in 49 alcohol dependent patients and found an improvement in the Frontal Assessment Battery (FAB) and reduced auditory event-related potentials (alcohol-related words) after anodal stimulation of the left DLPFC with 1 mA tDCS (extracephalic reference electrode) over 10 min compared to sham. Another randomized placebo controlled clinical trial in 13 patients with alcohol dependency (da Silva et al. 2013), anodal tDCS of the left DLPFC with 2 mA tDCS (extracephalic reference electrode) led to mood improvement and reduced craving as well as reduced event-related potentials after specific cue exposition in the active group compared to the sham tDCS group. Klauss et al. (2014) conducted a randomized placebo controlled trial with bilateral left cathodal/right anodal stimulation in 35 patients and found a significant lower relapse rate in the active group after 6 months. This study applied a different stimulation protocol in terms of electrode placement with a strengthening of the inhibitory cortical modulation by cathodal tDCS over the left DLPFC, possibly leading to block of the brain reward circuitry and therefore reducing relapse in alcohol consumption, which is an important predictor for treatment efficacy. However craving was not different between active and sham groups in this study. The effect of tDCS on craving was furthermore assessed in a randomized placebo controlled clinical trial by den Uyl et al. (2015) with anodal stimulation of the left DLPFC, right inferior frontal gyrus, and sham stimulation with the reference electrode over the right orbit in 41 patients. Anodal tDCS of the left DLPFC significantly reduced craving for alcohol compared to the other conditions.

The effect of tDCS on craving and decision making in patients with consumption of *illicit psychotropic drugs* was investigated in four studies so far. A randomized placebo controlled trial by Boggio et al. (2010) investigated the effects of tDCS on risk taking behavior and craving in marihuana users. 25 participants were randomized to either left anodal/right cathodal, left cathodal/right anodal, and sham tDCS (bilateral stimulation). Risk taking behavior was increased in bot active groups compared to the sham group, whereas craving was reduced after active stimulation compared to sham stimulation. The modulation of risk taking behavior was also assessed in another trial by Gorini et al. with the Balloon Analog Risk Task (BART) and a dice gaming task in 18 cocaine users compared to healthy controls (Gorini et al. 2014). Participants were randomized to receive either left anodal/right cathodal, left cathodal/right anodal, and sham stimulation (bilateral stimulation). Risk taking behavior in the BART was reduced after bot active stimulation conditions in cocaine users and healthy controls. Cocaine users showed a decrease in the risk taking in the dice gaming task after right anodal stimulation and an increase after left anodal stimulation. Contrarily, healthy controls showed decreased risk taking behavior after left anodal stimulation, pointing to an impairment of interhemispheric balance in cocaine users. A study by Conti et al. investigated the effects of tDCS on event-related potentials in crack cocaine users (2014). Participants were randomized to receive either left cathodal/right anodal and sham tDCS (bilateral stimulation). Active tDCS revealed a decrease of the P3 amplitude after presentation of a cocaine-specific cue and an increase of the amplitude after presentation of neutral cues. The sham group showed the contrary effects, pointing to changes in the processing of unspecific and specific stimuli by tDCS. Conti and Nakamura-Palacios (2014) conducted a second study in crack cocaine users with the same bilateral stimulation and could show that cathodal stimulation of the left DLPFC leads to a reduced cue-dependent activation in the anterior cingulate, whereas sham tDCS led to an increase of cue-dependent activation in this brain area. A randomized placebo-controlled study by Batista et al. in 36 crack cocaine dependent persons revealed a significant decrease in craving after 5 sessions of 2 mA anodal tDCS to the right DLPFC and cathodal tDCS to the left DLPFC (bilateral stimulation) compared to sham stimulation (Batista et al. 2015). Shahbabaie et al. (2014) investigated tDCS effects on craving in 30 users of methamphetamine after computer-based stimulus presentation in a randomized cross-over design. Anodal tDCS of the right DLPFC with the reference electrode over the left orbit significantly reduced craving after presentation of a specific cue compared to sham tDCS.

De Almeida Ramos et al. (2016) performed an open label trial with 11 users of crack cocaine (18–59 years) who were treated with bilateral 2 mA tDCS (anode: left DLPFC, cathode: right DLPFC, 10 sessions, 20 min each). They found a significant reduction of craving in the Cocaine Craving Questionnaire Brief (CCQB).

Over all there is some evidence that anodal stimulation of the right DLPFC and cathodal stimulation of the left DLPFC can prolong duration of abstinence and might reduce craving, however also studies with anodal tDCS over the left DLPFC have shown a reduction in craving (Table 15.3); however results are divergent and the specific role of tDCS on right and left DLPFC action for the modulation of craving and behavioral control is still unclear.

Adverse Events

No specific treatment-emergent adverse effects of tDCS in substance use studies have been reported so far.

Other Conditions

Anxiety Disorders

Negative perception bias plays a core role in depressive and anxiety disorders and impairs perception and memory that can be restored by anxiolytic and antidepressant drugs in healthy volunteers (Harmer et al. 2003) and depressed patients (Tranter et al. 2009). Furthermore attentional control is modulated by trait anxiety (Bishop et al. 2004). Trait anxiety negatively influences DLPFC activity in neuroimaging studies investigating attentional control over emotional (Bishop et al. 2007) and non-emotional (Bishop 2009) stimuli. Thus, DLPFC activity potentially modifies attentional control and influences trait anxiety.

A randomized cross-over trial in 60 healthy volunteers with anodal and sham stimulation of both DLPFC showed that attentional bias modification training to reduce attention to the threatening stimuli is improved by combination with left anodal tDCS (1 mA, 17 min) (Clarke et al. 2014). Another randomized parallel group study in 24 depressed patients showed a reduction of negative attentional bias after anodal tDCS of the left DLPFC compared to sham in the Emotional Stroop Task (Brunoni et al. 2013). Kelley, Hortensius, and Harmon-Jones (2013) found an increase in rumination after anodal stimulation of the right DLPFC compared to anodal stimulation of the left DLPFC and sham stimulation in a three-group parallel design with 115 healthy volunteers and suggest that enhanced right frontal activity increases inhibition rather anger expression and therefore results in increased rumination. These three studies indicate the modulating role of the left DLPFC in the attentional control over anxiety.

The treatment of generalized anxiety disorder with tDCS is described in a single case report of a 58 year-old woman. The cathode was placed over the right DLPFC, the anode over the left shoulder. 15 treatments with 2 mA tDCS over 30 min led to decrease in anxiety rating scales. The anxiolytic efficacy after inhibition of the right DLPFC is probably modulated by a change of activity in cortical and subcortical network structures, e.g. the medial prefrontal cortex, the amygdala, and the insula (Shiozawa et al. 2014).

Table 15.3 Summary of controlled tDCS trials in addiction disorders

Author	Sample (n)	Anode	Cathode	Current (mA)/ electrode size (cm²)	Number of sessions	Results
Tobacco						
Fregni et al. (2008) (Fregni et al.)	24	F3 (F4)	F4 (F3)	2/35 and 100	3 (cross-over, 3 conditions)	Positive
Boggio et al. (2009)(Boggio et al.)	27	F3	F4	2/35 and 100	5 (1×/day)	Positive
Fecteau et al. (2014)(Fecteau et al.)	12	F4	F3	2/35	5 (1×/day)	Positive
Xu et al. (2013) (Xu et al.)	24	F3	R SO	2/35	2 (cross-over, 2 conditions)	Mixed
Meng et al. (2014) (Meng et al.)	30	O1/O2/ L FPT	R FPT/L FPT	1/33	1	Positive
Pripfl et al. (2015) (Pripfl & Lamm)	17	F1-F3-Af1 (F4)	F4 (F2-F4-Af2)	0.45/5.3 and 35	3 (cross-over, 3 conditions)	Positive
Smith et al. (2015) (Smith et al.)	33	F3	R SO	2/5.1	5 (1×/day)	Negative
Alcohol						
Boggio et al. Boggio, Sultani, et al. (2008) (Boggio, Sultani, et al.)	13	F3 (F4)	F4 (F3)	2/35	3 (cross-over, 3 conditions)	Positive
Nakamura-Palacios et al. (2012) (Nakamura-Palacios et al.)	49	F3	R deltoid	1/35	1	Positive
da Silva et al. (2013) (da Silva et al.)	13	F3	R deltoid	2/35	5	Positive
Klauss et al. (2014) (Klauss et al.)	33	F4	F3	2/35	5 (1×/day)	Positive
den Uyl et al. (2015) (den Uyl et al.)	48	F3/IFG	R SO	1/35	1	Positive
Other substances						
Boggio et al. (2010) (Boggio et al.)	25	F3 (F4)	F4 (F3)	2/35	1	Positive
Gorini et al. (2014) (Gorini et al.)	36	F3 (F4)	F4 (F3)	1.5/32	3 (cross-over, 3 conditions)	Mixed

(continued)

Table 15.3 (continued)

Author	Sample (n)	Anode	Cathode	Current (mA)/ electrode size (cm^2)	Number of sessions	Results
Conti et al. (2014) (Conti et al.)	13	F4	F3	1/35	1	Positive
Conti et al. (2014) (Conti & Nakamura-Palacios)	13	F4	F3	1/35	5 (every other day)	Positive
Shahbabaie et al. (2014) (Shahbabaie et al.)	30	F4	L SO	2/35	1	Mixed
Batista et al. (2015) (Batista et al.)	36	F4	F3	2/35	5 (every other day)	Positive

R SO, L SO right and left supraorbital area, *F4* right dorsolateral prefrontal cortex, *FPT* frontal-parietal-temporal between F3, F7, C3, T3 (left) respectively F4, F8, C4, T4 (right), *IFG* inferior frontal gyrus, crossing between F7 and Cz and Fz and T3, *O1, O2* occipital, *Af1 Af2* anterior frontal, *R deltoid* right deltoid muscle

Posttraumatic Stress Disorder

Posttraumatic stress disorder (PTSD) includes various symptoms, including continuous expression of emotional symptoms to conditioned cues occurring after severe traumatic experiences. Several treatments, such as behavioral therapies and pharmacologic interventions, have been investigated. D-Cycloserine, a partial agonist of the N-methyl-D-aspartate (NMDA) receptor, facilitated fear extinction in clinical studies (Ressler et al. 2004) and the application of β-blockers leads to memory reconsolidation blockade; however there is still no pharmacologic standard intervention for oblivion. Rodent models suggest that the dorsal anterior cingulate cortex (dACC) is more involved in fear learning whereas the medial prefrontal cortex (mPFC) is more involved in fear extinction (Marin et al. 2014) Therefore superficial brain areas such as mPFC could serve as a target for non-invasive brain stimulation.

In addition to anxiety symptoms, working memory impairment occurs when these patients are exposed to stress (Honzel et al. 2014). tDCS of the prefrontal brain areas is known to improve working memory (Kuo & Nitsche, 2012), therefore it may also be used for reduction of stress-related cognitive impairment. Stress-related working memory deficits were reduced after anodal tDCS of the right DLPFC in 120 healthy adults, compared to cathodal or sham stimulation (Bogdanov & Schwabe, 2016). This points to the key role of the prefrontal cortex in anxiety control which could be used in disorders with stress-induced cognitive impairment. Saunders et al. (2015) investigated the effects of 5× 1 mA tDCS (20 min per sessions, anode over F3, cathode over Fp2) in four war veterans with PTSD (55–65 y). They found an increase of working memory performance in a standardized assessment battery and, to some extent, an improvement in emotional processing. EEG analyses revealed an increase of alpha peak frequency in both amplitude and frequency after stimulation.

Child and Adolescent Psychiatry

The investigation of tDCS in child and adolescent psychiatry is following the encouraging results in adults. tDCS or 'brain polarization' has a longer tradition for the treatment of neuropsychiatric and developmental disorders, especially in Russia (Pinchuk, Pinchuk, Sirbiladze, & Shugar, 2013). There is some evidence that tDCS improves motor deficits in cerebral palsy in combination with physiotherapeutic training. Also in childhood epilepsy, preliminary data suggest an efficacy of tDCS in suppressing epileptiform discharges (Auvichayapat et al. 2013). Furthermore, improvement of various symptoms of autism spectrum disorder (speech development, behavior, prefrontal EEG alpha activity) after anodal tDCS of the left DLPFC was suggested (Amatachaya et al. 2014, 2015; Schneider & Hopp, 2011). Application of tDCS in Attention Deficit/Hyperactivity Disorder (ADHD) was explored in several trials, and reported to improve accuracy in a go-no-go task (Soltaninejad, Nejati, & Ekhtiari, 2015), selective attention and to decrease error rate in an inhibitory control task (Bandeira et al. 2016), and to improve reaction time and memory performance via slow-oscillating tDCS during REM sleep stage 2 (Munz et al. 2015; Prehn-Kristensen et al. 2014); however the two latter studies should be interpreted with caution due to methodological and procedural shortcomings, e.g. lack of a control group.

Interestingly, frequent psychiatric disorders in adults are not yet investigated in children and adolescents, e.g. affective disorders, schizophrenia, and addiction disorders. Several studies addressed the feasibility and safety of tDCS in pediatric and adolescent patients, including a safety study in 12 patients with childhood onset schizophrenia (Mattai et al. 2011). Several studies investigated the peak current fields in children/adolescent head models and found increased peak electric fields when using the same parameters that are usually applied in adults (e.g. 2 mA, 20–30 min duration) (Kessler et al. 2013; Minhas et al. 2012; Parazzini et al. 2014). Therefore most authors conclude to halve the current strength. However several studies used standard parameters for application in adults without reporting adverse effects in children (Amatachaya et al. 2015; Mattai et al. 2011). Physiological effects of tDCS in children and adolescents seem to partially differ from those in adults, as shown in a study by Moliadze et al. 2015. These authors demonstrated age-specific influences of transcranial direct current stimulation on cortical excitability. 1 mA tDCS resulted in an excitability enhancement after both, cathodal and anodal stimulation. Reduction of cathodal tDCS intensity to 0.5 mA however resulted in an excitability reduction (Moliadze et al. 2015). The results of this study show non-linear intensity-dependent effects of cathodal tDCS also known from studies in adults (Batsikadze et al. J Physiol 2013).

Bipolar Disorder

The use of tDCS in bipolar depression has not been as yet sufficiently investigated, with only one open-label study comparing the efficacy of tDCS in unipolar vs. bipolar depressed patients and showing efficacy in both conditions (Brunoni et al. 2013; Brunoni et al. 2011). Another open study evaluated a sample of unipolar and bipolar patients for 3 months, but did not report results separately for the unipolar and bipolar groups (Dell'osso et al. 2012). Finally, Pereira-Junior et al. 2015 report pilot results from a double-blinded study in progress, in which 5 patients with bipolar depression received active tDCS. Response and remission rates were respectively 40% and 20% (Pereira Junior Bde et al. 2015). Regarding efficacy in mania, the evidence is limited to one single case report showing improvement of manic symptoms after 5 sessions of tDCS that was applied with the anode over the right and the cathode over the left DLPFC (Schestatsky et al. 2013).

Other Psychiatric Disorders

Restoring prefrontal control by anodal stimulation of the left DLPFC has been postulated in a variety of disorders that include impairment of insight, attention and stimulus control, e.g. eating disorders and attention deficit/hyperactivity disorder.

The treatment of anorexia nervosa was investigated by Khedr, Elfetoh, Ali, and Noamany (2014) in 25 patients receiving 10 stimulations (2 mA, anode over left DLPFC) in an open label design. It was postulated that anodal tDCS of left prefrontal areas restores cognitive control over eating behavior. Khedr et al. found mixed results concerning mood improvement and insight facilitation into eating behavior.

Attention Deficit/Hyperactivity Disorder (ADHD) in adults was assessed in two studies so far. Cosmo, Baptista et al. (2015) conducted a randomized placebo controlled trial in 30 ADHD patients undergoing a single session of 1 mA tDCS (anode F3; cathode F4) for 20 min. They found no difference between active and sham stimulation in the go-no-go task (behavioral performance). In another randomized placebo controlled trial, Cosmo, Ferreira et al. (2015) investigated the effect of a single active or sham tDCS application (1 mA, 20 min, anode F3, cathode F4) on EEG functional cortical networks in 60 ADHD patients. The weighted node degree, a measure for connectivity of the brain area under an electrode to another during a given time period, showed a significant increase for active stimulation compared to sham for the left frontal area.

Adverse Events

No specific treatment-emergent adverse effects of tDCS for other psychiatric conditions have been reported so far.

Concluding Remarks

This chapter provided an overview of the clinical evidence of tDCS efficacy in psychiatric disorders. In many cases, tDCS is investigated either due to its relative safety and tolerability (particularly when compared to pharmacotherapy) or as an augmentative option to standard treatments in order to boost their response. Other reasons presented to use tDCS in psychiatry include the possibility of home-use, its affordable price, and its ease of use.

TDCS clinical trials generally presented good methodology, in terms of randomization, blinding, sham control and definition of primary outcomes. However, except for a few studies in depression, virtually all clinical trials had very small sample sizes. Therefore, many non-significant findings might have occurred due to a type II error, i.e., a false negative finding, due to an underpowered trial.

The design of a large tDCS trial is challenging due to various aspects, such as logistic reasons (the need for the patient to return daily to a clinical center as well as the necessity of having a clinical center that can receive patients daily), funding issues, due to the lack of private funding (i.e., virtually no sponsorship of tDCS trials by industry), and sample selection, as the sample profile where tDCS would be used as an augmentative therapy (i.e., treatment-resistant sample) is different from a sample where tDCS would be used as a substitutive therapy. Moreover, it is still unknown which tDCS parameters (e.g., dose, session duration, number of sessions) are associated to optimal efficacy.

Nonetheless, there are several clinical trials ongoing, including large trials investigating tDCS efficacy in depression, as it can be seen in the online database clinicaltrials.gov. More recent trials are also aiming to investigate the therapeutic mechanisms of action of tDCS according to the treated disorder; which is important to design further trials.

To conclude, in the past years the amount of clinical trials investigating tDCS efficacy in psychiatry has grown exponentially. Results have been particularly promising in depression and schizophrenia. Nevertheless, major issues in the current scenario are the lack of large, sufficiently powered trials and the relative uncertainty regarding its therapeutic mechanisms at the neurobiological level.

References

Agarwal, S. M., Bose, A., Shivakumar, V., Narayanaswamy, J. C., Chhabra, H., Kalmady, S. V., … Gangadhar, B. N. (2016). Impact of antipsychotic medication on transcranial direct current stimulation (tDCS) effects in schizophrenia patients. *Psychiatry Research, 235*, 97–103.

Allan, C. L., & Ebmeier, K. P. (2011). The use of ECT and MST in treating depression. *International Review of Psychiatry, 23*(5), 400–412.

Allen, S. J., & Dawbarn, D. (2006). Clinical relevance of the neurotrophins and their receptors. *Clinical Science (London, England), 110*(2), 175–191.

Alonso, P., Cuadras, D., Gabriels, L., Denys, D., Goodman, W., Greenberg, B. D., … Menchon, J. M. (2015). Deep brain stimulation for obsessive-compulsive disorder: A meta-analysis of treatment outcome and predictors of response. *PLoS One, 10*(7), e0133591.

Amatachaya, A., Auvichayapat, N., Patjanasoontorn, N., Suphakunpinyo, C., Ngernyam, N., Aree-Uea, B., … Auvichayapat, P. (2014). Effect of anodal transcranial direct current stimulation on autism: A randomized double-blind crossover trial. *Behavioural Neurology, 2014*, 173073–173077.

Amatachaya, A., Jensen, M. P., Patjanasoontorn, N., Auvichayapat, N., Suphakunpinyo, C., Janjarasjitt, S., … Auvichayapat, P. (2015). The short-term effects of transcranial direct current stimulation on electroencephalography in children with autism: A randomized crossover controlled trial. *Behavioural Neurology, 2015*, 928631–928611.

Anderson, I. M., Ferrier, I. N., Baldwin, R. C., Cowen, P. J., Howard, L., Lewis, G., … Tylee, A. (2008). Evidence-based guidelines for treating depressive disorders with antidepressants: A revision of the 2000 British Association for Psychopharmacology guidelines. *Journal of Psychopharmacology (Oxford, England), 22*(4), 343–396.0269881107088441 [pii].

Antal, A., Chaieb, L., Moliadze, V., Monte-Silva, K., Poreisz, C., Thirugnanasambandam, N., … Paulus, W. (2010). Brain-derived neurotrophic factor (BDNF) gene polymorphisms shape cortical plasticity in humans. *Brain Stimulation, 3*(4), 230–237.

Arul-Anandam, A. P., Loo, C., & Mitchell, P. (2010). Induction of hypomanic episode with transcranial direct current stimulation. *The Journal of ECT, 26*(1), 68–69.

Auvichayapat, N., Rotenberg, A., Gersner, R., Ngodklang, S., Tiamkao, S., Tassaneeyakul, W., & Auvichayapat, P. (2013). Transcranial direct current stimulation for treatment of refractory childhood focal epilepsy. *Brain Stimulation, 6*(4), 696–700.

Baccaro, A., Brunoni, A. R., Bensenor, I. M., & Fregni, F. (2010). Hypomanic episode in unipolar depression during transcranial direct current stimulation. *Acta Neuropsychiatrica, 22*(6), 316–318.

Bajwa, S., Bermpohl, F., Rigonatti, S. P., Pascual-Leone, A., Boggio, P. S., & Fregni, F. (2008). Impaired interhemispheric interactions in patients with major depression. *The Journal of Nervous and Mental Disease, 196*(9), 671–677. 00005053-200809000-00003 [pii].

Bandeira, I. D., Guimaraes, R. S., Jagersbacher, J. G., Barretto, T. L., de Jesus-Silva, J. R., Santos, S. N., … Lucena, R. (2016). Transcranial direct current stimulation in children and adolescents with attention-deficit/hyperactivity disorder (ADHD): A Pilot Study. *J Child Neurol, 31*, 918–924.

Bation, R., Poulet, E., Haesebaert, F., Saoud, M., & Brunelin, J. (2016). Transcranial direct current stimulation in treatment-resistant obsessive-compulsive disorder: An open-label pilot study. *Progress in Neuro-Psychopharmacology & Biological Psychiatry, 65*, 153–157.

Batista, E. K., Klauss, J., Fregni, F., Nitsche, M. A., & Nakamura-Palacios, E. M. (2015). A randomized placebo-controlled trial of targeted prefrontal cortex modulation with bilateral tDCS in patients with crack-cocaine dependence. *The International Journal of Neuropsychopharmacology, 18*, pyv066.

Batsikadze, G., Moliadze, V., Paulus, W., Kuo, M. F., & Nitsche, M. A. (2013). Partially non-linear stimulation intensity-dependent effects of direct current stimulation on motor cortex excitability in humans. *The Journal of Physiology, 591*(7), 1987–2000.

Bennabi, D., Nicolier, M., Monnin, J., Tio, G., Pazart, L., Vandel, P., & Haffen, E. (2015). Pilot study of feasibility of the effect of treatment with tDCS in patients suffering from treatment-resistant depression treated with escitalopram. *Clinical Neurophysiology, 126*(6), 1185–1189.
Berlim, M. T., Neufeld, N. H., & Van den Eynde, F. (2013). Repetitive transcranial magnetic stimulation (rTMS) for obsessive-compulsive disorder (OCD): An exploratory meta-analysis of randomized and sham-controlled trials. *Journal of Psychiatric Research, 47*(8), 999–1006.
Berlim, M. T., & Turecki, G. (2007). Definition, assessment, and staging of treatment-resistant refractory major depression: A review of current concepts and methods. *Canadian Journal of Psychiatry, 52*(1), 46–54.
Bishop, S., Duncan, J., Brett, M., & Lawrence, A. D. (2004). Prefrontal cortical function and anxiety: Controlling attention to threat-related stimuli. *Nature Neuroscience, 7*(2), 184–188.
Bishop, S. J. (2009). Trait anxiety and impoverished prefrontal control of attention. *Nature Neuroscience, 12*(1), 92–98.
Bishop, S. J., Jenkins, R., & Lawrence, A. D. (2007). Neural processing of fearful faces: Effects of anxiety are gated by perceptual capacity limitations. *Cerebral Cortex, 17*(7), 1595–1603.
Blumberger, D. M., Tran, L. C., Fitzgerald, P. B., Hoy, K. E., & Daskalakis, Z. J. (2012). A randomized double-blind sham-controlled study of transcranial direct current stimulation for treatment-resistant major depression. *Frontiers in Psychiatry/Frontiers Research Foundation, 3*, 74.
Bogdanov, M., & Schwabe, L. (2016). Transcranial stimulation of the dorsolateral prefrontal cortex prevents stress-induced working memory deficits. *The Journal of Neuroscience, 36*(4), 1429–1437.
Boggio, P. S., Liguori, P., Sultani, N., Rezende, L., Fecteau, S., & Fregni, F. (2009). Cumulative priming effects of cortical stimulation on smoking cue-induced craving. *Neuroscience Letters, 463*, 82–86S0304-3940(09)00979-3 [pii].
Boggio, P. S., Rigonatti, S. P., Ribeiro, R. B., Myczkowski, M. L., Nitsche, M. A., Pascual-Leone, A., & Fregni, F. (2008). A randomized, double-blind clinical trial on the efficacy of cortical direct current stimulation for the treatment of major depression. *The International Journal of Neuropsychopharmacology, 11*(2), 249–254.S1461145707007833 [pii].
Boggio, P. S., Sultani, N., Fecteau, S., Merabet, L., Mecca, T., Pascual-Leone, A., … Fregni, F. (2008). Prefrontal cortex modulation using transcranial DC stimulation reduces alcohol craving: A double-blind, sham-controlled study. *Drug & Alcohol Dependence, 92*(1–3), 55–60. S0376-8716(07)00250-5 [pii].
Boggio, P. S., Zaghi, S., Villani, A. B., Fecteau, S., Pascual-Leone, A., & Fregni, F. (2010). Modulation of risk-taking in marijuana users by transcranial direct current stimulation (tDCS) of the dorsolateral prefrontal cortex (DLPFC). *Drug & Alcohol Dependence, 112*(3), 220–225. S0376-8716(10)00248-6 [pii].
Bora, E., Fornito, A., Pantelis, C., & Yucel, M. (2012). Gray matter abnormalities in major depressive disorder: A meta-analysis of voxel based morphometry studies. *Journal of Affective Disorders, 138*(1–2), 9–18.
Bose, A., Sowmya, S., Shenoy, S., Agarwal, S. M., Chhabra, H., Narayanaswamy, J. C., & Venkatasubramanian, G. (2015). Clinical utility of attentional salience in treatment of auditory verbal hallucinations in schizophrenia using transcranial direct current stimulation (tDCS). *Schizophrenia Research, 164*(1–3), 279–280.
Brunelin, J., Hasan, A., Haesebaert, F., Nitsche, M. A., & Poulet, E. (2015). Nicotine smoking prevents the effects of frontotemporal transcranial direct current stimulation (tDCS) in hallucinating patients with schizophrenia. *Brain Stimulation, 8*(6), 1225–1227.
Brunelin, J., Jalenques, I., Trojak, B., Attal, J., Szekely, D., Gay, A., … Poulet, E. (2014). The efficacy and safety of low frequency repetitive transcranial magnetic stimulation for treatment-resistant depression: The results from a large multicenter French RCT. *Brain Stimulation, 7*(6), 855–863.
Brunelin, J., Mondino, M., Gassab, L., Haesebaert, F., Gaha, L., Suaud-Chagny, M. F., … Poulet, E. (2012). Examining transcranial direct-current stimulation (tDCS) as a treatment for hallucinations in schizophrenia. *The American Journal of Psychiatry, 169*(7), 719–724.

Brunoni, A. R., Boggio, P. S., De Raedt, R., Bensenor, I. M., Lotufo, P. A., Namur, V., … Vanderhasselt, M. A. (2014). Cognitive control therapy and transcranial direct current stimulation for depression: A randomized, double-blinded, controlled trial. *Journal of Affective Disorders, 162*, 43–49.

Brunoni, A. R., Ferrucci, R., Bortolomasi, M., Scelzo, E., Boggio, P. S., Fregni, F., … Priori, A. (2013). Interactions between transcranial direct current stimulation (tDCS) and pharmacological interventions in the major depressive episode: Findings from a naturalistic study. *European Psychiatry, 28*(6), 356–361.

Brunoni, A. R., Ferrucci, R., Bortolomasi, M., Vergari, M., Tadini, L., Boggio, P. S., … Priori, A. (2011). Transcranial direct current stimulation (tDCS) in unipolar vs. bipolar depressive disorder. *Progress in Neuro-Psychopharmacology & Biological Psychiatry, 35*(1), 96–101. S0278-5846(10)00361-1 [pii].

Brunoni, A. R., Kemp, A. H., Dantas, E. M., GOulart, A. C., Nunes, M. A., Boggio, P. S., … Bensenor, I. M. (2013). Heart rate variability is a trait marker of major depressive disorder: Evidence from the sertraline vs. Electric Current Therapy to Treat Depression Clinical Study. *The International Journal of Neuropsychopharmacology*, 2013;70(4):383–91. [Epub ahead of print].

Brunoni, A. R., Kemp, A. H., Shiozawa, P., Cordeiro, Q., Valiengo, L. C., Goulart, A. C., … Bensenor, I. M. (2013). Impact of 5-HTTLPR and BDNF polymorphisms on response to sertraline versus transcranial direct current stimulation: Implications for the serotonergic system. *European Neuropsychopharmacology, 23*(11), 1530–1540.

Brunoni, A. R., Lopes, M., & Fregni, F. (2008). A systematic review and meta-analysis of clinical studies on major depression and BDNF levels: Implications for the role of neuroplasticity in depression. *The International Journal of Neuropsychopharmacology, 11*(8), 1169–1180. S1461145708009309 [pii].

Brunoni, A. R., Machado-Vieira, R., Zarate, C. A., Jr., Vieira, E. L., Valiengo, L., Bensenor, I. M., … Teixeira, A. L. (2014). Assessment of non-BDNF neurotrophins and GDNF levels after depression treatment with sertraline and transcranial direct current stimulation in a factorial, randomized, sham-controlled trial (SELECT-TDCS): An exploratory analysis. *Progress in Neuro-Psychopharmacology & Biological Psychiatry, 56C*, 91–96.

Brunoni, A. R., Machado-Vieira, R., Zarate, C. A., Jr., Vieira, E. L., Vanderhasselt, M. A., Nitsche, M. A., … Teixeira, A. L. (2014). BDNF plasma levels after antidepressant treatment with sertraline and transcranial direct current stimulation: Results from a factorial, randomized, sham-controlled trial. *European Neuropsychopharmacology: the Journal of the European College of Neuropsychopharmacology, 24*, 1144–1151.

Brunoni, A. R., Valiengo, L., Baccaro, A., Zanao, T. A., Oliveira, A. C., Goulart, A. C., … Fregni, F. (2013). The sertraline versus electrical current therapy for treating depression clinical study: Results from a factorial, randomized, controlled trial. *JAMA Psychiatry, 70*(4), 383–391.

Brunoni, A. R., Valiengo, L., Zanao, T., de Oliveira, J. F., Bensenor, I. M., & Fregni, F. (2011). Manic psychosis after sertraline and transcranial direct-current stimulation. *The Journal of Neuropsychiatry and Clinical Neurosciences, 23*(3), E4–E5.

Brunoni, A. R., Zanao, T. A., Vanderhasselt, M. A., Valiengo, L., de Oliveira, J. F., Boggio, P. S., … Fregni, F. (2013). Enhancement of affective processing induced by Bifrontal transcranial direct current stimulation in patients with major depression. *Neuromodulation: Journal of the International Neuromodulation Society*., [Epub ahead of print].

Campbell, S., & Macqueen, G. (2004). The role of the hippocampus in the pathophysiology of major depression. *Journal of Psychiatry & Neuroscience, 29*(6), 417–426.

Charvet, L. E., Kasschau, M., Datta, A., Knotkova, H., Stevens, M. C., Alonzo, A., … Bikson, M. (2015). Remotely-supervised transcranial direct current stimulation (tDCS) for clinical trials: Guidelines for technology and protocols. *Frontiers in Systems Neuroscience, 9*, 26.

Cipriani, A., La Ferla, T., Furukawa, T. A., Signoretti, A., Nakagawa, A., Churchill, R., … Barbui, C. (2010). Sertraline versus other antidepressive agents for depression. *Cochrane Database of Systematic Reviews, 4*, CD006117.

Clarke, P. J., Browning, M., Hammond, G., Notebaert, L., & MacLeod, C. (2014). The causal role of the dorsolateral prefrontal cortex in the modification of attentional bias: Evidence from transcranial direct current stimulation. *Biological Psychiatry, 76*(12), 946–952.

Collier, D. A., Stober, G., Li, T., Heils, A., Catalano, M., Di Bella, D., … Lesch, K. P. (1996). A novel functional polymorphism within the promoter of the serotonin transporter gene: Possible role in susceptibility to affective disorders. *Molecular Psychiatry, 1*(6), 453–460.

Conti, C. L., Moscon, J. A., Fregni, F., Nitsche, M. A., & Nakamura-Palacios, E. M. (2014). Cognitive related electrophysiological changes induced by non-invasive cortical electrical stimulation in crack-cocaine addiction. *The International Journal of Neuropsychopharmacology, 17*(9), 1465–1475.

Conti, C. L., & Nakamura-Palacios, E. M. (2014). Bilateral transcranial direct current stimulation over dorsolateral prefrontal cortex changes the drug-cued reactivity in the anterior cingulate cortex of crack-cocaine addicts. *Brain Stimulation, 7*(1), 130–132.

Cosmo, C., Baptista, A. F., de Araujo, A. N., do Rosario, R. S., Miranda, J. G., Montoya, P., & de Sena, E. P. (2015). A randomized, double-blind, sham-controlled trial of transcranial direct current stimulation in attention-deficit/hyperactivity disorder. *PLoS One, 10*(8), e0135371.

Cosmo, C., Ferreira, C., Miranda, J. G., do Rosario, R. S., Baptista, A. F., Montoya, P., & de Sena, E. P. (2015). Spreading effect of tDCS in individuals with attention-deficit/hyperactivity disorder as shown by functional cortical networks: A randomized, double-blind, sham-controlled trial. *Frontiers in Psychiatry/Frontiers Research Foundation, 6*, 111.

da Silva, M. C., Conti, C. L., Klauss, J., Alves, L. G., do Nascimento Cavalcante, H. M., Fregni, F., … Nakamura-Palacios, E. M. (2013). Behavioral effects of transcranial direct current stimulation (tDCS) induced dorsolateral prefrontal cortex plasticity in alcohol dependence. Journal of Physiology, Paris, 107(6), 493–502.

de Almeida Ramos, R., Taiar, I., Trevizol, A. P., Shiozawa, P., & Cordeiro, Q. (2016). Effect of a eten-day prefrontal transcranial direct current stimulation protocol for crack Craving: A proof-of-concept trial. *The Journal of ECT*.

de Wit, S. J., de Vries, F. E., van der Werf, Y. D., Cath, D. C., Heslenfeld, D. J., Veltman, E. M., … van den Heuvel, O. A. (2012). Presupplementary motor area hyperactivity during response inhibition: A candidate endophenotype of obsessive-compulsive disorder. *The American Journal of Psychiatry, 169*(10), 1100–1108.

Degenhardt, L., Stockings, E., Patton, G., Hall, W. D., & Lynskey, M. (2016). The increasing global health priority of substance use in young people. *Lancet Psychiatry, 3*(3), 251–264.

Dell'osso, B., Zanoni, S., Ferrucci, R., Vergari, M., Castellano, F., D'Urso, N., … Altamura, A. C. (2012). Transcranial direct current stimulation for the outpatient treatment of poor-responder depressed patients. *European Psychiatry: The Journal of the Association of European Psychiatrists, 27*(7), 513–517.

den Uyl, T. E., Gladwin, T. E., & Wiers, R. W. (2015). Transcranial direct current stimulation, implicit alcohol associations and craving. *Biological Psychology, 105*, 37–42.

Dunlop, K., Hanlon, C. A., & Downar, J. (2016). Noninvasive brain stimulation treatments for addiction and major depression. *Annals of the New York Academy of Sciences*.

D'Urso, G., Brunoni, A. R., Anastasia, A., Micillo, M., de Bartolomeis, A., & Mantovani, A. (2016). Polarity-dependent effects of transcranial direct current stimulation in obsessive-compulsive disorder. *Neurocase, 22*(1), 60–64.

Dutra, L., Stathopoulou, G., Basden, S. L., Leyro, T. M., Powers, M. B., & Otto, M. W. (2008). A meta-analytic review of psychosocial interventions for substance use disorders. *The American Journal of Psychiatry, 165*(2), 179–187.

Fecteau, S., Agosta, S., Hone-Blanchet, A., Fregni, F., Boggio, P., Ciraulo, D., & Pascual-Leone, A. (2014). Modulation of smoking and decision-making behaviors with transcranial direct current stimulation in tobacco smokers: A preliminary study. *Drug & Alcohol Dependence, 140*, 78–84.

Fitzgerald, P. B., McQueen, S., Daskalakis, Z. J., & Hoy, K. E. (2014). A negative pilot study of daily bimodal transcranial direct current stimulation in schizophrenia. *Brain Stimulation, 7*(6), 813–816.

Foa, E. B., Liebowitz, M. R., Kozak, M. J., Davies, S., Campeas, R., Franklin, M. E., … Tu, X. (2005). Randomized, placebo-controlled trial of exposure and ritual prevention, clomipramine, and their combination in the treatment of obsessive-compulsive disorder. *The American Journal of Psychiatry, 162*(1), 151–161.

Fregni, F., Boggio, P. S., Nitsche, M. A., Marcolin, M. A., Rigonatti, S. P., & Pascual-Leone, A. (2006). Treatment of major depression with transcranial direct current stimulation. *Bipolar Disorders, 8*(2), 203–204.BDI291 [pii].

Fregni, F., Boggio, P. S., Nitsche, M. A., Rigonatti, S. P., & Pascual-Leone, A. (2006). Cognitive effects of repeated sessions of transcranial direct current stimulation in patients with depression. *Depression & Anxiety, 23*(8), 482–484.

Fregni, F., Liguori, P., Fecteau, S., Nitsche, M. A., Pascual-Leone, A., & Boggio, P. S. (2008). Cortical stimulation of the prefrontal cortex with transcranial direct current stimulation reduces cue-provoked smoking craving: A randomized, sham-controlled study. *The Journal of Clinical Psychiatry, 69*(1), 32–40.

Fritsch, B., Reis, J., Martinowich, K., Schambra, H. M., Ji, Y., Cohen, L. G., & Lu, B. (2010). Direct current stimulation promotes BDNF-dependent synaptic plasticity: Potential implications for motor learning. *Neuron, 66*(2), 198–204. S0896-6273(10)00238-2 [pii].

Frohlich, F., Burrello, T. N., Mellin, J. M., Cordle, A. L., Lustenberger, C. M., Gilmore, J. H., & Jarskog, L. F. (2016). Exploratory study of once-daily transcranial direct current stimulation (tDCS) as a treatment for auditory hallucinations in schizophrenia. *European Psychiatry, 33*, 54–60.

Galvez, V., Alonzo, A., Martin, D., Mitchell, P. B., Sachdev, P., & Loo, C. K. (2011). Hypomania induction in a patient with bipolar II disorder by transcranial direct current stimulation (tDCS). *The Journal of ECT, 27*(3), 256–258.

Gartner, A., & Staiger, V. (2002). Neurotrophin secretion from hippocampal neurons evoked by long-term-potentiation-inducing electrical stimulation patterns. *Proceedings of the National Academy of Sciences of the United States of America, 99*(9), 6386–6391.

Göder, R., Baier, P. C., Beith, B., Baecker, C., Seeck-Hirschner, M., Junghanns, K., & Marshall, L. (2013). Effects of transcranial direct current stimulation during sleep on memory performance in patients with schizophrenia. *Schizophrenia Research, 144*(1–3), 153–154.

Gomes, J. S., Shiozawa, P., Dias, A. M., Valverde Ducos, D., Akiba, H., Trevizol, A. P., … Cordeiro, Q. (2015). Left dorsolateral prefrontal cortex anodal tDCS effects on negative symptoms in schizophrenia. *Brain Stimulation, 8*(5), 989–991.

Goncalves, O. F., Carvalho, S., Leite, J., Pocinho, F., Relvas, J., & Fregni, F. (2011). Obsessive compulsive disorder as a functional interhemispheric imbalance at the thalamic level. *Medical Hypotheses, 77*(3), 445–447.

Gorini, A., Lucchiari, C., Russell-Edu, W., & Pravettoni, G. (2014). Modulation of risky choices in recently abstinent dependent cocaine users: A transcranial direct-current stimulation study. *Frontiers in Human Neuroscience, 8*, 661.

Greenberg, B. D., Murphy, D. L., & Rasmussen, S. A. (2000). Neuroanatomically based approaches to obsessive-compulsive disorder. Neurosurgery and transcranial magnetic stimulation. *The Psychiatric Clinics of North America, 23*(3), 671–686. xii.

Group, U. E. R. (2003). Efficacy and safety of electroconvulsive therapy in depressive disorders: A systematic review and meta-analysis. *Lancet, 361*(9360), 799–808. S0140-6736(03)12705-5 [pii].

Hamilton, J. P., Siemer, M., & Gotlib, I. H. (2008a). Amygdala volume in major depressive disorder: A meta-analysis of magnetic resonance imaging studies. *Molecular Psychiatry, 13*, 993–1000.

Hamilton, J. P., Siemer, M., & Gotlib, I. H. (2008b). Amygdala volume in major depressive disorder: A meta-analysis of magnetic resonance imaging studies. *Molecular Psychiatry, 13*(11), 993–1000. mp200857 [pii].

Harmer, C. J., Hill, S. A., Taylor, M. J., Cowen, P. J., & Goodwin, G. M. (2003). Toward a neuropsychological theory of antidepressant drug action: Increase in positive emotional bias after potentiation of norepinephrine activity. *The American Journal of Psychiatry, 160*(5), 990–992.

Hasan, A., Falkai, P., Wobrock, T., Lieberman, J., Glenthoj, B., Gattaz, W. F., … Moller, H. J. (2012). World Federation of Societies of Biological Psychiatry (WFSBP) Guidelines for Biological Treatment of Schizophrenia, part 1: update 2012 on the acute treatment of schizophrenia and the management of treatment resistance. *The World Journal of Biological Psychiatry: The Official Journal of the World Federation of Societies of Biological Psychiatry, 13*(5), 318–378.

Hasan, A., Guse, B., Cordes, J., Wolwer, W., Winterer, G., Gaebel, W., … Wobrock, T. (2015). Cognitive effects of high-frequency rTMS in schizophrenia patients with predominant negative Symptoms: Results from a multicenter randomized sham-controlled trial. *Schizophrenia Bulletin.*

Honzel, N., Justus, T., & Swick, D. (2014). Posttraumatic stress disorder is associated with limited executive resources in a working memory task. *Cognitive, Affective, & Behavioral Neuroscience, 14*(2), 792–804.

Hoy, K. E., Arnold, S. L., Emonson, M. R., Daskalakis, Z. J., & Fitzgerald, P. B. (2014). An investigation into the effects of tDCS dose on cognitive performance over time in patients with schizophrenia. *Schizophrenia Research, 155*(1–3), 96–100.

Janocha, A., Pilecki, W., Bolanowski, M., Malyszczak, K., Salomon, E., Laszki-Szczachor, K., … Sobieszczanska, M. (2009). Interhemispheric cerebral asymmetry detected by VEPS in diabetic patients with recognized depression. *Neuro Endocrinology Letters, 30*(1), 119–124.

Jardri, R., Pouchet, A., Pins, D., & Thomas, P. (2011). Cortical activations during auditory verbal hallucinations in schizophrenia: A coordinate-based meta-analysis. *The American Journal of Psychiatry, 168*(1), 73–81.

Kay, S. R., Fiszbein, A., & Opler, L. A. (1987). The positive and negative syndrome scale (PANSS) for schizophrenia. *Schizophrenia Bulletin, 13*(2), 261–276.

Keeser, D., Meindl, T., Bor, J., Palm, U., Pogarell, O., Mulert, C., … Padberg, F. (2011). Prefrontal transcranial direct current stimulation changes connectivity of resting-state networks during fMRI. *The Journal of Neuroscience, 31*(43), 15284–15293.

Kelley, N. J., Hortensius, R., & Harmon-Jones, E. (2013). When anger leads to rumination: Induction of relative right frontal cortical activity with transcranial direct current stimulation increases anger-related rumination. *Psychological Science, 24*(4), 475–481.

Kemp, A. H., Quintana, D. S., Gray, M. A., Felmingham, K. L., Brown, K., & Gatt, J. (2010). Impact of depression and antidepressant treatment on heart rate variability: A review and meta-analysis. *Biological Psychiatry, 67*(11), 1067–1074. S0006-3223(09)01449-8 [pii].

Kessler, S. K., Minhas, P., Woods, A. J., Rosen, A., Gorman, C., & Bikson, M. (2013). Dosage considerations for transcranial direct current stimulation in children: A computational modeling study. *PLoS One, 8*(9), e76112.

Khedr, E. M., Elfetoh, N. A., Ali, A. M., & Noamany, M. (2014). Anodal transcranial direct current stimulation over the dorsolateral prefrontal cortex improves anorexia nervosa: A pilot study. *Restorative Neurology and Neuroscience, 32*(6), 789–797.

Kilts, C. D., Gross, R. E., Ely, T. D., & Drexler, K. P. (2004). The neural correlates of cue-induced craving in cocaine-dependent women. *The American Journal of Psychiatry, 161*(2), 233–241.

Klauss, J., Penido Pinheiro, L. C., Silva Merlo, B. L., de Almeida Correia Santos, G., Fregni, F., Nitsche, M. A., & Miyuki Nakamura-Palacios, E. (2014). A randomized controlled trial of targeted prefrontal cortex modulation with tDCS in patients with alcohol dependence. *The International Journal of Neuropsychopharmacology, 17*(11), 1793–1803.

Kuo, H. I., Paulus, W., Batsikadze, G., Jamil, A., Kuo, M. F., & Nitsche, M. A. (2015). Chronic enhancement of serotonin facilitates excitatory transcranial direct current stimulation-induced neuroplasticity. *Neuropsychopharmacology*.

Kuo, M. F., & Nitsche, M. A. (2012). Effects of transcranial electrical stimulation on cognition. *Clinical EEG and Neuroscience, 43*(3), 192–199.

Kurimori, M., Shiozawa, P., Bikson, M., Aboseria, M., & Cordeiro, Q. (2015). Targeting negative symptoms in schizophrenia: Results from a proof-of-concept trial assessing prefrontal anodic tDCS protocol. *Schizophrenia Research, 166*(1–3), 362–363.

Lawrie, S. M., Buechel, C., Whalley, H. C., Frith, C. D., Friston, K. J., & Johnstone, E. C. (2002). Reduced frontotemporal functional connectivity in schizophrenia associated with auditory hallucinations. *Biological Psychiatry, 51*(12), 1008–1011.

Lefaucheur, J. P., Andre-Obadia, N., Antal, A., Ayache, S. S., Baeken, C., Benninger, D. H., … Garcia-Larrea, L. (2014). Evidence-based guidelines on the therapeutic use of repetitive transcranial magnetic stimulation (rTMS). *Clinical Neurophysiology: Official Journal of the International Federation of Clinical Neurophysiology, 125*, 2150–2206.

Li, Q., Wang, Y., Zhang, Y., Li, W., Yang, W., Zhu, J., … Tian, J. (2012). Craving correlates with mesolimbic responses to heroin-related cues in short-term abstinence from heroin: An event-related fMRI study. *Brain Research, 1469*, 63–72.

Liebetanz, D., Nitsche, M. A., Tergau, F., & Paulus, W. (2002). Pharmacological approach to the mechanisms of transcranial DC-stimulation-induced after-effects of human motor cortex excitability. *Brain, 125*(Pt 10), 2238–2247.

Loo, C. K., Alonzo, A., Martin, D., Mitchell, P. B., Galvez, V., & Sachdev, P. (2012). Transcranial direct current stimulation for depression: 3-week, randomised, sham-controlled trial. *The British Journal of Psychiatry, 200*(1), 52–59.

Loo, C. K., Sachdev, P., Martin, D., Pigot, M., Alonzo, A., Malhi, G. S., … Mitchell, P. (2010). A double-blind, sham-controlled trial of transcranial direct current stimulation for the treatment of depression. *The International Journal of Neuropsychopharmacology, 13*(1), 61–69. S1461145709990411 [pii].

Maeda, F., Keenan, J. P., & Pascual-Leone, A. (2000). Interhemispheric asymmetry of motor cortical excitability in major depression as measured by transcranial magnetic stimulation. *The British Journal of Psychiatry, 177*, 169–173.

Magill, M., & Ray, L. A. (2009). Cognitive-behavioral treatment with adult alcohol and illicit drug users: A meta-analysis of randomized controlled trials. *Journal of Studies on Alcohol and Drugs, 70*(4), 516–527.

Maia, T. V., Cooney, R. E., & Peterson, B. S. (2008). The neural bases of obsessive-compulsive disorder in children and adults. *Development and Psychopathology, 20*(4), 1251–1283.

Mantovani, A., Rossi, S., Bassi, B. D., Simpson, H. B., Fallon, B. A., & Lisanby, S. H. (2013). Modulation of motor cortex excitability in obsessive-compulsive disorder: An exploratory study on the relations of neurophysiology measures with clinical outcome. *Psychiatry Research*.

Mantovani, A., Simpson, H. B., Fallon, B. A., Rossi, S., & Lisanby, S. H. (2010). Randomized sham-controlled trial of repetitive transcranial magnetic stimulation in treatment-resistant obsessive-compulsive disorder. *The International Journal of Neuropsychopharmacology/ Official Scientific Journal of the Collegium Internationale Neuropsychopharmacologicum, 13*(2), 217–227.

Marin, M. F., Camprodon, J. A., Dougherty, D. D., & Milad, M. R. (2014). Device-based brain stimulation to augment fear extinction: Implications for PTSD treatment and beyond. *Depression & Anxiety, 31*(4), 269–278.

Mattai, A., Miller, R., Weisinger, B., Greenstein, D., Bakalar, J., Tossell, J., … Gogtay, N. (2011). Tolerability of transcranial direct current stimulation in childhood-onset schizophrenia. *Brain Stimulation, 4*(4), 275–280.

Mayberg, H. S., Brannan, S. K., Tekell, J. L., Silva, J. A., Mahurin, R. K., McGinnis, S., & Jerabek, P. A. (2000). Regional metabolic effects of fluoxetine in major depression: Serial changes and relationship to clinical response. *Biological Psychiatry, 48*(8), 830–843.

Meng, Z., Liu, C., Yu, C., & Ma, Y. (2014). Transcranial direct current stimulation of the frontal-parietal-temporal area attenuates smoking behavior. *Journal of Psychiatric Research, 54*, 19–25.

Meron, D., Hedger, N., Garner, M., & Baldwin, D. S. (2015). Transcranial direct current stimulation (tDCS) in the treatment of depression: Systematic review and meta-analysis of efficacy and tolerability. *Neuroscience and Biobehavioral Reviews, 57*, 46–62.

Minhas, P., Bikson, M., Woods, A. J., Rosen, A. R., & Kessler, S. K. (2012). Transcranial direct current stimulation in pediatric brain: A computational modeling study. *Conference Proceedings: Annual International Conference of the IEEE Engineering in Medicine and Biology Society, 2012*, 859–862.

Moeller, S. J., Tomasi, D., Woicik, P. A., Maloney, T., Alia-Klein, N., Honorio, J., … Goldstein, R. Z. (2012). Enhanced midbrain response at 6-month follow-up in cocaine addiction, association with reduced drug-related choice. *Addiction Biology, 17*(6), 1013–1025.

Moliadze, V., Schmanke, T., Andreas, S., Lyzhko, E., Freitag, C. M., & Siniatchkin, M. (2015). Stimulation intensities of transcranial direct current stimulation have to be adjusted in children and adolescents. *Clinical Neurophysiology, 126*(7), 1392–1399.

Mondino, M., Brunelin, J., Palm, U., Brunoni, A. R., Poulet, E., & Fecteau, S. (2015). Transcranial direct current stimulation for the treatment of refractory symptoms of schizophrenia. Current evidence and future directions. *Current Pharmaceutical Design, 21*(23), 3373–3383.

Monte-Silva, K., Kuo, M. F., Thirugnanasambandam, N., Liebetanz, D., Paulus, W., & Nitsche, M. A. (2009). Dose-dependent inverted U-shaped effect of dopamine (D2-like) receptor activation on focal and nonfocal plasticity in humans. *The Journal of Neuroscience, 29*(19), 6124–6131. 29/19/6124 [pii].

Moreno, M. L., Vanderhasselt, M. A., Carvalho, A. F., Moffa, A. H., Lotufo, P. A., Bensenor, I. M., & Brunoni, A. R. (2015). Effects of acute transcranial direct current stimulation in hot and cold working memory tasks in healthy and depressed subjects. *Neuroscience Letters, 591*, 126–131.

Munz, M. T., Prehn-Kristensen, A., Thielking, F., Molle, M., Goder, R., & Baving, L. (2015). Slow oscillating transcranial direct current stimulation during non-rapid eye movement sleep improves behavioral inhibition in attention-deficit/hyperactivity disorder. *Frontiers in Cellular Neuroscience, 9*, 307.

Murphy, B. P., Chung, Y. C., Park, T. W., & McGorry, P. D. (2006). Pharmacological treatment of primary negative symptoms in schizophrenia: A systematic review. *Schizophrenia Research, 88*(1–3), 5–25.

Murray, C. J., & Lopez, A. D. (1997). Alternative projections of mortality and disability by cause 1990-2020: Global burden of disease study. *Lancet, 349*(9064), 1498–1504. S0140-6736(96)07492-2 [pii].

Nakamura-Palacios, E. M., de Almeida Benevides, M. C., da Penha Zago-Gomes, M., de Oliveira, R. W., de Vasconcellos, V. F., de Castro, L. N., … Fregni, F. (2012). Auditory event-related potentials (P3) and cognitive changes induced by frontal direct current stimulation in alcoholics according to Lesch alcoholism typology. *The International Journal of Neuropsychopharmacology/Official Scientific Journal of the Collegium Internationale Neuropsychopharmacologicum, 15*(5), 601–616.

Narayanaswamy, J. C., Jose, D., Chhabra, H., Agarwal, S. M., Shrinivasa, B., Hegde, A., … Reddy, Y. C. (2015). Successful application of add-on transcranial direct current stimulation (tDCS) for treatment of SSRI resistant OCD. *Brain Stimulation, 8*(3), 655–657.

Nemeroff, C. B. (2007). Prevalence and management of treatment-resistant depression. *The Journal of Clinical Psychiatry, 68*(Suppl 8), 17–25.

Nestler, E. J. (2005). Is there a common molecular pathway for addiction? *Nature Neuroscience, 8*(11), 1445–1449.

Nienow, T. M., MacDonald, A. W., 3rd, & Lim, K. O. (2016). TDCS produces incremental gain when combined with working memory training in patients with schizophrenia: A proof of concept pilot study. *Schizophrenia Research, 172*, 218–219.

Nieratschker, V., Kiefer, C., Giel, K., Kruger, R., & Plewnia, C. (2015). The COMT Val/Met polymorphism modulates effects of tDCS on response inhibition. *Brain Stimulation, 8*(2), 283–288.

Nitsche, M. A., Boggio, P. S., Fregni, F., & Pascual-Leone, A. (2009). Treatment of depression with transcranial direct current stimulation (tDCS): A review. *Experimental Neurology, 219*(1), 14–19. S0014-4886(09)00129-0 [pii].

Nitsche, M. A., Kuo, M. F., Grosch, J., Bergner, C., Monte-Silva, K., & Paulus, W. (2009). D1-receptor impact on neuroplasticity in humans. *The Journal of Neuroscience, 29*(8), 2648–2653. 29/8/2648 [pii].

Nitsche, M. A., Kuo, M. F., Karrasch, R., Wachter, B., Liebetanz, D., & Paulus, W. (2009). Serotonin affects transcranial direct current-induced neuroplasticity in humans. *Biological Psychiatry, 66*(5), 503–508. S0006-3223(09)00422-3 [pii].

Nitsche, M. A., & Paulus, W. (2000). Excitability changes induced in the human motor cortex by weak transcranial direct current stimulation. *The Journal of Physiology, 527*(Pt 3), 633–639. PHY_1055 [pii].

Nobler, M. S., & Sackeim, H. A. (2008). Neurobiological correlates of the cognitive side effects of electroconvulsive therapy. *The Journal of ECT, 24*(1), 40–45. 00124509-200803000-00008 [pii].

Palm, U., Fintescu, Z., Obermeier, M., Schiller, C., Reisinger, E., Keeser, D., … Padberg, F. (2013). Serum levels of brain-derived neurotrophic factor are unchanged after transcranial direct current stimulation in treatment-resistant depression. *Journal of Affective Disorders, 150*(2), 659–663.

Palm, U., Hasan, A., Kupka, M. J., Blautzik, J., Kaymakanova, F., Unger, I., … Padberg, F. (2016). Prefrontal transcranial direct current stimulation (tDCS) for treatment of schizophrenia with predominant negative symptoms: A double-blind, sham-controlled proof-of-concept study. *Schizophrenia Bulletin, 42*, 1253–1261.

Palm, U., Schiller, C., Fintescu, Z., Obermeier, M., Keeser, D., Reisinger, E., … Padberg, F. (2012). Transcranial direct current stimulation in treatment resistant depression: A randomized double-blind, placebo-controlled study. *Brain Stimulation, 5*(3), 242–251.

Parazzini, M., Fiocchi, S., Liorni, I., Priori, A., & Ravazzani, P. (2014). Computational modeling of transcranial direct current stimulation in the child brain: Implications for the treatment of refractory childhood focal epilepsy. *International Journal of Neural Systems, 24*(2), 1430006.

Pereira Junior Bde, S., Tortella, G., Lafer, B., Nunes, P., Bensenor, I. M., Lotufo, P. A., … Brunoni, A. R. (2015). The bipolar depression electrical treatment trial (BETTER): Design, rationale, and objectives of a randomized, sham-controlled trial and data from the pilot study phase. *Neural Plasticity, 2015*, 684025.

Pinchuk, D., Pinchuk, O., Sirbiladze, K., & Shugar, O. (2013). Clinical effectiveness of primary and secondary headache treatment by transcranial direct current stimulation. *Frontiers in Neurology, 4*, 25.

Player, M., Taylor, J., Weickert, C. S., Alonzo, A., Sachdev, P., Martin, D., … Loo, C. K. (2014). Increase in PAS-induced neuroplasticity after a treatment course of transcranial direct current stimulation for depression. *Journal of Affective Disorders, 167*, 140–147.

Plewnia, C., Zwissler, B., Langst, I., Maurer, B., Giel, K., & Kruger, R. (2013). Effects of transcranial direct current stimulation (tDCS) on executive functions: Influence of COMT Val/Met polymorphism. *Cortex; A Journal Devoted to the Study of the Nervous System and Behavior, 49*(7), 1801–1807.

Prehn-Kristensen, A., Munz, M., Goder, R., Wilhelm, I., Korr, K., Vahl, W., … Baving, L. (2014). Transcranial oscillatory direct current stimulation during sleep improves declarative memory consolidation in children with attention-deficit/hyperactivity disorder to a level comparable to healthy controls. *Brain Stimulation, 7*(6), 793–799.

Prendergast, M., Podus, D., Finney, J., Greenwell, L., & Roll, J. (2006). Contingency management for treatment of substance use disorders: A meta-analysis. *Addiction, 101*(11), 1546–1560.

Priori, A., Berardelli, A., Rona, S., Accornero, N., & Manfredi, M. (1998). Polarization of the human motor cortex through the scalp. *Neuroreport, 9*(10), 2257–2260.

Priori, A., Hallett, M., & Rothwell, J. C. (2009). Repetitive transcranial magnetic stimulation or transcranial direct current stimulation? *Brain Stimulation, 2*(4), 241–245. S1935-861X(09)00012-6 [pii].

Pripfl, J., Neumann, R., Köhler, U., & Lamm, C. (2013). Effects of transcranial direct current stimulation on risky decision making are mediated by 'hot' and 'cold' decisions, personality, and hemisphere. *The European Journal of Neuroscience, 38*(12), 3778–3785.

Pripfl, J., & Lamm, C. (2015). Focused transcranial direct current stimulation (tDCS) over the dorsolateral prefrontal cortex modulates specific domains of self-regulation. *Neuroscience Research, 91*, 41–47.

Rassovsky, Y., Dunn, W., Wynn, J., Wu, A. D., Iacoboni, M., Hellemann, G., & Green, M. F. (2015). The effect of transcranial direct current stimulation on social cognition in schizophrenia: A preliminary study. *Schizophrenia Research, 165*(2–3), 171–174.

Reinhart, R. M., Zhu, J., Park, S., & Woodman, G. F. (2015). Synchronizing theta oscillations with direct-current stimulation strengthens adaptive control in the human brain. *Proceedings of the National Academy of Sciences of the United States of America, 112*(30), 9448–9453.

Ressler, K. J., Rothbaum, B. O., Tannenbaum, L., Anderson, P., Graap, K., Zimand, E., … Davis, M. (2004). Cognitive enhancers as adjuncts to psychotherapy: Use of D-cycloserine in phobic individuals to facilitate extinction of fear. *Archives of General Psychiatry, 61*(11), 1136–1144.

Ribolsi, M., Lisi, G., Di Lorenzo, G., Koch, G., Oliveri, M., Magni, V., … Siracusano, A. (2013). Perceptual pseudoneglect in schizophrenia: Candidate endophenotype and the role of the right parietal cortex. *Schizophrenia Bulletin, 39*(3), 601–607.

Rigonatti, S. P., Boggio, P. S., Myczkowski, M. L., Otta, E., Fiquer, J. T., Ribeiro, R. B., … Fregni, F. (2008). Transcranial direct stimulation and fluoxetine for the treatment of depression. *European Psychiatry, 23*(1), 74–76. S0924-9338(07)01392-2 [pii].

Risinger, R. C., Salmeron, B. J., Ross, T. J., Amen, S. L., Sanfilipo, M., Hoffmann, R. G., … Stein, E. A. (2005). Neural correlates of high and craving during cocaine self-administration using BOLD fMRI. *NeuroImage, 26*(4), 1097–1108.

Ruscio, A. M., Stein, D. J., Chiu, W. T., & Kessler, R. C. (2010). The epidemiology of obsessive-compulsive disorder in the National Comorbidity Survey Replication. *Molecular Psychiatry, 15*(1), 53–63.

Rush, A. J., Trivedi, M. H., Wisniewski, S. R., Nierenberg, A. A., Stewart, J. W., Warden, D., … Fava, M. (2006). Acute and longer-term outcomes in depressed outpatients requiring one or several treatment steps: A STAR*D report. *Am J Psychiatry, 163*(11), 1905–1917. 163/11/1905 [pii].

Sanfilipo, M., Lafargue, T., Rusinek, H., Arena, L., Loneragan, C., Lautin, A., … Wolkin, A. (2000). Volumetric measure of the frontal and temporal lobe regions in schizophrenia: Relationship to negative symptoms. *Archives of General Psychiatry, 57*(5), 471–480.

Saunders, N., Downham, R., Turman, B., Kropotov, J., Clark, R., Yumash, R., & Szatmary, A. (2015). Working memory training with tDCS improves behavioral and neurophysiological symptoms in pilot group with post-traumatic stress disorder (PTSD) and with poor working memory. *Neurocase, 21*(3), 271–278.

Schestatsky, P., Janovik, N., Lobato, M. I., Belmonte-de-Abreu, P., Schestatsky, S., Shiozawa, P., & Fregni, F. (2013). Rapid therapeutic response to anodal tDCS of right dorsolateral prefrontal cortex in acute mania. *Brain Stimulation, 6*(4), 701–703.

Schmitt, A., Hasan, A., Gruber, O., & Falkai, P. (2011). Schizophrenia as a disorder of disconnectivity. *European Archives of Psychiatry and Clinical Neuroscience, 261*(Suppl 2), S150–S154.

Schneider, H. D., & Hopp, J. P. (2011). The use of the bilingual aphasia test for assessment and transcranial direct current stimulation to modulate language acquisition in minimally verbal children with autism. *Clinical Linguistics & Phonetics, 25*(6–7), 640–654.

Segrave, R. A., Arnold, S., Hoy, K., & Fitzgerald, P. B. (2013). Concurrent cognitive control training augments the antidepressant efficacy of tDCS: A pilot study. *Brain Stimulation*.

Segrave, R. A., Arnold, S., Hoy, K., & Fitzgerald, P. B. (2014). Concurrent cognitive control training augments the antidepressant efficacy of tDCS: a pilot study. *Brain Stimulation, 7*(2), 325–331.

Serretti, A., Kato, M., De Ronchi, D., & Kinoshita, T. (2007). Meta-analysis of serotonin transporter gene promoter polymorphism (5-HTTLPR) association with selective serotonin reuptake inhibitor efficacy in depressed patients. *Molecular Psychiatry, 12*(3), 247–257.

Shah, D. B., Pesiridou, A., Baltuch, G. H., Malone, D. A., & O'Reardon, J. P. (2008). Functional neurosurgery in the treatment of severe obsessive compulsive disorder and major depression: Overview of disease circuits and therapeutic targeting for the clinician. *Psychiatry, 5*(9), 24–33.

Shahbabaie, A., Golesorkhi, M., Zamanian, B., Ebrahimpoor, M., Keshvari, F., Nejati, V., … Ekhtiari, H. (2014). State dependent effect of transcranial direct current stimulation (tDCS) on methamphetamine craving. *The International Journal of Neuropsychopharmacology, 17*(10), 1591–1598.

Shergill, S. S., Murray, R. M., & Mcguire, P. K. (1998). Auditory hallucinations: A review of psychological treatments. *Schizophrenia Research, 32*(3), 137–150.

Shiozawa, P., Leiva, A. P., Castro, C. D., da Silva, M. E., Cordeiro, Q., Fregni, F., & Brunoni, A. R. (2014). Transcranial direct current stimulation for generalized anxiety disorder: A case study. *Biological Psychiatry, 75*(11), e17–e18.

Smith, R. C., Boules, S., Mattiuz, S., Youssef, M., Tobe, R. H., Sershen, H., … Davis, J. M. (2015). Effects of transcranial direct current stimulation (tDCS) on cognition, symptoms, and smoking in schizophrenia: A randomized controlled study. *Schizophrenia Research, 168*(1–2), 260–266.

Soltaninejad, Z., Nejati, V., & Ekhtiari, H. (2015). Effect of anodal and cathodal transcranial direct current stimulation on DLPFC on modulation of inhibitory control in ADHD. *Journal of Attention Disorders.*

Stitzer, M., & Petry, N. (2006). Contingency management for treatment of substance abuse. *Annual Review of Clinical Psychology, 2*, 411–434.

Subramaniam, A., Agarwal, S. M., Kalmady, S., Shivakumar, V., Chhabra, H., Bose, A., … Venkatasubramanian, G. (2015). Effect of transcranial direct current stimulation on prefrontal inhibition in schizophrenia patients with persistent auditory hallucinations: A study on antisaccade task performance. *Indian journal of psychological medicine, 37*(4), 419–422.

Tranter, R., Bell, D., Gutting, P., Harmer, C., Healy, D., & Anderson, I. M. (2009). The effect of serotonergic and noradrenergic antidepressants on face emotion processing in depressed patients. *Journal of Affective Disorders, 118*(1–3), 87–93.

Valiengo, L., Bensenor, I. M., Goulart, A. C., de Oliveira, J. F., Zanao, T. A., Boggio, P. S., … Brunoni, A. R. (2013). The sertraline versus electrical current therapy for treating depression clinical study (SELECT-TDCS): Results of the crossover and follow-up phases. *Depression & Anxiety, 30*(7), 646–653.

Vercammen, A., Rushby, J. A., Loo, C., Short, B., Weickert, C. S., & Weickert, T. W. (2011). Transcranial direct current stimulation influences probabilistic association learning in schizophrenia. *Schizophrenia Research, 131*(1–3), 198–205.

Volpato, C., Piccione, F., Cavinato, M., Duzzi, D., Schiff, S., Foscolo, L., & Venneri, A. (2013). Modulation of affective symptoms and resting state activity by brain stimulation in a treatment-resistant case of obsessive-compulsive disorder. *Neurocase, 19*(4), 360–370.

Whiteford, H. A., Degenhardt, L., Rehm, J., Baxter, A. J., Ferrari, A. J., Erskine, H. E., … Vos, T. (2013). Global burden of disease attributable to mental and substance use disorders: Findings from the global burden of disease study 2010. *Lancet, 382*(9904), 1575–1586.

WHO. (2016). Management of substance abuse. Retrieved from http://www.who.int/substance_abuse/facts/en/

Wobrock, T., Guse, B., Cordes, J., Wolwer, W., Winterer, G., Gaebel, W., … Hasan, A. (2015). Left prefrontal high-frequency repetitive transcranial magnetic stimulation for the treatment of schizophrenia with predominant negative symptoms: A sham-controlled, randomized multicenter trial. *Biological Psychiatry, 77*(11), 979–988.

Wolkenstein, L., & Plewnia, C. (2013). Amelioration of cognitive control in depression by transcranial direct current stimulation. *Biological Psychiatry, 73*(7), 646–651.

Xia, G., Gajwani, P., Muzina, D. J., Kemp, D. E., Gao, K., Ganocy, S. J., & Calabrese, J. R. (2008). Treatment-emergent mania in unipolar and bipolar depression: Focus on repetitive transcranial magnetic stimulation. *The International Journal of Neuropsychopharmacology, 11*(1), 119–130. S1461145707007699 [pii].

Xu, J., Fregni, F., Brody, A. L., & Rahman, A. S. (2013). Transcranial direct current stimulation reduces negative affect but not cigarette craving in overnight abstinent smokers. *Frontiers in Psychiatry, 4*, 112.

Yucel, M., Harrison, B. J., Wood, S. J., Fornito, A., Wellard, R. M., Pujol, J., … Pantelis, C. (2007). Functional and biochemical alterations of the medial frontal cortex in obsessive-compulsive disorder. *Archives of General Psychiatry, 64*(8), 946–955.

Zanao, T. A., Moffa, A. H., Shiozawa, P., Lotufo, P. A., Bensenor, I. M., & Brunoni, A. R. (2014). Impact of two or less missing treatment sessions on tDCS clinical efficacy: Results from a factorial, randomized, controlled trial in major depression. *Neuromodulation: Journal of the International Neuromodulation Society*.

Chapter 16
The Use and Efficacy of Transcranial Direct Current Stimulation in Individuals with Neurodegenerative Dementias

Annalise Rahman-Filipiak, Jaclyn M. Reckow, Adam J. Woods, Michael A. Nitsche, and Benjamin M. Hampstead

Introduction

Dementia, defined as subjective and objective cognitive and behavioral deficits that disrupt functioning (e.g., social, occupational) and represents a significant decline from previous level of functioning, constitutes a significant healthcare burden in middle and older aged adults. In a recent population-based sample of 856 American older adults drawn from the Health and Retirement Study, 13.9% of individuals over the age of 70 met criteria for dementia (Plassman et al. 2007). Global estimates of dementia range from 5% to 7% in most regions, with a significantly higher prevalence of 8.5% in Latin America and lower prevalence of 2–4% in sub-Saharan Africa (Prince et al. 2013). Rates of dementia diagnosis are also growing exponentially, with an estimated 115.4 million individuals worldwide expected to meet criteria by the year 2050 (Prince et al. 2013). The costs of dementia are notable; compared to individuals with heart disease, cancer, or other medical causes, individuals with dementia spend significantly more towards healthcare in their final 5 years of life, averaging $287,038 (Kelley et al. 2015). Among the

A. Rahman-Filipiak · J. M. Reckow · B. M. Hampstead (✉)
Department of Mental Health Services, Veterans Affairs Ann Arbor Healthcare Systems, Ann Arbor, MI, USA

Department of Psychiatry, University of Michigan, Ann Arbor, MI, USA
e-mail: bhampste@med.umich.edu

A. J. Woods
Center for Cognitive Aging and Memory (CAM), McKnight Brain Institute, Department of Clinical and Health Psychology, College of Public Health and Health Professions, University of Florida, Gainesville, FL, USA

M. A. Nitsche
Department of Psychology and Neurosciences, Leibniz Research Centre for Working Environment and Human Factors, Dortmund, Germany

University Medical Hospital Bergmannsheil, Bochum, Germany

H. Knotkova et al. (eds.), *Practical Guide to Transcranial Direct Current Stimulation*, https://doi.org/10.1007/978-3-319-95948-1_16

neurodegenerative diseases, Alzheimer's disease, Parkinson's disease dementia, Lewy Body dementia, and frontotemporal dementia, make up the vast majority. Although grouped together under the general concept of dementia, there are important differences in the underlying etiologies that result in unique patterns of neuropsychological, behavioral/emotional, and functional disturbance. This chapter aims to provide a brief summary of each of the neurodegenerative dementias, accompanied by a review of the existing literature on the use of transcranial direct current stimulation (tDCS) as an intervention for the associated behavioral and cognitive sequelae.

Alzheimer's Disease

Clinical Criteria

Among neurodegenerative dementias, dementia – Alzheimer's type (DAT) or Alzheimer's disease (AD) is the most common, occurring in 5.4 million Americans and one-in-nine U.S. adults aged 65 years or older (Alzheimer's Association 2016). Alzheimer's disease is characterized by a prominent memory impairment for recent information and events, most often experienced as forgetfulness in everyday life (Welsh-Bohmer and Warren 2006). Although histological confirmation is the gold standard for validating dementia subtype diagnosis, increased knowledge of AD-specific biomarkers (McKhann et al. 2011) and more robust measurement of cognitive impairment (Edmonds et al. 2015) have resulted in improved clinical criteria for diagnosing and staging AD (McKhann et al. 2011). A diagnosis of probable DAT requires evidence of an insidious onset, subjective decline, and a pattern of cognitive deficits not better accounted for by another dementia. While the "amnestic" (involving memory) subtype is most common, DAT can also manifest as primary dysfunction in the language, visuospatial, or executive domain (McKhann et al. 2011).

Neuropathology

The cardinal neuropathological characteristics of DAT include neurofibrillary tangles and senile beta-amyloid plaques that are ultimately accompanied by marked synaptic damage and neuronal loss. Neurofibrillary tangles (NFTs) are abnormal fibrous inclusions consisting primarily of hyper-phosphorylated tau protein, found within the perikaryal cytoplasm of pyramidal cells (Perl 2010; Serrano-Pozo et al. 2011). Although NFTs are present in other neuropathological processes (e.g., post-encephalitic parkinsonism, cognitive impairment after brain injury, amyotrophic lateral sclerosis), DAT is marked by a characteristic distribution of NFTs that begins in the transentorhinal (perirhinal, entorhinal) cortex of the medial temporal lobes. NFT distribution generally then progresses into the CA1 and subicular subregions of the hippocampus, followed by the deep layers of the neocortex, and finally affect the primary motor and somatosensory cortices during the final disease stages (Perl 2010; Serrano-Pozo et al. 2011). The other characteristic pathology is dense-core beta amyloid plaques, which consist of extracellular deposits with a core of amyloid beta (Aβ) surrounded by dystrophic neuritis (Serrano-Pozo et al. 2011). In contrast to NFTs, Aβ plaques are initially distributed in the basal portions of the frontal, temporal, and parietal/occipital lobes (Stage A), then in all isocortical association areas with minimal deposition in the hippocampi and primary sensory, motor, and visual cortex (Stage B), and finally in all areas of the isocortex, as well as some subcortical regions (Stage C; Braak and Braak 1991). Amyloid angiopathy in the leptomeningeal arteries and small arteries and vessels of the posterior cortex is also evident in approximately 80% of adults with DAT. As may be expected by the distribution of the above pathologies, DAT is marked by synaptic loss in the limbic system, neocortex, and basal forebrain (Serrano-Pozo et al. 2011) through early damage to synapses and retrograde degeneration of the axons and dendritic trees.

Neuropsychological Profile

The precise pattern of neuropsychological deficit often depends on the time at which patients present for evaluation, with more advanced patients demonstrating greater and more pervasive cognitive deficits (see Welsh-Bohmer and Warren 2006). The general consensus is that decline in the ability to learn and remember new information (i.e. declarative or episodic memory) is an early characteristic feature of DAT. Deficient learning is often detectable via a relatively flat learning curve across multiple presentation trials. Recall of recently learned information (i.e., memory) is poor and generally unaided via enhanced structure or cueing on recognition measures. Semantic memory tends to be preserved in early stages of the disease, with gradual decline corresponding to disease progression. Although simple attention is preserved, working memory (i.e., the ability to mentally hold and manipulate information) is variably deficient. Patients with DAT also demonstrate deficits in executive functioning, specifically in problem solving, abstract reasoning, inhibition, and mental flexibility. Language deficits are also common; in particular, word-finding and confrontation naming difficulties, reduced fluency and difficulty comprehending complex information are experienced. With the exception of posterior onset variants of DAT, visuospatial abilities are preserved early in the disease course but gradually decline.

tDCS in DAT

Given the pattern of deficits, a wide range of neocortical and cognitive targets could be considered when developing tDCS research. To date, we are not aware of any studies that have explicitly examined disease severity; rather, existing research has examined effects at the group level. A summary of published studies assessing effectiveness of tDCS for the treatment of cognitive impairments in DAT is provided in Table 16.1. As described below, tDCS has shown neuro-enhancing effects on multiple cognitive abilities on both short- and long-term bases, which are organized based on the targeted cognitive domain.

General Cognitive Functioning

In one of the largest completed clinical trials of tDCS efficacy in DAT, Khedr and colleagues (2014) demonstrated the impact of tDCS on general cognitive and intellectual functioning in a sample of 34 patients. The study utilized 10 consecutive daily sessions of 25 min of 2 mA active (anode vs. cathode placed over target) or sham stimulation over the left dorsolateral prefrontal cortex (DLPFC; 6 cm anterior to M1) plus 2 months of maintenance on memantine. Outcomes on a range of cognitive tasks (MMSE and subtests of the Wechsler Adult Intelligence Scale – Third Edition (WAIS-III) as well as neurophysiological changes in EEG were evaluated directly after the last session and at one- and two-month follow-up. Results indicated that, relative to sham, active stimulation resulted in a gain of approximately two points immediately and an additional one point after one- and two-months on the MMSE. In contrast, only cathodal stimulation over this area augmented performance IQ scores on the WAIS-III (Khedr et al. 2014). The reasons for these changes are unclear, especially given the potential hyperpolarizing effect of stimulation under the cathode electrode on neural soma, but the authors posited that active stimulation of either polarity engaged remaining "cognitive reserve." Prior findings of "excitatory" effects under the cathode at 2 mA have been reported in the motor cortex (Batsikadze et al. 2013; Wiethoff et al. 2014) and may support the authors' posited explanation for their findings.

Other studies assessing global cognitive change have been less positive and reported no effect of tDCS over the left DLPFC (Suemoto et al. 2014) or left temporal lobe (Boggio et al. 2012). Suemoto and colleagues (2014) found no differences on the MMSE and the Alzheimer's Disease Assessment Scale – Cognitive subscale (ADAS-Cog) in 40 AD patients who received six 20-min sessions of 2 mA sham or active (anode) tDCS over the left DLPFC. Boggio and colleagues (2012) utilized a double-blind crossover design in which 15 DAT patients received either repeated sham or active tDCS at 2 mA for 30 min per day, for five consecutive days. All participants completed both active and sham conditions, with several weeks in between each set of sessions. Dual anode electrodes were placed over the bilateral temporal lobes (T3 and T4) with the cathode placed noncephalically on the participants' right arm. Participants demonstrated no change in global cognition, as measured by the MMSE and ADAS-Cog, after either set of sessions.

Overall then, there is little evidence that tDCS enhances global cognitive functioning, though several potential explanations exist for this finding. Critically, the stimulation montage should target the functional neuroanatomy of the targeted

Table 16.1 Summary of published tDCS studies in patients with Alzheimer's disease and Mild Cognitive Impairment

Ref	Diagnosis	*n*	Design	Current	Anode location (size)	Cathode location	Duration	Session schedule	Outcome measures	Measurement timing	Effect	Side effects	Adverse effects
Bystad et al. (2016)	Early AD	1	Case study	2.0 mA	Left temporal lobe (T3) [NA]	FP2 [NA]	30 min	2 sessions/day, 6 consecutive days	Neuropsychological performance and EEG	Offline - at 2 days and 2 months post-stimulation	Improved verbal recall at 2 days and 2 months; no significant EEG changes	None reported	None reported
Boggio et al. (2009)	AD	10	Randomized single-blind crossover (order of sham, active DLPFC, active temporal lobe)	2.0 mA	Left DLPFC (F3) or left temporal lobe (T7) [35 cm^2]	Right supraorbital area [35 cm^2]	30 min	1 session/day, 3 days separated by 48-h for washout	Working memory (Digit Span F & B), Selective Attention (Stroop), Visual Recognition Task	Online - during stimulation	Better visual recognition after either LDLPFC or temporal stimulation vs. sham; ns working memory or attention effects	None reported	None reported

(continued)

Table 16.1 (continued)

Ref	Diagnosis	*n*	Design	Current	Anode location (size)	Cathode location	Duration	Session schedule	Outcome measures	Measurement timing	Effect	Side effects	Adverse effects
Boggio et al. (2012)	AD	15	Randomized double-blind crossover (order of active, sham)	2.0 mA	Bilateral anodes (T3, T4) [35 cm^2]	Right deltoid muscle [64 cm^2]	30 d	1 session/day, 5 consecutive days	MMSE, Adas-Cog, Visual Recognition Task, Visual Attention Task (Coglab)	Offline - at end of day 5, and at 1 week and 4 weeks post-stimulation	Improved visual recognition from baseline to 1-month post-stimulation; ns MMSE, Adas-cog, visual attention effects	None reported	None reported
Cheng et al. (2015)	AD	TBD	Randomized double-blind group comparison (active + working memory training vs. active + general training vs. sham + working memory training)	2.0 mA	Bilateral anodes (T3, T4) [35cm^2]	Right deltoid muscle [35cm^2]	20 min	3 sessions/week, 4 consecutive weeks	Adaptive N-back, Adas-Cog, Language and Memory Tasks, Chinese Neuropsychiatric Inventory	Offline - at 5 min post-stimulation	TBD	TBD	TBD

Ferrucci et al. (2008)	AD	10	Randomized double-blind crossover (order of anodal, cathodal, sham)	1.5 mA	Bilateral anodal or cathodal temporoparietal stimulation (P3-T5; P6-T4) [25 cm^2], reference electrode over right deltoid [64cm^2]	Bilateral anodal or cathodal temporoparietal stimulation (P3-T5; P6-T4) [25 cm^2], reference electrode over right deltoid [64 cm^2]	15 min	1 session/day, 3 days separated by >=1 week	Word recognition task (Adas-cog), visual attention	Offline - before and 30 min post-stimulation	Word recognition memory increased after AtDCS, decreased after cathodal tDCS and did not change after sham; ns effect on visual attention reaction times	Headache (n, 1)	None reported
Khedr et al. (2014)	AD	34	Randomized double-blind group comparison (anodal vs. cathodal vs. sham)	2.0 mA	Bilateral anodal or cathodal stimulation of left DLPFC (6 cm anterior to M1) [24 cm^2], reference electrode over contralateral supraorbital region [100 cm^2]	Bilateral anodal or cathodal stimulation of left DLPFC (6 cm anterior to M1) [24 cm^2], reference electrode over contralateral supraorbital region [100 cm^2]	25 min	1 session/day, 10 consecutive days	MMSE, WAIS-III; motor cortical excitability, P300 ERP	Offline - cognitive measures after last session, and at 1-month and 2-months post-stimulation; physiologic measures after last stimulation only	AtDCS and CtDCS associated with increased MMSE and reduced P300 latency; CtDCS also associated with improved PIQ	Headache, itching, dizziness (n, 2)	None reported

(continued)

Table 16.1 (continued)

Ref	Diagnosis	*n*	Design	Current	Anode location (size)	Cathode location	Duration	Session schedule	Outcome measures	Measurement timing	Effect	Side effects	Adverse effects
Marceglia et al. (2016)	AD	7	Randomized double-blind crossover (order of anodal, cathodal)	1.5 mA	Bilateral anodal or cathodal temporoparietal stimulation (P3-T5; P6-T4) [25 cm^2], reference electrode over right deltoid [64 cm^2]	Bilateral anodal or cathodal temporoparietal stimulation (P3-T5; P6-T4) [25 cm^2], reference electrode over right deltoid [64 cm^2]	15 min	2 sessions, separated by >=1 week	Plasma nitrite and nitrate levels, word recognition, qEEG cortical activity	Plasma nitrite and nitrate levels, word recognition, qEEG cortical activity	Decreased diffuse cortical theta oscillations after CtDCS; increased alpha and beta oscillations, increased nitrous oxide concentrations, and improved word recognition after AtDCS	None reported	None reported
Suemoto et al. (2014)	AD	40	Randomized, double-blind, group comparison (active vs. sham)	2.0 mA	Left DLPFC [35 cm^2]	Right orbit [35 cm^2]	20 min	1 session every other day for a total of 6 sessions	Scores on the apathy scale, neuropsychiatric inventory scores, caregiver burden, Adas-cog, depressive symptoms	Offline - at the end of week 1, week 2, and at 1 week post-intervention	No effect of tDCS on any outcome	Greater scalp burning in active stimulation group	None reported

Meinzer et al. (2015)	MCI	18 MCI vs. 18 healthy controls	Randomized double-blind cross-over (order of sham, active)	1.0 mA	Left ventral IFG [35 cm^2]	Right supraorbital region [100 cm^2]	20 min	Sham and active session, separated by 1 week	Semantic word-retrieval, resting state and task-related activation in the bilateral prefrontal cortex, self-report measures of mood & affect	Online - word retrieval and action; offline - self-report measures	Active tDCS improves semantic word-retrieval to level of healthy controls	None reported	None reported

NA not available, *IP* study in progress, no results available, *AD* Alzheimer's diease, *MCI* Mild Cognitive Impairment, *AtDCS* stimulation under the anode, *CtDCS* stimulation under the cathode, *mA* miliamps, *DLPFC* dorsolateral prefrontal cortex, *PFC* prefrontal cortex, *IFG* inferior frontal gyrus, *EEG* electroencephalography, *qEEG* quantitative electroencephalography, *fMRI* functional magnetic resonance imaging, *ERP* event-related potentials, *MMSE* Mini-Mental State Examination, *Adas-Cog* Alzheimer's Disease Assessment Scale – Cognitive, *WAIS* Wechsler Adult Intelligence Scale, *PIQ* Performance Intellectual Quotient

cognitive abilities. In this sense, global screening measures like the MMSE and ADAS-Cog may be too gross of tools to evaluate change in more selected brain regions/networks. As suggested below, there is some evidence that tDCS can enhance specific cognitive abilities as measured by more sensitive tasks. Additionally, the stimulation dose may have been insufficient to induce change at this global level. In this sense, the results of Khedr and colleagues (2014) are intriguing as they raise the possibility that tDCS may augment pharmacologic effects.

Memory

Several studies have demonstrated the beneficial effects of tDCS on memory using montages that targeted the frontal, parietal, and/or temporal lobes. Boggio and colleagues (2009) examined the memory performance of 10 DAT patients after a single 30-min session in which the anode was placed over either the left DLPFC (F3) or left temporal lobe (T3). Both locations resulted in improved visual recognition memory for animals, people, and objects when evaluated during stimulation (i.e., online task performance). Conversely, there was no effect on working memory (Digit Span subtest from the WAIS) or selective attention/inhibition (Stroop Color Word Test). The same group later reported enhanced visual recognition memory, which persisted at a 1 month follow-up after five consecutive daily 30-min sessions of 2 mA stimulation when the anode was placed over the bilateral temporal lobes (T3 & T4; cathode on right shoulder), relative to sham stimulation (Boggio et al. 2012).

Similar positive effects have been reported with verbal memory. In a double-blind randomized crossover design, Ferrucci et al. (2008) compared the effects of single 15-min sessions of anodal current, cathodal current, and sham stimulation on word recognition and visual attention in 10 DAT patients. This study used a bitemporal target location (P3-T5 and P6-T4) with non-cephalic placement of the other electrodes on the right shoulder, which was accomplished using dual tDCS units to each administer 1.5 mA. Placing the anodes over the target location significantly increased word recognition memory, whereas performance declined when cathodes were placed over the target location and remained stable following sham. These general results were recently replicated by Marceglia and colleagues (2016), who utilized the same study design and montage. In addition to demonstrating the enhancing effects of placing the anode, but not the cathode, over the targeted region on word recognition, the authors evaluated the neurophysiological effects of stimulation by electroencephalography (EEG). Patients with DAT generally demonstrate higher low-frequency theta oscillations in the temporoparietal cortex, a finding associated with poorer encoding in the hippocampal-cortical loops. Furthermore, DAT is associated with lower high-frequency alpha and beta oscillations in the frontal and temporoparietal cortex that underlies poorer search and retrieval of information. Marceglia and colleagues (2016) demonstrated that anodal tDCS specifically increased high-frequency alpha and beta oscillations in the temporoparietal area on EEG completed 30-min post-stimulation and posited that this effect drove the previously noted word recognition improvement (Marceglia et al. 2016).

tDCS may also have positive effects on verbal memory in early onset Alzheimer's disease, a diagnosis given when the patient meets criteria for DAT before age 65, likely due to a genetic mutation. In a case study of early onset DAT, Bystad et al. (2016) administered 2.0 mA stimulation with the anode over the left temporal lobe (T3) for 12 (2 per day over 6 days), 30-min sessions. Primary outcomes included neuropsychological testing and EEG monitoring with data acquired at baseline, 2 days after the last stimulation session, and again at a two-month follow-up. The participant exhibited a statistically significant improvement in delayed verbal recall at both post-stimulation time points. EEG was re-evaluated only at 2 months but there were no significant changes relative to baseline. These findings highlight a potentially interesting dichotomy between the behaviors/cognitive functions of interest and the underlying neurophysiology but also suggest that such measures need to be consistently paired across evaluation time points.

Thus, placing the anode over the temporal lobe(s) appears to consistently enhance memory performance in patients with DAT with the effects of multiple daily sessions persist for a month or more. These findings highlight the importance of aligning the disease process (e.g., temporal lobes in DAT), cognitive abilities (e.g., memory), and stimulation montage (e.g., targeting the temporal cortex). However, considerably more work is needed to clarify dose-response relationships and the neurophysiological changes mediating the behavioral effects.

Attention

The previously described study by Ferrucci and colleagues (2008) also evaluated visual attention, given the vital contribution of the parietal lobes in this process. However, there were no effects of either tDCS polarity relative to sham. Ferrucci and colleagues attributed this lack of effect to two hypotheses: (a) that the visual attention system required for task performance is too complex to be affected by a single session of stimulation, and (b) that the particular montage utilized in the study failed to sufficiently stimulate posterior parietal regions implicated in visual attention. It is also reasonable to consider a lack of task sensitivity and inappropriate target location to these potential explanations. Thus, the attentional system is clearly an understudied target for tDCS in those with dementia.

Neuropsychiatric Symptoms

The cognitive sequelae of DAT are often accompanied by a constellation of neuropsychiatric symptoms that include mood disorders, apathy, social isolation, and "personality" changes associated with impulsivity or reduced inhibitory control. Currently, only one study has assessed the impact of tDCS on such symptoms. Suemoto and colleagues (2014) evaluated the effect of six sessions of sham or 1.5 mA stimulation where the anode was over the left DLPFC (10/20 location not listed) on apathy, depression, caregiver burden, and other neuropsychiatric symptoms in a sample of 40 moderate DAT patients. There was some general improvement in mood over the two-week period that was comparable in those receiving active and sham tDCS. Therefore, while tDCS has shown promise in treating symptoms of mood and anxiety disorders (Tortella et al. 2015), additional work is clearly needed to evaluate whether this promise extends to those with DAT (or other forms of dementia). As with all studies, the inclusion criteria for both patients and caregivers should be carefully evaluated to ensure sufficient symptoms.

Overall, tDCS shows promise for the treatment of the primary cognitive deficit in DAT patients: memory. In contrast, the few existing studies of tDCS targeting attention, working memory, and neuropsychiatric symptoms have found no significant effect. These conclusions should be viewed as preliminary given the relatively small number of studies in DAT in general. Additional targets, montages, and doses should be investigated in the future. Pharmacologic trials have recently begun investigating efficacy in earlier disease stages given the limited effects in more advanced DAT stages. Thus, it is also possible that tDCS would have optimal effects if implemented earlier in the disease course, such as during the clinical precursor stage of mild cognitive impairment (MCI).

Mild Cognitive Impairment

Clinical Criteria

The transitional phase of MCI offers an ideal point in which treatments that enhance or prolong cognitive functioning can be administered, though we have previously discussed several methodological challenges in this regard (Hampstead et al. 2014). For the purpose of this chapter, the term MCI will be used in reference to the clinical precursor phase of DAT. In 2011, a workgroup commissioned by the National Institute on Aging and Alzheimer's Association published updated criteria defining MCI due to DAT (Albert et al. 2011) in order to facilitate the early identification of the conversion from cognitively asymptomatic to symptomatic. These revised criteria include (a) subjective report of cognitive decline via the patient, an informant, or skilled clinician, (b) objective evidence of impairment beyond expectations for the patient's age and educational attainment in at least one cognitive domain and, (c) preserved functional independence (Albert et al. 2011). Recognizing that multiple medical conditions could result in the above cognitive phenotype, the criteria also specify that a diagnosis of MCI is inappropriate if symptoms arise from a different underlying pathophysiologic process (e.g., traumatic brain injury) or a different neurodegenerative dementia.

Neuropathology

The above noted clinical criteria were accompanied by a list of potential biomarkers that may inform etiology and prognosis of MCI due to DAT (Albert et al. 2011). These biomarkers closely mirror the known neuropathology in AD, including amyloid beta (Aβ) levels in the cerebrospinal fluid, positron emission tomography (PET) scanning with ligands to detect fibrillar Aβ, hippocampal volume loss, or glucose hypometabolism and hypoperfusion in the posterior temporal and parietal cortex via PET and single positron emission computerized tomography (SPECT) imaging. The presumed temporal order of DAT biomarker progression (i.e., Stage 1: cerebral amyloid accumulation; Stage 2: neurodegeneration; Stage 3 subtle cognitive decline Sperling et al. 2011) has recently been challenged (Edmonds et al. 2015) but may be a critical factor to consider as it relates to tDCS efficacy.

Neuropsychological Performance

As with DAT, the severity and extent of cognitive impairment varies as a function of when individuals present clinically. Impairments generally parallel those seen in DAT. Patients with MCI due to DAT most often demonstrate impairments in memory (i.e., amnestic MCI) but may also have difficulty with aspects of language or executive functioning. Patients may also demonstrate impairments across multiple domains, particularly as they are advancing towards a DAT diagnosis.

tDCS in MCI

To date, only one randomized controlled trial has been published using tDCS in patients with MCI due to DAT. Meinzer et al. (2015) utilized a randomized double-blind crossover design to evaluate the effects of a single 20-min session of 1 mA stimulation where the anode was placed over the left lateral PFC. During each session, participants performed a semantic word retrieval task during stimulation (or sham) while undergoing fMRI (note that resting state fMRI was also acquired; Meinzer et al. 2013). Active, but not sham, stimulation enhanced patient performance to levels comparable to those of healthy older adults who took part in an earlier study (Meinzer et al. 2013). These behavioral findings were reflected by the fMRI data where bilateral PFC hyperactivation during sham tDCS was significantly reduced after active tDCS to levels comparable to those of healthy older adults. These changes were not only evident in the PFC, but also the left basal ganglia and thalamus and right middle temporal gyrus. The authors interpreted these findings as evidence of increased neural efficiency and top-down control of task performance (Meinzer et al. 2015); a pattern that fits with a "restorative" model of tDCS effects.

Additional studies of the impact of tDCS on behavior and functional activity in MCI are ongoing. Cheng and colleagues (2015) have published the protocol for a randomized double-blind study that compares three intervention conditions: sham tDCS plus adaptive N-back cognitive training, active tDCS plus adaptive N-back training, and active tDCS plus general cognitive training. The proposed montage utilizes 35cm^2 pad anode electrodes placed over the temporal lobes (T3 & T4), with a 35cm^2 pad cathode placed on the right deltoid muscle. Each group will undergo 4 weeks of three training sessions per week, with primary outcome measures of working memory (Adaptive N-back task performance) and general cognitive functioning (Alzheimer's Disease Assessment Scale – Cognitive subscale; ADAS-Cog) assessed at baseline and at 5 min post-stimulation during the fourth, eighth, and twelfth week sessions. Additional measures of language, memory, and neuropsychiatric symptoms will be assessed at baseline and after stimulation at week four, eight, and 12 to determine if tDCS and/or either cognitive training modality demonstrate far transfer effects.

We are currently performing a 2 (active vs. sham HD-tDCS) × 2 (mnemonic strategy training vs. autobiographical memory recall) double blind RCT in patients with MCI (NCT02155946). This trial builds on our earlier work that found mnemonic strategies not only enhanced long-term retention of learned information but were also accompanied by increased activation in the lateral PFC and other memory network regions in those with MCI (e.g., Hampstead et al. 2008, 2011, 2012a, b). However, two problems emerged in our earlier studies: (1) not all patients benefitted from mnemonic strategy training and (2) patients had difficulty transferring the skills to novel types of information. Thus, our ongoing study targets the lateral PFC using HD-tDCS (center anode at F5) in order to enhance the neuroplasticity of the network of interest and then capitalize on this process by pairing stimulation with mnemonic strategy training. Participants are randomized to active or sham HD-tDCS and to either mnemonic strategy training or the active control condition of autobiographical recall (analogous to reminiscence therapy). The four resulting groups are run in parallel. Participants complete baseline cognitive testing and fMRI during both task- and resting-state, followed by five consecutive daily training in which HD-tDCS (2 mA for 30 min) is performed concurrent with training. Cognitive and fMRI outcome measures are performed 3–4 days after the final stimulation session and again at 3-months. The primary outcome measures are ecologically relevant memory tasks (face-name and object-location associations) while secondary outcome measures include self-report of memory change (via the Multifactorial Memory Questionnaire) and objective evidence of near- and far-transfer (route memory and medical instructions from the Ecological Memory Simulations).

Parkinson's Disease Dementia

Clinical Characteristics

Parkinson's disease (PD) is the second most common neurodegenerative disease after DAT (de Lau and Breteler 2006). While diagnostic confirmation is performed post-mortem, probable PD requires the presence of two of the following symptoms: resting tremor, bradykinesia, rigidity or postural imbalance (Litvan et al. 2003). Symptoms typically have an asymmetric onset and are responsive to medications such as levodopa (Litvan et al. 2003). For cases in which cognitive impairments significantly interfere with instrumental activities of daily living (beyond the disturbance caused by motor symptoms), Parkinson's disease dementia (PDD) is diagnosed. The prevalence of PDD varies; however, it is estimated that between 26% and 28% of newly diagnosed PD patients develop PDD in the three-to-five years after initial diagnosis (Reid et al. 1996).

Neuropathology

PD is characterized by degeneration of dopaminergic neurons in the substantia nigra (Lehéricy et al. 2012). PDD and dementia with Lewy Bodies (DLB) share the underlying neuropathology of accumulation of alpha-synuclein embedded in Lewy bodies (Yousuf and Daniyal 2012), but differ in the clinical presentation (i.e., DLB has onset of cognitive impairments before motor symptoms). There is associated atrophy of the cerebral grey matter in bilateral frontal and temporal lobes in patients with PDD but the medial temporal lobes are generally intact relative to DAT (Burton et al. 2004).

Neuropsychological Profile

Early cognitive changes in PD are associated with dysfunction in frontostriatal and dopaminergic systems (Kehagia et al. 2010) with cognitive impairment developing in 20% to 57% of patients in three-to-five years after diagnosis (Kehagia et al. 2010). The neuropsychological profile in PD includes executive dysfunction, as evidenced by impairments in executive abilities like working memory, cognitive flexibility, response inhibition and attention (Kehagia et al. 2010). These abilities are generally believed mediated by the dorsolateral prefrontal cortex (DLPFC) and associated subcortical circuits. As the disease progresses to non-dopaminergic neuronal systems, cognitive dysfunction may develop in visuospatial abilities, memory, and verbal fluency (Kehagia et al. 2010).

Medication management, such as dopaminergic agonists or levodopa, is the first line of treatment for PD symptoms given its ability to enhance dopamine availability. Such dopaminergic enhancement can improve executive functioning and is accompanied by increased bloodflow to the DLPFC (Cools et al. 2002). However, levodopa has a range of side effects (see Boravac 2016) and generally becomes less effective with disease progression (Advokat et al. 2014). Deep brain stimulation (DBS) has promising effects for treating PD motor symptoms as it provides direct electrical stimulation to the ventral intermediate nucleus, subthalamic nucleus, or the internal segment of the globus pallidus (Perlmutter and Mink 2006). Thus, there is precedent for the success of electrical stimulation in PD using invasive methods; a critical question is whether the weak electric currents associated with non-invasive in tDCS are sufficient to mitigate motor or cognitive impairment.

tDCS in Parkinson's Disease

Improvements in motor symptoms have been found when the anode is placed over motor cortical regions (Benninger et al. 2015; Kaski et al. 2014) or the cerebellum (Ferrucci et al. 2015). However, this chapter focuses on cognitive changes associated with tDCS, a summary of which can be found in Table 16.2. Eleven studies have examined tDCS in PD, and only one study of other related Parkinsonism dementias (i.e., corticobasal syndrome). Of the 11 studies in PD, six have targeted cognition and five of these applied tDCS to the DLPFC as a method of enhancing executive functioning. These studies implemented slight variations in anode placement; three studies used F3 or F4, one study placed it halfway between F3/F4 and F7/F8, and one study did not specify the location. Regarding dose, current intensity at 1–2 mA, session duration was in the typical 20–25 min range for between one and 16 sessions. As with DAT, there is insufficient data to guide dose-response relationships. Only one of the studies measures outcomes online (Boggio et al. 2006) while the remainder tested participants offline and immediately following stimulation and up to a 16-week follow-up (Biundo et al. 2015). We discuss the efficacy of these studies below based on cognitive domain.

Executive Functioning

In one of the first tDCS studies in PD, Boggio and colleagues (2006) compared the effect of 1 mA, 2 mA, and sham stimulation with anode placement over the left DLPFC (F3) on n-back working memory task performance. Whereas no changes in 3-back performance were observed after sham or 1 mA of stimulation, 2 mA stimulation significantly increased accuracy. Critically, performance was unchanged when the anode was placed over M1. Together, these results highlight the importance of both stimulation location and electrical current intensity for tDCS efficacy in PD.

Pereira and colleagues (2013) used a randomized cross-over design with 2.0 mA stimulation where the anode was over the left DLPFC (F3) or left temporo-parietal cortex (P3-T5). Participants completed semantic and phonemic fluency tasks during fMRI immediately after stimulation. All participants completed both stimulation locations, which were counterbalanced and separated by a 2 h break. The results revealed significant improvements in phonemic fluency compared to baseline in both conditions. Functional neuroimaging during the tasks demonstrated increased connectivity in the frontal, parietal, and fusiform areas, which are associated with verbal fluency tasks in the DLPFC condition, but not the left temporo-parietal condition. The study completed both stimulations on the same day (2 h apart), which may have confounded the active tDCS results; however, the researchers questioned whether a single session of stimulation would have realistically have persisting effects over this time period.

Doruk and colleagues (2014) used a double-blind randomized procedure in which 18 PD patients received stimulation with either the anode over the left DLPFC

Table 16.2 Summary of published tDCS studies in patients with Parkinson's Disease Dementia

Refs (yr)	Diagnosis	*n*	Design	Current	Anode location (10–2-site [size])	Cathode location (10–20 site) [size]	Duration	Session schedule	Outcome measures	Measurement timing	Results summary	Side effects	Adverse effects
Benninger et al. (2015)	PD	25	Randomized double-blind group comparison (active motor vs. active premotor vs. sham)	2.0 mA	(A) Premotor and motor (10 cm anterior to Cz); (B) prefrontal (forehead above eyebrows) [97.5 cm^2]	Mastoids [25 cm^2]	20 min	8 sessions (each target area 4 times) within 2.5 weeks	Timed test of gait; bradykinesia; serial reaction time; BDI-II and SF-12v2	Offline - baseline, 24 h, 1 month and 3 months	Decreased walking time and decreased bradykinesia in tDCS vs. sham	None reported	First-degree burns (n = 1)
Bianchi et al. (2015)	Possible CBS	14	Randomized double-blind crossover (order of active left parietal, active right parietal, sham)	2.0 mA	(A) Left parietal cortex; (B) right parietal cortex [5 cm × 5 cm]	Contralateral deltoid muscle [6 cm × 8 cm]	7 min	3 sessions (1 per condition)	De Renzi ideomotor apraxia test	Offline - baseline, immediately after	Improved De Renzi scores for left AtDCS but not for right or sham	None reported	None reported

(continued)

Table 16.2 (continued)

Refs (yr)	Diagnosis	*n*	Design	Current	Anode location (10–2-site [size])	Cathode location (10–20 site) [size]	Duration	Session schedule	Outcome measures	Measurement timing	Results summary	Side effects	Adverse effects
Biundo et al. (2015)	PD-MCI	24	Randomized double-blind group comparison (active tDCS + cognitive training vs. sham)	2.0 mA	Left DLPFC [NA]	Contralateral supraorbital region [NA]	20 min	4 days/ week for 4 weeks	Unified PD Rating Scale-III (UPDRS-III), State Trait Anxiety Inventory-Y (STAI-Y), Parkinsons Disease Questionnaire-8 (PD-8), BDI-II, MoCA, RBANS	Offline - baseline, after 4 wk treatment, 16 wk	After 4 weeks: Poorer coding in active vs. sham; at 16 week follow-up: Better perfor-mance in story learning and immediate memory index in active vs. sham	None reported	None reported
Boggio et al. (2006)	PD	18	Randomized single-blind crossover (order of 1 mA, 2 mA), group comparison (active left DLPFC vs. active M1 vs. sham)	1.0 mA; 2.0 mA	(A) F3; (B) left M1 [35 cm^2]	Contralateral right orbit [35 cm^2]	20 min	3 sessions separated by 48 h	3-back letter	Online	AtDCS of LDLPFC at 2.0 mA improved accuracy compared to 1.0 mA at same location and the placebo and sham conditions	None reported	None reported

Doruk et al. (2014)	PD	18	Randomized double-blind group comparison (active left DLPFC vs. active right DLPFC vs. sham)	2.0 mA	(A) F3; (B) F4 [35 cm²]	Contralateral supraorbital region [35 cm²]	20 min	10 sessions over 2 weeks (Mon-Fri);	TMT-A & B; WCST; probabilistic classification learning; working Mmeory test; Stroop test; Hooper visual organization test; colored progressive matrices	Offline - baseline, after 2 week treatment, 1 month	TMT-B: All groups reduced time at end of 10 sessions; at 1-month follow-up both active (R and L DLPFC) had better TMT-B time than sham; no other signfiicant cognitive effects	Tingling (50%), sleepiness (55%), mild headache (22%), neck pain (11%), skin redness (22%), trouble concentrating (22%)	None reported
Ferrucci et al. (2015)	PD	9	Randomized double-blind crossover (order of active cerebellar, active M1 and sham)	2.0 mA	(A) Cerebellum (1–2 cm below the inion); (B) bilateral M1 (C3 and C4); (C) sham (half cerebellar, half M1 montage) [5 × 7 cm]	Cerebellar: Not specified; right deltoid [5 × 7 cm]	20 min	5 sessions over 5 consecutive days (1-month 'wash-out')	UPDRS; Parkinson's disease Questionnaire-8 (PDQ-8); Beck depression inventory (BDI); word recall, visual attention task (VAT), serial reaction time task (SRTT)	Offline - baseline, end of treatment, 1 wk., 4 wk	UPDRS dyskinesia score improved in both cerebellar and M1 only immediately following tDCS; no other significant effects	None reported	None reported

(continued)

Table 16.2 (continued)

Refs (yr)	Diagnosis	*n*	Design	Current	Anode location (10–2-site [size])	Cathode location (10–20 site) [size]	Duration	Session schedule	Outcome measures	Measurement timing	Results summary	Side effects	Adverse effects
Fregni et al. (2006)	PD	1	Double-blind crossover (active, sham) case study	2.0 mA	10–20% anterior to Cz [10 × 4 cm]	Inion [4 cm × 4 cm]	6.9; 5 min	Two sessions (active or sham; 2 h apart) during two 3.45 min tango dances (repeated 1 week later); 2 weeks later two 5-min sessions active or sham (1 week apart)	Trunk velocity, 6 meter walk; TUG	Online	Less trunk rigidity and faster gait velocity during tDCS tango; reduced time in TUG in tDCS vs sham	None reported	None reported

Kaski et al. (2014)	PD	1	Double-blind crossover (active, sham) case study	2.0 mA	10–20% anterior to Cz [10 × 4 cm]	Inion [4 cm × 4 cm]	6.9; 5 min	Two sessions (active or sham; 2 h apart) during two 3.45 min tango dances (repeated 1 week later); 2 weeks later two 5-min sessions active or sham (1 week apart)	Trunk velocity, 6 meter walk; TUG	Online	Less trunk rigidity and faster gait velocity during tDCS tango; reduced time in TUG in tDCS vs sham	None reported	None reported
Manenti et al. (2016)	PD	20	Double-blind covariate (age, side of stimulation) -adaptive randomized group comparison (AtDCS + phyiscal therapy vs. CtDCS + physical therapy)	2.0 mA	DLPFC: Halfway between F3 and F7 or halfway between F4 and F8 contralateral to most affected side [7 cm × 5 cm]	Contralateral supraorbital region [35 cm^2]	25 min	10 sessions over 2 weeks	Neuropsychological assessment	Offline - basline, posttreat-ment, 3 months	AtDCS group improved in PD-CRS, verbal fluency and TMT-B. Stable effects at 3 months in all except TMT-B	None reported	None reported

(continued)

Table 16.2 (continued)

Refs (yr)	Diagnosis	*n*	Design	Current	Anode location (10–2-site [size])	Cathode location (10–20 site) [size]	Duration	Session schedule	Outcome measures	Measurement timing	Results summary	Side effects	Adverse effects
Pereira et al. (2013)	PD	16	Randomized cross-over (order of DLPFC, TPC)	2.0 mA	(A) DLPFC (F3); (B) TPC (P3-T5) [35 cm^2]	Right supraorbital [35 cm^2]	20 min	1 session targeting DLPFC, 1 targeting TPC with 2-hr break between	Verbal fluency; fMRI	Offline - immediately after	AtDCS at DLPFC improved phonemic but not semantic fluency	None reported	None reported
Valentino et al. (2014)	PD	10	Randomized double-blind crossover (order of AtDCS, sham)	2.0 mA	Anteroposterior orientation over M1 (side associated with first leg to move after FOG episode) [NA]	Contralateral orbitofrontal cortex [NA]	20 min	5 sessions over 5 consecu-tive days (3-month 'wash-out')	Italian-validated MDS-UPDRS, SWS, FOG-Q	Offline - baseline, 2 days, 2wk and 4 wk	Total and part III of MDS-UPDRS, FOG-Q and gait and falls question-naire improved in active tDCS	None reported	None reported
Verheyden et al. (2013)	PD	20	Double-blind cross-over (active, sham)	1.0 mA	M1 cortex (C3) [NA]	Contralateral supraorbital region [NA]	15 min	1 session	Sit-to-stand, functional reach, standing start 180-degree turn, TUG, 10-m walk	Online	No effect, possible deleterious immediate effects	None reported	None reported

Note. *NA* not available, *PD* Parkinson's disease, *PD-MCI* Mild Cognitive Impairment due to Parkinson's disease, *tDCS* transcranial direct current stimulation, *AtDCS* stimulation under the anode, *CtDCS* stimulation under the cathode, *mA* milliamps, *DLPFC* dorsolateral prefrontal cortex, *TPC* temporoparietal cortex, *M1* primary motor cortex, *FOG* freezing of gait, *FOG-Q* Freezing of Gait Questionnaire, *TUG* timed up-and-go task, *SWS* Sit-Walk-Stand Test, *MDS-UPDRS* Movement Disorders Society - Unified Parkinson's Disease Rating Scale, *PD-CRS* Parkinson's Disease - Cognitive Rating Scale, *TMT* Trail-Making Test, *BDI-II* Beck Depression Inventory, Second Edition, *SF-12v2* Short-Form 12, Version 2, *MEP* motor-evoked potential, *fMRI* functional magnetic resonance imaging

(F3), the right DLPFC (F4), or sham. Each group completed ten 20-min sessions over two consecutive weeks (5 sessions per week). The participants completed a variety of executive functioning neuropsychological tasks before stimulation, post-stimulation, and at 1-month follow-up, including the Trail-Making Tests A & B (TMT), Wisconsin Card Sorting Task (WCST), Probabilistic Classification Learning (PCL), Working Memory (WM) Test, and the Stroop Color-Word Test. All groups demonstrated significant improvement on TMT-B immediately after the 10 sessions, which suggests general practice effects. However, these gains persisted at 1 month only in participants who received active stimulation over the DLPFC – regardless of hemisphere. There were no significant changes in any other cognitive measure. While these findings suggest some delayed benefits on select cognitive abilities, they may represent a spurious finding related to multiple comparisons and limited statistical power; therefore, replication is critical for validating these effects.

Manenti and colleagues (2016) examined the synergistic effects of physical therapy and tDCS in 20 patients with cognitive impairment associated with PD, examining both motor and cognitive outcomes. Since there is generally an asymmetric symptom presentation in PD, patients were randomized into active or sham groups using a covariate adaptive method based on age and side of motor symptoms. Specifically, the anode was placed over the DLPFC (8 cm frontally and 6 cm laterally from the scalp vertex) contralateral to the individual's most affected limb. Each group completed ten 25-min sessions over 2 weeks (five consecutive days per week) while completing physical therapy exercises. Relative to sham, active stimulation resulted in significant post-treatment improvement on the Parkinson's Disease Cognitive Rating Scale (PD-CRS), semantic fluency, and TMT-B tasks. Impressively, PD-CRS and semantic fluency gains persisted at a three-month follow-up.

Learning and Memory

A single study has evaluated the effects of tDCS on learning and memory in PD patients. Biundo and colleagues (2015) compared 4 weeks (16 total sessions) of concurrent computer-based cognitive training and active or sham tDCS with anode placement over the left DLPFC (F3) in 24 PD patients with memory deficits. Neuropsychological tests (e.g., Montreal Cognitive Assessment; Repeatable Battery for the Assessment of Neuropsychological Status [RBANS]) were administered at baseline, following the 4-week treatment, and at a 16-week follow-up. The active tDCS group showed significantly worse performance on a measure of psychomotor processing speed immediately post-training relative to sham but performances were comparable at 16 weeks. There were no statistically significant beneficial effects of active tDCS. However, there were encouraging trends at the follow-up wherein medium to large effect sizes suggested beneficial effects of active tDCS on the Story Learning subtest ($p = 0.077$; Cohen's $d = 0.9$) and Immediate Memory Index ($p = 0.075$; Cohen's $d = 0.7$) of the RBANS. Thus, additional work is clearly needed to determine whether these promising effect sizes represent actual improvement.

Corticobasal Syndrome

Corticobasal syndrome (CBS) is a neurodegenerative process characterized by insidious onset of stiffness, dystonia, and clumsiness resistant to levodopa treatment (Armstrong et al. 2013). Characteristic clinical presentation includes asymmetric onset of motor symptoms, “alien limb” syndrome, and apraxia (Boeve 2011). CBS is a collection of symptoms that are generally associated with corticobasal degeneration (CBD), a Parkinson’s plus syndrome; however, neuropathological studies have revealed that CBS is non-specific to CBD, but can be found in Alzheimer’s disease, progressive supranuclear palsy, and frontotemporal lobar degeneration (Lee et al. 2011). As levodopa is not efficacious in treating CBS, and genetic or neuropathological substrates for treatment have not been defined, tDCS may present an option for managing the symptoms of CBS.

tDCS in CBS

To date, only one study has examined tDCS as an intervention in CBS. Bianchi and colleagues (2015) used a double-blind randomized, sham-controlled crossover design with 14 individuals with bilateral or asymmetric limb apraxia and possible CBS. Seven min of 2.0 mA stimulation was administered with the anode over the right (about halfway between P4 and P8) or left parietal cortex (about halfway between P3 and P7) and the cathode on the contralateral deltoid muscle. Each participant completed the three conditions over 2 days (i.e., sham, then active condition on 1 day; active condition on another day). The results revealed a significant improvement in ideomotor praxis following stimulation over the left parietal cortex. No significant changes in praxis were found following sham stimulation or stimulation over the right parietal cortex. The findings provide interesting preliminary evidence that builds on decades of functional neuroanatomic work linking the left parietal cortex and ideomotor apraxia; however, larger and more homogenous samples are required to verify these findings and the clinical application of tDCS in this population.

Frontotemporal Dementia

Clinical Characteristics

Frontotemporal dementia (FTD) is a heterogeneous group of disorders characterized by progressive neurodegeneration of the frontal and temporal lobes (Bott et al. 2014). Age of onset is typically younger than other dementias with the average most commonly between 50 and 60 years old (Saykin and Rabin 2014). Approximately half of all FTD cases are behavioral variant (bvFTD), which is characterized by early changes in personality and impaired social functioning (Bott et al. 2014). In bvFTD there is focal atrophy bilaterally in the frontal lobes (Bott et al. 2014). The remaining half of FTD cases are classified as subtypes of primary progressive aphasia (PPA) and are characterized by focal language deficits (Bott et al. 2014). The semantic variant (svPPA) presents with loss of semantic knowledge and associated atrophy in the anterior temporal lobes bilaterally (Bott et al. 2014). The nonfluent variant/agrammatic (nfvPPA or avPPA) presents with motor-speech difficulties and agrammatism with associated atrophy in the left inferior frontal and insular regions (Bott et al. 2014). Logopenic variant (lvPPA) is characterized by slowed speech and frequent word-finding pauses and has cortical atrophy in the left temporoparietal junction area (Gorno-Tempini et al. 2011) (Table 16.3).

tDCS in FTD

Nine studies have examined tDCS effects in FTD, three of which have been case studies. Since there is great heterogeneity in clinical presentations of FTD and associated differential cortical atrophy, the majority of studies have focused on a specific FTD subtypes (i.e., one case study with behavioral variant, four studies with nonfluent PPA, and study study with semantic variant PPA). Three studies combined FTD subtypes; one combined behavioral variant ($n = 9$) and language variant ($n = 1$; Huey et al. 2007) and the others combined participants with nonfluent variant and logopenic variant PPA (Gervits et al. 2016; Tsapkini et al. 2014). Given this heterogeneity, tDCS studies have varied greatly in the montages focusing on the left DLPFC (Cotelli et al. 2014, 2016), language cortical areas (crosspoint between T3/P3 and C3/T5 or crosspoint between T3/Fz and F7/Cz; Wang et al. 2013), F7 and F3 (Huey et al. 2007), and on the temporal pole using MRI guidance. The stimulation intensities varied from 1 mA to 2 mA and sessions lasted for 20–25 min. The studies greatly varied in the duration of treatment ranging from single-session to 20 sessions over 4 weeks. With the exception of one study, all outcomes were measured offline and time points ranged from immediately following tDCS to 48 weeks after stimulation.

tDCS in Advanced FTD

Huey and colleagues (2007) used a double-blind sham-controlled design to examine the effects of anodal tDCS in advanced FTD. Ten participants that met criteria for FTD (nine with primarily behavioral symptoms and one with language symptoms) completed one 40-min session with 2 mA stimulation with the anode at F3. No significant differences were found between the active and sham conditions. The

Table 16.3 Summary of published tDCS studies in patients with Frontotemporal Dementia

Ref (yr)	Diagnosis	*n*	Design	Current	Anode location (10–2-site [size])	Cathode location (10–20 site) [size]	Duration	Session schedule	Outcome measures	Measurement timing	Results summary	Side effects	Adverse effects
Agarwal et al. (2016)	bvFD	1	Case study	2.0 mA	Between F3 and FP1 [NA]	Right supraorbital area [NA]	20 min	2 sessions per day (separated by 3 h) for 5 days	Observed functional abilities; FTD rating scale	Offline	Improved speech output, began cooking, washing clothes; FRS logit score improved	None reported	None reported
Cotelli et al. (2016)	nfvPPA	18	Within subjects comparison (AtDCS + individualized computerized training [ICAT])	2.0 mA	Left DLPFC (8 cm frontally and 6 cm laterally of scalp vertex) [5 cm × 5 cm]	Right arm [6 cm × 10 cm]	25 min	10 sessions over 2 weeks	Neuropsychological assessment	Offline - baseline, posttreatment, 3 months	Improved naming of treated and untreated objects at post-treatment and at 3-month follow-up	Marginal perceptual sensations	None reported
Cotelli et al. (2014)	nfvPPA	16	Randomized double-blind group comparison (AtDCS vs. sham + individualized computerized training [ICAT])	2.0 mA	Left DLPFC (8 cm frontally and 6 cm laterally from scalp vertex) [5 cm × 5 cm]	Right shoulder [6 cm × 10 cm]	25 min	10 sessions over 2 weeks	Neuropsychological assessment	Offline - baseline, post-treatment, 12 weeks	Naming improved in both AtDCS and sham with greater effects in AtDCS which remained at 12 weeks; analysis of daily living language improved in AtDCS only	None reported	None reported

Gervits et al. (2016)	PPA	6	Within subjects comparison	1.5 mA	F7 [5 cm × 5 cm]	Left occipito-parietal region [5 cm × 5 cm]	20 min	10 sessions over 2 weeks	Linguistic assessment battery	Offline - baseline, post-treatment, 6 weeks	Improvements in speech production and grammatical comprehension sustained for 3 months	None reported	None reported
Huey et al. (2007)	FTD	10	Randomized double-blind crossover (order of active vs. sham)	2.0 mA	F3 [25 cm^2]	Right supraorbital area [25 cm^2]	40 min	1 session anodal, 1 sham	Verbal fluency	Online	No signficant changes	None reported	None reported
Teichmann et al. (2016)	svPPA	12 clinical; 15 controls	Double-blind cross-over (AtDCS, CtDCS, sham)	1.59 mA	(A) Stimulation under the anode over MRI-guided left temporal pole; cathode over FT8 to FT10 [25 cm^2]; (B) stimulation under cathode over MRI-guided right temporal pole, anode placed over AF8 [25 cm^2]	(A) Stimulation under the anode over MRI-guided left temporal pole; cathode over FT8 to FT10 [25 cm^2]; (B) stimulation under cathode over MRI-guided right temporal pole, anode placed over AF8 [25 cm^2]	20 min	1 session per montage separated by 1 week	Semantic matching	Offline - baseline, immediately after stimulation	Left AtDCS and right CtDCS improved semantic accuracy; right CtDCS also improved processing speed	None reported	None reported

(continued)

Table 16.3 (continued)

Ref (yr)	Diagnosis	*n*	Design	Current	Anode location (10–2-site [size])	Cathode location (10–20 site) [size]	Duration	Session schedule	Outcome measures	Measurement timing	Results summary	Side effects	Adverse effects
Tsapkini et al. (2014)	PPA	6	Double-blind cross-over (active + spelling intervention vs sham + spelling intervention)	1–2 mA	F7 [2 inch × 2 inch]	NA	20 min	15 sessions (3–5 per week) conditions separated by 2 months	# Correct phoneme-grapheme correspon-dences and # correctly spelled word prompts	Offline - baseline, post-treatment, 2 weeks, 2 months	Untrained items improved in tDCS but not in sham	None reported	None reported
Wang et al. (2013)	nfvPPA	1	Cross-over case study (AtDCS at left Wernicke's point + AtDCS at left Broca's point vs. sham)	1.2 mA	(A) Crosspoint between T3-P3 and C3-T5 (left Wernicke's point); (B) cross point between T3-Fz and F7-Cz (left Broca's point)	Right shoulder	20 min	2 sessions per day for 5 days (Wernicke's in morning, Broca's in afternoon) per phase; phases: Sham1-Active1-Sham2-Active2	Subtests of the psycholin-guistic assess-ment in Chinese aphasia (PACA)	Offline - before and after each stimulation	Accuracy improved after AtDCS of Wernicke's area; no other significant differences	None reported	None reported

NA not available, *FTD* Frontotemporal Dementia, *bvFTD* behavioral variant FTD, *PPA* Primary Progressive Aphasia, *svPPA* semantic variant PPA, *nfvPPA* Nonfluent Variant PPA, *AtDCS* stimultion under the anode, *CtDCS* stimulation under the cathode, *mA* milliamps, *DLPFC* dorsolateral prefrontal cortex, *MRI* magnetic resonance imaging

authors hypothesized that this lack of effect resulted from the current being impacted by increased CSF secondary to brain atrophy of the targeted region. While reasonable, the authors assumed atrophy to be present and did not confirm its presence using neuroimaging. Equally plausible explanations are the heterogeneity of the group, small sample size, and use of a single session design.

tDCS in bvFTD

A single case study has been performed with tDCS in bvFTD (Agarwal et al. 2016). A female 45-year-old patient diagnosed with probable bvFTD 4 months prior completed a total of ten, 20-min sessions that were administered twice per day (separated by 3 h) over five consecutive days. Stimulation was performed at 2 mA with the anode placed between F3 and FP1 and the cathode placed over the right supraorbital region. The patient demonstrated significant improvements in the FTD Rating Scale and in subjectively observed functional activities (i.e., speech output, cooking, washing clothes). Improvements persisted in follow-up appointments throughout the following 7 months (Agarwal et al. 2016).

tDCS in PPA

Gervits and colleagues (2016) studied the effects of tDCS with the anode placed over the left frontotemporal region (F7) in a case series of six un-blinded participants with PPA (two with nfvPPA, four with lvPPA). Participants received ten, 20-min stimulation sessions at 1.5 mA and were asked to narrate wordless picture books during stimulation. The participants completed a one-to-two hour linguistic assessment that measured a wide range of linguistic abilities that yielded four composite measures (Speech Production, Grammatical Comprehension, Repetition, and Semantic Processing) and one global composite score. Improvements were found in speech production and grammatical comprehension composite scores, and the effects persisted at 3 months; however, without sham control or comparison group, the role of expectation or placebo cannot be quantified.

Tsapkini and colleagues (2014) used a sham-controlled cross-over design with six patients with PPA (two nfvPPA; four lvPPA) to compare the effects of stimulation concurrent with spelling training. Here, the anode was placed over F7 since this area overlies the left inferior frontal gyrus, which is implicated in phoneme-to-grapheme translations. The participants completed 15 sessions (3–5 sessions per week) with a two-month washout period between conditions. The results revealed significant improvements in spelling ability for trained items in both sham and active tDCS; however, untrained item spelling improved only in the active tDCS condition and persisted at two-week and two-month follow-ups (Tsapkini et al. 2014).

A single case study has examined nfvPPA and demonstrated long-lasting language improvements. In a case study using a cross-over sham-controlled design, a 67-year-old nfvPPA patient completed two 20-min sessions of 1.2 mA stimulation where the anode was placed over "Wernicke's area" (crosspoint between T3-P3 and C3-T5) in the morning, and over "Broca's area" (cross point between T3-Fz and F7-Cz) in the afternoon (Wang et al. 2013). The conditions were completed in the following order: $Sham_1$, $Active_1$, $Sham_2$, $Active_2$. The individual demonstrated improvements on the Psycholinguistic Assessment in Chinese Aphasia (PACA), with particular improvement in naming (2/30 items correct at baseline, 11/30 items correct post-stimulation) after the first active stimulation session only. No further gains were demonstrated after the second active condition.

Cotelli and colleagues (2014) used a randomized sham-controlled design to evaluate the effect of tDCS on naming in 16 patients with nfvPPA. Participants completed 10 (five session per week for 2 weeks) 25-min sessions of stimulation with the anode over the left DLPFC (8 cm frontally and 6 cm laterally from vertex) and cathode on the right shoulder. Stimulation was applied during anomia training. No control group was used; instead, pre-post analyses were completed, with naming performance measured at baseline, after the last stimulation session, and at three-month follow-up. Significant naming improvement was found post-intervention and persisted at the three-month follow-up. The authors also examined the impact of structural compromise on naming improvement and found that change in performance on trained object naming was positively correlated with baseline grey matter volume in the left fusiform, left middle temporal, and right inferior temporal gyri. Cotelli and colleagues (2016) later replicated the persistent effect of tDCS in 18 patients with nfvPPA who underwent the same montage, session schedule, and anomia training program. There were significant improvements in naming for both trained and untrained items that persisted at the three-month follow-up. Together, these results suggest that earlier intervention may promote greater benefit from tDCS and that tDCS may pair well with other behavioral interventions for the treatment of nfvPPA. Future studies must include control groups to determine (a) whether improvements can be can attributed to the intervention, as opposed to practice effects, and (b) whether tDCS specifically enhances the positive effects of behavioral interventions, such as anomia training.

Only one study has examined tDCS in svPPA. Teichmann and colleagues (2016) used a double-blind sham-controlled cross-over design to evaluate the effect of stimulation on semantic matching in 12 patients and 15 healthy controls. Participants completed one 20-min stimulation session for each of three montages (2 active; 1 sham). Electrode location was guided by baseline MRI scans that identified: 1) the left temporal pole, over which the anode was placed and stimulation applied in Condition 1, and 2) the right temporal pole, over which the cathode was placed and stimulation applied in Condition 2. Both stimulation conditions improved semantic matching relative to sham but only condition 2 (cathode over the right temporal pole) improved processing speed. While MRI guided electrode placement is atypical in tDCS, these findings provide interesting preliminary evidence that such methods also hold promise in this area of neuromodulation.

Conclusions and Future Directions

In summary, early trials of tDCS (both controlled and uncontrolled) as an intervention for neurodegenerative dementias demonstrate mixed but promising findings without the deleterious side effects of some pharmacological interventions. The efficacy of tDCS varies greatly across dementia subtype and cognitive domain, at least in part due to heterogeneity in study design. To date, no study has systematically varied important study design elements like comparison method (e.g. crossover vs. parallel groups), montage details (e.g., electrode size, placement), electrical current intensity, session schedule (e.g., number, duration, and spacing of sessions), or outcome measurement timing (e.g., online vs. offline measurement). Furthermore, outcome measures varied widely across studies and may not have always been optimally matched to montage or cognitive construct. The gross majority of studies also utilize traditional pad-based approaches to tDCS, with our ongoing RCT being the only study to our knowledge to use the more focal HD-tDCS approach. Such dose-response information is essential for better understanding tDCS effects.

A second potential explanation for the mixed findings relates to the inter-individual variability seen both within and across dementia subtypes. As noted above, neurodegeneration characterizes these conditions and may dramatically affect electrical current flow given evidence that inter-individual variability in skull and brain morphology impacts current density, flow, and localization in even healthy adults (Bikson et al. 2012; Datta et al. 2012). Thus, the traditional use of the 10/20 system may be insufficient even for tDCS targeting. Computational modeling and, possibly, MRI guided electrode placement may allow for more individualized montages that optimize results.

Finally, most published studies and clinical trials using tDCS for dementia have small and often heterogeneous samples comprised of patients with varying neuropathological burden and neuropsychological deficits. Larger trials are needed to elucidate whether a 'critical period' of maximal benefit from tDCS exists for healthy adults and those with cognitive impairment. Despite these limitations, tDCS offers a cost-effective, safe, and well-tolerated option that warrants further study.

References

Advokat, C. D., Comaty, J. E., & Julien, R. M. (2014). *Julien's primer of drug action*. New York, NY: Worth Publishers.

Agarwal, S. M., Rajur, S., Bose, A., Shenoy, S., Miriyala, S., Shivakkumar, V., & Venkatasubramanian, G. (2016). Use of transcranial direct current stimulation (tDCS) in a woman with behavioral variant fronto-temporal dementia. *Asian Journal of Psychiatry, 21*, 31–32.

Albert, M. S., DeKosky, S. T., Dickson, D., Dubois, B., Feldman, H. H., Fox, B. C., ... Phelps, C. H. (2011). The diagnosis of mild cognitive impairment due to Alzheimer's disease: Recommendations for the National Institute on Aging-Alzheimer's Association workgroups on diagnostic guidelines for Alzheimer's disease. *Alzheimer's Dementia, 7*(3), 270–279.

Alzheimer's Association. (2016). 2016 Alzheimer's disease facts and figures. *Alzheimer's & Dementia, 12*(4), 1–84.

Armstrong, M. J., Litvan, I., Lang, A. E., Bak, T. H., Bhatia, K. P., Borroni, B., … Winer, W. J. (2013). Criteria for the diagnosis of corticobasal degeneration. *Neurology, 80*(5), 496–503.

Batsikadze, G., Moliadze, V., Paulus, W., Kuo, M. F., & Nitsche, M. A. (2013). Partially non-linear stimulation intensity-dependent effects of direct current stimulation on motor cortex excitability in humans. *Journal of Physiology, 51*(7), 1987–2000.

Benninger, D. H., Lomarev, M., Lopez, G., Wassermann, E. M., Li, X., Considine, E., & Hallett, M. (2015). Transcranial direct current stimulation for the treatment of Parkinson's disease. *J Neurol Neurosurg Psychiatry, 81*, 1105–1111.

Bianchi, M., Cosseddu, M., Manenti, R., Brambilla, M., Rizzetti, C., Padovani, A., & Borroni, B. (2015). Left parietal cortex transcranial direct current stimulation enhances gesture processing in corticobasal syndrome. *European Journal of Neurology, 22*, 1317–1322.

Bikson, M., Rahman, A., Datta, A., Fregni, F., & Merabet, L. (2012). High-resolution modeling assisted design of customized and individualized transcranial direct current stimulation protocols. *Neuromodulation, 15*, 306–315.

Biundo, R., Fiorenzato, E., Gentile, G., Martinez-Martin, P., & Bisiacchi, P. (2015). Double-blind randomized trial of t-DCS versus sham in Parkinson patients with mild cognitive impairment receiving cognitive training. *Brain Stimulation, 8*, 1223–1240.

Boeve, B. F. (2011). The multiple phenotypes of corticobasal syndrome and corticobasal degeneration: Implications for further study. *Journal of Molecular Neuroscience, 45*, 350–353.

Boggio, P. S., Ferrucci, R., Mameli, F., Martins, D., Martins, O., Vergari, M., … Priori, A. (2012). Prolonged visual memory enhancement after direct current stimulation in Alzheimer's disease. *Brain Stimulation, 5*, 223–230.

Boggio, P. S., Ferrucci, R., Rigonatti, S. P., Covre, P., Nitche, M., Pascual-Leone, A., & Fregni, F. (2006). Effects of transcranial direct current stimulation on working memory in patients with Parkinson's disease. *Journal of Neurological Sciences, 249*, 31–38.

Boggio, P. S., Khoury, L. P., Martins, D. C. S., Martins, O. E. M. S., Macedo, E. C., & Fregni, F. (2009). Temporal cortex direct current stimulation enhances performance on a visual recognition memory task in Alzheimer's disease. *Journal of Neurology, Neurosurgery, & Psychiatry, 80*, 444–447.

Boravac, J. A. (2016). Side effects of a dopamine agonist therapy for Parkinson's disease: A mini-review of clinical pharmacology. *Yale Journal of Biology and Medicine, 89*(1), 37–47.

Bott, N. T., Radke, A., Stephens, M. L., & Kramer, J. H. (2014). Frontotemporal dementia: diagnosis, deficits and management. *Neurodegenerative disease management, 4*(6), 439–454.

Braak, H., & Braak, E. (1991). Neuropathological stageing of Alzheimer-related changes. *Acta Neuropathologica, 82*(4), 239–259.

Burton, E. J., McKeith, I. G., Burn, D. J., Williams, D., & O'Brien, J. T. (2004). Cerebral atrophy in Parkinson's disease with the without dementia: A comparison with Alzheimer's disease, dementia with Lewy bodies and controls. *Brain, 127*, 791–800.

Bystad, M., Rasmussen, I. D., Abeler, K., & Aslaksen, P. M. (2016). Accelerated direct current stimulation in Alzheimer's disease: A case study. *Brain Stimulation, 9*, 634–635.

Cheng, C. P. W., Chan, S. S. M., Mak, A. D. P., Chan, W. C., Cheng, S. T., Shi, L., … Lam, L. (2015). Would transcranial direct current stimulation (tDCS) enhance the effects of working memory training in older adults with mild neurocognitive disorder due ot Alzheimer's disease: Study protocol for a randomized controlled trial. *Trials, 16*, 479–486.

Cools, R., Stefanova, E., Barker, R. A., Robbins, T. W., & Owen, A. M. (2002). Dopaminergic modulation of high-level cognition in Parkinson's disease: The role of the prefrontal cortex revealed by PET. *Brain, 125*, 584–594.

Cotelli, M., Manenti, R., Paternico, D., Cosseddu, M., Brambilla, M., Petesi, M., … Borroni, B. (2016). Grey matter density predicts the improvement of naming abilities after tDCS intervention in agrammatic variant of primary progressive aphasia. *Brain Topography, 29*, 738–751.

Cotelli, M., Manenti, R., Petesi, M., Brambilla, M., Cosseddu, M., Zanetti, O., … Borroni, B. (2014). Treatment of primary progressive aphasias by transcranial direct current stimulation combined with language training. *Journal of Alzhemier's Disease, 39*, 779–808.

Datta, A., Truong, D., Minhas, P., Parra, L. C., & Bikson, M. (2012). Inter-individual variation during transcranial direct current stimulation and normalization of dose using MRI-derived computational models. *Frontiers in Psychiatry, 3*(91), 1–8.

De Lau, L. M., & Breteler, M. M. (2006). Epidemiology of Parkinson's disease. *Lancet Neurology, 5*(6), 525–535.

Doruk, D., Gray, Z., Bravo, G. L., Pascual-Leone, A., & Fregni, F. (2014). Effects of tDCS on executive function in Parkinson's disease. *Neuroscience Letters, 582*, 27–31.

Edmonds, E. C., Delano-Wood, L., Galasko, D. R., Salmon, D. P., & Bondi, M. W. (2015). Subtle cognitive decline and biomarker staging in preclinical Alzheimer's disease. *Journal of Alzheimer's Disease, 47*, 231–242.

Ferrucci, R., Cortese, F., Bianchi, M., Pittera, D., Turrone, R., Bocci, T., … Priori, A. (2015). Cerebellar and motor cortical transcranial stimulation decrease Levodopa-induced dyskinesias in Parkinson's disease. *Cerebellum, 15*(1), 43–47.

Ferrucci, R., Mameli, F., Guidi, I., Mrakic-Sposta, S., Vergari, M., Marceglia, S., … Priori, A. (2008). Transcranial direct current stimulation improves recognition memory in Alzheimer's disease. *Neurology, 71*, 493–498.

Fregni, F., Boggio, P. S., Santos, M. C., Lima, M., Vieira, A. L., Rigonatti, S. P., … Pascual-Leone, A. (2006). Noninvasive cortical stimulation with transcranial direct current stimulation in Parkinson's disease. *Movement Disorders, 21*(10), 1693–1702.

Gervits, F., Ash, S., Coslett, H. B., Rascovsky, K., & Grossman, M. (2016). Transcranial direct current stimulation for the treatment of primary progressive aphasia: An open-label pilot study. *Brain & Language, 162*, 35–41.

Gorno-Tempini, M. L., Hillis, A. E., Weintraub, S., Kertesz, A., Mendez, M., Cappa, S. F., … Grossman, M. (2011). Classification of primary progressive aphasia and its variants. *Neurology, 76*(11), 1006–1014.

Hampstead, B. M., Gillis, M. M., & Stringer, A. Y. (2014). Cognitive rehabilitation of memory for mild cognitive impairment: A methodological review and model for future research. *Journal of the International Neuropsychological Society, 20*(2), 135–151.

Hampstead, B. M., Sathian, K., Moore, A. B., Nalisnick, C., & Stringer, A. Y. (2008). Explicit memory training leads to improved memory for face-name pairs in patients with mild cognitive impairment: Results of a pilot investigation. *Journal of the International Neuropsychological Society, 14*(5), 883–889.

Hampstead, B. M., Sathian, K., Phillips, P. A., Amaraneni, A., Delaune, W. R., & Stringer, A. Y. (2012a). Mnemonic strategy training improves memory for object location associations in both healthy elderly and patients with amnestic mild cognitive impairment: A randomized, single-blind study. *Neuropsychology, 26*(3), 385–399.

Hampstead, B. M., Stringer, A. Y., Stilla, R. F., Deshpande, G., Hu, X., Moore, A. B., … Sathian, K. (2011). Activation and effective connectivity changes following explicit-memory training for face-name pairs in patients with mild cognitive impairment: A pilot study. *Neurorehabilitation and Neural Repair, 25*(3), 210–222.

Hampstead, B. M., Stringer, A. Y., Stilla, R. F., & Sathian, K. (2012b). Mnemonic strategy training partially restores hippocampal activity in patients with mild cognitive impairment. *Hippocampus, 22*(8), 1652–1658.

Huey, E. D., Probasco, J. C., Moll, J., Stocking, J., Ko, M.-H., Grafman, J., & Wassermann, E. M. (2007). No effect of DC brain polarization on verbal fluency in patients with advanced ftronto-temporal dementia. *Clinical Neurophysiology, 118*(6), 1417–1418.

Kaski, D., Allum, J. H., Bronstein, A. M., & Dominguez, R. O. (2014). Applying anodal tDCS during tango dancing in a patient with Parkinson's disease. *Neuroscience Letters, 568*, 39–43.

Kehagia, A. A., Barker, R. A., & Robbins, T. W. (2010). Neuropsychological and clinical heterogeneity of cognitive impairment and dementia in patients with Parkinson's disease. *Lancet Neurology, 9*, 1200–1213.

Kelley, A. S., McGarry, K., Gorges, R., & Skinner, J. S. (2015). The burden of health care costs for patients with dementia in the last 5 years of life. *Annals of Internal Medicine, 163*(10), 729–736.

Khedr, E. M., El Gamel, N. F., El-Fetoh, N. A., Khalifa, H., Ahmed, E. M., Ali, A. M., … Karim, A. A. (2014). A double-blind randomized clinical trial on the efficacy of cortical direct current stimulation for the treatment of Alzheimer's disease. *Frontiers in Aging Neuroscience, 6*(275), 1–12.

Lee, S. E., Rabinovici, G. D., Mayo, M. C., Wilson, S. M., Seeley, W. W., DeArmond, S. J., … Sidhu, M. (2011). Clinicopathological correlations in corticobasal degeneration. *Annals of Neurology, 70*, 327–340.

Lehéricy, S., Sharman, M. A., Longo Dos Santos, C., Paquin, R., & Gallea, C. (2012). Magnetic resonance imaging of the substantia nigra in Parkinson's disease. *Movement Disorders, 27*(7), 822–830.

Litvan, I., Bhatia, K. P., Burn, D. J., Goetz, C. G., Lang, A. E., McKeith, I., … Wenning, G. K. (2003). Movement Disorder Society Scientific Issues Committee report: SIC Task Force appraisal of clinical diagnostic criteria for Parkinsonian disorders. *Movement Disorders, 18*, 467–486.

Manenti, R., Brambilla, M., Benussi, A., Rosini, S., Cobelli, C., Ferrari, C., … Cotelli, M. (2016). Mild cognitive impairment in Parkinson's disease is improved by transcranial direct current stimulation combined with physical therapy. *Movement Disorders, 31*(5), 715–724.

Marceglia, S., Mrakic-Sposta, S., Rosa, M., Ferrucci, R., Mameli, F., Vergari, M., … Priori, A. (2016). Transcranial direct current stimulation modulates cortical neuronal activity in Alzheimer's disease. *Frontiers in Neuroscience, 10*(134), 1–11.

McKhann, G. M., Knopman, D. S., Chertkow, H., Hyman, B. T., Jack, C. R., Kawas, C. H., … Phelps, C. H. (2011). The diagnosis of dementia due to Alzheimer's disease: Recommendations from the National Institute on Aging-Alzheimer's Association workgroups on diagnostic guidelines for Alzheimer's disease. *Alzheimer's Dementia, 7*(3), 263–269.

Meinzer, M., Lindenberger, R., Antonenko, D., Flaisch, T., & Floel, A. (2013). Anodal transcranial direct current stimulation temporarily reverses age-associated cognitive decline and functional brain activity changes. *Journal of Neuroscience, 33*, 12470–12478.

Meinzer, M., Lindenberger, R., Phan, M. T., Ulm, L., Volk, C., & Floel, A. (2015). Transcranial direct current stimulation in mild cognitive impairment: Behavioral effects and neural mechanisms. *Alzheimer's and Dementia, 11*, 1032–1040.

Pereira, J. B., Junque, C., Bartres-Faz, D., Marti, M., Sala-Llonch, R., Compta, Y., … Tolosa, E. (2013). Modulation of verbal fluency networks by transcranial direct current stimulation (tDCS) in Parkinson's disease. *Brain Stimulation, 6*, 16–24.

Perl, D. P. (2010). Neuropathology of Alzheimer's disease. *Mount Sinai Journal of Medicine, 77*(1), 32–42.

Perlmutter, J. S., & Mink, J. W. (2006). Deep brain stimulation. *Annual Review of Neuroscience, 29*, 229–257.

Plassman, B. L., Langa, K. M., Fisher, G. G., Heeringa, S. G., Weir, D. R., Ofstedal, M. B., … Wallace, R. B. (2007). Prevalence of dementia in the United States: The aging, demographics, and memory study. *Neuroepidemiology, 29*, 125–132.

Prince, M., Bryce, R., Albanese, E., Wimo, A., Ribeiro, W., & Ferri, C. P. (2013). The global prevalence of dementia: A systematic review and metaanalysis. *Alzheimer's and Dementia, 9*, 63–75.

Reid, W. G. J., Hely, M. A., Morris, J. G. L., Broe, G. A., Adena, M., Sullivan, D. J. O., & Williamson, P. M. (1996). A longitudinal study of Parkinson's disease: Clinical and neuropsychological correlates of dementia. *Journal of Clinical Neuroscience, 3*, 327–333.

Saykin, A. J., & Rabin, L. A. (2014). Dementias and neurodegenerative diseases. In M. W. Parsons & T. A. Hammeke (Eds.), *Clinical neuropsychology: A pocket handbook for assessment* Washington, DC, US: American Psychological Association. (pp. 266–286). http://dx.doi.org/10.1037/14339-012

Serrano-Pozo, A., Frosch, M. P., Masliah, E., & Hyman, B. T. (2011). Neuropathological alterations in Alzheimer's disease. *Cold Spring Harbor Perspectives in Medicine, 1*(1), 1–23.

Sperling, R. A., Aisen, P. S., Beckett, D. A., Craft, S., Fagan, A. M., Iwatsubo, T., … Phelps, C. H. (2011). Toward defining the preclinical stages of Alzheimer's disease: Recommendations from the National Institute on Aging-Alzheimer's Association workgroups on diagnostic guidelines for Alzheimer's disease. *Alzheimer's Dementia, 7*(3), 280–292.

Suemoto, C. K., Apolinario, D., Nakamura-Palacios, E. M., Lopes, L., Paraizo Leite, R. E., Castro Sales, M., … Fregni, F. (2014). Effects of a non-focal plasticity protocol on apathy in moderate Alzheimer's disease: A randomized, double-blind, sham-controlled trial. *Brain Stimulation, 7*, 308–313.

Teichmann, M., Lesoil, C., Godard, J., Vernet, M., Bertrand, A., Levy, R., … Kas, A. (2016). Direct current stimulation over the anterior temporal areas boosts semantic processing in primary progressive aphasia. *Annals of Neurology*.

Tortella, G., Casati, R., Aparicio, L. V. M., Mantovani, A., Senco, N., D'Urso, G., … Brunoni, A. R. (2015). Transcranial direct current stimulation in psychiatric disorders. *World Journal of Psychiatry, 5*(1), 88–102.

Tsapkini, K., Frangakis, C., Gomez, Y., Davis, C., & Hillis, A. E. (2014). Augmentation of spelling therapy with transcranial direct current stimulation in primary progressive aphasia: Preliminary results and challenges. *Aphasiology, 28*(8–9), 1112–1130.

Valentino, F., Cosentino, G., Brighina, F., Pozzi, N. G., Sandrini, G., Fierro, B., … Pacchetti, C. (2014). Transcranial direct current stimulation for treatment of freezing of gait: a cross-over study. *Movement Disorders, 29*(8), 1064–1069.

Verheyden, G., Purdey, J., Burnett, M., Cole, J., & Ashburn, A. (2013). Immediate effect of transcranial direct current stimulation on postural stability and functional mobility in Parkinson's disease. *Movement Disorders, 28*(14), 2040–2041.

Wang, J., Wu, D., Chen, Y., Yuan, Y., & Zhang, M. (2013). Effects of transcranial direct current stimulation on language improvement and cortical activation in nonfluent variant primary progressive aphasia. *Neuroscience Letters, 549*, 29–33.

Welsh-Bohmer, K. A., & Warren, L. H. (2006). Neurodegenerative dementias. In D. K. Attix & K. A. Welsh-Bohmer (Eds.), *Geriatric neuropsychology: Assessment and intervention* (pp. 56–88). New York, NY: The Guilford Press.

Wiethoff, S., Hamada, M., & Rothwell, J. C. (2014). Variability in response to transcranial direct current stimulation of the motor cortex. *Brain Stimulation, 7*, 468–475.

Yousuf, M. S., & Daniyal, U. (2012). Dementia in Parkinson's disease – A comprehensive review. *Journal of Parkinsonism & Restless Legs Syndrome, 21*(1), 6–10.

Chapter 17
Transcranial Direct Current Stimulation in Stroke Rehabilitation: Present and Future

Oluwole O. Awosika and Leonardo G. Cohen

Introduction

Stroke is a leading cause of serious longtime disability around the world (Bernhardt et al. 2016; Dobkin 2005; Dobkin and Dorsch 2013; Langhorne et al. 2011; Mead et al. 2012). New training-based neurorehabilitative techniques have been applied in the subacute and chronic stage after stroke [constraint-induced movement therapy, robot-assisted devices, functional electrical stimulation, body weight supported treadmill, over ground walking, and neuropharmaceuticals (i.e. selective serotonin reuptake inhibitors, amphetamines, dopamine and neurostimulants)] (Dimyan and Cohen 2010, 2011; Winstein et al. 2016). Despite these advances, most patients remain disabled, and unlikely to achieve premorbid function and independence (Dimyan and Cohen 2011; Mozaffarian et al. 2015). Preliminary information seems consistent with the view that more therapy than currently given or allowed is needed to further ameliorate the impairment burden cause by stroke (Lohse et al. 2014).

With steadily increasing life expectancy and rising costs of healthcare, it is important to develop interventions to facilitate the rate and trajectory of recovery and enhance long-term functional outcome. Work over the past several decades has investigated the use of transcranial direct current stimulation (tDCS) as an adjuvant neuromodulatory strategy to enhance the beneficial effects of the gold-

O. O. Awosika
Human Cortical Physiology and Stroke Neurorehabilitation Section,
National Institutes of Health, Bethesda, MD, USA

Department of Neurology and Rehabilitation Medicine,
University of Cincinnati College of Medicine, Cincinnati, OH, USA
e-mail: oluwole.awosika@uc.edu

L. G. Cohen
Human Cortical Physiology and Stroke Neurorehabilitation Section,
National Institutes of Health, Bethesda, MD, USA

H. Knotkova et al. (eds.), *Practical Guide to Transcranial Direct Current Stimulation*, https://doi.org/10.1007/978-3-319-95948-1_17

standard in neurorehabilitation, physical therapy. Due to its relatively favorable safety profile (Woods et al. 2016), low cost and ability to blind (Gandiga et al. 2006), tDCS has been proposed as a useful investigational tool and a potential therapeutic adjunct to stroke rehabilitation (Dayan et al. 2013).

Mechanisms Underlying Motor Disability after Stroke

The mechanisms underlying motor disability after stroke are incompletely understood (Auriat et al. 2015a; Cassidy and Cramer 2016; Duque et al. 2005; Murase et al. 2004). Previous work demonstrated that the premovement level of inhibition from the primary motor cortex in the contralesional primary motor cortex ($M1_{contralesional}$) directed at the ipsilesional motor cortex ($M1_{ipsilesional}$) relates to the Medical Research Council (MRC) Scale scores and to performance on a finger-tapping task in chronic stroke patients with substantial motor recovery (Duque et al. 2005a; Murase et al. 2004). In this situation, the $M1_{ipsilesional}$ may experience an overactive inhibitory drive from the contralesional M1 resulting in an imbalance in interhemispheric inhibitory interactions (Butefisch et al. 2008; Gerloff et al. 2006; Hummel et al. 2005, 2006; Hummel and Cohen 2005a, b, 2006; Ward and Cohen 2004), Fig. 17.1.

This phenomenon, described in patients with relatively good motor recovery is referred to as the "interhemispheric inhibition model" (Butefisch et al. 2007, 2008; Cicinelli et al. 2003; Di Pino et al. 2014; Dimyan et al. 2014; Duque et al. 2005a, b; Harris-Love et al. 2015, 2016; Kinsbourne 1977, 1980; Kirton et al. 2010; Mansur et al. 2005; Mello et al. 2015; Nair et al. 2006, 2007; Perez and Cohen 2008, 2009; Vines et al. 2006). Neuroimaging investigations demonstrated consistent interhemispheric differences after stroke (Auriat et al. 2015; Baron et al. 2004; Cramer and Riley 2008; Cramer et al. 2011; Grefkes et al. 2008, 2010; Hodics et al. 2006; Nowak et al. 2009). Most of the available work on tDCS and stroke has focused on upregulating and downregulating activity in the ipsilesional and contralesional M1 with anodal or cathodal tDCS, respectively (Feng and Belagaje 2014; Feng et al. 2013; Kang et al. 2016; Schlaug and Cohen 2010; Schlaug and Renga 2008). Overall, effects sizes reported in these studies either have not been reported or have been modest (Tables 17.1a and 17.1b), but see also (Khedr et al. 2013; Kim et al. 2010), thus leading to continuing the search for mechanistic understanding of motor disability (Cramer et al. 2011; Fritsch et al. 2010) and optimization of interventions (Bernhardt et al. 2016; Di Pino et al. 2014; Otal et al. 2016). Recent work in combination with previous reports suggest that neurobiological mechanisms associated with movements of a paretic hand in patients may differ depending on the degree of impairment, with an adaptive role of the contralesional hemisphere (Buch et al. 2012; Harris-Love et al. 2015, 2016; Johansen-Berg et al. 2002; Lotze et al. 2006) in patients with more severe impairment and a contributory role of the ipsilesional motor structures in patients with lesser impair-

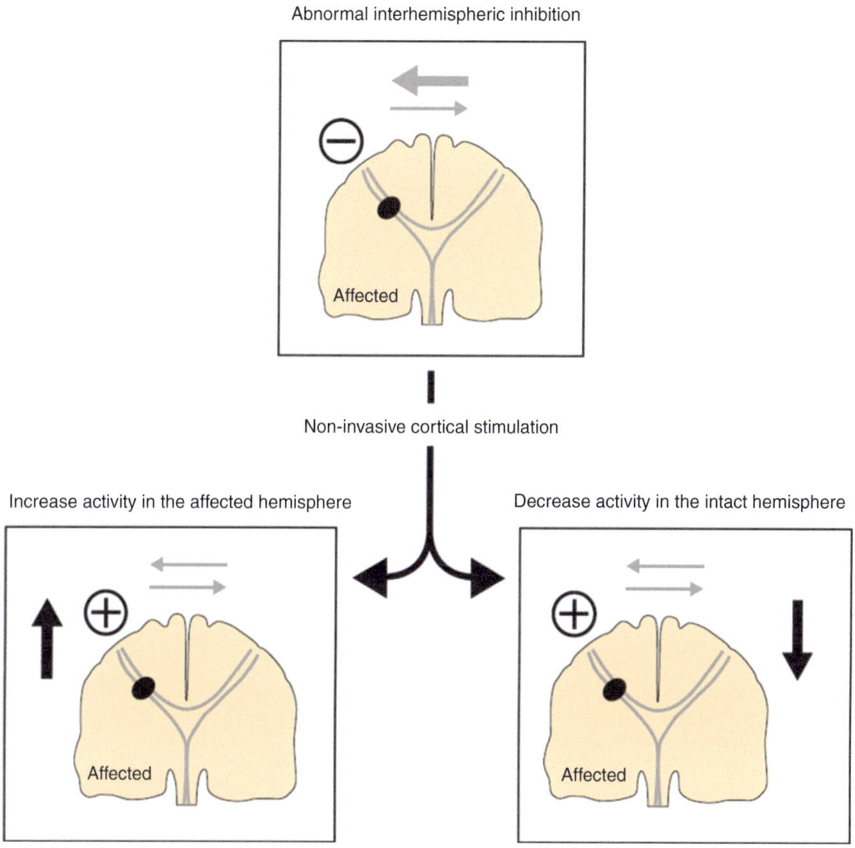

Fig. 17.1 Hypothesis for interventional strategies based on the finding that movements of the paretic hand are associated with unbalanced interhemispheric inhibition in patients with subcortical stroke. Two interventional approaches have been proposed and tested to improve motor function: upregulation of activity in the ipsilesional motor cortex and downregulation of activity of the contralesional motor cortex. (Reproduced with permission from Hummel and Cohen (2006))

ment (Fridman et al. 2004; Group et al. 2008; Johansen-Berg et al. 2002; Nudo et al. 1996). Di Pino et al. suggested a bimodal recovery model that links interhemispheric balancing (Murase et al. 2004) and the structural reserve spared by the lesion (Byblow and Stinear 2015; Feng et al. 2015; Schambra et al. 2015; Stinear et al. 2012, 2014), Fig. 17.2. This approach links with a developing understanding of the need to improve biomarkers of functional recovery (Bernhardt et al. 2016) and develop more individualized strategies for neurorehabilitation (Di Pino et al. 2014; Otal et al. 2016). One goal of these models is to enable NIBS to be tailored to the needs of individual patients, if proven efficacious. More work is required to merge these different models with others recently proposed (Stinear et al. 2014).

Table 17.1a Summary of tDCS post stroke studies on motor function (upper)

Study design							Stimulation parameters						Outcome measures					
Study	N	Mean age, y	Recovery stages	Mean impairment	Type	Concurrent task	Control	mA	Location	Duration, min	Pad size	Current density	Charge density	Sessions, n	Length of follow-up	Scale	Outcome (+,o,−)	Effect size
Hummel and Cohen (2005)	1	84	Chronic	2 (RUE-MRC)	A	None	S	1	A: IL M1	20	25	0.04	0.01	1	Immediate	JTT/ SRT/PF	A(+)	N/A
Fregni et al. (2005)	6	53.7	Chronic	N/A	A/C	None	S	1	A: IL M1; C:CL M1 (FDI Hot Spot)	20	35	0.028	0.009	1	Immediate	JTT	A(+) < C(+)	N/A
Hummel et al. (2005)	6	62.2	Chronic	95% (FMA)	A	None	S	1	A: IL M1	20	25	0.04	0.01	1	Immediate (10 days)	JTT/ SRT/PF	(A(+) immediate, A(o) at day 10	N/A
Hummel et al. (2006)	11	57	Chronic	90.7% (FMA)	A	None	S	1	A: IL M1	20	25	0.04	0.01	1	Immediate	SRT and PF	A(+)	N/A
Boggio et al. (2007) (Exp 1)	4	N/A	Chrnoic	N/A	A/C	None	S	1	A: IL M1; C: CL M1	20	N/A	N/A	N/A	4 (1 per week)	Immediate	JTT	A(+) = C(+)	0.16
Boggio et al. (2007) (Exp 2)	5	N/A	Chronic	N/A	C	None	N	1	C:ILM1S1	20	N/A	N/A	N/A	5	Immediate (2 wk)	JTT	C(+)	N/A
Hesse et al. (2007)	10	663	Subacute	7.2 (FMA)	A	RAT (20 min)	N	1.5	A: IL M1; C: CL M1	7	35	0.04	0.005	30	Immediate	FMA/ MRC	A(+)	MRC
Celnik et al. (2009)	9	55.3	Chronic	62.0/66 (FMA)	A	PNS (120 min)	S + PNS	1	A: IL M1 (APB Hot Spot)	20	57.8	0.11	0.04	1	Immediate: 6 days	Movement accuracy?	A(+)	0.18
Kim et al. (2009)	10	62.8	Subacute	MRC ≥ 3 < 5	A	1	S	1	A: IL M1 (FDI Hot Spot)	20	25	0.04	0.03	1	Immediate: 1 hr	BTT/FA	A(+)	N/A

Qu et al. (2009)	50	45	Subacute-chronic	MAS = 2	C*	None	S	0.5	C:ILM1S1	20	18	0.03	0.01	20	Immediate (4 wk)	MAS/ FMA/BI	C*(+)	N/A
Kim et al. (2010)	18	57.8	Subacute	37.2/66 (FMA)	AC	OT (30 min)	S	2	A: IL M1; C:CL M1 (FDI Hot Spot)	20	25	0.08	0.03	10	Immediate (24 wk)	FMA	A (−)/C(+)	1.39 (C)
Lindenberg et al. (2010)	20	58.8	Chronic	39.0/66 (FMA)	Bi	OT (60 min)	S	1.5	A: IL M1; C: CL M1	30	16.3	0.09	0.05	5	Immediate (1 wk)	FMA/ WFMT	Bi(+)	0.68
Hesse et al. (2011)	96	65	Subacute	8.0/66 (FMA)	A/C	RAMT (20 min)	S + AMT	2	A: IL M1; C: CL M1	20	35	0.057	0.02	30	Immediate (12 wk)	FMA	A (−)/C(−)	Neg 0.01/ Neg 0.02
Bolognini et al. (2011)	14	46.7	Chronic	26.0/66 (FMA)	Bi	CIT	S + CIT	2	A: IL M1; C: CL M1	40	35	0.057	0.04	10	Immediate (4 wk)	FMA/MAL (AOU) //HG/JTT	Bi(+)	0.98
Nair et al. (2011)	14	46.7	Chronic	26.0/66 (FMA)	Bi	CIT	S + CIT	2	A: IL M1; C: CL M1	40	35	0.057	0.04	10	Immediate (4 wk)	FMA/MAL (AOU) //HG/JTT	Bi(+)	0.98
Mahmoudi et al. (2011)	10	60.8	Subacute-chronic	12.3 (JTT)	A/C/ Bi	None	S	1	A: IL M1; C: CL M1	20	35	0.057	0.02	1	Immediate	JTT	A (+)/C(+)/ Bi(+)	N/A
Lindenberg et al. (2012)	10	58.8	Chronic	39.0/66 (FMA)	Bi	PT + OT (60 min)	S	1.5	A: IL M1; C: CL M1	30	16.3	0.092	0.05	5	Immediate	FMA	Bi(+)	0.29
Zimerman et al. (2012)	12	58.3	Chronic	64.0/66 (FMA)	C	MSL	S	1	C: CL M1	20	25	0.04	0.01	1	90 min–24 hr	MSC	C(+)	N/A
Stagg et al. (2012)	13	64	Chronic	36.6/66 (FMA)	A/C	None	S	1	A: IL M1; C: CL M1	20	35	0.057	0.02	1	Immediate	MRT	A(+) > C(+)	N/A

(continued)

Table 17.1a (continued)

Study design							Stimulation parameters						Outcome measures					
Study	1	Mean age, y	Recovery stages	Mean impairment	Type	Concurrent task	Control	mA	Location	Duration, min	Pad size	Current density	Charge density	Sessions, n	Length of follow-up	Scale	Outcome (+,o,−)	Effect size
Rossi et al. (2013)	50	66.1	Acute	15/42 (NIHSS)	A	None	S	2	A: IL M1	20	35	0.057	0.02	5	Immediate: 3 mo	FMA/ NIHSS	A(−)	0.16–1.54 (FMA)/ 0.20–0.21 (NIHSS)
Khedr et al. (2013)	40	58.3	Subacute	10.7/42 (NIHSS)	A/C	Rehab	S + rehab	2	A: IL M1; C: CL M1	25	35	0.047	0.02	6	Immediate: 3 mo	NIHSS	A(+)	1.59(A)/ 1.08(S)
Lefebvre et al. (2013)	18	61	Chronic	7.1/25 (PPT)	Bi	MSL	S	1	A: IL M1 (Hand muscle Hot Spot); C:CL M1 (FDI Hot Spot)	30	35	0.028	0.01	1	Immediate: 1 wk	MSL Learning Index	Bi(+)	0.93
Wu et al. (2013)	90	47.6	Subacute-chronic	10.0./66 (FMA)	C*	PT(after tDCS)	S	1.2	C:ILM1S1	20	24.8	0.26	0.09	20	Immediate (4 wk)	MAS	C*(+)	–
Viana et al. (2014)	20	55.5	Chronic	40/66(FMA)	A	VRT	S + VRT	2	A: IL M1	13	35	0.057	0.01	15	Immediate	FMA/ WMFT/ MAS/HG/ SSQOL	A(o)	N/A
Di Lazzaro et al. (2014) (Exp. 1)	14	77.1	Acute	7/42 (NIHSS)	Bi	None	S	2	A: IL M1; C: CL M1	40	35	0.057	0.04	5	1 wk–12 wk	NIHSS/ mRS/ARAT/ HG/MAL (AOU)/ MAL (QOM), NHPT	Bi(o)	0.36

Di Lazzaro et al. (2014) (Exp. 2)	14	77.1	Acute	7/42 (NIHSS)	Bi	None	S	2	A: IL M1; C: CL M1	40	35	0.057	0.04	5	1 wk	NIHSS/ mRS/ ARAT/HG/ MAL (AOU)/ MAL (QOM), NHPT	Bi(o)	N/A
Fusco et al. (2014)	11	58.4	Acute	24.7/66 (FMA)	C	Rehab	S + Rehab	1.5	C: CL M1	10	35	0.043	0.01	10	10 days–4 wk	ADL/ Manual Dexterirty and Force, Locomotion	C(o)	0.08
Lefebvre et al. (2014)	19	65	Chronic	7.4/25 (PPT)	A/C	MSL	S	1	A: IL M1 (Hand muscle Hot Spot); C:CL M1 (FDI Hot Spot)	30	35	0.028	0.01	1	Immediate (1 wk)	MSL Learning Index	Bi (+)	0.82
Triccas et al. (2015)	23	63.4	Subacute-chronic	32.3 (FMA)	A	RAT (1 h)	S	1	A: IL M1	20	35	0.028	0.01	18	Immediate: 12 wk	FMA	A(o)	N/A
Sattler et al. (2015)	20	65.2	Acute	48.0/66 (FMA)	A	RPNS +Rhab	S + RPNS+ Rhab	1.2	A: IL M1	13	35	0.03	0.01	5	Immediate (4 wk)	JTT	A(+)	0.65
Park et al. (2015)	24	61.6	Chronic	N/A	A	TRT (30 min)	S + TRT/ TRT alone	2	A:Cz of left parietal lobe	15	N/A	N/A	N/A	12	Immediate	Gait velocity, stance, length, symmetry	A(+)	N/A
Mortensen et al. (2015)	15	63.1	Chronic	15.5/25 (SIS, hand)	A	OT	S	1.5	A: IL M1	20	35	0.04	0.01	5	Immediate (1 wk)	JTT	A(+)	0.61

(continued)

Table 17.1a (continued)

Study design							Stimulation parameters						Outcome measures					
Study	1	Mean age, y	Recovery stages	Mean impairment	Type	Concurrent task	Control	mA	Location	Duration, min	Pad size	Current density	Charge density	Sessions, n	Length of follow-up	Scale	Outcome (+,o,−)	Effect size
Rocha et al. (2016)	21	58.5	Chronic	49.1/66 (FMA)	A/C	CIT(after tDCS)	S + CIT	2	A: IL M1; C: CL M1	13 A; 9 C	35	0.057	0.01(A)/ 0.009 (C)	12	Immediate (4 wk)	FMA/MAL/ HG	A(+), C(o)	0.94
Straudi et al. (2016)	23	58.2	Subacute-chronic	22.83 (FMA)/8.56 (BBT)	Bi	RAT	S-RAT	1	A: IL M1; C: CL M1	30	35	0.028	0.01	10	Immediate	FMA/BBT/ MAL	Bi(o)	0.07 Neg (FMA)/ 0.03 (BBT)/ 0.16 (MAL-AOM)/ 0.15 (MALQOM)

ADL Activities of Daily Living, *ARAT* Action Research Arm Test, *BI* Barthel Index Score, *FA* finger acceleration, *FMA* Fugl-Meyer Assessment, *JTT* Jebsen Taylor test, *HG* handgrip force, *LEFMA* lower extremity Fugl-Meyer Assessment, *LEIS* lower extremity impairment strength, *MAS* Modified Ashworth Scale, *MRC* Medical Research Council, *mRS* modified Rankin Scale, *MRT* motor response time, *MST* motor sequence training; NIHSS, National Institutes of Health Stroke Scale, *OT* occupational therapy, *PT* physical therapy, *RAMT* robotic arm motor training, *SIS* Supports Intensity Scale, *SRT* single reaction time, *SSS* Scandinavian Neurological Stroke Scale, *WMFT* Wolf Motor Function Test

*C signifies instances when the cathode was placed over the lesioned hemisphere, as opposed to the contralesional

Table 17.1b Summary of tDCS post stroke studies on motor function (lower)

Study design							Stimulation parameters						Outcome measures					
Study	N	Mean age, y	Recovery stages	Mean impairment	Type	Concurrent task	Control	mA	Location	Duration, min	Pad size	Current density	Charge density	Sessions, n	Length of follow-up	Scale	Outcome (+,o,–)	Effect size
Madhavan et al. (2010)	9	65.4	Chronic	25.2/30 (LEFMA)	A	Motor Practice (Tracking Task sinusoidal waveform)	S	2	A: IL M1 (leg); C: CL M1 (leg)	15	35	0.057	0.01	1	Immediate	Movement accuracy	A(+)	N/A
Tanaka et al. (2011)	8	59.6	Chronic	N/A	A	None	S	2	A: IL M1 (TA Hot Spot)	10	50	0.06	0.01	1	During – 30 min	Knee extensor force	A(+) durring and immediate, A(o) at 30 min	1.11
Geroin et al. (2011)	30	62.1	Subacute-chronic	79.9/100 (ESS)	A	RGT (50 min)	S or OGW	1.5	A: IL M1 (leg)	7	35	0.057	0.01	10	Immediate (2 wk)	6MWT/ 10MWT	A (o), A and S > OVW	0.38
Sohn et al. (2013)	11	58.5	Subacute	N/A	A	PT	S	2	A: IL M1 (QF Hot Spot)	10	25	0.08	0.01	1	Immediate	SPS/LEIS	A(+)	A/A
Danzl et al. (2013)	8	67.8	Chronic	N/A	A	RGT	S + RGT	2	A:Vertex	20	35	0.08	0.03	12	Immediate	Gait	A(o)	N/A
Tahtis et al. (2014)	14	56.4	Subacute	17.89 s (TUGT)	Bi	None	S	2	A: IL M1; C: CL M1	15	25	0.08	0.02	1	Immediate	TGUT	Bi(+)	N/A
Chang et al. (2015)	24	63	Acute	3.3 (mRS)	A	PT	S + PT	2	A: IL M1 (TA Hot Spot)	10	28	0.28	0.05	10	Immediate	Impairment Score	A(+)	N/A
Saeys et al. (2015)	31	63	Subacute	N/A	Bi	PT and OT	S+ PT/OT	1.5	A: IL M1; C: CL M1	20	35	0.04	0.01	16	Immediate: 8 wks	Tinetti	Bi(+)	N/A
van Asseldonk et al. (2016)	10	58	Chronic	25.8 (FMA)	A/C/ Bi	Treadmill	S + Treadmill	2	A: IL M1; C: CL M1	10	35	0.057	0.01	1	15–45 min	Force production	A(o)/C(o)/ Bi(o)	N/A

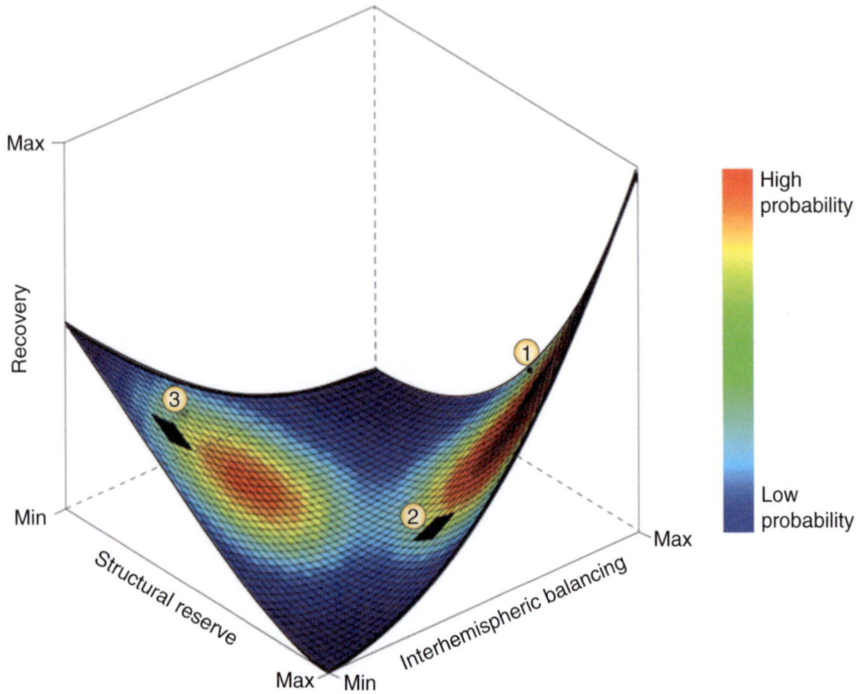

Fig. 17.2 The bimodal balance–recovery model. Structural reserve is the quantity of strategic neural pathways and relays that are spared by the lesion and can reallocate previous or outsource new functions. Patients with high structural reserve often achieve better functional recovery. In such cases, the balance of activity between the two hemispheres tends toward the previous equilibrium (1), whereas persistence of interhemispheric imbalance is a predictor of worse outcome (2). When structural reserve is low—such as in a subclass of patients with more-severe impairment—and the sensorimotor network is far from reaching a physiological restitution "ad integrum", persistence of interhemispheric imbalance promotes vicarious activity of the unaffected hemisphere (3), allowing compensatory plasticity. Colour code indicates frequency distribution of an event in a population of stroke patients, which is equivalent to the probability that a given individual is represented by that point of the surface. 'Hot' colours indicate higher probability than 'cold' colours. The probability distribution presented here follows a bimodal statistical distribution, which arises from the superimposed distributions of two populations: patients with high reserve and high balancing versus patients with low reserve and low balancing. (Reproduced with permission (Di Pino et al. 2014))

tDCS Applied to the Motor Cortex

tDCS can modulate cortical excitability (Chhatbar et al. 2016; Feng and Belagaje 2014; Lang et al. 2004; Nitsche et al. 2002) but see also (Horvath et al. 2016) and has been reported to improve motor learning in young (Ciechanski and Kirton 2016; Kincses et al. 2004; Reis et al. 2008, 2009; Schambra et al. 2011; Stagg et al. 2011; Tanaka et al. 2011) and older adults (Heise et al. 2014; Meinzer et al. 2013, 2014; Perceval et al. 2016; Zimerman et al. 2013).

Upper Extremity Motor Function

We reviewed 34 studies on effects of tDCS on upper limb motor function (Tables 17.1a and 17.1b).

Anodal tDCS over ipsilesional M1 Initial reports on the effects of tDCS on upper limb motor performance date back to 2005 (Hummel et al. 2005, 2006; Hummel and Cohen 2005a, b). Other studies found beneficial effects of both anodal and cathodal tDCS (Boggio et al. 2007; Fregni et al. 2005). Overall, 26 studies reported positive effects on different endpoint measures like the Jebsen Taylor test (JTT) (Boggio et al. 2007; Fregni et al. 2005), simple reaction time, SRT (Hummel et al. 2005, 2006; Stagg et al. 2012), Box and Block Test (BBT) (Kim et al. 2009) and Fugl-Meyer Assessment (FMA) (Kim et al. 2009) and pinch strength (Stagg et al. 2012). Multiple applications of anodal tDCS were reported to have longer lasting effects compared to single application (Allman et al. 2016; Hesse et al. 2007), consistent with results in healthy volunteers (Hashemirad et al. 2016). For example, Allman and colleagues tested the effects of anodal tDCS paired with daily motor training over 9 days, and found improvements in the Action Research Arm Test (ARAT) and Wolf Motor Function Test (WMFT), up to 3 months post training. However, it is worth noting that this lasting effect was not seen for the upper extremity FMA. One meta-analysis study on the effects of anodal tDCS on motor function found that this polarity may benefit motor function of the paretic upper limb in patients suffering from chronic stroke (Butler et al. 2013).

Cathodal tDCS over the contralesional M1 15 studies have reported the effects of cathodal tDCS on upper extremity motor function (Tables 17.1a and 17.1b). Initial studies date back to 2005 (Fregni et al. 2005). The investigators suggested that a single application of c- tDCS was slightly more advantageous than a-tDCS, although both were superior to sham. Additionally, multiple applications of c-tDCS with simultaneous occupational therapy (OT) over 5 consecutive daily sessions resulted in significant improvement in range of motion in multiple joints of the paretic upper extremity and in the Upper-Extremity FMA scores relative to sham tDCS+OT, and the effects lasted at least 1 week post-stimulation (Nair et al. 2011). It has been proposed that cathodal tDCS applied to the ipsilesional sensorimotor cortex may result in functional gains in both spasticity and impairment scores (Qu et al. 2009; Wu et al. 2013). *Bihemispheric stimulation*: We reviewed 8 studies which reported effects of Bi-hemispheric tDCS on different endpoint measures including the FMA, WMFT, JTT and MAL (Tables 17.1a and 17.1b). Lindenberg and colleagues (2010) applied bihemispheric tDCS stimulation positioning the anode over ipsilesional M1 and the cathode over contralesional M1 in combination with occupational(OT)/physical therapy(PT) in chronic stroke patients for five daily sessions and reported greater improvement of motor function (20.7% in FM and 19.1% in WMFT scores) in the active stimulation group, compared to sham (3.2% in FM and 6.0% in WMFT). They indicated that these effects outlasted the stimulation period for at least 1 week. Following this study, the same group of patients underwent another

5 days of bihemispheric stimulation + OT/PT, and were found to have benefited from the second series of stimulation (2012).

In sum, of the 34 studies to date on upper extremity motor recovery after stroke (see Kang et al. 2016), 8 have found very little to null effects (see also Ward 2016). As an example of a study with a null result, a multicenter randomized clinical trial of 96 patients, paring tDCS (anodal, cathodal, sham) with robot assisted arm training, found improvement across groups; however, there were no between group differences, (Hesse et al. 2011) (see also Rocha et al. 2016). It is likely that the number of reports with null findings is underestimated given the publication bias (Hummel et al. 2008; Mancuso et al. 2016; Shiozawa et al. 2014; Vannorsdall et al. 2016).

Lower Extremity Motor Function

Lower limb function, crucial for posture, stance and locomotion, experiences commonly better recovery than upper limb function (Lee et al. 2015; Paci et al. 2016). Lower limb motor deficits after stroke, when present, relate closely to morbidity and mortality due to the risk of falls, fractures, and venous thromboembolism related to immobility. We reviewed 9 studies to date which have reported the effects of tDCS on lower limb function. Outcome measures in lower limb trials included lower extremity strength (Sohn et al. 2013; Tanaka et al. 2011), motor control, posture (Madhavan et al. 2010), balance and gait (Geroin et al. 2011; Saeys et al. 2015; Tahtis et al. 2014).

Anodal tDCS over ipsilesional M1 One report using anodal tDCS demonstrated that a single 15 min session of anodal tDCS at a low intensity of 0.5 mA improved performance on a tracking task involving reciprocal dorsiflexion and plantar flexion (Madhavan et al. 2010), and improved knee extensor force production (2 mA, 10 min) in another (Tanaka et al. 2011). Multiple sessions of anodal tDCS over the midline, resulted in improvements in postural stability and balance relative to sham after subacute stroke (Sohn et al. 2013). Similarly, anodal tDCS+physiotherapy resulted in between-group improvements in lower-limb function, following 10 days relative to sham after chronic stroke (Chang et al. 2015). We found no reports of cathodal tDCS on leg motor function after stroke.

Bihemispheric stimulation 3 studies reported effects of bihemispheric tDCS on lower extremity function. Tahtis and colleagues report improvements in the Timed Up and Go task (a measure of gait performance), compared to the sham group (Tahtis et al. 2014). Similarly, one study found that bihemispheric stimulation resulted in significantly greater improvement in total Tinetti score (assessment of functional balance and gait), compared to sham up to 4 weeks post stimulation (Saeys et al. 2015).

As is the case with tDCS in upper extremity motor function, results for anodal tDCS and lower extremity function have not been consistently positive. For example, a randomized parallel design controlled pilot study (Geroin et al. 2011) combined anodal tDCS with robot-assisted gait training (RAGT) in patients with chronic stroke (n = 10/group). Subjects received 10–50 min sessions of RAGT with concurrent stimulation (anodal or sham) or over ground walking exercises. Although both anodal and sham groups improved, no between group differences was seen. Overall, the feasibility of positioning electrodes over the lower extremity region of M1 with tDCS is still in question given its relative depth (van Asseldonk and Boonstra 2016). Additionally, the relative role of the motor cortex vs subcortical structures in automatic locomotion is not fully understood (Jeffery et al. 2007; Madhavan and Shah 2012; Madhavan and Stinear 2010).

Meta-Analysis of TDCS and Motor Function

Although the majority of small, single-center studies have reported positive results, some larger multicenter studies have failed to show significant differences between active tDCS and sham stimulation, such as the study by Hesse and colleagues (2011). A critical look at the most recent reviews and meta-analysis suggest that tDCS has a modest effect on improving motor outcome after stroke (Butler et al. 2013; Chhatbar et al. 2016; Elsner et al. 2016; Kang et al. 2016). A Cochrane review of randomized controlled trials and cross-over trials (N = 32, 748 participants) that compared tDCS versus control after stroke found evidence of "very low" to "low quality" evidence supporting tDCS effectiveness in improving performance on activities of daily living (Elsner et al. 2016). On the other hand, Kang and colleagues (2016) published a comprehensive review and meta-analysis investigating the effects of tDCS coupled with standard or task-specific motor training on long term motor learning. Importantly, this report included a wide range of studies (N = 21, positive and null). The authors found an overall tDCS effect size of 0.59 (moderately positive) in favor of improving long term motor learning after stroke (size effect for efficacy of antidepressants is approximately 0.3 as per (Spielmans and Kirsch 2014; Turner et al. 2008; Turner and Rosenthal 2008). Kang et al.'s finding is also consistent with results from other recent meta-analysis (Chhatbar et al. 2016; Butler et al. 2013). No significant differences were found documenting superiority of anodal vs sham vs bihemispheric stimulation, application in the subacute vs chronic stage, application before or during training, or application during specific types of training).

Another meta-analysis by Chhatbar et al. (2016) evaluated dosing (intensity, duration electrode size, current density, and charge density), stroke stage, and tDCS protocol (ipsileasional anodal, contralesional sham, bihemisperic), on motor recovery, Fig. 17.3. Importantly, the authors found a positive dose response relationship for current and charge density but not for stimulation intensity. Results suggest that smaller electrodes result in stronger tDCS effects. In contrast to Kang et al. (2016), bihemispheric stimulation was found in this study to have a more robust effect (Hedge's g = 1.30) compared to anodal or cathodal tdCS, and patients with chronic stroke responded better than those with acute and subacute strokes (Hedge's g = 1.23).

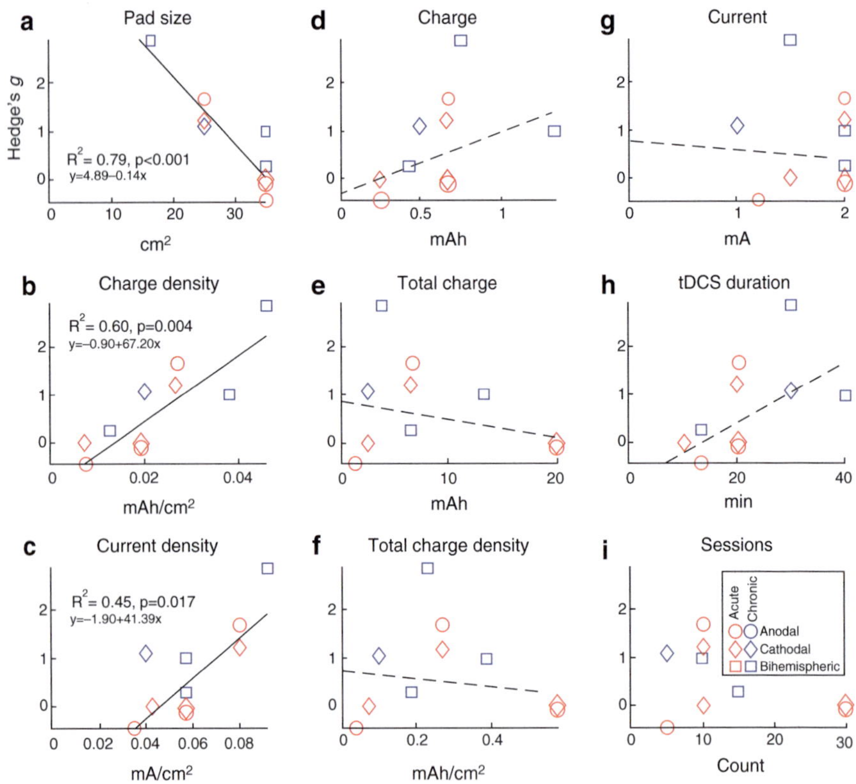

Fig. 17.3 Dose–response relationship. Plots showing that the improvement in FM-UE scores after tDCS relative to the sham group (Hedge's g) exhibited a positive correlation with current and charge density, and a negative one with electrode size. Inverse-variance-weighted linear meta-regression of Hedge's g against dose-related parameters revealed statistical significance for pad size (**a**), charge density (**b**) and current density (**c**) as shown by solid regression line with coefficient of determination (R2), significance value (p) and equation shown next to the line (**a–c**). No statistical significance was found for any other derived (**d–f**) or primary (**g–i**) dose-related parameters, as shown by dashed regression line. (Reproduced with permission (Chhatbar et al. 2016))

Hemineglect

Hemineglect is the failure to respond or orient to meaningful or novel stimuli on the contralesional side of space (Vallar 1998). Hemineglect is seen in approximately two thirds of right hemispheric strokes, and is usually related to lesions of the right parietal lobe. It has a negative influence on rehabilitation, limited mobility, longer hospitalizations, increased functional disability and family burden (Marshall 2009; Müri et al. 2013; Pedersen et al. 1997). Similar to post stroke motor deficit or aphasia, tDCS has been investigated as a therapy for neglect, either solely or in addition to conventional therapy (Adeyemo et al. 2012; Fasotti and van Kessel 2013; Mylius et al. 2012). tDCS has been applied to either facilitate the affected hemisphere or suppress the unaffected posterior parietal cortex (Ko et al. 2008; Làdavas et al. 2015; Sparing et al. 2009; Sunwoo et al. 2013).

Ko and colleagues investigated the effect of 1 session of anodal tDCS applied over the right posterior parietal cortex (PPC) (intensity of 2.0 mA for 20 min) on visuospatial scanning in subacute stroke patients with spatial neglect. Patients underwent two neglect tests (figure cancellation and line bisection) before and immediately after anodal tDCS or sham in a double-blind protocol. The study found that anodal but not sham tDCS, led to a significant improvement in neglecting the figure cancellation and failing line bisection tests (Ko et al. 2008). Similarly, Sparing and collaborators, found that a single session of either anodal tDCS over the lesioned PCC or contralesional cathodal tDCS (intensity of 1.0 mA for 10 min) resulted in significant improvements, compared to sham tDCS (Sparing et al. 2009).

Most recently, Ladavas and colleagues evaluated the effects of multiple sessions of anodal or cathodal tDCS on the beneficial effects of prism adaptation (PA) treatment in neglect patients. 30 neglect patients were recruited and underwent 10 daily sessions of PA treatment with concurrent stimulation lasting 20 min. This study found that anodal tDCS+PA induced stronger improvement on the Behavioral Inattention Test (measure of neglect). However, little improvement was reported in the cathodal tDCS+PA and sham+PA group (Làdavas et al. 2015).

Bihemispheric stimulation The effects of bihemispheric tDCS over the parietal cortices was investigated in a double-blind random-order cross-over investigation by Sunwoo and colleagues. 10 chronic right hemispheric stroke patients underwent three randomly ordered tDCS (1 mA, 20 min) sessions: bihemispheric (anode and cathode over right and left PPC respectively), cathodal tDCS over L PPC, and sham tDCS. Outcome measures were pre and post-performance on the line bisection and star cancelation tests. The study found that both active stimulation groups improved in the line bisection test. Further analysis also suggested that bihemispheric tDCS was superior to cathodal stimulation alone (Sunwoo et al. 2013).

Overall, the studies on tDCS and neglect appear promising. However, given the relatively small number of published reports, caution should be taken in interpreting these findings.

Aphasia

Aphasia is an acquired deficit of language, typically resulting from damage to the left hemisphere of the brain, and is a common cause of morbidity, affecting approximately 20% of stroke patients (Saur and Hartwigsen 2012). The syndrome typically involves the left perisylvian circuit, where anterior frontal lesions typically result in nonfluent (Broca's) aphasia, whereas more posterior and temporal lesions results in fluent (Wernicke's) fluent aphasia. Approximately 12% of post stroke survivors are left with some degree of communication deficits (Brady et al. 2012; Lazar et al. 2010; Otal et al. 2016; Wade et al. 1986). Current speech and language therapy has limited effectiveness in aphasia treatment. Studies to date in healthy individuals suggest that tDCS over language –related brain regions can modulate linguistic abilities (Cohen-Maximov et al. 2015; Hussey et al. 2015; Rosso et al. 2014; Wirth et al. 2011). Based on this information, tDCS has been tested in patients with aphasia.

Non-fluent (Broca's) Aphasia

Monti et al. (2008) evaluated the effect of tDCS (anodal, cathodal, or sham) over the left frontotemporal areas in 8 chronic non-fluent post-stroke aphasic patients. The study consisted of the assessment of picture naming (accuracy and response time) before and immediately after ipsilesional anodal or contralesional cathodal tDCS (2 mA, 10 min) and sham stimulation. They found that cathodal tDCS significantly improved the accuracy of picture naming by 33.6% (SEM 13.8%) in the absence of differences between anodal tDCS and sham (Monti et al. 2008). The authors postulated as a mechanism cathodal tDCS-mediated downregulation of cortical inhibitory interneurons (disinhibition) in the lesioned regions (Monti et al. 2008). In a small cohort of 6 subjects with chronic Broca's aphasia Vines and colleagues, investigated the effects of tDCS (over the right inferior frontal gyrus) paired with melodic intonation therapies (MIT), on speech recovery in a randomized crossover design fashion. All patients, who had moderate to severe non-fluent aphasia, underwent three consecutive days of anodal-tDCS + MIT, and an equivalent series of sham-tDCS + MIT allowing for a 1 week washout period between sessions. The authors found that anodal-tDCS + MIT led to significant improvements in fluency of speech, relative to sham (Vines et al. 2011).

Kang and colleagues evaluated the hypothesis that cathodal tDCS applied over the right Broca's homologue area during concurrent word-retrieval training could improve picture naming in patients with post-stroke aphasia. 10 right-handed patients with post-stroke aphasia were randomized to cathodal tDCS (2 mA for 20 min) and sham tDCS daily for 5 consecutive days, in a crossover design. Picture naming at 1 h following the last training session improved only in the cathodal tDCS group (Kang et al. 2011). Likewise, Fiori et al. (2011) investigated the effects of anodal tDCS over the left posterior perisylvian area over 5 sessions (1 mA, 20 mins) in 3 chronic non-fluent aphasics. Anodal tDCS improved speed and accuracy on the picture-naming task immediately after application and 1 and 3 weeks post intervention (2 of 3 subjects) relative to sham (Fiori et al. 2011).

Bihemispheric stimulation Marangolo and colleagues reported the first published study of bihemispheric tDCS in aphasia (Marangolo et al. 2013), where 8 aphasic patients with apraxia of speech underwent intensive language therapy in two different conditions (crossover design): bihemispheric (anodal and cathodal electrodes over the ipsilesional Broca's area and contralesional homologue, respectively) and sham tDCS, with concurrent language therapy over 10 days. Performance was superior in the bihemispheric than sham tDCS sessions and the effects persisted for at least 1 week after stimulation (Marangolo et al. 2013). In a follow up investigation the authors reported that bihemispheric stimulation for 15 days elicited stronger functional connectivity in the left hemisphere compared to sham (Marangolo et al. 2016).

Fluent (Wernike's) Aphasia

One study evaluated the effects of tDCS on comprehension in stroke in 21 aphasic patients with subacute stroke (You et al. 2011). Participants were divided into 3 groups (2 mA, 30 min): anodal tDCS over the left superior temporal gyrus+ speech therapy (SLP), cathodal tDCS over the right superior temporal gyrus +SLP, or sham tDCS+SLP, for 10 daily sessions. The study found significant improvement in auditory verbal comprehension with cathodal tDCS compared to both anodal tDCS and sham. In contrast, Floel and colleagues applied 3 different stimulus conditions (anodal, cathodal, or sham tDCS) over the right superior temporal gyrus (homologue to Wernike's area) and found that anodal tDCS improved performance relative to both cathodal and sham stimulation, and this effect persisted 2 week after treatment (Flöel et al. 2011).

Interestingly, a previously referenced study (Hesse et al. 2007) designed to test the effects of ipsilesional anodal tDCS on the M1 on upper limb motor impairment, incidentally found improvement in speech in 5 of 7 study participants with large cortical strokes. This finding raises the question of topographic specificity of tDCS effects, in lieu of the close anatomical relationship between the hand motor area and language areas (Harnish et al. 2014; Meinzer et al. 2014; Primaßin et al. 2015). With this said, the broad spatial resolution may be more beneficial than a more focused stimulation, particularly given that aphasia recovery has been demonstrated to involve a complex network, involving multiple regions, during language activation (Turkeltaub et al. 2011); hence, more of these regions could be targeted.

A recent Cochrane review and meta-analysis involving 12 randomized control trials on aphasia (N = 136 participants) reported minimal effect size of the intervention (0.37), due to heterogeneity among study protocols and insufficient power for most studies (Elsner et al. 2015).

Dysphagia

Dysphagia is defined as difficulty or discomfort swallowing. Dysphagia affects approximately 50% of stroke patients and influence morbidity and mortality through increased risk for aspiration (Hamdy 2010). Only 3 studies on effects of tDCS on dysphagia have been reported (Kumar et al. 2011; Shigematsu et al. 2013; Yang et al. 2012).

Kumar and colleagues investigated the effects of contralesional anodal tDCS applied over putative pharyngeal motor representations (2 mA, 30 min × 5 consecutive days) simultaneously with swallowing (SLP). Dysphagia Outcome and Severity scale (DOSS) scores improved more in the anodal tDCS group that in the sham group (Kumar et al. 2011). Using a different stimulation montage, Yang and colleagues evaluated the effects of ipsilesional anodal tDCS on swallowing. In their protocol, subjects received anodal or sham tDCS (1 mA, 20 min, × 10 daily sessions) placed over the affected pharyngeal motor cortex with concurrent SLP. At 3 month follow-up, the anodal tDCS group performed better than the sham group, in spite of a transient worsening immediately post stimulation (Yang et al. 2012). Shigematsu and colleagues also found that anodal tDCS resulted in significantly greater improvement in DOSS scores up to 1 month post intervention (Shigematsu et al. 2013).

A recent meta-analysis evaluated the effects of noninvasive brain stimulation (NIBS), including rTMS) on post-stroke dysphagia, and found a significant moderate pooled effect size (0.55). Subgroup analysis demonstrated that studies stimulating the ipsilesional hemisphere had a slightly smaller effect size (0.46), compared to protocols stimulating the contralesional hemisphere (0.65). Of note, pooled analysis for tDCS also was not performed because of the limited number of studies available in literature (Pisegna et al. 2016).

Critical Considerations

Of the over 872 stroke patients that underwent tDCS in the framework of reported clinical trials to date, none has reported seizures. Of the 43 clinical trials to date on tDCS effects on motor impairment in stroke, relatively few reported null results (Tables 17.1a and 17.1b). Ways to strengthen research in this area include: use of double-blind designs, positive controls (stimulation of cortical regions not hypothesized to have an effect), a clear statement on whether a study is exploratory (not requiring preregistration) or hypothesis-driven (ideally preregistered) (Finkel et al. 2015). The field should collectively work to reduce the problem of p-hacking particularly in studies geared to power subsequent larger clinical trials. Preregistration in these cases is particularly useful (see for example: https://blogs.royalsociety.org/publishing/registered-reports/). Consideration should be given, when appropriate, to prepublish and share materials (Lauer et al. 2015; Morey et al. 2016) as well as implement postpublication data sharing (Campbell et al. 2002; Nosek et al. 2015). Implementation of within trial replications would go a long way towards improving the rate of false positives and negatives in this area of research (Anderson et al. 2016; Cohen et al. 1997; Gilbert et al. 2016; Open Science, 2015). Across the board, detailed description of methodologies is important to allow replication. It should be kept in mind that so far publication bias may have led to under-reporting of negative or null results in this field as in others (Mancuso et al. 2016; Shiozawa et al. 2014; Vannorsdall et al. 2016).

Of note, most of these issues are relevant to all clinical and basic science research and not solely to tDCS, see for review (Kaplan and Irvin 2015; Nosek et al. 2015). A challenge ahead of us in improving tDCS interventions after stroke is to identify the best way to address these points in trials of tDCS for stroke recovery. Another important area of work in the future is the optimization of techniques. In the reviewed reports, we encountered a substantial heterogenity of stimulus intensity, placement of reference electrode, sham setting, electrode size, stimulation duration, and application of double blinding procedures and frequency of stimulation, Fig. 17.4. Finally, inter-individual variability (age, genetics, comorbidities, stroke

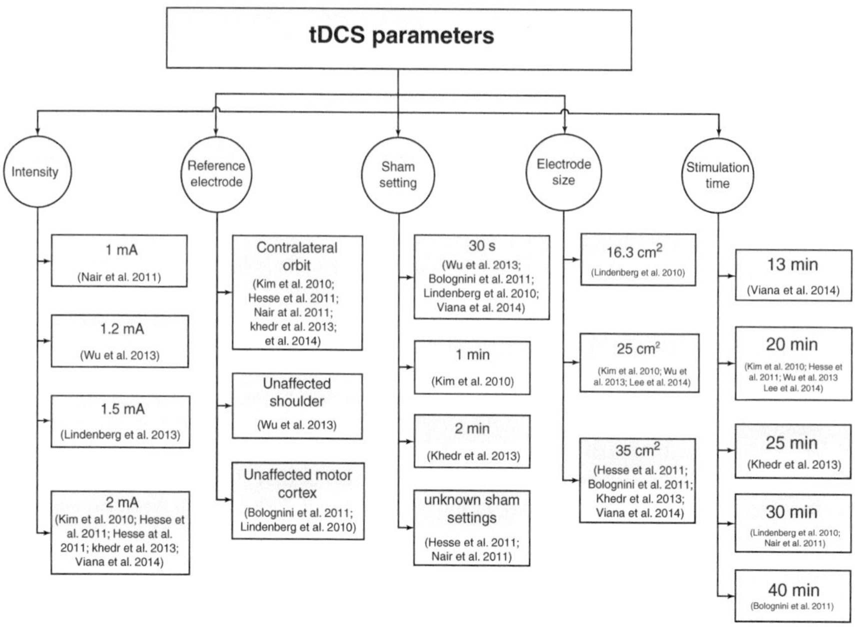

Fig. 17.4 A flow diagram displaying the different tDCS parameters of select studies in literature. (Reproduced with permission (Triccas et al. 2016))

etiology, size, location, and level of disability), also vary study outcomes. More work is needed to understand how to individualize interventions to optimize response and fundamentally understand the mechanisms by which tDCS influence functional recovery after stroke.

In summary, the encouraging yet conflicting results on effects of tDCS on motor recovery to date highlight the need for a better understanding of the mechanisms underlying tDCS effects, of optimal stimulation parameters, of interindividual variability in response and overall better interventional designs. Additionally, as general requirements for basic and clinical science, there is a need for more transparency, better powered designs, preregistered trials, and longer-term follow-ups.

References

Adeyemo, B. O., Simis, M., Macea, D., & Fregni, F. (2012). Systematic review of parameters of stimulation, clinical trial design characteristics, and motor outcomes in non-invasive brain stimulation in stroke. *Frontiers in Psychiatry, 3*, 88.

Allman, C., Amadi, U., Winkler, A. M., Wilkins, L., Filippini, N., Kischka, U., … Johansen-Berg, H. (2016). Ipsilesional anodal tDCS enhances the functional benefits of rehabilitation in patients after stroke. *Science Translational Medicine, 8*(330), 330re1.

Anderson, C. J., Bahnik, S., Barnett-Cowan, M., Bosco, F. A., Chandler, J., Chartier, C. R., … Zuni, K. (2016). Response to comment on "Estimating the reproducibility of psychological science". *Science, 351*(6277), 1037.

Auriat, A. M., Neva, J. L., Peters, S., Ferris, J. K., & Boyd, L. A. (2015). A review of transcranial magnetic stimulation and multimodal neuroimaging to characterize post-stroke neuroplasticity. *Frontiers in Neurology, 6*, 226.

Baron, J. C., Cohen, L. G., Cramer, S. C., Dobkin, B. H., Johansen-Berg, H., Loubinoux, I., … Ward, N. S. (2004). Neuroimaging in stroke recovery: A position paper from the first international workshop on neuroimaging and stroke recovery. *Cerebrovascular Diseases, 18*(3), 260–267. Retrieved from http://www.ncbi.nlm.nih.gov/entrez/query.fcgi?cmd=Retrieve&db=PubMed&dopt=Citation&list_uids=15484327

Bernhardt, J., Borschmann, K., Boyd, L., Carmichael, T. S., Corbett, D., Cramer, S. C., … Ward, N. (2016). Moving rehabilitation research forward: Developing consensus statements for rehabilitation and recovery research. *International Journal of Stroke, 11*(4), 454–458.

Boggio, P. S., Rigonatti, S. P., Ribeiro, R. B., Myczkowski, M. L., Nitsche, M. A., Pascual-Leone, A., & Fregni, F. (2007). A randomized, double-blind clinical trial on the efficacy of cortical direct current stimulation for the treatment of major depression. *The International Journal of Neuropsychopharmacology/Official Scientific Journal of the Collegium Internationale Neuropsychopharmacologicum (CINP), 11*(2), 249–254. Retrieved from http://www.ncbi.nlm.nih.gov/pubmed/17559710

Bolognini, N., Rossetti, A., Casati, C., Mancini, F., & Vallar, G. (2011). Neuromodulation of multisensory perception: A tDCS study of the sound-induced flash illusion. *Neuropsychologia, 49*(2), 231–237.

Brady, M. C., Kelly, H., Godwin, J., & Enderby, P. (2012). Speech and language therapy for aphasia following stroke. *The Cochrane Library, 5*.

Buch, E. R., Modir Shanechi, A., Fourkas, A. D., Weber, C., Birbaumer, N., & Cohen, L. G. (2012). Parietofrontal integrity determines neural modulation associated with grasping imagery after stroke. *Brain* awr331 [pii], *135*, 596–614.

Butefisch, C. M., Wessling, M., Netz, J., Seitz, R. J., & Homberg, V. (2008). Relationship between interhemispheric inhibition and motor cortex excitability in subacute stroke patients. *Neurorehabilitation and Neural Repair, 22*(1), 4–21. 1545968307301769 [pii].

Butefisch, C. M., Wessling, M. M., Netz, J., Seitz, R. J., & Homberg, V. (2007). Relationship between interhemispheric inhibition and motor cortex excitability in subacute stroke patients. *Neurorehabilitation and Neural Repair* Retrieved from http://www.ncbi.nlm.nih.gov/entrez/query.fcgi?cmd=Retrieve&db=PubMed&dopt=Citation&list_uids=17507644

Butler, A. J., Shuster, M., O'Hara, E., Hurley, K., Middlebrooks, D., & Guilkey, K. (2013). A meta-analysis of the efficacy of anodal transcranial direct current stimulation for upper limb motor recovery in stroke survivors. *Journal of Hand Therapy, 26*(2), 162–171.

Byblow, W. D., & Stinear, C. M. (2015). Proportional upper limb recovery after stroke is predicated upon corticospinal tract integrity. *Brain Stimulation, 8*(2), 429–430.

Campbell, E. G., Clarridge, B. R., Gokhale, M., Birenbaum, L., Hilgartner, S., Holtzman, N. A., & Blumenthal, D. (2002). Data withholding in academic genetics: Evidence from a national survey. *JAMA, 287*(4), 473–480. Retrieved from http://www.ncbi.nlm.nih.gov/pubmed/11798369

Cassidy, J. M., & Cramer, S. C. (2016). Spontaneous and therapeutic-induced mechanisms of functional recovery after stroke. *Translational Stroke Research., 8*, 33–46.

Celnik, P., Paik, N.-J. J., Vandermeeren, Y., Dimyan, M., & Cohen, L. G. (2009). Effects of combined peripheral nerve stimulation and brain polarization on performance of a motor sequence task after chronic stroke. *Stroke; A Journal of Cerebral Circulation, 40*(5), 1764–1771.

Chang, W.-J., Bennell, K. L., Hodges, P. W., Hinman, R. S., Liston, M. B., & Schabrun, S. M. (2015). Combined exercise and transcranial direct current stimulation intervention for knee osteoarthritis: Protocol for a pilot randomised controlled trial. *BMJ Open, 5*(8).

Chhatbar, P. Y., Ramakrishnan, V., Kautz, S., George, M. S., Adams, R. J., & Feng, W. (2016). Transcranial direct current stimulation post-stroke upper extremity motor recovery studies exhibit a dose–response relationship. *Brain Stimulation, 9*(1), 16–26.

Cicinelli, P., Pasqualetti, P., Zaccagnini, M., Traversa, R., Oliveri, M., & Rossini, P. M. (2003). Interhemispheric asymmetries of motor cortex excitability in the postacute stroke stage: A paired-pulse transcranial magnetic stimulation study. *Stroke, 34*(11), 2653–2658. Retrieved from http://www.ncbi.nlm.nih.gov/entrez/query.fcgi?cmd=Retrieve&db=PubMed&dopt=Citation&list_uids=14551397

Ciechanski, P., & Kirton, A. (2016). Transcranial direct-current stimulation can enhance motor learning in children. *Cerebral Cortex (New York, NY 1991).*

Cohen, L. G., Celnik, P., Pascual-Leone, A., Corwell, B., Falz, L., Dambrosia, J., … Hallett, M. (1997). Functional relevance of cross-modal plasticity in blind humans. *Nature, 389*(6647), 180–183. Retrieved from http://www.ncbi.nlm.nih.gov/entrez/query.fcgi?cmd=Retrieve&db=PubMed&dopt=Citation&list_uids=9296495

Cohen-Maximov, T., Avirame, K., Flöel, A., & Lavidor, M. (2015). Modulation of gestural-verbal semantic integration by tDCS. *Brain Stimulation, 8*(3), 493–498.

Cramer, S. C., & Riley, J. D. (2008). Neuroplasticity and brain repair after stroke. *Current Opinion in Neurology, 21*(1), 76–82.

Cramer, S. C., Sur, M., Dobkin, B. H., O'Brien, C., Sanger, T. D., Trojanowski, J. Q., … Vinogradov, S. (2011). Harnessing neuroplasticity for clinical applications. *Brain: A Journal of Neurology, 134*(Pt 6), 1591–1609. awr039 [pii].

Danzl, M. M., Chelette, K. C., Lee, K., Lykins, D., & Sawaki, L. (2013). Brain stimulation paired with novel locomotor training with robotic gait orthosis in chronic stroke: A feasibility study. *NeuroRehabilitation, 33*(1), 67–76.

Dayan, E., Censor, N., Buch, E. R., Sandrini, M., & Cohen, L. G. (2013). Noninvasive brain stimulation: From physiology to network dynamics and back. *Nature Neuroscience, 16*(7), 838–844.

Di Lazzaro, V., Dileone, M., Capone, F., Pellegrino, G., Ranieri, F., Musumeci, G., … Fregni, F. (2014). Immediate and late modulation of interhemipheric imbalance with bilateral transcranial direct current stimulation in acute stroke. *Brain Stimulation, 7*(6), 841–848.

Di Pino, G., Pellegrino, G., Assenza, G., Capone, F., Ferreri, F., Formica, D., … Di Lazzaro, V. (2014). Modulation of brain plasticity in stroke: A novel model for neurorehabilitation. *Nature Reviews. Neurology, 10*(10), 597–608.

Dimyan, M. A., & Cohen, L. G. (2010). Contribution of transcranial magnetic stimulation to the understanding of functional recovery mechanisms after stroke. *Neurorehabilitation and Neural Repair, 24*(2), 125–135. 1545968309345270 [pii].

Dimyan, M. A., & Cohen, L. G. (2011). Neuroplasticity in the context of motor rehabilitation after stroke. *Nature Reviews Neurology, 7*(2), 76–85. nrneurol.2010.200 [pii].

Dimyan, M. A., Perez, M. A., Auh, S., Tarula, E., Wilson, M., & Cohen, L. G. (2014). Nonparetic arm force does not overinhibit the paretic arm in chronic poststroke hemiparesis. *Archives of Physical Medicine and Rehabilitation, 95*(5), 849–856.

Dobkin, B. H. (2005). Rehabilitation after stroke. *The New England Journal of Medicine, 352*(16), 1677–1684.

Dobkin, B. H., & Dorsch, A. (2013). New evidence for therapies in stroke rehabilitation. *Current Atherosclerosis Reports, 15*(6), 331.

Duque, J., Hummel, F., Celnik, P., Murase, N., Mazzocchio, R., & Cohen, L. G. (2005a). Transcallosal inhibition in chronic subcortical stroke. *NeuroImage, 28*(4), 940–946. S1053-8119(05)00480-5 [pii].

Duque, J., Mazzocchio, R., Dambrosia, J., Murase, N., Olivier, E., & Cohen, L. G. (2005b). Kinematically specific interhemispheric inhibition operating in the process of generation of a voluntary movement. *Cerebral Cortex, 15*(5), 588–593. Retrieved from http://www.ncbi.nlm.nih.gov/entrez/query.fcgi?cmd=Retrieve&db=PubMed&dopt=Citation&list_uids=15342437

Elsner, B., Kugler, J., Pohl, M., & Mehrholz, J. (2015). Transcranial direct current stimulation (tDCS) for improving aphasia in patients with aphasia after stroke. *The Cochrane Library, 5*.

Elsner, B., Kugler, J., Pohl, M., & Mehrholz, J. (2016). Transcranial direct current stimulation (tDCS) for improving activities of daily living, and physical and cognitive functioning, in people after stroke. *The Cochrane Database of Systematic Reviews, 3*.

Fasotti, L., & van Kessel, M. (2013). Novel insights in the rehabilitation of neglect. *Frontiers in Human Neuroscience, 7*, 780.

Feng, W., & Belagaje, S. (2014). Recent advances in stroke recovery and rehabilitation. *Seminars in Neurology, 33*(05), 498–506.

Feng, W., Bowden, M. G., & Kautz, S. (2013). Review of transcranial direct current stimulation in poststroke recovery. *Topics in Stroke Rehabilitation, 20*(1), 68–77.

Feng, W., Wang, J., Chhatbar, P. Y., Doughty, C., Landsittel, D., Lioutas, V. A., … Schlaug, G. (2015). Corticospinal tract lesion load: An imaging biomarker for stroke motor outcomes. *Annals of Neurology, 78*(6), 860–870.

Finkel, E. J., Eastwick, P. W., & Reis, H. T. (2015). Best research practices in psychology: Illustrating epistemological and pragmatic considerations with the case of relationship science. *Journal of Personality and Social Psychology, 108*(2), 275–297.

Fiori, V., Coccia, M., Marinelli, C. V., Vecchi, V., Bonifazi, S., Ceravolo, G. M., … Marangolo, P. (2011). Transcranial direct current stimulation improves word retrieval in healthy and nonfluent aphasic subjects. *Journal of Cognitive Neuroscience, 23*(9), 2309–2323.

Flöel, A., Meinzer, M., Kirstein, R., Nijhof, S., Deppe, M., Knecht, S., & Breitenstein, C. (2011). Short-term anomia training and electrical brain stimulation. *Stroke, 42*(7), 2065–2067.

Fregni, F., Boggio, P. S., Mansur, C. G., Wagner, T., Ferreira, M. J., Lima, M. C., … Pascual-Leone, A. (2005). Transcranial direct current stimulation of the unaffected hemisphere in stroke patients. *Neuroreport, 16*(14), 1551–1555. Retrieved from http://www.ncbi.nlm.nih.gov/entrez/query.fcgi?cmd=Retrieve&db=PubMed&dopt=Citation&list_uids=16148743

Fridman, E. A., Hanakawa, T., Chung, M., Hummel, F., Leiguarda, R. C., & Cohen, L. G. (2004). Reorganization of the human ipsilesional premotor cortex after stroke. *Brain: A*

Journal of Neurology, 127(Pt 4), 747–758. Retrieved from http://www.ncbi.nlm.nih.gov/pubmed/14749291

Fritsch, B., Reis, J., Martinowich, K., Schambra, H. M., Ji, Y., Cohen, L. G., & Lu, B. (2010). Direct current stimulation promotes BDNF-dependent synaptic plasticity: Potential implications for motor learning. *Neuron, 66*(2), 198–204.

Fusco, A., Assenza, F., Iosa, M., Izzo, S., Altavilla, R., Paolucci, S., & Vernieri, F. (2014). The ineffective role of cathodal tDCS in enhancing the functional motor outcomes in early phase of stroke rehabilitation: An experimental trial. *BioMed Research International, 2014*, 547290.

Gandiga, P. C., Hummel, F. C., & Cohen, L. G. (2006). Transcranial DC stimulation (tDCS): A tool for double-blind sham-controlled clinical studies in brain stimulation. *Clinical Neurophysiology, 117*(4), 845–850. Retrieved from http://www.ncbi.nlm.nih.gov/entrez/query.fcgi?cmd=Retrieve&db=PubMed&dopt=Citation&list_uids=16427357

Gerloff, C., Bushara, K., Sailer, A., Wassermann, E. M., Chen, R., Matsuoka, T., … Hallett, M. (2006). Multimodal imaging of brain reorganization in motor areas of the contralesional hemisphere of well recovered patients after capsular stroke. *Brain, 129*(Pt 3), 791–808. Retrieved from http://www.ncbi.nlm.nih.gov/entrez/query.fcgi?cmd=Retrieve&db=PubMed&dopt=Citation&list_uids=16364955

Geroin, C., Picelli, A., Munari, D., Waldner, A., Tomelleri, C., & Smania, N. (2011). Combined transcranial direct current stimulation and robot-assisted gait training in patients with chronic stroke: A preliminary comparison. *Clinical Rehabilitation, 25*(6), 537–548.

Gilbert, D. T., King, G., Pettigrew, S., & Wilson, T. D. (2016). Comment on "Estimating the reproducibility of psychological science". *Science, 351*(6277), 1037.

Grefkes, C., Eickhoff, S. B., Nowak, D. A., Dafotakis, M., & Fink, G. R. (2008). Dynamic intra- and interhemispheric interactions during unilateral and bilateral hand movements assessed with fMRI and DCM. *NeuroImage, 41*(4), 1382–1394. S1053-8119(08)00283-8 [pii].

Grefkes, C., Nowak, D. A., Wang, L. E., Dafotakis, M., Eickhoff, S. B., & Fink, G. R. (2010). Modulating cortical connectivity in stroke patients by rTMS assessed with fMRI and dynamic causal modeling. *NeuroImage, 50*(1), 233–242. S1053-8119(09)01317-2 [pii].

Group, C., Cheeran, B., Cohen, L., Dobkin, B., Ford, G., Greenwood, R., … Wolf, S. (2008). The future of restorative neurosciences in stroke: Driving the translational research pipeline from basic science to rehabilitation of people after stroke. *Neurorehabilitation and Neural Repair, 23*(2), 97–107.

Hamdy, S. (2010). Role of neurostimulation and neuroplasticity in the rehabilitation of dysphagia after stroke. *SIG 13 Perspectives on Swallowing and Swallowing Disorders (Dysphagia), 19*(1), 3–9.

Harnish, S., Meinzer, M., Trinastic, J., Fitzgerald, D., & Page, S. (2014). Language changes coincide with motor and fMRI changes following upper extremity motor therapy for hemiparesis: A brief report. *Brain Imaging and Behavior, 8*(3), 370–377.

Harris-Love, M. L., Chan, E., Dromerick, A. W., & Cohen, L. G. (2015). Neural substrates of motor recovery in severely impaired stroke patients with hand paralysis. *Neurorehabilitation and Neural Repair, 30*, 328–338.

Harris-Love, M. L., Chan, E., Dromerick, A. W., & Cohen, L. G. (2016). Neural substrates of motor recovery in severely impaired stroke patients with hand paralysis. *Neurorehabilitation and Neural Repair, 30*(4), 328–338.

Hashemirad, F., Zoghi, M., Fitzgerald, P. B., & Jaberzadeh, S. (2016). The effect of anodal transcranial direct current stimulation on motor sequence learning in healthy individuals: A systematic review and meta-analysis. *Brain and Cognition, 102*, 1–12.

Heise, K. F., Niehoff, M., Feldheim, J. F., Liuzzi, G., Gerloff, C., & Hummel, F. C. (2014). Differential behavioral and physiological effects of anodal transcranial direct current stimulation in healthy adults of younger and older age. *Frontiers in Aging Neuroscience, 6*, 146.

Hesse, S., Waldner, A., Mehrholz, J., Tomelleri, C., Pohl, M., & Werner, C. (2011). Combined transcranial direct current stimulation and robot-assisted arm training in subacute stroke patients: An exploratory, randomized multicenter trial. *Neurorehabilitation and Neural Repair, 25*(9), 838–846.

Hesse, S., Werner, C., Schonhardt, E. M., Bardeleben, A., Jenrich, W., & Kirker, S. G. B. (2007). Combined transcranial direct current stimulation and robot-assisted arm training in subacute stroke patients: A pilot study. *Restorative Neurology and Neuroscience, 25*(1), 9–15. Retrieved from http://www.ncbi.nlm.nih.gov/pubmed/17473391. http://content.iospress.com/articles/restorative-neurology-and-neuroscience/rnn00347

Hodics, T., Cohen, L. G., & Cramer, S. C. (2006). Functional imaging of intervention effects in stroke motor rehabilitation. *Archives of Physical Medicine and Rehabilitation, 87*(12 Suppl 2), S36–S42. Retrieved from http://www.ncbi.nlm.nih.gov/entrez/query.fcgi?cmd=Retrieve&db=PubMed&dopt=Citation&list_uids=17140878

Horvath, J., Vogrin, S. J., Carter, O., Cook, M. J., & Forte, J. D. (2016). Effects of a common transcranial direct current stimulation (tDCS) protocol on motor evoked potentials found to be highly variable within individuals over 9 testing sessions. *Experimental Brain Research, 234*, 2629–2642.

Hummel, F., Celnik, P., Giraux, P., Floel, A., Wu, W.-H. H., Gerloff, C., & Cohen, L. G. (2005). Effects of non-invasive cortical stimulation on skilled motor function in chronic stroke. *Brain: A Journal of Neurology, 128*(Pt 3), 490–499. Retrieved from http://www.ncbi.nlm.nih.gov/entrez/query.fcgi?cmd=Retrieve&db=PubMed&dopt=Citation&list_uids=15634731

Hummel, F., & Cohen, L. G. (2005a). Improvement of motor function with noninvasive cortical stimulation in a patient with chronic stroke. *Neurorehabilitation and Neural Repair, 19*(1), 14–19. Retrieved from http://www.ncbi.nlm.nih.gov/entrez/query.fcgi?cmd=Retrieve&db=PubMed&dopt=Citation&list_uids=15673839

Hummel, F. C., Celnik, P., Pascual-Leone, A., Fregni, F., Byblow, W. D., Buetefisch, C. M., … Gerloff, C. (2008). Controversy: Noninvasive and invasive cortical stimulation show efficacy in treating stroke patients. *Brain Stimulation, 1*(4), 370–382.

Hummel, F. C., & Cohen, L. G. (2005b). Drivers of brain plasticity. *Current Opinion in Neurology, 18*(6), 667–674. Retrieved from http://www.ncbi.nlm.nih.gov/entrez/query.fcgi?cmd=Retrieve&db=PubMed&dopt=Citation&list_uids=16280678

Hummel, F. C., & Cohen, L. G. (2006). Non-invasive brain stimulation: A new strategy to improve neurorehabilitation after stroke? *Lancet Neurology, 5*(8), 708–712. Retrieved from http://www.ncbi.nlm.nih.gov/entrez/query.fcgi?cmd=Retrieve&db=PubMed&dopt=Citation&list_uids=16857577

Hummel, F. C., Voller, B., Celnik, P., Floel, A., Giraux, P., Gerloff, C., & Cohen, L. G. (2006). Effects of brain polarization on reaction times and pinch force in chronic stroke. *BMC Neuroscience, 7*(1), 73. Retrieved from http://www.ncbi.nlm.nih.gov/entrez/query.fcgi?cmd=Retrieve&db=PubMed&dopt=Citation&list_uids=17083730

Hussey, E. K., Ward, N., Christianson, K., & Kramer, A. F. (2015). Language and memory improvements following tDCS of left lateral prefrontal cortex. *PLoS One, 10*(11), e0141417.

Jeffery, D. T., Norton, J. A., Roy, F. D., & Gorassini, M. A. (2007). Effects of transcranial direct current stimulation on the excitability of the leg motor cortex. *Experimental Brain Research, 182*(2), 281–287.

Johansen-Berg, H., Rushworth, M. F., Bogdanovic, M. D., Kischka, U., Wimalaratna, S., & Matthews, P. M. (2002). The role of ipsilateral premotor cortex in hand movement after stroke. *Proceedings of the National Academy of Sciences of the United States of America, 99*(22), 14518–14523. Retrieved from http://www.ncbi.nlm.nih.gov/entrez/query.fcgi?cmd=Retrieve&db=PubMed&dopt=Citation&list_uids=12376621

Kang, E. K., Kim, Y. K., Sohn, H. M., Cohen, L. G., & Paik, N. J. (2011). Improved picture naming in aphasia patients treated with cathodal tDCS to inhibit the right Broca's homologue area. *Restorative Neurology and Neuroscience, 29*(3), 141–152.

Kang, N., Summers, J. J., & Cauraugh, J. H. (2016). Transcranial direct current stimulation facilitates motor learning post-stroke: A systematic review and meta-analysis. *Journal of Neurology, Neurosurgery & Psychiatry, 87*(4), 345–355.

Kaplan, R. M., & Irvin, V. L. (2015). Likelihood of null effects of large NHLBI clinical trials has increased over time. *PLoS One, 10*(8), e0132382.

Khedr, E. M., Shawky, O. A., El-Hammady, D. H., Rothwell, J. C., Darwish, E. S., Mostafa, O. M., & Tohamy, A. M. (2013). Effect of anodal versus cathodal transcranial direct current

stimulation on stroke rehabilitation: A pilot randomized controlled trial. *Neurorehabilitation and Neural Repair, 27*(7), 592–601.
Kim, D.-Y., Lim, J.-Y., Kang, E., You, D., Oh, M.-K., Oh, B.-M., & Paik, N.-J. (2010). Effect of transcranial direct current stimulation on motor recovery in patients with subacute stroke. *American Journal of Physical Medicine & Rehabilitation, 89*(11), 879–886.
Kim, D. Y., Ohn, S. H., Yang, E. J., Park, C.-I. I., & Jung, K. J. (2009). Enhancing motor performance by anodal transcranial direct current stimulation in subacute stroke patients. *American Journal of Physical Medicine & Rehabilitation/Association of Academic Physiatrists, 88*(10), 829–836.
Kincses, T. Z., Antal, A., Nitsche, M. A., Bartfai, O., & Paulus, W. (2004). Facilitation of probabilistic classification learning by transcranial direct current stimulation of the prefrontal cortex in the human. *Neuropsychologia, 42*(1), 113–117. Retrieved from http://www.ncbi.nlm.nih.gov/entrez/query.fcgi?cmd=Retrieve&db=PubMed&dopt=Citation&list_uids=14615081
Kinsbourne, M. (1977). Hemi-neglect and hemisphere rivalry. *Advances in Neurology, 18*, 41–49. Retrieved from http://www.ncbi.nlm.nih.gov/entrez/query.fcgi?cmd=Retrieve&db=PubMed&dopt=Citation&list_uids=920524
Kinsbourne, M. (1980). Dichotic imbalance due to isolated hemisphere occlusion or directional rivalry? *Brain and Language, 11*(1), 221–224. Retrieved from http://www.ncbi.nlm.nih.gov/entrez/query.fcgi?cmd=Retrieve&db=PubMed&dopt=Citation&list_uids=7427722
Kirton, A., Deveber, G., Gunraj, C., & Chen, R. (2010). Cortical excitability and interhemispheric inhibition after subcortical pediatric stroke: Plastic organization and effects of rTMS. *Clinical Neurophysiology, 121*(11), 1922–1929. S1388-2457(10)00374-3 [pii].
Ko, M.-H. H., Han, S.-H. H., Park, S.-H. H., Seo, J.-H. H., & Kim, Y.-H. H. (2008). Improvement of visual scanning after DC brain polarization of parietal cortex in stroke patients with spatial neglect. *Neuroscience Letters, 448*(2), 171–174.
Kumar, S., Wagner, C. W., Frayne, C., Zhu, L., Selim, M., Feng, W., & Schlaug, G. (2011). Noninvasive brain stimulation may improve stroke-related dysphagia a pilot study. *Stroke, 42*(4), 1035–1040.
Làdavas, E., Giulietti, S., Avenanti, A., Bertini, C., Lorenzini, E., Quinquinio, C., & Serino, A. (2015). a-tDCS on the ipsilesional parietal cortex boosts the effects of prism adaptation treatment in neglect. *Restorative Neurology and Neuroscience, 33*(5), 647–662.
Lang, N., Nitsche, M. A., Paulus, W., Rothwell, J. C., & Lemon, R. N. (2004). Effects of transcranial direct current stimulation over the human motor cortex on corticospinal and transcallosal excitability. *Experimental Brain Research, 156*(4), 439–443. Retrieved from http://www.ncbi.nlm.nih.gov/entrez/query.fcgi?cmd=Retrieve&db=PubMed&dopt=Citation&list_uids=14745467
Langhorne, P., Bernhardt, J., & Kwakkel, G. (2011). Stroke rehabilitation. *The Lancet, 377*(9778), 1693–1702.
Lauer, M. S., Krumholz, H. M., & Topol, E. J. (2015). Time for a prepublication culture in clinical research? *Lancet, 386*(10012), 2447–2449.
Lazar, R. M., Minzer, B., Antoniello, D., Festa, J. R., Krakauer, J. W., & Marshall, R. S. (2010). Improvement in aphasia scores after stroke is well predicted by initial severity. *Stroke, 41*(7), 1485–1488.
Lee, K., Lim, S., Kim, K., Kim, K., Kim, Y., Chang, W., … Hwang, B. (2015). Six-month functional recovery of stroke patients: A multi-time-point study. *International Journal of Rehabilitation Research, 38*(2), 173–180.
Lefebvre, S., Laloux, P., Peeters, A., Desfontaines, P., Jamart, J., & Vandermeeren, Y. (2013). Dual-tDCS enhances online motor skill learning and long-term retention in chronic stroke patients. *Frontiers in Human Neuroscience, 6*, 343.
Lefebvre, S., Thonnard, J.-L., Laloux, P., Peeters, A., Jamart, J., & Vandermeeren, Y. (2014). Single session of dual-tDCS transiently improves precision grip and dexterity of the paretic hand after stroke. *Neurorehabilitation and Neural Repair, 28*(2), 100–110.
Lindenberg, R., Renga, V., Zhu, L. L., Nair, D., & Schlaug, G. (2010). Bihemispheric brain stimulation facilitates motor recovery in chronic stroke patients. *Neurology, 75*(24), 2176–2184.

Lindenberg, R., Zhu, L. L., & Schlaug, G. (2012). Combined central and peripheral stimulation to facilitate motor recovery after stroke: The effect of number of sessions on outcome. *Neurorehabilitation and Neural Repair, 26*(5), 479–483.

Lohse, K. R., Lang, C. E., & Boyd, L. A. (2014). Is more better? Using metadata to explore dose-response relationships in stroke rehabilitation. *Stroke, 45*(7), 2053–2058.

Lotze, M., Markert, J., Sauseng, P., Hoppe, J., Plewnia, C., & Gerloff, C. (2006). The role of multiple contralesional motor areas for complex hand movements after internal capsular lesion. *The Journal of Neuroscience, 26*(22), 6096–6102. Retrieved from http://www.ncbi.nlm.nih.gov/entrez/query.fcgi?cmd=Retrieve&db=PubMed&dopt=Citation&list_uids=16738254

Madhavan, S., & Shah, B. (2012). Enhancing motor skill learning with transcranial direct current stimulation – A concise review with applications to stroke. *Frontiers in Psychiatry, 3*, 66.

Madhavan, S., & Stinear, J. W. (2010). Focal and bidirectional modulation of lower limb motor cortex using anodal transcranial direct current stimulation. *Brain Stimulation, 3*(1), 42–50.

Madhavan, S., Weber, K. A., & Stinear, J. W. (2010). Non-invasive brain stimulation enhances fine motor control of the hemiparetic ankle: Implications for rehabilitation. *Experimental Brain Research, 209*(1), 9–17.

Mahmoudi, H., Haghighi, A., Petramfar, P., Jahanshahi, S., Salehi, Z., & Fregni, F. (2011). Transcranial direct current stimulation: Electrode montage in stroke. *Disability and Rehabilitation, 33*(15–16), 1383–1388.

Mancuso, L. E., Ilieva, I. P., Hamilton, R. H., & Farah, M. J. (2016). Does transcranial direct current stimulation improve healthy working memory?: A meta-analytic review. *Journal of Cognitive Neuroscience, 28*, 1–27.

Mansur, C. G., Fregni, F., Boggio, P. S., Riberto, M., Gallucci-Neto, J., Santos, C. M., … Pascual-Leone, A. (2005). A sham stimulation-controlled trial of rTMS of the unaffected hemisphere in stroke patients. *Neurology, 64*(10), 1802–1804.

Marangolo, P., Fiori, V., Cipollari, S., Campana, S., Razzano, C., Paola, M., … Caltagirone, C. (2013). Bihemispheric stimulation over left and right inferior frontal region enhances recovery from apraxia of speech in chronic aphasia. *European Journal of Neuroscience, 38*(9), 3370–3377.

Marangolo, P., Fiori, V., Sabatini, U., Pasquale, G., Razzano, C., Caltagirone, C., & Gili, T. (2016). Bilateral transcranial direct current stimulation language treatment enhances functional connectivity in the left hemisphere: Preliminary data from aphasia. *Journal of Cognitive Neuroscience, 28*(5), 1–15.

Marshall, R. S. (2009). Rehabilitation approaches to Hemineglect. *The Neurologist, 15*(4), 185–192.

Mead, G., Bernhardt, J., & Kwakkel, G. (2012). Stroke: Physical fitness, exercise, and fatigue. *Stroke Research and Treatment, 2012*, 632531.

Meinzer, M., Lindenberg, R., Antonenko, D., Flaisch, T., & Floel, A. (2013). Anodal transcranial direct current stimulation temporarily reverses age-associated cognitive decline and functional brain activity changes. *The Journal of Neuroscience, 33*(30), 12470–12478.

Meinzer, M., Lindenberg, R., Sieg, M. M., Nachtigall, L., Ulm, L., & Floel, A. (2014). Transcranial direct current stimulation of the primary motor cortex improves word-retrieval in older adults. *Frontiers in Aging Neuroscience, 6*, 253.

Mello, E. A., Cohen, L. G., Monteiro Dos Anjos, S., Conti, J., Andrade, K. N., Tovar Moll, F., … Conforto, A. B. (2015). Increase in short-interval Intracortical facilitation of the motor cortex after low-frequency repetitive magnetic stimulation of the unaffected hemisphere in the subacute phase after stroke. *Neural Plasticity, 2015*, 407320.

Monti, A., Cogiamanian, F., Marceglia, S., Ferrucci, R., Mameli, F., Mrakic-Sposta, S., … Priori, A. (2008). Improved naming after transcranial direct current stimulation in aphasia. *Journal of Neurology, Neurosurgery & Psychiatry, 79*(4), 451–453.

Morey, R. D., Chambers, C. D., Etchells, P. J., Harris, C. R., Hoekstra, R., Lakens, D., … Zwaan, R. A. (2016). The peer reviewers' openness initiative: Incentivizing open research practices through peer review. *Royal Society Open Science, 3*(1), 150547.

Mortensen, J., Figlewski, K., & Andersen, H. (2015). Combined transcranial direct current stimulation and home-based occupational therapy for upper limb motor impairment following intracerebral hemorrhage: A double-blind randomized controlled trial. *Disability and Rehabilitation, 38*(7), 637–643.

Mozaffarian, D., Benjamin, E. J., Go, A. S., Arnett, D. K., Blaha, M. J., Cushman, M., … Subcommittee, A. (2015). Heart disease and stroke statistics—2016 update. *Circulation, 133*(4), e38–e360.

Murase, N., Duque, J., Mazzocchio, R., & Cohen, L. G. (2004). Influence of interhemispheric interactions on motor function in chronic stroke. *Annals of Neurology, 55*(3), 400–409. Retrieved from

Müri, R., Cazzoli, D., Nef, T., Mosimann, U. P., Hopfner, S., & Nyffeler, T. (2013). Non-invasive brain stimulation in neglect rehabilitation: An update. *Frontiers in Human Neuroscience, 7*.

Mylius, V., Ayache, S. S., Zouari, H. G., Aoun-Sebaïti, M., Farhat, W. H., & Lefaucheur, J. -P. (2012). Stroke rehabilitation using noninvasive cortical stimulation: Hemispatial neglect. *Expert Review of Neurotherapeutics, 12*(8), 983–991. Retrieved from http://www.ncbi.nlm.nih.gov/pubmed/23002941. http://www.tandfonline.com/doi/pdf/10.1586/ern.12.78

Nair, D. G., Hutchinson, S., Fregni, F., Alexander, M., Pascual-Leone, A., & Schlaug, G. (2006). Imaging correlates of motor recovery from cerebral infarction and their physiological significance in well-recovered patients. *NeuroImage* Retrieved from http://www.ncbi.nlm.nih.gov/entrez/query.fcgi?cmd=Retrieve&db=PubMed&dopt=Citation&list_uids=17070707

Nair, D. G., Hutchinson, S., Fregni, F., Alexander, M., Pascual-Leone, A., & Schlaug, G. (2007). Imaging correlates of motor recovery from cerebral infarction and their physiological significance in well-recovered patients. NeuroImage, 34(1), 253–263. Retrieved from Documents%20and%20Settings/cohenl1/Local%20Settings/Application%20Data/Quosa/Data/My%20Citations/a1a7nvmt52dkf8usi7407m7aig.qpw. http://www.ncbi.nlm.nih.gov/entrez/query.fcgi?cmd=Retrieve&db=pubmed&dopt=Citation&list_uids=17070707

Nair, D. G., Renga, V., Lindenberg, R., Zhu, L., & Schlaug, G. (2011). Optimizing recovery potential through simultaneous occupational therapy and non-invasive brain-stimulation using tDCS. *Restorative Neurology and Neuroscience, 29*(6), 411–420.

Nitsche, M. A., Liebetanz, D., Tergau, F., & Paulus, W. (2002). Modulation of cortical excitability by transcranial direct current stimulation. *Nervenarzt, 73*(4), 332–335. Retrieved from http://www.ncbi.nlm.nih.gov/entrez/query.fcgi?cmd=Retrieve&db=PubMed&dopt=Citation&list_uids=12040980

Nosek, B. A., Alter, G., Banks, G. C., Borsboom, D., Bowman, S. D., Breckler, S. J., … Yarkoni, T. (2015). Scientific standards. Promoting an open research culture. *Science, 348*(6242), 1422–1425.

Nowak, D. A., Grefkes, C., Ameli, M., & Fink, G. R. (2009). Interhemispheric competition after stroke: Brain stimulation to enhance recovery of function of the affected hand. *Neurorehabilitation and Neural Repair* 1545968309336661 [pii], *23*, 641–656.

Nudo, R. J., Wise, B. M., SiFuentes, F., & Milliken, G. W. (1996). Neural substrates for the effects of rehabilitative training on motor recovery after ischemic infarct. *Science (New York, NY), 272*(5269), 1791–1794.

Open Science, C. (2015). Psychology. Estimating the reproducibility of psychological science. *Science, 349*(6251), aac4716.

Otal, B., Dutta, A., Foerster, Á., Ripolles, O., Kuceyeski, A., Miranda, P. C., … Ruffini, G. (2016). Opportunities for guided multichannel non-invasive transcranial current stimulation in post-stroke rehabilitation. *Frontiers in Neurology, 7*, 21.

Paci, M., Nannetti, L., Casavola, D., & Lombardi, B. (2016). Differences in motor recovery between upper and lower limbs: Does stroke subtype make the difference? *International Journal of Rehabilitation Research. Internationale Zeitschrift fur Rehabilitationsforschung. Revue internationale de recherches de readaptation., 39*, 185–187.

Park, S., Kim, J., & Song, H. (2015). Effect of application of transcranial direct current stimulation during task-related training on gait ability of patients with stroke. *Journal of Physical Therapy Science, 27*(3), 623–625.

Pedersen, P. M., Jørgensen, H. S., Nakayama, H., Raaschou, H. O., & Olsen, T. S. (1997). Hemineglect in acute stroke--incidence and prognostic implications. The Copenhagen Stroke Study. *American Journal of Physical Medicine & Rehabilitation/Association of Academic Physiatrists, 76*(2), 122–127. Retrieved from http://www.ncbi.nlm.nih.gov/pubmed/9129518

Perceval, G., Floel, A., & Meinzer, M. (2016). Can transcranial direct current stimulation counteract age-associated functional impairment? *Neuroscience and Biobehavioral Reviews, 65*, 157–172.

Perez, M. A., & Cohen, L. G. (2008). Mechanisms underlying functional changes in the primary motor cortex ipsilateral to an active hand. *The Journal of Neuroscience, 28*(22), 5631–5640. 28/22/5631 [pii].

Perez, M. A., & Cohen, L. G. (2009). Interhemispheric inhibition between primary motor cortices: What have we learned? *The Journal of Physiology, 587*(Pt 4), 725–726. jphysiol.2008.166926 [pii].

Pisegna, J. M., Kaneoka, A., Pearson, W. G., Kumar, S., & Langmore, S. E. (2016). Effects of non-invasive brain stimulation on post-stroke dysphagia: A systematic review and meta-analysis of randomized controlled trials. *Clinical Neurophysiology, 127*(1), 956–968.

Primaßin, A., Scholtes, N., Heim, S., Huber, W., Neuschäfer, M., Binkofski, F., & Werner, C. J. (2015). Determinants of concurrent motor and language recovery during intensive therapy in chronic stroke patients: Four single-case studies. *Frontiers in Neurology, 6*.

Qu, Y. P., Wu, D. Y., Tu, X. Q., Quian, L., Yang, Y. B., & Geng, H. (2009). Effect of transcranial direct current stimulation on relieving upper-limb spasticity after stroke (in Chinese). *Chinese Journal of Cerebrovascular Disease, 6*, 586–589.

Reis, J., Robertson, E. M., Krakauer, J. W., Rothwell, J., Marshall, L., Gerloff, C., … Cohen, L. G. (2008). Consensus: Can transcranial direct current stimulation and transcranial magnetic stimulation enhance motor learning and memory formation? *Brain Stimulation, 1*(4), 363–369. S1935-861X(08)00325-2 [pii].

Reis, J., Schambra, H. M., Cohen, L. G., Buch, E. R., Fritsch, B., Zarahn, E., … Krakauer, J. W. (2009). Noninvasive cortical stimulation enhances motor skill acquisition over multiple days through an effect on consolidation. *Proceedings of the National Academy of Sciences of the United States of America, 106*(5), 1590–1595. 0805413106 [pii].

Rocha, S., Silva, E., Foerster, Á., Wiesiolek, C., Chagas, A. P., Machado, G., … Monte-Silva, K. (2016). The impact of transcranial direct current stimulation (tDCS) combined with modified constraint-induced movement therapy (mCIMT) on upper limb function in chronic stroke: A double-blind randomized controlled trial. *Disability and Rehabilitation, 38*(7), 653–660.

Rossi, C., Sallustio, F., Legge, D. S., Stanzione, P., & Koch, G. (2013). Transcranial direct current stimulation of the affected hemisphere does not accelerate recovery of acute stroke patients. *European Journal of Neurology, 20*(1), 202–204.

Rosso, C., Valabregue, R., Arbizu, C., Ferrieux, S., Vargas, P., Humbert, F., … Lehéricy, S. (2014). Connectivity between right inferior frontal gyrus and supplementary motor area predicts after-effects of right frontal cathodal tDCS on picture naming speed. *Brain Stimulation, 7*(1), 122–129.

Saeys, W., Vereeck, L., Lafosse, C., Truijen, S., Wuyts, F. L., & Heyning, P. (2015). Transcranial direct current stimulation in the recovery of postural control after stroke: A pilot study. *Disability and Rehabilitation, 37*(20), 1857–1863.

Sattler, V., Acket, B., Raposo, N., Albucher, F. J., Thalamas, C., Loubinoux, I., … Simonetta-Moreau, M. (2015). Anodal tDCS combined with radial nerve stimulation promotes hand motor recovery in the acute phase after ischemic stroke. *Neurorehabilitation and Neural Repair, 29*(8), 743–754.

Saur, D., & Hartwigsen, G. (2012). Neurobiology of language recovery after stroke: Lessons from neuroimaging studies. *Archives of Physical Medicine and Rehabilitation, 93((*1), S15–S25.
Schambra, H. M., Abe, M., Luckenbaugh, D. A., Reis, J., Krakauer, J. W., & Cohen, L. G. (2011). Probing for hemispheric specialization for motor skill learning: A transcranial direct current stimulation study. *Journal of Neurophysiology, 106*(2), 652–661. jn.00210.2011 [pii].
Schambra, H. M., Ogden, T. R., Martínez-Hernández, I. E., Lin, X., Chang, B. Y., Rahman, A., … Krakauer, J. W. (2015). The reliability of repeated TMS measures in older adults and in patients with subacute and chronic stroke. *Frontiers in Cellular Neuroscience, 9*, 335.
Schlaug, G., & Cohen, L. G. (2010). *Brain repair after stroke* (pp. 207–218). Cambridge.
Schlaug, G., & Renga, V. (2008). Transcranial direct current stimulation: A noninvasive tool to facilitate stroke recovery. *Expert Review of Medical Devices, 5*(6), 759–768.
Shigematsu, T., Fujishima, I., & Ohno, K. (2013). Transcranial direct current stimulation improves swallowing function in stroke patients. *Neurorehabilitation and Neural Repair, 27*(4), 363–369.
Shiozawa, P., Fregni, F., Benseñor, I. M., Lotufo, P. A., Berlim, M. T., Daskalakis, J. Z., … Brunoni, A. R. (2014). Transcranial direct current stimulation for major depression: An updated systematic review and meta-analysis. *The International Journal of Neuropsychopharmacology/ Official Scientific Journal of the Collegium Internationale Neuropsychopharmacologicum (CINP), 17*(9), 1443–1452.
Sohn, M., Jee, S., & Kim, Y. (2013). Effect of transcranial direct current stimulation on postural stability and lower extremity strength in hemiplegic stroke patients. *Annals of Rehabilitation Medicine, 37*(6), 759–765.
Sparing, R., Thimm, M., Hesse, M. D., Küst, J., Karbe, H., & Fink, G. R. (2009). Bidirectional alterations of interhemispheric parietal balance by non-invasive cortical stimulation. *Brain: A Journal of Neurology, 132*(Pt 11), 3011–3020.
Spielmans, G. I., & Kirsch, I. (2014). Drug approval and drug effectiveness. *Annual Review of Clinical Psychology, 10*(1), 741–766.
Stagg, C., Bachtiar, V., O'Shea, J., Allman, C., Bosnell, R., Kischka, U., … Johansen-Berg, H. (2012). Cortical activation changes underlying stimulation-induced behavioural gains in chronic stroke. *Brain, 135*(1), 276–284.
Stagg, C. J., Jayaram, G., Pastor, D., Kincses, Z. T., Matthews, P. M., & Johansen-Berg, H. (2011). Polarity and timing-dependent effects of transcranial direct current stimulation in explicit motor learning. *Neuropsychologia, 49*(5), 800–804. S0028-3932(11)00071-6 [pii].
Stinear, C., Barber, A., Petoe, M., Answar, S., & Byblow, W. (2012). Predicting potential for motor recovery after stroke. *Annals of Physical and Rehabilitation Medicine, 55*.
Stinear, C. M., Byblow, W. D., & Ward, S. H. (2014). An update on predicting motor recovery after stroke. *Annals of Physical and Rehabilitation Medicine, 57*(8), 489–498.
Straudi, S., Fregni, F., Martinuzzi, C., Pavarelli, C., Salvioli, S., & Basaglia, N. (2016). tDCS and robotics on upper limb stroke rehabilitation: Effect modification by stroke duration and type of stroke. *BioMed Research International, 2016*, 1–8.
Sunwoo, H., Kim, Y.-H., Chang, W., Noh, S., Kim, E.-J., & Ko, M.-H. (2013). Effects of dual transcranial direct current stimulation on post-stroke unilateral visuospatial neglect. *Neuroscience Letters, 554*, 94–98.
Tahtis, V., Kaski, D., & Seemungal, B. M. (2014). The effect of single session bi-cephalic transcranial direct current stimulation on gait performance in sub-acute stroke: A pilot study. *Restorative Neurology and Neuroscience, 32*(4), 527–532.
Tanaka, S., Sandrini, M., & Cohen, L. G. (2011). Modulation of motor learning and memory formation by non-invasive cortical stimulation of the primary motor cortex. *Neuropsychological Rehabilitation, 21*(5), 650–675.
Triccas, T. L., Burridge, J. H., Hughes, A. M., Pickering, R. M., Desikan, M., Rothwell, J. C., & Verheyden, G. (2016). Multiple sessions of transcranial direct current stimulation and upper extremity rehabilitation in stroke: A review and meta-analysis. *Clinical Neurophysiology, 127*(1), 946–955.

Triccas, T. L., Burridge, J. H., Hughes, A., Verheyden, G., Desikan, M., & Rothwell, J. (2015). A double-blinded randomised controlled trial exploring the effect of anodal transcranial direct current stimulation and uni-lateral robot therapy for the impaired upper limb in sub-acute and chronic stroke. *NeuroRehabilitation, 37*(2), 181–191.

Turkeltaub, P. E., Messing, S., Norise, C., & Hamilton, R. H. (2011). Are networks for residual language function and recovery consistent across aphasic patients? *Neurology, 76*(20), 1726–1734.

Turner, E. H., Matthews, A. M., Linardatos, E., Tell, R. A., & Rosenthal, R. (2008). Selective publication of antidepressant trials and its influence on apparent efficacy. *The New England Journal of Medicine, 358*(3), 252–260.

Turner, E. H., & Rosenthal, R. (2008). Efficacy of antidepressants. *BMJ (Clinical Research Ed.), 336*(7643), 516–517.

Vallar, G. (1998). Spatial hemineglect in humans. *Trends in Cognitive Sciences, 2*(3), 87–97.

van Asseldonk, E., & Boonstra, T. A. (2016). Transcranial direct current stimulation of the leg motor cortex enhances coordinated motor output during walking with a large inter-individual variability. *Brain Stimulation, 9*(2), 182–190.

Vannorsdall, T. D., van Steenburgh, J. J., Schretlen, D. J., Jayatillake, R., Skolasky, R. L., & Gordon, B. (2016). Reproducibility of tDCS results in a randomized trial: Failure to replicate findings of tDCS-induced enhancement of verbal fluency. *Cognitive and Behavioral Neurology, 29*(1), 11–17.

Viana, R. T., Laurentino, G. E. C., Souza, R. J. P., Fonseca, J. B., Filho, S. E. M., Dias, S. N., … Monte-Silva, K. K. (2014). Effects of the addition of transcranial direct current stimulation to virtual reality therapy after stroke: A pilot randomized controlled trial. *NeuroRehabilitation, 34*(3), 437–446.

Vines, B. W., Nair, D. G., & Schlaug, G. (2006). Contralateral and ipsilateral motor effects after transcranial direct current stimulation. *Neuroreport, 17*(6), 671–674. Retrieved from http://www.ncbi.nlm.nih.gov/entrez/query.fcgi?cmd=Retrieve&db=PubMed&dopt=Citation&list_uids=16603933

Vines, B. W., Norton, A. C., & Schlaug, G. (2011). Non-invasive brain stimulation enhances the effects of melodic intonation therapy. *Frontiers in Psychology, 2*, 230.

Wade, D. T., Hewer, R. L., David, R. M., & Enderby, P. M. (1986). Aphasia after stroke: Natural history and associated deficits. *Journal of Neurology, Neurosurgery & Psychiatry, 49*(1), 11–16.

Ward, N. S. (2016). Non-invasive brain stimulation for stroke recovery: Ready for the big time? *Journal of Neurology, Neurosurgery, and Psychiatry, 87*(4), 343–344.

Ward, N. S., & Cohen, L. G. (2004). Mechanisms underlying recovery of motor function after stroke. *Archives of Neurology, 61*(12), 1844–1848. Retrieved from http://www.ncbi.nlm.nih.gov/entrez/query.fcgi?cmd=Retrieve&db=PubMed&dopt=Citation&list_uids=15596603

Winstein, C. J., Stein, J., Arena, R., Bates, B., Cherney, L. R., Cramer, S. C., … Zorowitz, R. D. (2016). Guidelines for adult stroke rehabilitation and recovery. *Stroke, 47*, e98–e169.

Wirth, M., Rahman, R., Kuenecke, J., Koenig, T., Horn, H., Sommer, W., & Dierks, T. (2011). Effects of transcranial direct current stimulation (tDCS) on behaviour and electrophysiology of language production. *Neuropsychologia, 49*(14), 3989–3998.

Woods, A. J., Antal, A., Bikson, M., Boggio, P. S., Brunoni, A. R., Celnik, P., … Nitsche, M. A. (2016). A technical guide to tDCS, and related non-invasive brain stimulation tools. *Clinical Neurophysiology, 127*(2), 1031–1048.

Wu, D., Qian, L., Zorowitz, R. D., Zhang, L., Qu, Y., & Yuan, Y. (2013). Effects on decreasing upper-limb poststroke muscle tone using transcranial direct current stimulation: A randomized sham-controlled study. *Archives of Physical Medicine and Rehabilitation, 94*(1), 1–8.

Yang, E., Baek, S.-R., Shin, J., Lim, J., Jang, H., Kim, Y., & Paik, N.-J. (2012). Effects of transcranial direct current stimulation (tDCS) on post-stroke dysphagia. *Restorative Neurology and Neuroscience, 30*(4), 303–311.

You, D., Kim, D.-Y., Chun, M., Jung, S., & Park, S. (2011). Cathodal transcranial direct current stimulation of the right Wernicke's area improves comprehension in subacute stroke patients. *Brain and Language, 119*(1), 1–5.

Zimerman, M., Heise, K. F., Hoppe, J., Cohen, L. G., Gerloff, C., & Hummel, F. C. (2012). Modulation of training by single-session transcranial direct current stimulation to the intact motor cortex enhances motor skill acquisition of the paretic hand. *Stroke; a Journal of Cerebral Circulation, 43*(8), 2185–2191.

Zimerman, M., Nitsch, M., Giraux, P., Gerloff, C., Cohen, L. G., & Hummel, F. C. (2013). Neuroenhancement of the aging brain: Restoring skill acquisition in old subjects. *Annals of Neurology, 73*(1), 10–15.

Chapter 18
Transcranial Direct Current Stimulation Potential for Pain Management

Helena Knotkova, Jeffrey J. Borckardt, Alexa Riggs, and Alexandre F. DaSilva

Introduction

The anatomical and functional components of pain processing network represent viable targets for neuromodulation. Building on early findings from invasive neurostimulation, such as deep brain stimulation or motor cortex stimulation, analgesic effects of tDCS have been explored in both acute and chronic pain conditions in research settings as well as in clinic. Neurophysiological and neuroimaging studies in the past decades have shown that the pain processing network in the brain is more complex than traditionally thought (Hemington et al. 2016).

Determining the areas of the brain that might serve as the best clinical targets is somewhat challenging to date. Pain is a complex experience that has sensory-discriminatory, motivational-affective and cognitive-evaluative dimensions (Gatchel et al. 2007). Experimental and clinical fMRI findings suggest that parietal areas, including the primary somatosensory cortex (SI), are mainly involved in the sensory-discriminative dimension of pain experience and frontolimbic networks are

H. Knotkova (✉)
MJHS Institute for Innovation in Palliative Care, New York, NY, USA

Department of Family and Social Medicine, Albert Einstein College of Medicine, Bronx, NY, USA
e-mail: HKnotkov@mjhs.org

J. J. Borckardt
Departments of Psychiatry, Anesthesia, and Stomatology, Medical University of South Carolina, Charleston, SC, USA

A. Riggs
MJHS Institute for Innovation in Palliative Care, New York, NY, USA

A. F. DaSilva
The Molecular & Behavioral Neuroscience Institute (MBNI), Ann Arbor, MI, USA

Biologic & Materials Sciences, School of Dentistry, Ann Arbor, MI, USA

H. Knotkova et al. (eds.), *Practical Guide to Transcranial Direct Current Stimulation*, https://doi.org/10.1007/978-3-319-95948-1_18

involved in the affective dimension (Greer and Hoyt 1990; Treede et al. 1999). Activation of SI tends to be limited to activation contralateral to the side of stimulation, whereas the SII tends to demonstrate bilateral activation (Crue et al. 1976; Dyck et al. 1976). There is evidence supporting the involvement of the anterior cingulate cortex (ACC) in the affective dimension of pain experience (Burns et al. 2003; Greer and Hoyt 1990; Staud et al. 2003; Treede et al. 1999). Other brain structures that appear to be involved in the affective component of pain experience include the lateral and medial thalamus, insular cortex, and the prefrontal cortex (Atkinson et al. 1999; Brooks et al. 2002; Davis 2003; Giardino et al. 2003). The role of the left prefrontal cortex in pain control is unclear. However, there is evidence to support the concept that left prefrontal activation is negatively correlated with pain unpleasantness (Lorenz et al. 2003) suggesting a possible governing role of the left prefrontal cortex on the affective dimension of pain experience (Seminowicz and Davis 2006). There is evidence that activation of the left prefrontal cortex is associated with analgesic effects, presumably by modulating limbic response to pain. There is also evidence that deactivation of the right prefrontal cortex is associated with improvement in clinical pain (Sampson et al. 2006) suggesting a distinct laterality with respect to the role(s) of the prefrontal cortex in pain modulation. However, imaging studies and numerous cortical stimulation studies in humans suggest that motor cortex stimulation can significantly reduce pain as well by modulating activity in networks of brain areas involved in pain processing, such as the thalamus and by facilitating descending pain inhibitory mechanisms (Garcia-Larrea et al. 1997, 1999; Peyron et al. 2007).

When managing pain with tDCS, the goal is to modulate activity in the areas of the brain that are involved in pain processing. tDCS with anode placed over a cortical target results in a raised level of excitability under the electrode, whereas cathodal stimulation appears to decrease local cortical excitability (Nitsche et al. 2008). While most tDCS-pain studies to date have focused on anodal stimulation of the motor cortex, there is accumulating evidence to suggest that the prefrontal cortex and the somatosensory cortex may be reasonable tDCS cortical targets for pain management as well (Antal et al. 2008, and others).

TDCS for Acute Post-operative Pain

The proper control of acute pain is one of the most important areas in health care. Despite the profound advances in neuroscience over the past 20 years, medicine still largely resorts to opiate narcotics, however this strategy is not without considerable risk, and is only marginally effective in many cases. Non-invasive brain stimulation techniques like tDCS may have a role in both acute and chronic pain management by modulating circuits involved with pain perception and pain inhibition in the brain. However, little is known about optimal stimulation strategies (e.g., cortical targets, stimulation parameters, duration of treatment) that can produce robust analgesic effects. One unique, yet largely under-studied potential application of tDCS, is in the perioperative arena. While pain is often a complaint that precedes certain surgical procedures such as lumbar surgery and knee replacement surgery, the procedures themselves are associated with considerable post-operative pain lasting days to weeks, and adequate postoperative pain control is an important factor in determining recovery time and hospital length of stay (Capdevila et al. 1999; Chelly et al. 2001; Wang et al. 2002).

Primary methods used to manage post-operative pain in general involve systemic opioid or other analgesic drug delivery, and regional blocks. Despite these pain-management strategies, patients still report considerable post-operative pain, and often struggle to complete post-operative physical therapy regimens (when indicated). Systemic opioid analgesic use has associated side-effects that can lead to post-operative complications including but not limited to mental-clouding, confusion, respiratory depression, interactions with other medications, addiction in some cases, fatigue, and gastric motility problems. Further, surgical procedures along with the associated intraoperative anesthesia protocols have been associated with increased risk for post-operative cognitive problems (Deo et al. 2011) especially among the elderly (Talmo et al. 2010). For obese patients, apnea is a real concern that post-operative systemic opioid use can complicate (Samson et al. 2010; Talmo et al. 2010).

As more and more novel brain stimulation technologies including transcranial magnetic stimulation (TMS) and tDCS are beginning to demonstrate promise as treatments for a variety of pain conditions (Barker et al. 1985, 1989; Fregni et al. 2007; George et al. 2003; Rosen et al. 2009; Williams et al. 2009), the notion of neurostimulation for post-operative pain is becoming viable and promising for exploration. Electricity has no metabolite or other residue, and can be delivered with minimal discomfort and without problems associated with drug-drug interactions. These advantages help support the idea that non-invasive brain stimulation techniques may play a role in a multi-modal post-operative pain management regimen.

The development of tDCS protocols for management of acute postoperative pain builds on evidence and experience from applications of other non-invasive brain stimulation methods that were introduced to medicine earlier, such as Transcranial Magnetic Stimulation. An example including findings that facilitated use of tDCS to manage post-procedural pain is discussed below.

Post-operative Pain Following Gastric Bypass Surgery

The first study of neurostimulation to manage post-operative pain was conducted using transcranial magnetic stimulation in gastric bypass patients. In 2002, there were 63,000 bariatric surgeries in the US. The number of bariatric surgeries increased to 196,000 in 2015 according to the American Society for Metabolic and Bariatric Surgery (asmbs.org). Opioid medications are the most commonly used drugs for pain relief in the perioperative setting, however there are, of course, risks and problems associated with opioid use (Morgan et al. 2006). Many of the side-effects of opioid medications are particularly problematic in gastric-bypass surgery patients who tend to have respiratory problems (like obstructive sleep apnea), right ventricular dysfunction, pulmonary hypertension, and for whom post-operative vomiting could result in serious complications.

In the first studies of TMS for post-operative pain (Borckardt et al. 2008), subjects were randomly assigned to receive real TMS or sham TMS over the left dorsolateral prefrontal cortex. Subjects received 20 min of 10 Hz rTMS at 100% of resting motor threshold (10-s stimulation trains with 20-s inter-stimulus intervals) for a total of 4000 pulses. Subjects that received real TMS used an average of 39.59 mg (SD = 19.33) of morphine and subjects receiving sham TMS used 62.27 (SD = 40.44). Real TMS was associated with a 36% decrease in total morphine usage at the time of discharge (Cohen's d = 0.70) in 40 participants (see Fig. 18.1). There was a significant effect for TMS condition (sham versus real; $F(6,31) = 3.06$, $p < .05$). Subjects that received real TMS reported lower ratings of "pain on average", "pain at its worst" and reported better "mood at its worst" than did subjects receiving sham TMS (see Fig. 18.2). Interestingly, these subjective reports of less pain and better mood occurred in the treatment group despite them using significantly less

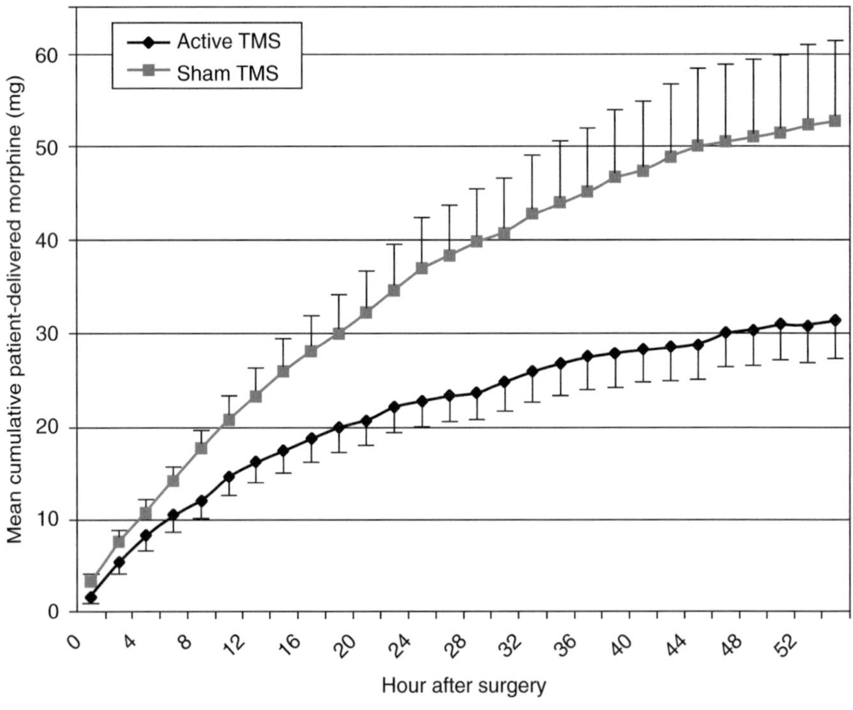

Fig. 18.1 Mean (& Std Err) cumulative PCA morphine use after surgery for patients receiving sham versus real prefrontal TMS

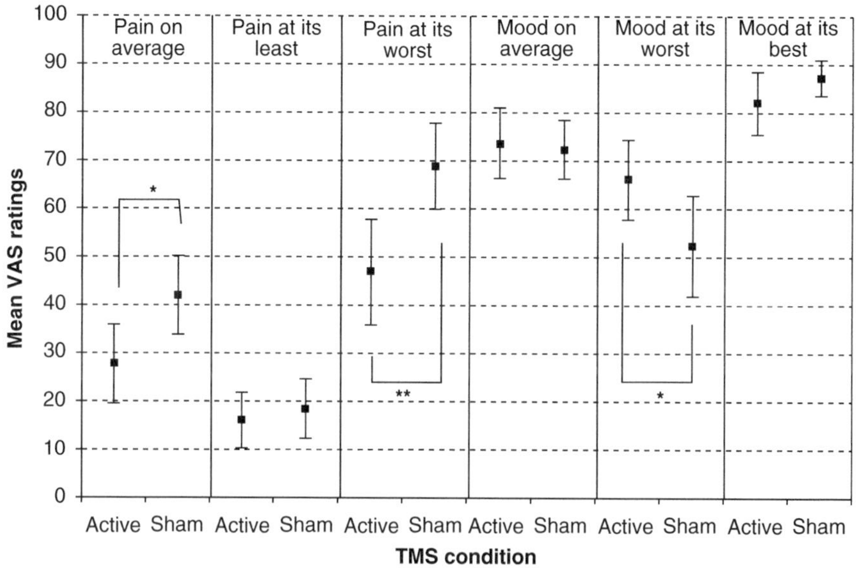

Fig. 18.2 Mean VAS ratings (and 95% CI) for pain and mood among patients receiving real versus sham left prefrontal TMS postoperatively (*p < .05; **p < .01)

PCA morphine. While these findings were promising, from a practical standpoint, TMS has limitations compared to tDCS as the dosing procedures are complicated, the machine is cumbersome, the procedure is uncomfortable for some, the stimulation is loud, there is a documented risk of seizure, and patients cannot move their heads during treatment. tDCS is simple, portable, silent, painless and is much better suited to managing pain in post-anesthesia care units.

tDCS for Post-procedural Pain Following Endoscopic Retrograde Cholangiopancreatography (ERCP)

Abdominal pain and irritable bowel syndrome (IBS) are a growing indication for endoscopy. An international study showed 18% of IBS patients are now treated with narcotics (Drossman et al. 2007). When patients with this profile undergo endoscopy, they frequently have post-endoscopy pain, partially due to the stretch of bowel by the endoscope and because of air added during the procedure. The pain is generally transient, but can be confused with an early complication, and can prompt an admission for observation or a return to the emergency dept. Pain can be severe during and after ERCP in these patients, mimicking early pancreatitis, or even perforation, in the recovery bay. There is growing evidence supporting the role of central mechanisms in gut-related pain. Hyperexcitability of the pain neuromatrix in the brain and failure of pain inhibitory cortical circuits may contribute to the gut-pain experience and exacerbation. Direct targeting of these cortical circuits might make it possible for transient pain to be reduced to something tolerable with oral pain medication.

In the first-ever pilot study on the effects of tDCS on post-ERCP pain (Borckardt et al. 2011), 19 Caucasian females underwent post-ERCP tDCS. After ERCP was completed, participants were randomly assigned to receive 20-min of 2 mA tDCS with anode over the left-prefrontal cortex and cathode over the gut representation of the sensory cortex (electrode size 4 cm × 4 cm). There were no serious adverse events associated with tDCS, and the side-effects of tDCS were limited to tingling (42%), itching (47%) and mild stinging (11%) under the electrodes. Patients that received real tDCS used 22% less total hydromorphone than those that received sham at the end of the 24-h inpatient post-procedural period (Cohen's $d = .38$). The slope of the cumulative PCA usage curve was significantly steeper in the sham tDCS group compared to real ($t(355) = 10.80$, $p < .0001$). VAS pain scores suggested an arithmetic advantage for real tDCS compared to sham. Results from this pilot feasibility study suggest that tDCS is safe, well-tolerated, and may be able to reduce post-ERCP opioid requirements without increasing subjective pain ratings. Since this pilot only tested a low dose of tDCS (a single 20-min session), and given that the observed analgesic/opioid-sparing effect was mild, it may be that more tDCS sessions could produce more robust post-operative analgesic effects.

tDCS in the Management of Knee Arthroplasty Post-procedural Pain

Total knee arthroplasty (TKA) is one of the most common orthopedic procedures, and according to the Agency for Healthcare Research and Quality (AHRQ), more than 600,000 knee replacements are performed each year in the United States. Because the prevalence of arthritis is expected to grow substantially as the population ages (Acheson and Collart 1975; Peyron 1986), TKA procedures are likely to become even more common. The rate of revision total knee arthroplasties is increasing by approximately 6 procedures per 100,000 persons per decade. TKA has been shown to improve functional status, and relieve pain, and the number and the rate of total knee arthroplasties is increasing steadily. Between 1990 and 2002, the rate of primary total knee arthroplasties per 100,000 persons almost tripled. While knee pain is often a complaint that precedes TKA, the procedure itself is associated with considerable post-operative pain lasting days to weeks post-operatively.

As with many surgical procedures, adequate postoperative pain control in TKA is an important factor in determining recovery time and hospital length of stay (Capdevila et al. 1999; Chelly et al. 2001; Wang et al. 2002). Many of the side-effects of opioid medications for post-operative pain control are problematic in TKA patients who tend to be overweight and/or elderly (Deo et al. 2011; Samson et al. 2010; Talmo et al. 2010). While the risk of opioid patient-controlled analgesia (PCA) pump usage leading to future opioid abuse appears to be relatively small (1%) (Greer et al. 2001), opioid abuse is on the rise in the United States (Compton and Volkow 2006). In many cases, both patients and physicians worry about the potential for dependence and abuse of opioid medications, and this sometimes results in undertreatment of acute and chronic pain (Greer et al. 2001). Despite the use of regional blocks and patient administered opioid medication, patients still report considerable post-operative pain, exhibit decreased functioning, and often struggle to complete post-operative physical therapy regimens.

In a preliminary pilot study (Borckardt et al. 2013), we randomly assigned 40 patients undergoing unilateral TKA to receive a total of 80 min of real (n = 20) or sham tDCS (n = 20) with the anode over the knee representation of the motor strip and cathode over the right dorsolateral prefrontal cortex. Twenty-minute tDCS treatments were delivered: (1) in the PACU, (2) 4-h later, (3) the morning of post-operative day-1, and (4) the afternoon of post-operative day-1. VAS pain and mood ratings were collected every 4 h following surgery provided that patients were awake. The slopes of the cumulative PCA usage curves were significantly different between groups, and those TKA in the real tDCS group used 44% less PCA dilaudid at 48-h post-op ($p = .007$; Cohen's $d = 1.0$). Despite significantly lower PCA dilaudid levels, VAS ratings of pain-on-average were also significantly lower in the real tDCS group ($t(37) = 2.28$, $p = .029$). No adverse events or serious adverse events were encountered. There were no cases in which tDCS needed to be discontinued due to patient discomfort or tDCS-related complications (Fig. 18.3).

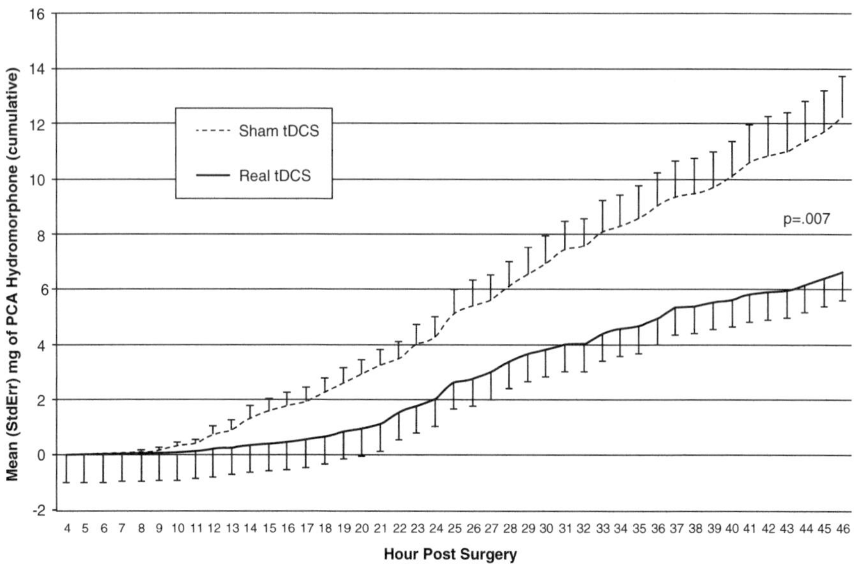

Fig. 18.3 Cumulative PCA hydromorphone use following TKA among participants receiving 80-min of either real or sham tDCS

In a follow-up, randomized, sham-controlled trial (Borckardt, under editorial consideration), we enrolled 61 TKA patients and randomly assigned them to receive 4 post-operative sessions of tDCS with electrode placements of: (1) anode-motor cortex, cathode-right prefrontal cortex; (2) anode-left prefrontal cortex, cathode sensory cortex; (3) anode-left temporal-occipital junction, cathode-medial anterior pre-motor area (active-sham condition); and a zero-current sham condition. There were no differences in PCA opioid usage between the active-sham and the zero-current-sham groups. Prefrontal placement was associated with a 26% decrease in PCA opioid usage compared to sham, however, motor stimulation was associated with a 24% increase compared to sham. The slopes of the PCA usage curves in both the prefrontal ($t(2979) = -6.5$, $p < .0001$) and motor cortex ($t(2979) = 9.9$, $p < .0001$) stimulation groups were significantly different from sham.

tDCS for Post-operative Pain Following Lumbar Surgery

In a recent randomized, double-blind, sham-controlled pilot clinical trial (Glaser et al. 2016), 4 sessions of tDCS were delivered for pain and patient controlled analgesia (PCA) opioid usage control among patients receiving spine surgery. Twenty-seven patients undergoing lumbar spine procedures that required at least one-night hospitalization for parenteral pain medication were enrolled in the present study.

Immediately after surgery, participants were randomly assigned to undergo 20-min-long sessions of real or sham tDCS (2 mA, anode placed over the superior motor cortex (corresponding to the low-back/trunk area) and cathode over the right dorsolateral prefrontal cortex. Electrode placement was determined using the EEG 10–20 system (positions Cz and F4). At total of four sessions of tDCS (all real or all sham) were administered (Session 1 – approximately 30 min following surgery, Session 2–4 h later, Session 3 – on the morning of post-operative day-1 and Session 4–4-h later). In order to monitor for adverse events directly associated with tDCS, participants were asked to report any sensations they experienced during each of the 4 tDCS stimulation sessions at 1-, 10- and 20-min into the sessions.

The mean numerical rating scale (NRS) average-pain rating of the sample was 6.6 ($SD = 1.5$) out of 10 at the time of admission. Fourteen (14) participants were randomized to receive real tDCS and 13 received sham. There were no differences between the real and sham tDCS groups at baseline with respect to age, chronic opioid therapy status, pain at its worst, pain at its least, pain on average, weight, or sex. No adverse events were observed with the tDCS.

The effect of tDCS (real versus sham) on the slope of the cumulative PCA hydromorphone curve was significant ($F(238,2879) = 5.06$, $p < .001$). At the time of discharge, participants who received real tDCS used an average of 12.6 mg ($SD = 9.9$) of hydromorphone and subjects receiving sham tDCS used an average of 16.5 mg ($SD = 12.7$) suggesting that tDCS was associated with a 23% reduction in PCA usage (effect-size Cohen's $d = 0.3$). Participants were unable to correctly guess whether they received real or sham tDCS at a rate better than chance (52% correct guess rate; $p = .84$, ns). Independent t-test analysis of NRS scores from the BPI at admission and discharge indicated no significant differences between tDCS groups at admission for pain on average, pain at its least or pain at its worst ($p = .24$, $p = .22$, $p = .27$, respectively) nor at discharge ($p = .58$, $p = .47$, $p = .72$). In the real tDCS group a significant 31% reduction was observed in pain-at-its-least ratings from admission (mean = 4.5 SD = 2.5) to discharge (mean = 3.2 SD = 2.2; $t(12) = 2.52$, $p = .027$), but no other changes in pain ratings were significant in either group.

In another study examining the effects of tDCS on post-lumbar surgery pain and opioid use, the prefrontal cortex was targeted (Dubois et al. 2013); participants received either anodal, cathodal or sham stimulation over the left DLPFC. This study found no difference between groups on any of the outcomes of interest.

tDCS for Management of Chronic Pain

tDCS applications in chronic pain syndromes build on findings that indicate that the development and maintenance of chronic pain is associated with multitude of persisting dynamic changes in the pain-processing neural network as well as altered functional connectivity with other cerebral networks (Apkarian et al. 2013; Hemington et al. 2016; Liu et al. 2012; Moseley and Flor 2012; Saab 2012). In chronic pain patients, altered cortical functioning within the default mode network and salience network has been observed (Hemington et al. 2016), and functional connectivity between the networks was affected as well. As compared to healthy subjects, patients with chronic pain present with a decrease in the functional connectivity between the default mode network and salience network, and the degree of this abnormality parallels pain reports and disease-related symptoms (Hemington et al. 2016). Overall, research evidence suggests that in chronic pain, maladaptive neuroplasticity plays a role in functional and/or structural changes in the brain that may be associated with persistence of pain beyond healing and the development and maintenance of chronic pain (DeSouza et al. 2016; Flor 2003; Frost et al. 2003; Hemington et al. 2016; Jain et al. 2008; Kelly and Garavan 2005; López-Solà et al. 2016; and others). Importantly, research conducted over the pasts decades provide evidence that reversal of the maladaptive changes in brain function is possible and can be associated with an improvement of symptoms, including chronic pain (Juottonen et al. 2002; MacIver et al. 2008; Maihöfner et al. 2003, 2004, 2006; Napadow et al. 2009, 2012; Pleger et al. 2005; and others). Up to date, tDCS effects on chronic pain have been explored in numerous controlled clinical trials supported by pilot studies and clinical reports in a variety of pain conditions, including difficult-to-treat pain syndromes such as multiple sclerosis-related pain, fibromyalgia, complex regional pain syndrome, central pain due to spinal cord injury, phantom-limb pain, painful peripheral diabetic neuropathy and others (Knotkova et al. 2013, 2015). Illustratory examples are discussed below.

Fibromyalgia

Fibromyalgia (FM) is a chronic pain syndrome characterized by bilateral pain above and below waist, axial skeletal pain and at least 11 of 18 tender points (Arnold et al. 2008). Other symptoms of FM include fatigue, difficulty sleeping, headaches, and mood disorders (McCarthy 2016). FM affects about 2% of the population, and women are diagnosed at a ratio of 9:1 compared to men (Bartels et al. 2009; Lawrence et al. 2008). FM is thought to have several causal components including a genetic component, as well as a predisposition to central pain processing abnormalities leading to central sensitization (Ablin and Buskila 2015; Chinn et al. 2016; Rossi et al. 2015). Treatment strategies consists of a multifaceted array of techniques including medications, exercise, or life-style adjustments (Goldenberg et al. 2016; Kibar et al. 2015; McCarthy 2016; Rossi et al. 2015).

Effects of tDCS on pain and related symptoms in FM have been examined in multiple studies (Castillo-Saavedra et al. 2016; Fagerlund et al. 2015; Fregni et al. 2006a, b; Mendonca et al. 2016; Riberto et al. 2011; Roizenblatt et al. 2007; Valle et al. 2009; Villamar et al. 2013). The studies evaluated tDCS applications involving M1 as well as DLPFC montages, and stimulations on 5 or more days (Fregni et al. 2006a, b; Roizenblatt et al. 2007; Valle et al. 2009), as well as a combination of tDCS with other supportive treatment strategies, such as rehabilitation or exercise (Mendonca et al. 2016; Riberto et al. 2011).

In a randomized sham controlled trial by Fregni and colleagues 2006a, b, 32 FM patients received either sham, or real tDCS with anode over the M1 or over the left DLPFC at 2 mA on 5 consecutive days. M1 tDCS yielded significantly greater pain relief than DLPFC tDCS or sham ($p < 0.0001$), and the analgesic effect was still significant after 3 weeks of follow up ($p = 0.004$). In addition, the M1 stimulation resulted in a small improvement of quality of life. Similar results of M1 tDCS on 5 consecutive days were observed by Fagerlund et al. (2015) in a randomized sham controlled trial involving 48 patients. In a longer stimulation protocol (10 consecutive sessions of M1 or DLPFC tDCS at 2 mA, or sham; $n = 41$) by Valle et al. (2009), both M1 and DLPFC stimulation led to improvements of pain and quality of life by the end of the 10-day treatment, but only M1 tDCS yielded long-lasting benefits that persisted through the follow-up at 30 and 60 days after the treatment.

Further, a combination of M1 tDCS with weekly sessions of multidisciplinary rehabilitation program (Riberto et al. 2011, $n = 23$) resulted in significantly better pain relief ($p = 0.006$) as compared to rehabilitation paired with sham, and also showed trending ($p = 0.056$) toward better improvement of FM burden. Similarly, a combination of the anodal M1 tDCS with aerobic exercise (Mendonca et al. 2016; $n = 45$) resulted is significantly greater FM pain relief than each individual intervention ($p = 0.0056$ and $p = .007$ respectively), and the combined intervention had significantly greater benefiting effects on mood and anxiety.

Other studies in fibromyalgia examined outcomes from high-definition tDCS (HD-tDCS) stimulation, in a single (Villamar et al. 2013) or multiple sessions (Castillo-Saavedra et al. 2016) aiming for tDCS dose optimization in order to achieve FM-related pain relief at clinically meaningful degree. In a double-blind sham controlled RCT by Villamar et al. (2013) 18 patients were randomized to undergo single 20-min sessions of sham, anodal and cathodal HD-tDCS at 2.0 mA in a cross-over counterbalanced manner, using the 4 × 1-ring configuration, with the center electrode positioned over the left primary motor cortex. The results have shown that both active stimulation conditions led to significant reduction in overall perceived pain as compared to sham, and the effects were present at 30 min after the stimulation. In addition, active anodal stimulation induced a significant bilateral increase in mechanical detection thresholds. A follow-up open-label study from the same group aimed to establish the number of HD-tDCS sessions required to achieve a 50% reduction of FM pain (Castillo-Saavedra et al. 2016). The pre-defined 50% pain reduction was achieved in 7 of 14 patients, with both responders and non-responders benefiting from a cumulative effect of treatment, reflected in significant pain reduction ($p = .035$) as well as improved quality of life ($p = .001$) over time. The authors also reported an aggregate 6-week response rate of 50% of patients, and median number of 15 HD-tDCS sessions to reach clinically meaningful outcomes. This study provided evidence supporting an optimization of stimulation protocol toward individualized patient-tailored tDCS treatment of FM pain.

Central Pain Due to Multiple Sclerosis

Multiple sclerosis (MS) is a demyelinating disease in which the insulating covers of nerve cells in the brain and spinal cord are damaged (Berer and Krishnamoorthy 2014). MS has a relatively low age of onset, on average 25.3 years of age (Berer and Krishnamoorthy 2014). Women are diagnosed more than men at a ratio of about 2:1 (Marrie et al. 2016). A variety of neurological and physical symptoms include motor weakness, sensory problems, fatigue, visual disturbances, balance problems and pain. The prevalence of pain in MS patients is estimated to range from 29% to 86% (Clifford and Trotter 1984; Foley et al. 2013; Solaro et al. 2013; Stenager et al. 1995) and the pain is more likely for those that are older, and have been diagnosed for longer (Foley et al. 2013; Solaro et al. 2013). MS pain may include continuous central pain, intermittent central pain, musculoskeltal pain, or mixed neuropathic and non-neuropathic pain. The central MS pain is thought to be the most prevalent type of pain reported by MS patients (Solaro et al. 2013). Pain management in MS includes pharmacological treatment with tricyclic antidepressants, antiepileptic drugs, opioids, or cannabinoids, but results remain unsatisfactory for many patients (Solaro et al. 2013). Therefore, explorations of adjunctive non-pharmacological approaches in MS are of high clinical importance, and there is a limited but encouraging evidence on MS pain relief by tDCS.

In a randomized controlled study by Mori et al. (2010), patients received 5 days of sham tDCS or real anodal tDCS over the motor cortex at 2 mA, with electrodes 5 × 7 cm. Following anodal tDCS over the motor cortex but not sham, there was a significant ($p < 0.05$) pain improvement as assessed by VAS for pain and McGill questionnaire, and an improvement of overall quality of life. The magnitude of pain improvement on last day of a 3-week follow-up relative to the baseline was 63.17% on VAS for pain scores, indicating clinically relevant pain relief.

Phantom Limb Pain

It is estimated that phantom limb pain (PLP) may occur after limb amputation at a prevalence as high as 61% (Bekrater-Bodmann et al. 2015; Hsu and Cohen 2013). PLP is distinct from other phenomena that may occur after amputation, such as telescoping. PLP is multifaceted and includes peripheral, spinal and supraspinal mechanisms (Flor et al. 2013; and others).

Medical treatment for PLP include NSAIDs, anti-depressants, tricyclic antidepressants, anticonvulsants including gabapentin and pregabalin, NMDA receptor antagonists, or opioids (Knotkova et al. 2012). Supportive treatment strategies include occupational therapy, visualization techniques or non-invasive neurostimulation using a mirror-box technique (Foell et al. 2014).

Bolognini and colleagues (2013) examined analgesic effects of a single tDCS session on PLP, stump pain, non-painful phantom limb sensations and telescoping in 8 patients with unilateral lower or upper limb amputation (Bolognini et al. 2013). Sham, or tDCS at 2 mA for 15 min with anode or cathode over the primary motor cortex (M1) and over the posterior parietal cortex (PPC) were applied in 2 double-blind cross-over experiments. Anodal tDCS of M1 resulted in a selective short-lasting decrease of PLP; other montage configurations had no effect on PLP.

A follow-up study by the same group (Bolognini et al. 2015) examined the effects of 5-day tDCS treatment. Sham or anodal tDCS over M1 for 15 min at 1.5 mA on 5 consecutive days was delivered in cross-over manner in 8 subjects with unilateral lower or upper limb amputation and chronic PLP. Immediately after completion of the 5-day real tDCS treatment, the patients reported a significant ($p = 0.04$) decrease of overall PLP as compared to sham and an improvement in the phantom limb movement ($p = 0.05$). Further, the real tDCS as compared to sham resulted in a sustained decrease of background PLP ($p = 0.04$) and a decrease of the frequency of PLP paroxysms ($p = 0.04$). The improvements were present at a follow-up 1 week after the end of treatment. The average degree of PLP relief after the active tDCS was 41%, with 4 patients among 8 reporting a reduction greater than 30%. The frequency of PLP paroxysms decreased at an average of 33%, with a reduction greater than 30% in 4 of 8 patients.

Central Post-stroke Pain

Stoke, either hemorrhagic or ischemic, is one of the leading causes of death in the United States (American Heart Association, 2015). About 19–74% of stroke survivors report pain (Kim 2014). Post stroke pain may include musculoskeletal or central component. Central post stroke pain (CPSP) generally develops days to months after stroke (Flaster et al. 2013) and is described as stabbing, burning pain, often with hyperpathia and allodynia; and mostly in arms, legs, trunk and face (Flaster et al. 2013; Hansen et al. 2012; Kumar et al. 2009). Medical treatments for post stroke central pain include anticonvulsants, tricyclic antidepressants, opioid antagonists, and NMDA blockers (Kim 2014; Mulla et al. 2015), but despite the medications, the CPSP is difficult to manage.

Non-invasive neuromodulation, including tDCS, in stroke survivors has been explored mostly for the purpose of neurorehabilitation to restore mobility and other functions, such as speech. An initial evidence on tDCS for the CPSP (Bae et al. 2014) arises from a RCT involving 14 CPSP patients. Sham or real anodal tDCS at 2 mA over the primary motor cortex were delivered for 20 min 3 days per week, for a period of 3 weeks. Subjective pain was measured using the visual analogue scale (VAS), and in addition pain elicited by cold and heat stimuli were quantified to examine analgesic effects. The sham-tDCS group showed no statistically significant differences over time, while tDCS group showed decreased VAS scores and skin temperature ($p < 0.05$). The threshold temperatures for the sense of cold and pain from cold increased ($p < 0.05$), and those for the sense of warmth and pain from heat decreased ($p < 0.05$).

Diabetic Polyneuropathy

Diabetes is one of the most common chronic illnesses, it is estimated that 592 million people will have diabetes by 2035 (Guariguata et al. 2014). A complication from diabetes is peripheral diabetic neuropathy also known as distal symmetrical polyneuropathy, which is extremely prevalent in the diabetic population over the age of 65, and 61.5% of patients report pain (Jones et al. 2016). As people living with diabetes age and as the duration of illness persists, the likelihood of peripheral diabetic neuropathy increases (Fischer and Waxman 2010; Jones et al. 2016).

The pathology of the pain is not fully understood, yet it's theorized that high blood sugar over time contributes to nerve injuries and that poor insulin regulation contributes to abnormalities in the dorsal root ganglion. Treatment for peripheral diabetic neuropathy include pancreas transplant, diet and exercise, physical therapy, and pharmaceuticals. Medications to treat peripheral neuropathy include tricyclic antidepressants, SNRIs, anticonvulsants, opioids, intravenous alpha-lipoic acid, capsaicin and lidocaine.

In a RCT of patients with painful diabetic polyneuropathy (Kim et al. 2013; n = 60), 20-min tDCS stimulation on five consecutive days resulted in significant decrease of pain intensity ($p < 0.001$) as compared to sham and the analgesic effects were present and significant at 4-week follow-up ($p = 0.007$).

Migraine

Among various types of primary headaches distinguished by the International Classification of Headache Disorders (2013), tDCS has been applied to manage symptoms in migraine. Migraine is a disorder that impairs the life of nearly 1 in 4 American households, with annual direct economic burden with Healthcare and lost productivity estimated to be as high as $36 billion annually in the U.S according to the Migraine Research Foundation (Edmeads and Mackell 2002). Moreover, some migraine sufferers can develop a progressive state of this disease with more than 15 attacks per month. This state is referred to as chronic migraine (CM), a disorder whose patients experience significantly greater headache impact on daily life and have a large potential for substance abuse, especially opiates (Adams et al. 2014; Bigal et al. 2009; Buse et al. 2012). This is arguably one of the neuromechanisms most centrally involved in pain regulation, affecting multiple elements of the pain experience (Zubieta et al. 2002). Moreover, MRI-based reports have found that those findings co-localize with neuroplastic changes in migraine patients (DaSilva et al. 2007a, b).

Conventional therapies are unable to selectively target those dysfunctional brain regions, and there is a paucity of data on how to reverse embedded neuroplastic molecular mechanisms when available medications and surgical therapies fail. Interestingly, several studies with motor cortex stimulation (MCS) have shown that epidural electrodes in the primary motor cortex (M1) are effective in providing analgesia in patients with refractory central pain (Lima and Fregni 2008). The rationale for MCS stimulation is based in part on the thalamic dysfunction noticed in chronic pain and migraine (Lenz et al. 2004), and also on studies demonstrating that MCS significantly changes thalamic activity (Garcia-Larrea et al. 1999). Obviously, the surgical nature of such a procedure limits its indication to more severe chronic pain disorders. tDCS, can now non-invasively modulate and activate the μOR system (DosSantos et al. 2012, 2014), providing relatively lasting pain relief in chronic pain patients and migraine (DaSilva et al. 2011a, b). Hitherto, the molecular information on the dysfunctional μ-opioid system in episodic and chronic patients and how it responds to neuromodulation is scarce. The continuous modulation of this neurotransmitter system, intimately involved in the pain experience could be related to migraine and chronic pain symptomatology, and to brain molecular neuroplasticity in humans. While understanding central mechanisms of pain using molecular neuroimaging is important, equally important is developing novel concepts for future clinical application to provide much needed relief for those patients. tDCS may be one feasible therapeutic options to modulate our endogenous analgesic resources. In this section we will discuss the rationale and endogenous mechanisms associated with tDCS use in migraine.

Dysfunction μ-Opioid Activity in Migraine Patients

There is now direct evidence of endogenous μ-opioid activation during spontaneous migraine and allodynia by measuring μOR non-displaceable binding potential (BP_{ND}) *in vivo* with [^{11}C]carfentanil (DaSilva et al. 2014). The authors noticed a reduction in μOR BP_{ND}, calculated as an increase in endogenous μ-opioid receptor-mediated neurotransmission (RM), during a spontaneous migraine attack compared to baseline in pain-modulatory regions of the opioid system, including the thalamus and PAG (Fig. 18.4). The authors evaluated *in vivo* the μ-opioid system during spontaneous episodic migraine headaches. Seven patients were scanned at interictal and ictal phases using the selective μ-opioid receptor (μOR) radiotracer [^{11}C]carfentanil**.** In the ictal phase there was dysfunctional μOR activation in the medial prefrontal cortex (mPFC), an area highly related to clinical pain processing. Furthermore, μ-opioid binding changes in mPFC showed moderate negative correlation with the combined extension and severity of the attacks. These results indicated for the first time that there is higher endogenous μ-opioid neurotransmission interacting with μOR in migraineurs (DaSilva et al. 2014).

When challenged for sustained thermal stimulus on the trigeminal ophthalmic region (STPTS) during the ictal and interictal phases, six of those migraineurs showed ictal allodynia that was concurrent and positively correlated with μOR activation in the midbrain, extending from red nucleus to vlPAG. These findings demonstrate *in vivo* the high μOR activation in the migraineurs' brains in response to their allodynic experience (Nascimento et al. 2014).

Management of Migraine Symptoms with tDCS

Recently, one study with tDCS was shown to induce a significant decrease in pain in CM patients following 10 non-invasive sessions of anodal M1 and cathodal supraorbital cortex (SO) (DaSilva et al. 2011a)**,** here described as M1-tDCS (Fig. 18.5). Notwithstanding the several studies exploring and challenging the clinical outcomes produced by tDCS (O'Connell et al. 2010, 2014), its beneficial effect in migraine has consistently been reproduced since that study (Antal et al. 2011; Auvichayapat et al. 2012; Cosentino et al. 2014; Vigano et al. 2013; Wickmann et al. 2015). Based on a concept of cortical hyperexcitability in migraine, the primary visual cortex (V1) has also been used as a target for tDCS in prophylactic treatment of migraine. Repetitive application of cathodal stimulation of V1

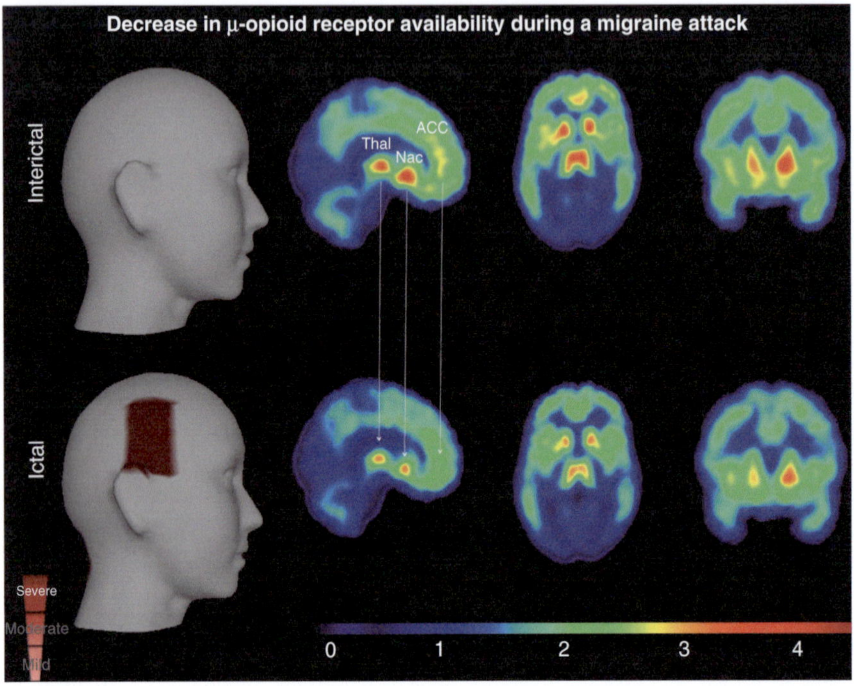

Fig. 18.4 PET during ictal and interictal phases of migraine. Images show decrease in μOR BPND during the ictal migraine phase in the Thal, PAG, ACC, NAc, and Ins. This result possibly represents an increase in endogenous μ-opioid release during the migraine attack due to the ongoing pain {DaSilva, 2014 #1205}. (Adapted from DaSilva et al. (2014); with permission)

significantly decreased the pain intensity of the migraine attacks (Antal et al. 2011). Auvichayapat and coworkers also showed that V1-tDCS significant reduced the attack frequency, pain intensity, and abortive medications (Auvichayapat et al. 2012).

Putative Neural Mechanisms of tDCS Analgesic Effects

Growing evidence suggests that several distinct neural mechanisms may contribute to tDCS analgesic effects. M1 tDCS is thought to modulate sensory-discriminative processing of pain by suppressing lateral thalamic activity, and possibly also by inhibition of the somatosensory cortex through direct cortico-cortical M1-S1 pathways (DosSantos et al. 2016). Further, direct inhibition of the somatosensory cortex via cathodal tDCS may contribute to the modulation of the somatosensory component of pain as well (Antal et al. 2008). The emotional/affective component of pain is thought to modulated mainly by tDCS targeting the dopaminergic and serotoninergic circuits of the frontal and prefrontal cortex and related subcortical areas that mediate

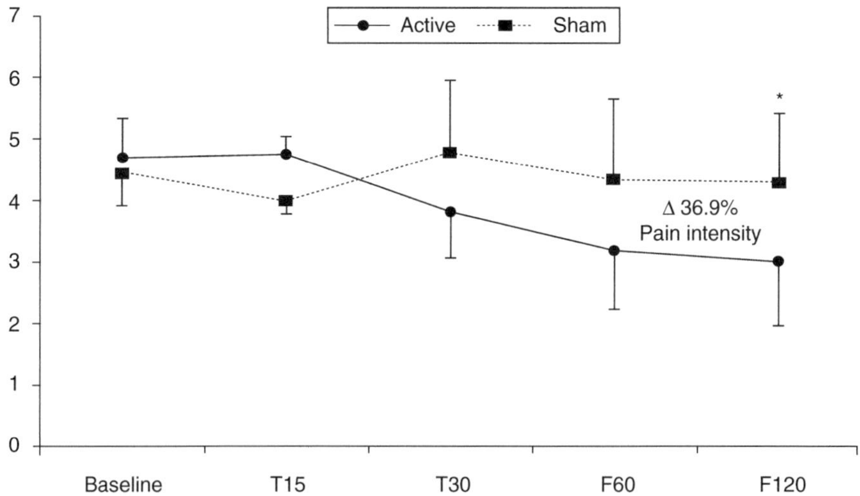

Fig. 18.5 Positive response of chronic migraine to M1-tDCS. Mean pain levels (as assessed by VAS) at baseline, T15 days, T30, F60, and F120 in the 2 groups of stimulation (active & sham tDCS). Error bars indicate standard error of the mean. (DaSilva et al. 2012; with permission)

emotional processing. In addition, results from epidural motor cortex stimulation (Garcia-Larrea et al. 1999; Peyron et al. 1995) suggest that M1 stimulation may also contribute to modulation of the emotional/affective component of pain. Indeed, activation of the brain structures associated with emotional appraisal of pain by epidural M1 stimulation correlated with subjectively reported pain relief (Garcia-Larrea et al. 1999; Peyron et al. 1995).

Another substantial mechanism contributing to modulation of both the somatosensory and emotional/affective component of pain includes the endogenous opioid system.

Interestingly, a recent work by DosSantos et al. (2012) has shown that a single session of anodal M1 tDCS results in reduction of mu opioid receptor binding of an exoge- nous receptor ligand in the pain processing network, suggesting that the analgesic effect of M1 tDCS may possibly be due to a direct increase of endogenous opioid release (DosSantos et al. 2012). The investigation with the μ-opioid specific radiotracer, [^{11}C]carfentanil, showed that the immediate effect of M1 tDCS application induced great μ-opioid system activation in the descending inhibitory system, including the PAG (DosSantos et al. 2014) (Fig. 18.6). The authors examined with PET nine healthy volunteers with no history of chronic pain or systemic disorders. The protocol consisted of two PET scans, using [^{11}C]carfentanil, a selective μOR radiotracer. The first PET provided a baseline evaluation of regional μOR BP_{ND}. During the second PET, placebo and active (2 mA) M1-tDCS sessions were delivered sequentially for 20 min each using the M1 tDCS montage. When analyzed separately, placebo and active tDCS were both associated with an acute reduction in μOR $BP_{ND,}$ indicating activation of this neurotransmitter system in the PAG. In addition, the initial sham tDCS phase induced immediate activation of μORs in the left

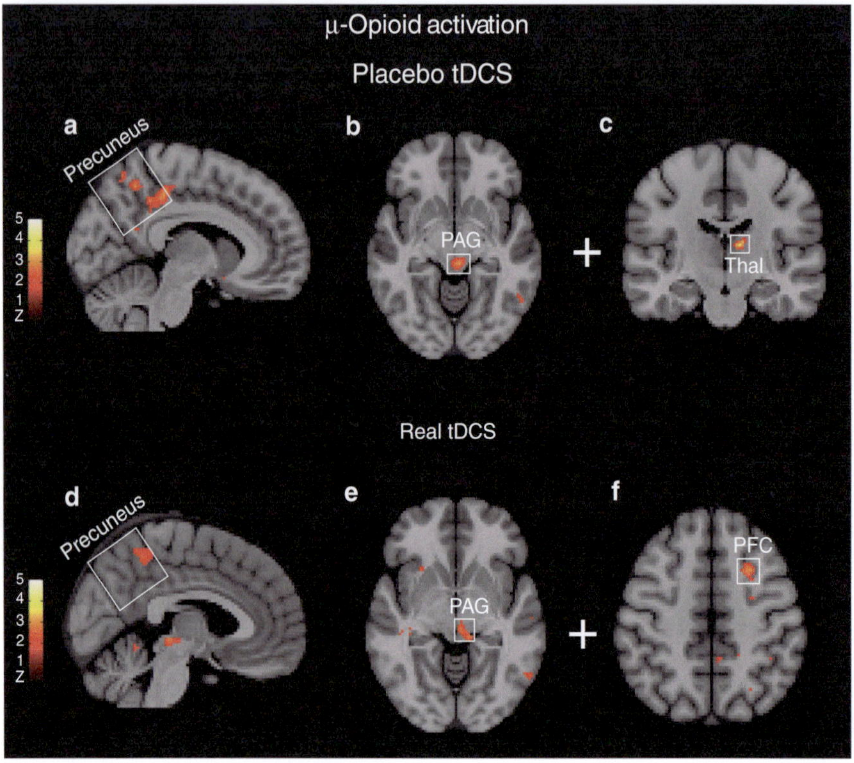

Fig. 18.6 The immediate effect of M1 tDCS application induced great μ-opioid system activation in the descending inhibitory system, including the PAG

thalamus (Thal) and post-cingulate cortex (PCC), and subsequently during the active tDCS phase in the left pre-frontal cortex (PreF) and precuneus (PreC). However, only after active tDCS was there significant improvement of pain thresholds measured by quantitative sensory testing, which were correlated with μOR system activation (DosSantos et al. 2014).

Moreover, there is now sufficient evidence that tDCS modulates not only the endogenous opioid system, but also other biochemical mechanisms related to pain modulation. In a study by Foerster and colleagues (2014), 12 patients with fibromyalgia who underwent 5 daily M1 tDCS had a clinical pain assessment and ^{1}H-MRS testing at baseline, the week of the post-sham tDCS trial, and the week of the post-active M1-tDCS trial. Although this was a cross-over trial, baseline anterior cingulate Glx levels correlated significantly with changes in pain score, both for the time period from baseline to sham tDCS and for the time period from baseline to active tDCS (Fig. 18.7). There was a decrease in pain between baseline-active tDCS time-points. In addition, Glx (glutamate and glutamine) decreased in the ACC and there was a trend towards decreased Glx in the thalamus for the sham-active tDCS

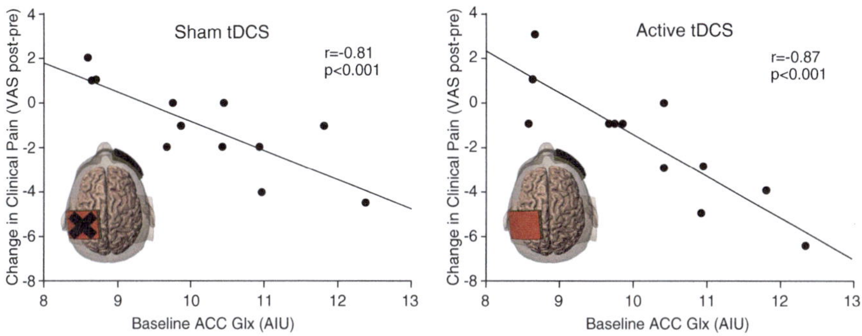

Fig. 18.7 Pretreatment Glx with the anterior cingulate predicts subsequent clinical response to sham and active tDCS

comparison. There was also a trend towards increased GABA in the anterior insula for the baseline-active tDCS comparison and significant linear regression coefficients between the ACC Glx levels and the clinical pain scale changes between the baseline-sham and the baseline-active tDCS.

Practical Considerations for tDCS in Pain Populations

Many practical issues that pertain to tDCS use in pain populations are guided by general principles of best practices in tDCS use that are addressed in various chapters of this book. However, a specific consideration should be given to montages that have been probed in pain populations. The most frequently used montage in tDCS pain studies is the excitability-enhancing ("anodal") tDCS over the primary motor cortex contralateral to the location of pain. In case of bilateral pain with uneven intensity, the anode can be placed contralaterally to the area with higher pain intensity. However, in cases with bilateral/spread pain of even intensity it is at the discretion of the investigator as there are no specific guidelines in place. Other montages probed in pain populations include the excitability-diminishing ("cathodal") tDCS over the somatosensory cortex (Antal et al. 2008; Knotkova et al. 2009) or the stimulation over the dorsolateral prefrontal cortex (DLPFC, anode left, cathode right or over the supraorbital region) (e.g. Riberto et al. 2011; Valle et al. 2009).

Further, as it has been discussed in preceding chapters, tDCS effects can be altered by various pharmacological agents. It may be ethically problematic to aim for a complete pain medication wash-out prior tDCS application, especially in studies involving patients with moderate/severe pain. However, the issue can be minimized for example by a partial wash-out or by switching patients to pre-selected classes of medication within the analgesic armamentarium.

Conclusions

The emerging application of tDCS for pain appears promising, however, it is still not clear how best to use tDCS in order to get the most robust analgesic results.

In the field of post-surgical acute pain, the evidence shows that targeting the motor cortex representation of the surgical/pain area with anodal tDCS might be a good strategy, but concomitant placement of the cathode over the right prefrontal cortex may also play some part in the observed analgesic effects. Stimulation with anode placed over the left prefrontal cortex may also be a promising approach, especially when there is no specific motor target associated with the surgical area (e.g., abdominal surgery). However, findings of prefrontal tDCS analgesic effects in the post-operative arena appear to be mixed.

Overall, it has been shown that stimulating areas of the human cortex involved in pain processing has the potential to significantly reduce post-operative opioid requirements without negatively impacting subjective pain ratings, and in some cases, it can significantly decrease pain ratings even though patients use less opioids. Conducting brain stimulation in the post-operative settings appears feasible and the risks appear minimal. At the very least, several promising, preliminary findings of novel brain stimulation technologies in the post-operative setting suggest that future studies are warranted.

In chronic pain, tDCS has been explored (with mixed success) in a variety of difficult-to-treat syndromes, using a large array of tDCS stimulation protocols and parameters. As a result, comparison of the findings is difficult and no uniform "optimal" stimulation protocol has been identified.

In summary, the field of non-invasive brain stimulation for pain is expanding rapidly. tDCS appears to have the potential to serve as an adjunct to pain management strategies, but better insight into neural mechanisms mediating the tDCS analgesic effects is needed to navigate the development of future larger-scale, well-controlled clinical trials. Further, more high-quality data is needed to evaluate the specificity of tDCS cortical targeting strategies to determine whether there is an optimal electrode placement array for the management of pain.

References

Ablin, J. N., & Buskila, D. (2015). Update on the genetics of the fibromyalgia syndrome. *Best Practice & Research. Clinical Rheumatology, 29*(1), 20–28.

Acheson, R. M., & Collart, A. B. (1975). New Haven survey of joint diseases XVII: Relationship between some systemic characteristics and osteoarthrosis in a general population. *Annals of the Rheumatic Diseases, 34*(5), 379–387.

Adams, A. M., Serrano, D., Buse, D. C., Reed, M. L., Marske, V., Fanning, K. M., & Lipton, R. B. (2014). The impact of chronic migraine: The Chronic Migraine Epidemiology and Outcomes (CaMEO) Study methods and baseline results. *Cephalalgia, 35*, 563–578.

American Heart Association. (2015). Heart disease and stroke statistics. *2015 Update, 131*(4), 29–322.
Antal, A., Brepohl, N., Poreisz, C., Boros, K., Csifcsak, G., & Paulus, W. (2008). Transcranial direct current stimulation over somatosensory cortex decreases experimentally induced acute pain perception. *The Clinical Journal of Pain, 24*(1), 56–63.
Antal, A., Kriener, N., Lang, N., Boros, K., & Paulus, W. (2011). Cathodal transcranial direct current stimulation of the visual cortex in the prophylactic treatment of migraine. *Cephalalgia, 31*, 820–828.
Apkarian, A. V., Baliki, M. N., & Farmer, M. A. (2013). Predicting transition to chronic pain. *Current Opinion in Neurology, 26*(4), 360–367.
Arnold, L. M., Bradley, L. A., Clauw, D. J., Glass, J. M., & Goldenberg, D. L. (2008). Multidisciplinary care and stepwise treatment for fibromyalgia. *The Journal of Clinical Psychiatry, 69*(12), 35–35.
Atkinson, J. H., Slater, M. A., Wahlgren, D. R., Williams, R. A., Zisook, S., Pruitt, S. D., … Garfin, S. R. (1999). Effects of noradrenergic and serotonergic antidepressants on chronic low back pain intensity. *Pain, 83*(2), 137–145.
Auvichayapat, P., Janyacharoen, T., Rotenberg, A., Tiamkao, S., Krisanaprakornkit, T., Sinawat, S., … Auvichayapat, N. (2012). Migraine prophylaxis by anodal transcranial direct current stimulation, a randomized, placebo-controlled trial. *Journal of the Medical Association of Thailand, 95*, 1003–1012.
Bae, S. H., Kim, G. D., & Kim, K. Y. (2014). Analgesic effect of transcranial direct current stimulation on central post-stroke pain. *The Tohoku Journal of Experimental Medicine, 234*(3), 189–195.
Barker, A., Freeston, I., Jarratt, J., & Jalinous, R. (1989). Magnetic stimulation of the human nervous system: An introduction and basic principles. In S. Chokroverty (Ed.), *Magnetic stimulation in clinical neurophysiology* (pp. 55–72). Boston, MA: Butterworth.
Barker, A. T., Jalinous, R., & Freeston, I. L. (1985). Non-invasive magnetic stimulation of human motor cortex. *Lancet, 1*(8437), 1106–1107.
Bartels, E. M., Dreyer, L., Jacobsen, S., Jespersen, A., Bliddal, H., & Danneskiold-Samsøe, B. (2009). Fibromyalgia, diagnosis and prevalence: Are gender differences explainable? *Ugeskrift for Laeger, 171*(49), 3588–3592.
Bekrater-Bodmann, R., Schredl, M., Diers, M., Reinhard, I., Foell, J., Trojan, J., … Flor, H. (2015). Post-amputation pain is associated with the recall of an impaired body representation in dreams-results from a nation-wide survey on limb amputees. *PLoS One, 10*(3), e0119552.
Berer, K., & Krishnamoorthy, G. (2014). Microbial view of central nervous system autoimmunity. *FEBS Letters, 588*(22), 4207–4213.
Bigal, M. E., Borucho, S., Serrano, D., & Lipton, R. B. (2009). The acute treatment of episodic and chronic migraine in the USA. *Cephalalgia, 29*, 891–897.
Bolognini, N., Olgiati, E., Maravita, A., Ferraro, F., & Fregni, F. (2013). Motor and parietal cortex stimulation for phantom limb pain and sensations. *Pain, 154*(8), 1274–1280.
Bolognini, N., Spandri, V., Ferraro, F., Salmaggi, A., Molinari, A. C., Fregni, F., & Maravita, A. (2015). Immediate and sustained effects of 5-day transcranial direct current stimulation of the motor cortex in phantom limb pain. *The Journal of Pain, 16*(7), 657–665.
Borckardt, J. J., Reeves, S. T., Robinson, S. M., May, J. T., Epperson, T. I., Gunselman, R. J., & George, M. S. (2013). Transcranial direct current stimulation (tDCS) reduces postsurgical opioid consumption in total knee arthroplasty (TKA). *The Clinical Journal of Pain, 29*(11), 925–928.
Borckardt, J. J., Reeves, S. T., Weinstein, M., Smith, A. R., Shelley, N., Kozel, F. A., … George, M. S. (2008). Significant analgesic effects of one session of postoperative left prefrontal cortex repetitive transcranial magnetic stimulation: A replication study. *Brain Stimulation, 1*(2), 122–127.
Borckardt, J. J., Romagnuolo, J., Reeves, S. T., Madan, A., Frohman, H., Beam, W., & George, M. S. (2011). Feasibility, safety, and effectiveness of transcranial direct current stimulation

for decreasing post-ERCP pain: A randomized, sham-controlled, pilot study. *Gastrointestinal Endoscopy, 73*(6), 1158–1164.

Brooks, J. C., Nurmikko, T. J., Bimson, W. E., Singh, K. D., & Roberts, N. (2002). fMRI of thermal pain: Effects of stimulus laterality and attention. *NeuroImage, 15*(2), 293–201.

Burns, J. W., Kubilus, A., & Bruehl, S. (2003). Emotion induction moderates effects of anger management style on acute pain sensitivity. *Pain, 106*(1–2), 109–118.

Buse, D., Manack, A., Serrano, D., Reed, M., Varon, S., Turkel, C., & Lipton, R. (2012). Headache impact of chronic and episodic migraine: Results from the American Migraine Prevalence and Prevention study. *Headache, 52*, 3–17.

Capdevila, X., Barthelet, Y., Biboulet, P., Ryckwaert, Y., Rubenovitch, J., & d'Athis, F. (1999). Effects of perioperative analgesic technique on the surgical outcome and duration of rehabilitation after major knee surgery. *Anesthesiology, 91*(1), 8–15.

Castillo-Saavedra, L., Gebodh, N., Bikson, M., Diaz-Cruz, C., Brandao, R., Coutinho, L., & Laufer, I. (2016). Clinically effective treatment of fibromyalgia pain with high-definition transcranial direct current stimulation: Phase II open-label dose optimization. *The Journal of Pain, 17*(1), 14–26.

Chelly, J. E., Greger, J., Gebhard, R., Coupe, K., Clyburn, T. A., Buckle, R., & Criswell, A. (2001). Continuous femoral blocks improve recovery and outcome of patients undergoing total knee arthroplasty. *The Journal of Arthroplasty, 6*(4), 436–445.

Chinn, S., Caldwell, W., & Gritsenko, K. (2016). Fibromyalgia pathogenesis and treatment options update. *Current Pain and Headache Reports, 20*(4), 1–10.

Clifford, D. B., & Trotter, J. L. (1984). Pain in multiple sclerosis. *Archives of Neurology, 41*, 1270–1272.

Compton, W. M., & Volkow, N. D. (2006). Major increases in opioid analgesic abuse in the United States: Concerns and strategies. *Drug and Alcohol Dependence, 81*(2), 103–107.

Cosentino, G., Brighina, F., Talamanca, S., Paladino, P., Vigneri, S., Baschi, R., … Fierro, B. (2014). Reduced threshold for inhibitory homeostatic responses in migraine motor cortex? A tDCS/TMS study. *Headache: The Journal of Head and Face Pain, 54*(4), 663–674.

Crue, B. L., Kenton, B., & Carregal, E. J. (1976). Neurophysiology of pain-peripheral aspects: Speculation concerning the possibility of a unitary peripheral cutaneous input system for pressure, hot, cold and tissue damage. *Bulletin of the Los Angeles Neurological Societies, 41*(1), 13–42.

DaSilva, A. F., Datta, A., Mendonca, M. E., Zaghi, S., Lopes, M., DosSantos, M. F., … Fregni, F. (2011a). Chronic migraine alleviation by tDCS is predicted to be associated with current flow through pain-related (sub) cortical regions. *Headache, 51*, 48–49.

DaSilva, A. F., Granziera, C., Snyder, J., & Hadjikhani, N. (2007a). Thickening in the somatosensory cortex of patients with migraine. *Neurology, 69*, 1990–1995.

DaSilva, A. F., Granziera, C., Tuch, D. S., Snyder, J., Vincent, M., & Hadjikhani, N. (2007b). Interictal alterations of the trigeminal somatosensory pathway and periaqueductal gray matter in migraine. *Neuroreport, 18*, 301–305.

DaSilva, A. F., Mendonca, M. E., Zaghi, S., Lopes, M., Dossantos, M. F., Spierings, E. L., … Fregni, F. (2012). tDCS-induced analgesia and electrical fields in pain-related neural networks in chronic migraine. *Headache., 52*(8), 1283–1295. Epub 2012 Apr 18.

DaSilva, A. F., Nascimento, T. D., DosSantos, M. F., Lucas, S., Van Holsbeeck, H., DeBoer, M., … Koeppe, R. A. (2014). μ-Opioid activation in the prefrontal cortex in migraine attacks – Brief report I. *Annals of Clinical Translational Neurology, 1*, 439–444.

DaSilva, A. F., Volz, M. S., Bikson, M., & Fregni, F. (2011b). Electrode positioning and montage in transcranial direct current stimulation. *Journal of Visualized Experiments, 51*, e2744–e2744.

Davis, K. D. (2003). Neurophysiological and anatomical considerations in functional imaging of pain. *Pain, 105*(1–2), 1–3.

Deo, H., West, G., Butcher, C., & Lewis, P. (2011). The prevalence of cognitive dysfunction after conventional and computer-assisted total knee replacement. *Knee, 18*(2), 117–120.

DeSouza, D. D., Hodaie, M., & Davis, K. D. (2016). Structural magnetic resonance imaging can identify trigeminal system abnormalities in classical trigeminal neuralgia. *Frontiers in Neuroanatomy, 10*, 95.

DosSantos, M. F., Ferreira, N., Toback, R. L., Carvalho, A. C., & DaSilva, A. F. (2016). Potential mechanisms supporting the value of motor cortex stimulation to treat chronic pain syndromes. *Frontiers in Neuroscience, 10*, 18.

DosSantos, M. F., Love, T. M., Martikainen, I. K., Nascimento, T. D., Fregni, F., Cummiford, C., … Dasilva, A. F. (2012). Immediate effects of tDCS on the μ-opioid system of a chronic pain patient. *Frontiers in Psychiatry, 3*, 93.

DosSantos, M. F., Martikainen, I. K., Nascimento, T. D., Love, T. M., DeBoer, M. D., Schambra, H. M., … DaSilva, A. F. (2014). Building up analgesia in humans via the endogenous μ-opioid system by combining placebo and active tDCS: A preliminary report. *PLoS One, 9*(7), e102350.

Drossman, D., Morris, C. B., Hu, Y., Toner, B. B., Diamant, N., Whitehead, W. E., … Bangdiwala, S. I. (2007). Characterization of health related quality of life (HRQOL) for patients with functional bowel disorder (FBD) and its response to treatment. *The American Journal of Gastroenterology, 102*(7), 1442–1453.

Dubois, P. E., Ossemann, M., de Fays, K., De Bue, P., Gourdin, M., Jamart, J., & Vandermeeren, Y. (2013). Postoperative analgesic effect of transcranial direct current stimulation in lumbar spine surgery: A randomized control trial. *The Clinical Journal of Pain, 29*(8), 696–601.

Dyck, P. J., Lambert, E. H., & O'Brien, P. C. (1976). Pain in peripheral neuropathy related to rate and kind of fiber degeneration. *Neurology, 26*(5), 466–471.

Edmeads, J., & Mackell, J. A. (2002). The economic impact of migraine: An analysis of direct and indirect costs. *Headache: The Journal of Head and Face Pain, 42*(6), 501–509.

Fagerlund, A. J., Hansen, O. A., & Aslaksen, P. M. (2015). Transcranial direct current stimulation as a treatment for patients with fibromyalgia: A randomized controlled trial. *Pain, 156*(1), 62–71.

Fischer, T. Z., & Waxman, S. G. (2010). Neuropathic pain in diabetes – Evidence for a central mechanism. *Nature Reviews. Neurology, 6*(8), 462–466.

Foerster, B. R., Nascimento, T. D., DeBoer, M., Bender, M. A., Rice, I. C., Truong, D. Q., Bikson, M., Clauw, D. J., Zubieta, J. K., Harris, R. E., & DaSilva, A. F. (2014). Excitatory and inhibitory brain metabolites as targets and predictors of effective motor cortex tDCS therapy in fibromyalgia. *Arthritis & Rheumatology*.

Flaster, M., Meresh, E., Rao, M., & Biller, J. (2013). Central poststroke pain: Current diagnosis and treatment. *Topics in Stroke Rehabilitation, 20*(2), 116–123.

Flor, H. (2003). Cortical reorganization and chronic pain: Implications for rehabilitation. *Journal of Rehabilitation Medicine, 41*, 66–72.

Flor, H., Diers, M., & Andoh, J. (2013). The neural basis of phantom limb pain. *Trends in Cognitive Sciences, 17*(7), 307–308.

Foell, J., Bekrater-Bodmann, R., Diers, M., & Flor, H. (2014). Mirror therapy for phantom limb pain: Brain changes and the role of body representation. *European Journal of Pain, 18*(5), 729–739.

Foley, P. L., Vesterinen, H. M., Laird, B. J., Sena, E. S., Colvin, L. A., Chandran, S., … Fallon, M. T. (2013). Prevalence and natural history of pain in adults with multiple sclerosis: Systematic review and meta-analysis. *Pain, 154*(5), 632–642.

Fregni, F., Boggio, P. S., Lima, M. C., Ferreira, M. J., Wagner, T., Rigonatti, S. P., … Pascual-Leone, A. (2006a). A sham-controlled, phase II trial of transcranial direct current stimulation for the treatment of central pain in traumatic spinal cord injury. *Pain, 122*(1–2), 197–209.

Fregni, F., Freedman, S., & Pascual-Leone, A. (2007). Recent advances in the treatment of chronic pain with non-invasive brain stimulation techniques. *Lancet Neurology, 6*(2), 188–191.

Fregni, F., Gimenes, R., Valle, A. C., Ferreira, M. J., Rocha, R. R., Natalle, L., … Boggio, P. S. (2006b). A randomized, sham-controlled, proof of principle study of transcranial direct current stimulation for the treatment of pain in fibromyalgia. *Arthritis and Rheumatism, 54*(12), 3988–3998.

Frost, S. B., Barbay, S., Friel, K. M., Plautz, E. J., & Nudo, R. J. (2003). Reorganization of remote cortical regions after ischemic brain injury: A potential substrate for stroke recovery. *Journal of Neurophysiology, 89*(6), 3205–3214.

Garcia-Larrea, L., Peyron, R., Mertens, P., Gregoire, M. C., Lavenne, F., Bonnefoi, F., … Sindou, M. (1997). Positron emission tomography during motor cortex stimulation for pain control. *Stereotactic and Functional Neurosurgery, 68*(1), 141–148.

Garcia-Larrea, L., Peyron, R., Mertens, P., Gregoire, M. C., Lavenne, F., Le Bars, D., … Laurent, B. (1999). Electrical stimulation of motor cortex for pain control: A combined PET-scan and electrophysiological study. *Pain, 83*(2), 259–273.

Gatchel, R. J., Peng, Y. B., Peters, M. L., Fuchs, P. N., & Turk, D. C. (2007). The biopsychosocial approach to chronic pain: Scientific advances and future directions. *Psychological Bulletin, 133*(4), 581–524.

George, M. S., Nahas, Z., Kozol, F. A., Li, X., Yamanaka, K., Mishory, A., & Bohning, D. E. (2003). Mechanisms and the current state of transcranial magnetic stimulation. *CNS Spectrums, 8*(7), 496–414.

Giardino, N. D., Jensen, M. P., Turner, J. A., Ehde, D. M., & Cardenas, D. D. (2003). Social environment moderates the association between catastrophizing and pain among persons with a spinal cord injury. *Pain, 106*(1–2), 19–25.

Glaser, J., Reeves, S. T., Stoll, W. D., Epperson, T. I., Hilbert, M., Madan, A., … Borckardt, J. J. (2016). Motor/prefrontal transcranial direct current stimulation (tDCS) following lumbar surgery reduces postoperative analgesia use. *Spine, 41*(10), 835–839.

Goldenberg, D. L., Clauw, D. J., Palmer, R. E., & Clair, A. G. (2016). Opioid use in fibromyalgia: A cautionary tale. *Mayo Clinic Proceedings, 91*(5), 640–648.

Granziera, C., DaSilva, A. F., Snyder, J., Tuch, D. S., & Hadjikhani, N. (2006). Anatomical alterations of the visual motion processing network in migraine with and without aura. *PLoS Medicine, 3*, e402.

Greer, K. R., & Hoyt, J. W. (1990). Pain: Theory, anatomy, and physiology. *Critical Care Clinics, 6*(2), 227–234.

Greer, S. M., Dalton, J. A., Carlson, J., & Youngblood, R. (2001). Surgical patients' fear of addiction to pain medication: The effect of an educational program for clinicians. *The Clinical Journal of Pain, 17*(2), 157–164.

Guariguata, L., Whiting, D. R., Hambleton, I., Beagley, J., Linnenkamp, U., & Shaw, J. E. (2014). Global estimates of diabetes prevalence for 2013 and projections for 2035. *Diabetes Research and Clinical Practice, 103*(2), 137–149.

Hansen, A. P., Marcussen, N. S., Klit, H., Andersen, G., Finnerup, N. B., & Jensen, T. S. (2012). Pain following stroke: A prospective study. *European Journal of Pain, 16*(8), 1128–1136.

Headache classification Subcommittee of the International Headache Society. (2013). *The international classification of headache disorders* (3rd ed., pp. 629–808). Cephalagia.

Hemington, K. S., Wu, Q., Kucyi, A., Inman, R. D., & Davis, K. D. (2016). Abnormal cross-network functional connectivity in chronic pain and its association with clinical symptoms. *Brain Structure & Function, 221*(8), 4203–4219.

Hsu, E., & Cohen, S. P. (2013). Postamputation pain: Epidemiology, mechanisms, and treatment. *Journal of Pain Research, 6*, 121–136.

Jain, N., Qi, H. X., Collins, C. E., & Kaas, J. H. (2008). Large-scale reorganization in the somatosensory cortex and thalamus after sensory loss in macaque monkeys. *The Journal of Neuroscience, 28*(43), 11042–11060.

Jones, M. R., Ehrhardt, K. P., Ripoll, J. G., Sharma, B., Padnos, I. W., Kaye, R. J., & Kaye, A. D. (2016). Pain in the elderly. *Current Pain and Headache Reports, 20*(4), 23.

Juottonen, K., Gockel, M., Silen, T., Hurri, H., Hari, R., & Forss, N. (2002). Altered central sensorimotor processing in patients with complex regional pain syndrome. *Pain, 98*, 315–323.

Kelly, C., & Garavan, H. (2005). Human neuroimaging of brain changes associated with practice. *Cerebral Cortex, 15*, 1089–1002.

Kibar, S., Yıldız, H. E., Ay, S., Evcik, D., & Ergin, E. S. (2015). New approach in fibromyalgia exercise program: A preliminary study regarding the effectiveness of balance training. *Archives of Physical Medicine and Rehabilitation, 96*(9), 1576–1582.

Kim, J. S. (2014). Pharmacological management of central post-stroke pain: A practical guide. *CNS Drugs, 28*(9), 787–797.

Kim, Y. J., Ku, J., Kim, H. J., Im, D. J., Lee, H. S., Han, K. A., & Kang, Y. J. (2013). Randomized, sham controlled trial of transcranial direct current stimulation for painful diabetic polyneuropathy. *Annals of Rehabilitation Medicine, 37*(6), 766–776.

Knotkova, H., Cruciani, R. A., Tronnier, V. M., & Rasche, D. (2012). Current and future options for the management of phantom-limb pain. *Journal of Pain Research, 5*, 39–49.

Knotkova, H., Greenberg, A., Soto, E., & Cruciani, R. A. (2015). Applications of neuromodulation in pain management. In H. Knotkova & D. Rasche (Eds.), *Textbook of neuromodulation* (pp. 113–126). New York, NY: Springer.

Knotkova, H., Homel, P., & Cruciani, R. A. (2009). Cathodal tDCS over the somatosensory cortex relieved chronic neuropathic pain in a patient with complex regional pain syndrome (CRPS/RSD). *Journal of Pain Management, 2*(3), 365–368.

Knotkova, H., Soto, E., Leuschner, Z., Greenberg, A., Stock, V., Das, D., & Cruciani, R. (2013). Transcranial direct current stimulation (tDCS) for the treatment of chronic pain. *Journal of Pain, 4*(14), 64.

Kumar, B., Kalita, J., Kumar, G., & Misra, U. K. (2009). Central poststroke pain: A review of pathophysiology and treatment. *Anesthesia & Analgesia, 108*(5), 1645–1657.

Lawrence, R. C., Felson, D. T., Helmick, C. G., Arnold, L. M., Choi, H., Deyo, R. A., … Wolfe, F. (2008). National Arthritis Data Workgroup. Estimates of the prevalence of arthritis and other rheumatic conditions in the United States: Part II. *Arthritis and Rheumatism, 58*(1), 26–35.

Lenz, F. A., Weiss, N., Ohara, S., Lawson, C., & Greenspan, J. D. (2004). The role of the thalamus in pain. *Supplements to Clinical Neurophysiology, 57*, 50–61.

Lima, M. C., & Fregni, F. (2008). Motor cortex stimulation for chronic pain: Systematic review and meta-analysis of the literature. *Neurology, 70*, 2329–2337.

Liu, J., Zhao, L., Li, G., Xiong, S., Nan, J., Li, J., … Tian, J. (2012). Hierarchical alteration of brain structural and functional networks in female migraine sufferers. *PLoS One, 7*(12), e51250.

López-Solà, M., Woo, C. W., Pujol, J., Deus, J., Harrison, B. J., Monfort, J., & Wager, T. D. (2016). Towards a neurophysiological signature for fibromyalgia. *Pain, 158*(1), 34–47.

Lorenz, J., Minoshima, S., & Casey, K. L. (2003). Keeping pain out of mind: The role of the dorsolateral prefrontal cortex in pain modulation. *Brain, 126*(5), 1079–1091.

MacIver, K., Lloyd, D. M., Kelly Roberts, S. N., & Nurmikko, T. (2008). Phantom limb pain, cortical reorganization and the therapeutic effect of mental imagery. *Brain, 131*(8), 2181–2191.

Maihöfner, C., Handwerker, H. O., Neundorfer, B., & Birklein, F. (2003). Patterns of cortical reorganization in complex regional pain syndrome. *Neurology, 61*, 1715–1717.

Maihöfner, C., Handwerker, H. O., Neundorfer, B., & Birklein, F. (2004). Cortical reorganization during recovery from complex regional pain syndrome. *Neurology, 63*, 693–601.

Maihöfner, C., Neundörfer, B., Birklein, F., & Handwerker, H. O. (2006). Mislocalization of tactile stimulation in patients with complex regional pain syndrome. *Journal of Neurology, 253*, 772–779.

Marrie, R. A., Patten, S. B., Tremlett, H., Wolfson, C., Warren, S., Svenson, L. W., … Yu, B. N. (2016). Sex differences in comorbidity at diagnosis of multiple sclerosis: A population-based study. *Neurology, 86*(14), 1279–1286.

McCarthy, J. (2016). Myalgias and myopathies: Fibromyalgia. *FP Essentials, 440*, 11–15.

Mendonca, M. E., Simis, M., Grecco, L. C., Battistella, L. R., Baptista, A. F., & Fregni, F. (2016). Transcranial direct current stimulation combined with aerobic exercise to optimize analgesic responses in fibromyalgia: A randomized placebo-controlled clinical trial. *Frontiers in Human Neuroscience, 10*, 68.

Morgan, D., Forst-Pineda, K., & Gold, M. (2006). Medical and nonmedical use of prescription opioids: Epidemiology and prevalence. *Psychiatric Annals, 36*(6), 404–409.

Mori, F., Codecà, C., Kusayanagi, H., Monteleone, F., Buttari, F., Fiore, S., … Centonze, D. (2010). Effects of anodal transcranial direct current stimulation on chronic neuropathic pain in patients with multiple sclerosis. *The Journal of Pain, 11*(5), 436–442.

Moseley, G. L., & Flor, H. (2012). Targeting cortical representations in the treatment of chronic pain: A review. *Neurorehabilitation and Neural Repair, 26*(6), 646–652.

Mulla, S. M., Wang, L., Khokhar, R., Izhar, Z., Agarwal, A., Couban, R., … Busse, J. W. (2015). Management of central poststroke pain systematic review of randomized controlled trials. *Stroke, 46*(10), 2853–2860.

Napadow, V., Dhond, R. P., Kim, J., LaCount, L., Vangel, M., Harris, R. E., … Park, K. (2009). (2009). Brain encoding of acupuncture sensation – Coupling on-line rating with fMRI. *NeuroImage, 47*(3), 1055–1065.

Napadow, V., Maeda, Y., Audette, J., & Kettner, N. (2012). Chapter IX. Neuroplasticity in carpal tunnel syndrome. In H. Knotkova, R. Cruciani, & J. Merrick (Eds.), *Neural plasticity in chronic pain* (pp. 153–184). New York, NY: Nova Science Publishers, Inc.

Nascimento, T. D., DosSantos, M. F., Lucas, S., Van Holsbeeck, H., DeBoer, M., Maslowski, E., … Smith, Y. R. (2014). μ-Opioid activation in the midbrain during migraine allodynia – Brief report II. *Annals of Clinical Translational Neurology, 1*, 445–450.

Nitsche, M. A., Cohen, L. G., Wassermann, E. M., Priori, A., Lang, N., Antal, A., … Pascual-Leone, A. (2008). Transcranial direct current stimulation: State of the art 2008. *Brain Stimulation, 1*(3), 206–223.

O'Connell, N. E., Wand, B. M., Marston, L., Spencer, S., & DeSouza, L. H. (2010). Non-invasive brain stimulation techniques for chronic pain. *The Cochrane Library, 8*(9): CD008208.

O'Connell, N. E., Wand, B. M., Marston, L., Spencer, S., & Desouza, L. H. (2014). Non-invasive brain stimulation techniques for chronic pain. *Cochrane Database of Systematic Reviews, 11*, 4.

Peyron, J. (1986). Osteoarthritis: The epidemiologic viewpoint. *Clinical Orthopaedics and Related Research, 213*, 13–19.

Peyron, R., Faillenot, I., Mertens, P., Laurent, B., & Garcia-Larrea, L. (2007). Motor cortex stimulation in neuropathic pain; correlations between analgesic effect and hemodynamic changes in the brain: A PET study. *NeuroImage, 34*(1), 310–321.

Peyron, R., Garcia-Larrea, L., Deiber, M. P., Cinotti, L., Convers, P., Sindou, M., … Laurent, B. (1995). Electrical stimulation of precentral cortical area in the treatment of central pain: Electrophysiological and PET study. *Pain, 62*(3), 275–286.

Pleger, B., Tegenthoff, M., Ragert, P., Forster, A. F., Dinse, H., Nicolas, P. V., & Maier, C. (2005). (2005). Sensorimotor returning in complex regional pain syndrome parallels pain reduction. *Annals of Neurology, 57*, 425–429.

Riberto, M., Marcon, A. F., Monteiro de Benedetto, P. K., Dini, L. V., Nemoto, K. H., Fregni, F., & Rizzo, B. L. (2011). Efficacy of transcranial direct current stimulation coupled with a multidisciplinary rehabilitation program for the treatment of fibromyalgia. *Open Rheumatology Journal, 5*, 45–50.

Roizenblatt, S., Fregni, F., Gimenez, R., Wetzel, T., Rigonatti, S. P., Tufik, S., … Valle, A. C. (2007). Site-specific effects of transcranial direct current stimulation on sleep and pain in fibromyalgia: A randomized, sham-controlled study. *Pain Practice, 7*(4), 297–206.

Rosen, A. C., Ramkumar, M., Nguyen, T., & Hoeft, F. (2009). Noninvasive transcranial brain stimulation and pain. *Current Pain and Headache Reports, 13*(1), 12–17.

Rossi, A., Di Lollo, A. C., Guzzo, M. P., Giacomelli, C., Atzeni, F., Bazzichi, L., & Di Franco, M. (2015). Fibromyalgia and nutrition: What news? *Clinical and Experimental Rheumatology, 33*(1), 117–125.

Saab, C. Y. (2012). Pain-related changes in the brain: Diagnostic and therapeutic potentials. *Trends in Neurosciences, 35*(10), 629–637.

Sampson, S. M., Rome, J. D., & Rummans, T. A. (2006). Slow-frequency rTMS reduces fibromyalgia pain. *Pain Medicine, 7*(2), 115–118.

Samson, A. J., Mercer, G. E., & Campbell, D. G. (2010). Total knee replacement in the morbidly obese: A literature review. *ANZ Journal of Surgery, 80*(9), 595–599.

Seminowicz, D. A., & Davis, K. D. (2006). Cortical responses to pain in healthy individuals depends on pain catastrophizing. *Pain, 120*(3), 297–206.

Solaro, C., Trabucco, E., & Messmer-Uccelli, M. (2013). Pain and multiple sclerosis: Pathophysiology and treatment. *Current Neurology and Neuroscience Reports, 13*(1), 1–9.

Staud, R., Robinson, M. E., Vierck, C. J., Cannon, R. C., Mauderli, A. P., & Price, D. D. (2003). Ratings of experimental pain and pain-related negative affect predict clinical pain in patients with fibromyalgia syndrome. *Pain, 105*(1–2), 215–222.

Stenager, E., Knudsen, L., & Jensen, K. (1995). Acute and chronic pain syndromes in multiple sclerosis: A 5-year follow-up study. *Italian Journal of Neurological Sciences, 16*, 629–632.

Talmo, C. T., Robbins, C. E., & Bono, J. V. (2010). Total joint replacement in the elderly patient. *Clinics in Geriatric Medicine, 26*(3), 517–529.

Treede, R. D., Kenshalo, D. R., Gracely, R. H., & Jones, A. K. (1999). The cortical representation of pain. *Pain, 79*(2–3), 105–111.

Valle, A., Roizenblatt, S., Botte, S., Zaghi, S., Riberto, M., Tufik, S., ... Fregni, F. (2009). Efficacy of anodal transcranial direct current stimulation (tDCS) for the treatment of fibromyalgia: Results of a randomized, sham-controlled longitudinal clinical trial. *Journal of Pain Management, 2*(3), 353–362.

Vigano, A., D'Elia, T. S., Sava, S. L., Auve, M., De Pasqua, V., Colosimo, A., ... Magis, D. (2013). Transcranial direct current stimulation (tDCS) of the visual cortex: A proof-of-concept study based on interictal electrophysiological abnormalities in migraine. *The Journal of Headache and Pain, 14*, 23.

Villamar, M. F., Wivatvongvana, P., Patumanond, J., Bikson, M., Truong, D. Q., Datta, A., & Fregni, F. (2013). Focal modulation of the primary motor cortex in fibromyalgia using 4× 1-ring high-definition transcranial direct current stimulation (HD-tDCS): Immediate and delayed analgesic effects of cathodal and anodal stimulation. *The Journal of Pain, 14*(4), 371–383.

Wang, H., Boctor, B., & Verner, J. (2002). The effect of single-injection femoral nerve block on rehabilitation and length of hospital stay after total knee replacement. *Regional Anesthesia and Pain Medicine, 27*(2), 139–144.

Wickmann, F., Stephani, C., Czesnik, D., Klinker, F., Timäus, C., Chaieb, L., ... Antal, A. (2015). Prophylactic treatment in menstrual migraine: A proof-of-concept study. *Journal of the Neurological Sciences, 354*(1), 103–109.

Williams, J. A., Imamura, M., & Fregni, F. (2009). Updates on the use of non-invasive brain stimulation in physical and rehabilitation medicine. *Journal of Rehabilitation Medicine, 41*(5), 305–311.

Zubieta, J. K., Smith, Y. R., Bueller, J. A., Xu, Y., Kilbourn, M. R., Jewett, D. M., ... Stohler, C. S. (2002). μ-Opioid receptor-mediated antinociceptive responses differ in men and women. *The Journal of Neuroscience, 22*, 5100–5107.

Chapter 19
Transcranial Direct Current Stimulation in Aging Research

Adam J. Woods, Daria Antonenko, Agnes Flöel, Benjamin M. Hampstead, David Clark, and Helena Knotkova

Introduction

The world population is aging. For example, the United States population of older adults is expected to double by the year 2050 (Bureau 2009; Brault 2012). With advanced age comes decline in both physical and cognitive function, as well as higher prevalence of chronic pain, co-morbid conditions, and depression (Anton et al. 2015; Woods et al. 2011, 2013). There is a significant need for new and improved intervention approaches for addressing the effects of aging on the body

A. J. Woods (✉)
Center for Cognitive Aging and Memory (CAM), McKnight Brain Institute, Department of Clinical and Health Psychology, College of Public Health and Health Professions, University of Florida, Gainesville, FL, USA
e-mail: ajwoods@phhp.ufl.edu

D. Antonenko
Department of Neurology, NeuroCure Clinical Research Center, Charité – Universitätsmedizin, Berlin, Germany

A. Flöel
Department of Neurology, University Medical Hospital Greifswald, Greifswald, Germany

B. M. Hampstead
Department of Mental Health Services, Veterans Affairs Ann Arbor Healthcare Systems, Ann Arbor, MI, USA

Department of Psychiatry, University of Michigan, Ann Arbor, MI, USA

D. Clark
Department of Aging and Geriatric Research, Brain Rehabilitation Research Center, Malcom Randall VA Medical Center, Gainesville, FL, USA

H. Knotkova
MJHS Institute for Innovation in Palliative Care, New York, NY, USA

Department of Family and Social Medicine, Albert Einstein College of Medicine, Bronx, NY, USA

H. Knotkova et al. (eds.), *Practical Guide to Transcranial Direct Current Stimulation*, https://doi.org/10.1007/978-3-319-95948-1_19

and the brain. Transcranial direct current stimulation (tDCS) has shown promise for treating symptoms associated with many of these age-related issues through non-invasive direct intervention on brain function (Ahn et al. 2017; Jones et al. 2015; Kuo and Nitsche 2012; Woods et al. 2016). This chapter will summarize the current state of tDCS in aging research and explore its potential application in aging populations. In addition, this chapter will discuss several special considerations for tDCS study design in aging populations.

The chapter will start by reviewing effects of tDCS on motor excitability in older adults. Mechanistically, much of what is known about the effects of tDCS is based on prior research in motor neurophysiology. This section will serve to review the basis for our knowledge of tDCS effects. We will then describe the use of tDCS in the context of EEG and fMRI in older adults, highlighting technical considerations for study design. The aforementioned section will provide the reader with knowledge of age-related effects of tDCS and practical considerations important for integration of tDCS with state-of-the-art neural measures. The chapter will then consider the effects of tDCS on functional outcomes in older adults and describe special considerations regarding population heterogeneity and individual differences. This material is intended to arm the reader with knowledge important for considering functional outcome measure selection in studies of older adults. The chapter will then describe the current state of research on the impact of tDCS on cognitive function, before discussing effects on motor and sensory function. These sections will serve to provide insight into potential areas of influence of tDCS that deserve future study as interventions targeting conditions common in older adults. Finally, the chapter will discuss practical considerations for tDCS research in older adults, including the consent process, polypharmacy and common medications in older adults that impact tDCS effects, and how age-related brain changes may impact current flow. Collectively, this chapter will provide critical information for the understanding the potential impact of tDCS in aging populations, carefully design investigations in this domain, and critically assess tDCS research in aging.

Motor Cortical Excitability in Aging

The use of tDCS in older adults requires special consideration of age-related changes in the brain that may affect optimal stimulation parameters and treatment outcomes. Aging often results in substantial alterations to cerebral structure and function, including smaller brain volume (Resnick et al. 2000), reduced cortical thickness (Salat et al. 2004), altered cortical excitability (McGinley et al. 2010), and functional lateralization of cortical activity (Coppi et al. 2014). Structural changes in the aging brain (i.e., reduced brain volume and cortical thickness) increase the distance between the cortex and the scalp, and also influences the volume and distribution of cerebrospinal fluid in the meninges of the skull. These factors can have a profound influence on the conduction of electrical current, which in turn may alter the relative impact of tDCS on the underlying neuronal tissue (Bikson et al. 2012). As with other populations, the effects of tDCS in older adults depend on the extent to which cortical excitability is modifiable. Evidence suggests that the motor cortex of older adults is inhibited relative to that of younger adults, possibly due to GABAergic inhibition (Heise et al. 2014; McGinley et al. 2010). As a possible result of this inhibited state, there is evidence that elderly adults require longer stimulation times to exhibit similar levels of motor cortical excitation as younger adults (Fujiyama et al. 2014). Nevertheless, a number of studies have found that tDCS increases cortical excitability in older adults, as indicated by larger motor evoked potentials with transcranial magnetic stimulation (Goodwill et al. 2013, 2015). The baseline state of cortical excitation prior to conducting tDCS experiments can also influence tDCS outcomes. Fujiyama and colleagues demonstrated this using an inhibitory pre-conditioning protocol in which stimulation with a cathode placed over the primary motor cortex was delivered for a short period of time to elicit a baseline state of inhibition. Elderly participants who received this pre-conditioning prior to a force training protocol with anodal tDCS showed greater improvements in skilled movement accuracy (Fujiyama et al. 2017). Differences in functional performance levels might also alter the responsiveness to tDCS. Learmonth and colleagues compared the effect of tDCS on elderly adults who performed better or worse on a baseline visuomotor task. Only the group who performed worse at baseline exhibited further detriments in performance when tDCS was delivered to the posterior parietal cortex (Learmonth et al. 2015). Even within samples of older adults with relatively homogeneous motor function, there is likely to be considerable inter-individual variability of brain structural and functional characteristics. Furthermore, genetic factors may be of importance, as some research suggests a beneficial influence of the BDNF Vall66Met polymorphism on corticospinal excitability, though this finding is not universal (Fujiyama et al. 2014; Puri et al. 2015; Puri and Hinder 2016; Shpektor 2015). Cumulatively, the evidence suggests that a 'one size fits all' approach for defining optimal tDCS parameters may not be prudent in older adults. Future research in this population will require careful attention to changes in the aging brain that may affect optimal parameters of tDCS dosage (Summers et al. 2015).

tDCS, Brain Waves and Functional Connectivity (EEG, FMRI) in Aging

Neuroscience research has shown that brain activity and connectivity patterns change with advancing age (Antonenko and Flöel 2013; Grady 2012; Sala-Llonch et al. 2015). Those changes are most often interpreted as disrupted neuronal efficiency and/or emergence of compensatory mechanisms (Goh 2011; Sala-Llonch et al. 2015). Particular because of their dynamic structure even on short time scales, those activity and connectivity measures have become a target of tDCS protocols in order to unveil the underlying neuronal mechanisms and define appropriate targets for intervention. The information about activity and connectivity alterations can then be useful for determining targets in training and pharmacological interventions. Few recent studies have investigated the effect of tDCS on task-related activity and task-independent functional connectivity patterns in healthy aged adults using electroencephalography (EEG) and functional magnetic resonance imaging (fMRI).

EEG Studies with tDCS in Aging

Only one study included EEG assessments in a group of older adults to study the effects of anodal tDCS over the motor cortex on upper limb function (Marquez et al. 2015). The authors found improved functional performance irrespective of stimulation site, but no tDCS effects on event-related components as assessed by EEG after stimulation. In particular, the analysis of the contingent negative variation component, indicating the level of readiness to respond to a predicted target, did not show differences between anodal and sham tDCS conditions. Here, the authors noted that timing of the EEG measurements may have been an issue as it was assessed 40 min after stimulation offset. In order to provide methodological considerations, more research is needed combining EEG and tDCS in aging.

fMRI Studies with tDCS in Aging

Few recent studies included fMRI assessments in older adults to study the effects of tDCS on task-related activity (Holland et al. 2011; Lindenberg et al. 2013; Martin et al. 2017; Meinzer et al. 2013, 2014) and resting state connectivity during stimulation (Antonenko et al. 2017; Lindenberg et al. 2013; Meinzer et al. 2013). Left prefrontal anodal tDCS led to faster picture naming performance and significantly reduced task-related blood oxygenation level-dependent (BOLD) signal compared to the sham tDCS condition (Holland et al. 2011). BOLD signal was significantly associated with reaction times in the task. This observed correlation of behavioral and neuronal effects further supported the efficiency-enhancing effect of tDCS. Similarly, Meinzer et al. (2013) compared the effects of anodal tDCS over the left prefrontal cortex during semantic word generation with performance of young controls, showing enhanced (compensatory) bilateral prefrontal activity in older adults that was associated with reduced performance under sham tDCS (Meinzer et al. 2013). Anodal tDCS improved performance up to a level of young controls and also led to reduced task-related activity in bilateral prefrontal areas, the anterior cingulate gyrus, and the precuneus in older adults. In addition, resting-state fMRI revealed widespread connectivity changes in older adults, characterized by increased frontotemporal and decreased posterior connectivity, using a hypothesis-free graph-based analysis approach (Lohmann et al. 2010). Anodal tDCS produced both increases and decreases of connectivity during stimulation, changing the overall pattern toward that of young controls (Meinzer et al. 2013). Lindenberg et al. supported this tDCS-induced reorganization of brain networks in older adults, observing a modulation of inter-hemispheric interactions. The authors observed several decreases in connectivity contralateral to the anode, such as of right hippocampus and motor cortex, and increases in connectivity ipsilateral to the anode, such as of prefrontal areas and motor cortex. Both anodal and dual tDCS counteracted age-related connectivity changes in this study, more precisely, they yielded connectivity decreases in right motor cortices compared to sham, indicating a functional decoupling of those areas (Lindenberg et al. 2013).

The pattern that emerges from the studies so far suggests that anodal tDCS in older adults may reduce task-related brain activity (in most cases, "hyperactivity" as compared to young adults), and alter resting-state connectivity towards patterns found in younger subjects; both processes paralleled by an increase in performance (Meinzer et al. 2013). Certainly, more research is needed to elucidate the neuronal mechanisms underlying tDCS in older adults, particularly because effects may be different to those in young adults (Martin et al. 2017; Prehn and Flöel 2015).

In sum, studies combining behavioral outcomes with investigations of brain neurophysiology and metabolism can unveil the neuronal mechanisms underlying tDCS effects in aging. The few studies to date suggest that tDCS-induced modulations in the aged brain are complex with both increases and decreases in regional BOLD signal and its inter-regional correlations, pointing towards a complex effect on brain networks. So despite the general assumption that tDCS-induced behavioral effects are reflective of the targets' function, evidence suggests that tDCS produces widespread alterations on a network level (Antonenko et al. 2017; Summers et al. 2015; Zheng et al. 2011).

Technical Considerations

From what we know so far, when studying brain activity and connectivity changes related to tDCS in older adults, it may be favorable to:

- Compare brain activity and connectivity patterns to those of young controls, in order to obtain "normal" levels and interpret the direction (i.e., increase versus decrease) of the tDCS effects;
- Assess changes in multiple brain regions or at the level of neuronal networks (Luft et al. 2014; Summers et al. 2015): As aging is accompanied by a range of activity and connectivity alterations in both directions (i.e., increases and decreases compared to young) (Grady 2012; Gutchess 2014), effects of tDCS may emerge in brain areas known to be recruited due to compensatory processes

or age-related disinhibition, for instance (Lindenberg et al. 2013), and in brain areas not directly targeted by stimulation (Meinzer et al. 2014).

Effects of TDCS on Functional Outcomes in Healthy Aging

A considerable amount of studies has shown that tDCS has the ability to counteract age-associated decline in various functional domains (Hsu et al. 2015; Perceval et al. 2016; Prehn and Flöel 2015; Summers et al. 2015).

Differential Effects of tDCS in Age Groups

Stimulation with tDCS of particular target regions may have distinct effects in young versus older adults due to alterations in neuronal mechanisms that mediate cognitive function in the course of aging (Gutchess 2014). It is possible that tDCS over identical regions leads to different functional effects and also that tDCS over different regions leads to identical effects, for instance, when applied in a group of young compared to one of older adults (Perceval et al. 2016).

First evidence for such differential effects in young and older adults have been demonstrated in the language (Fertonani et al. 2014; Ross et al. 2011) as well as in the memory domain (Manenti et al. 2013). Ross et al. observed that during a face naming task anodal tDCS over the dominant (right) hemisphere improved proper name recall in young, tDCS over the left hemisphere produced more pronounced performance-ameliorating effects in older adults (Ross et al. 2011). In this study, tDCS over both left and right anterior temporal lobes led to improvements of proper name recall in both age groups, but with different extents depending on the stimulated hemisphere. In addition, right tDCS improved place name recall only in older adults, which suggests that effects of anodal tDCS on functional outcomes may be broader in the healthy aged group. A study by Fertonani et al. revealed that while both online and offline tDCS effects were present in young adults, older adults benefitted only from (online) tDCS during naming performance (Fertonani et al. 2014). Manenti et al. argued that tDCS over stimulation targets effective in young adults were not present in an older sample. Here, tDCS effects on retrieval performance were observed irrespective of site (prefrontal versus parietal) or hemisphere in young, but only during left hemisphere tDCS in the healthy aged group (Manenti et al. 2013). These studies have directly compared functional outcomes between age groups, suggesting the presence of an interaction between age group and stimulation site. Thus, the extent of tDCS-induced performance-ameliorating effects may be dependent on the interplay on various factors such as age, stimulation site, but also functional domain under study as well as inter-individual factors. All these variables may contribute to and determine the effectiveness of tDCS.

Inter-individual Differences in Responsiveness to tDCS

Some recent studies have focused on the investigation of inter-individual differences in the responsiveness to tDCS that may account for differential effects on functional outcomes (Krause and Cohen Kadosh 2014). For instance, a recent study showed that tDCS in older adults produced electrical fields that were about 30% weaker compared to young adults (Laakso et al. 2015), emphasizing that age may also interfere with technical parameters. Furthermore, recent research has demonstrated altered levels of neuronal excitability, changes in balance between neurotransmitters as well as in baseline neuronal activations in aging (Bishop et al. 2010; Grady 2012). These alterations lead to inter-individually different degrees of age-associated neuronal network reorganization which may mediate the response to tDCS protocols (Krause and Cohen Kadosh 2014; Summers et al. 2015). Consequently, qualitatively different functional outcomes are expected when tDCS is applied to "intact" young versus "deviant" (as compared to the pattern of the young) neuronal networks (Hsu et al. 2015).

Learmonth et al. did not find tDCS effects of parietal stimulation on spatial attention performance in either young or older adults. However, when the authors considered baseline task performance in their analysis, they found that while tDCS had no effect in good performance, it had even a negative effect when performance was already poor (Learmonth et al. 2015). This study suggests the possibility of state-dependent effects of tDCS and underlines the importance to more precisely look into initial performance levels. Similarly, Berryhill and Jones did not observe any tDCS effect of frontal stimulation on neither visual nor verbal working memory (Berryhill and Jones 2012). However, when the authors considered education levels, they found tDCS-induced improvements in higher educated subjects. In lower educated subjects no beneficial or even detrimental effects emerged in the tDCS condition.

The inter-individual variability in the responsiveness to tDCS dependent on baseline performance that is seen across all age ranges may be particularly relevant in the course of aging because behavioral tasks may be more challenging here in general (Berryhill and Jones 2012; Summers et al. 2015). Lower task performance levels in older compared to young adults may imply larger gains by stimulation, so tDCS may be even more effective in older populations (cf. Hsu et al. 2015). Speculatively, differences to tDCS responsiveness may result from inter-individual variability, such as in baseline performance levels, instead of from age per se. If this is the case, high performing older and low performing young adults should respond similarly to tDCS interventions – an issue that has to be scrutinized in future studies.

In sum, distinct tDCS effects may not only emerge due to age, but also due to individual performance levels or baseline activation states. Noteworthy, all studies to date that investigated tDCS in aging included groups of older adults (most often above 65 years), with some but not all comparing tDCS-induced effects to a group of young adults. What effects emerge between these extremes of the age spectrum is not known yet. However, in order to infer whether or not tDCS exerts more or less beneficial effects in aging on functional outcomes, and unveil the factors underlying these possible differences, an integrative approach is needed that includes high- as well as lower-performing adults of various ages across the lifespan.

Technical Considerations

From what we know so far, when it comes to functional outcome selection for tDCS interventional studies with older adults, it may be favorable to:

- Carefully consider how demanding the task of interest is for the age group under study (Summers et al. 2015);
- Elaborate whether age-associated task performance decrease is expected and consider the underlying mechanisms (slowing of processing speed versus cognitive decline; compensatory versus detrimental recruitment of additional brain areas etc.).
- Consider baseline performance levels as additional covariate or grouping variable (Learmonth et al. 2015).

Cognitive Functions

Methodology is critical to consider when reviewing tDCS literature since factors such as electrode size, montage, intensity, and stimulation duration could affect the outcome. Likewise, cognition is a heterogeneous construct that must be dissected when considering the efficacy of tDCS. Therefore, the following sections are organized by cognitive domain and tables summarizing key methodological variables are provided at the start of each section.

Attention and Working Memory

Nilsson et al. (2015) performed a single-blind, crossover, sham controlled experiment in which they evaluated the effect of tDCS on spatial working memory (Nilsson et al. 2015) (Table 19.1). Participants each completed three sessions, two active (one at 1 mA, the other at 2 mA) and one sham, the order of which was randomized and counterbalanced. The anode was placed over the left dorsolateral prefrontal cortex during each session. Despite this electrode montage, the authors used a 3-back task with visuospatial stimuli that would be theoretically dependent on the right cerebral hemisphere (assuming typical language lateralization in the left hemisphere). Task duration was 5 min and performance was evaluated before tDCS, during tDCS (at 0–5, 10–15, 20–25 min), and after tDCS (at 5–10 and 30–35 min). There were no

Table 19.1 Attention and working memory: online effects

	Age	n	Anode location (size)	Cathode location (size)	Intensity	Duration (min)
Nilsson et al. (2015)	69	30	F3 (35 cm^2)	Contralateral supraorbit (100 cm^2)	1 mA, 2 mA, sham	25
Learmonth et al. (2015)	66.6	20	P3 or P4 (35 cm^2)	Contralateral supraorbit (35 cm^2)	1 mA	15

Table 19.2 Attention and working memory: offline effects

	Age	n	Anode location (size)	Cathode location (size)	Intensity	Duration (min)
Berryhill and Jones (2012)	63.7	25	F3 or F4 (35 cm^2)	Contralateral cheek (35 cm^2)	1.5 mA	10
Seo et al. (2011)	70.0	24	F3 (25 cm^2)	Left arm (25 cm^2)	2.0 mA	30

significant effects of stimulation at any time point. However, the interpretation of these results is difficult given the mismatch between the montage, which targeted the left prefrontal cortex, and the cognitive task, which was potentially more reliant on the right prefrontal cortex.

A study by Learmonth et al. (2015) used a lateralized visual detection task, which is a measure of visual attention, to evaluate the effects of tDCS over the posterior parietal cortex (PPC) (Learmonth et al. 2015). The team found small effects such that those with "good" baseline performances showed relative improvement with right anodal tDCS while those with "poor" baseline performances showed decline following left anodal tDCS. These subtle effects were evident regardless of age and suggest that the inter-individual variability following a single tDCS session response arises from the innate integrity of the targeted brain region(s).

Another cross-over study evaluated the effects of anodal stimulation over the left and right prefrontal cortex, relative to sham, as participants performed verbal and visuospatial n-back tasks (Berryhill and Jones 2012) (Table 19.2). Participants practiced the task during stimulation but outcome was evaluated after the electrodes had been removed. There was no overall effect of stimulation. However, significant differences emerged when the group was split based on median education (16.9 vs. 13.5 years) where the high education group responded to tDCS but the low education group did not. This beneficial effect was evident regardless of montage or task. In contrast, the low education group showed reduced visuospatial working memory performance when the anode was over the right prefrontal cortex; a finding that is rather counterintuitive. Like the Learmonth et al. (2015) study, these findings raise the possibility that cognitive and neural reserve may affect stimulation results; however, replication is clearly warranted given the post-hoc nature of the education analyses (Learmonth et al. 2015).

Using a parallel groups design, anodal tDCS over the left prefrontal cortex enhanced accuracy on a verbal working memory task relative to sham tDCS in older adults (Jeon and Han 2012). Importantly, there were no differences between the groups on a visuospatial working memory task that would be theoretically dependent on the right prefrontal cortex. Thus, the findings highlight the potential weakness of Nilsson and colleagues' design and reinforce the need to select tasks that are mediated by the targeted brain region(s) (Nilsson et al. 2015).

Dual Task Motor Control

Falls are a common problem in older age and may be associated with reduced cognitive control (Table 19.3). Thus, stimulation could enhance cognitive and motor control thereby mitigating fall risk. Two studies have evaluated the effects of tDCS on dual task performance. Manor and colleagues (2016) used a cross-over design to evaluate active versus sham tDCS over the left prefrontal cortex on single and dual task performance (Manor et al. 2016). In the single task condition, participants walked, stood, or verbally performed serial subtractions (while seated). The dual task condition required them to perform serial subtractions while either walking or standing. There were no effects of stimulation on single task performance, consonant with the easy nature of the tasks. However, active tDCS reduced dual task costs relative to sham. Likewise, Zhou et al. (2015) reported that active tDCS enhanced the capacity of the postural control system to adapt to stressors and reduced the cost of dual-task performance (Zhou et al. 2015). The effects of stimulation appear to be greatest in those with the poorest baseline postural control.

Cognitive training is a general class of interventions that are designed to enhance targeted cognitive abilities via rehearsal based exercises (Table 19.4). Working memory is a relatively fundamental cognitive ability on which other cognitive domains rely, yet it is known to decline during "normal" aging (Nissim et al. 2017). Thus, a growing body of research has investigated the ability of cognitive training to mitigate age-related decline. Park et al. (2014) extended this question by evaluating the synergistic effects of concurrent tDCS and cognitive training (Nilsson

Table 19.3 Dual task motor control: offline effects

	Age	n	Anode location (size)	Cathode location (size)	Intensity	Duration (min)
Manor et al. (2016)	61	37	F3 (35 cm^2)	Right supraorbit (35 cm^2)	2.0 mA	20
Zhou et al. (2015)	63	20	F3 (35 cm^2)	Fp2 (35 cm^2)	Average of 1.4 mA	20

Table 19.4 Cognitive training: online effects

	Age (SD)	n	Anode location (size)	Cathode location (size)	Intensity	Duration (min)
Park et al. (2014)	69.7	40	F3 and F4 (concurrently) (25 cm^2)	"Non-dominant" arm (25 cm^2)	2 mA	30

Table 19.5 Combined online and offline effects

	Age (SD)	n	Anode location (size)	Cathode location (size)	Intensity	Duration (min)
Jones et al. (2015)	64.4	72	F4, P4, or both (35 cm^2)	Contralateral cheek (35 cm^2)	1.5 mA	10

et al. 2017; Park et al. 2014). A total of 40 healthy older adults were randomized to active or sham tDCS over the PFC bilaterally (note that two tDCS units were used to accomplish the bilateral stimulation). All participants completed 10 cognitive training sessions (5 days per week for 2 weeks). Neuropsychological evaluations were performed at baseline and repeated on day 10 as well as 7 and 28 days after the final session. Active stimulation resulted in persistent improvements at all time points on a 2 back verbal working memory paradigm. Some evidence of near transfer was evident as this group also showed transient improvement on the digits forward task, though there was no evidence of far-transfer on the other 9 outcome measures. Thus, stimulation appeared to enhance performance on the trained task as there were no significant changes in the sham group.

Jones et al. (2015) also examined the combination of cognitive training and tDCS but focused these effects on visuospatial working memory (Jones et al. 2015) (Table 19.5). Participants were randomized to receive active tDCS over the right prefrontal, posterior parietal, or both locations (site alternated daily) or to a sham condition. All participants completed 10 days of training (5 days per week for 2 weeks). During each session, participants practiced each of 4 visuospatial paradigms while receiving stimulation (or sham) and then completed the tasks during the aftereffect period. Composite indices were calculated for the trained tasks as well as theoretically related transfer tasks, all of which were evaluated at baseline, on day 10, and at a 1-month follow-up. There were no effects of stimulation on day 10; however, significant effects were evident for both trained and transfer-indices at the 1-month time point regardless of stimulation site. Thus, active tDCS appeared to facilitate long-term gains that are interesting to consider in light of the effects on memory that are described below. A Phase III clinical trial of tDCS combined with cognitive training is currently underway (Woods et al. 2018).

Language

Ross et al. (2011) administered anodal tDCS over either lateral temporal lobe of healthy older adults during 2 separate sessions (Ross et al. 2011) (Table 19.6). Participants were asked to name famous faces and landmarks starting 2 min after stimulation started. There was no effect of stimulation when all trials were included. However, there was a significant effect of stimulation on trials that the authors retrospectively labeled as "difficult" (i.e., reaction time of >5 s). Specifically, there was a double dissociation where left stimulation enhanced face but not landmark recall whereas right stimulation enhanced landmark but not face recall. The findings reinforce the need for task-specific targeting and raises the intriguing question of

Table 19.6 Language: online effects during confrontation naming

	Age (SD)	n	Anode location (size)	Cathode location (size)	Intensity	Duration (min)
Ross et al. (2011)	65	14	T3 or T4 (35 cm^2)	Contralateral cheek (35 cm^2)	1.5 mA	15
Fertonani et al. (2014)	66.5	20	Left prefrontal: 8 cm frontally and 6 cm laterally to CZ (35 cm^2)	Right shoulder (35 cm^2)	2 mA	6–10 (depending on condition)

whether task difficulty is a critical mediating factor. Fertonani et al. (2014) reported that tDCS enhanced naming ability in young participants regardless of whether performance was measured online and offline. In contrast, this effect was only evident during online stimulation in older adults (Fertonani et al. 2014). Thus, the montage and timing of stimulation appear critical to consider in older adults.

Learning and Memory

Memory is widely known to decline with "normal" aging, at least partially due to decline in key medial temporal lobe regions (Small et al. 2011). However, such difficulty can arise with failure during any (or all) of the involved phases including encoding, consolidation, and retrieval. The neocortex plays an important role in the initial processing and subsequent reprocessing (or re-experiencing) of sensory information related to memories. Moreover, the lateral frontoparietal cognitive control network appears especially important in intentional memory formation (Hampstead et al. 2016; Spaniol et al. 2009). Thus, there may be important differences in the effects of tDCS based on memory phase as well as the targeted brain region. Therefore, we have separated the existing research in this area based on when tDCS was performed and have included the targeted regions in the tables contained within each section.

Remembering the location of objects is critical in everyday life and becomes more difficult with age. Flöel and colleagues (2012) used an object-location paradigm in which older participants were instructed to remember the location of buildings on a street-map (Flöel et al. 2012) (Table 19.7). Each participant completed 2 sessions that were separated by 1 week, using alternate test versions. Stimulation order was randomized so that half the participants received active tDCS and then sham tDCS, with the other half receiving the opposite order. Participants received 5 learning blocks of the object-location stimuli, which took approximately 45 min. Stimulation was delivered concurrently during the first 20 min of the task. Participants then completed a memory task immediately after the learning trial ended (roughly 25 min post-stimulation), at which point there were no significant differences between the groups. However, memory was reassessed 1 week after

Table 19.7 Learning and memory: online effects during encoding

	Mean Age	n	Anode location (size)	Cathode location (size)	Intensity	Duration (min)
Floel et al. (2012)	62.1	20	~T6 (35 cm^2)	Contralateral supraorbit (100 cm^2)	1 mA	20
Sandrini et al. (2016)	68.9	28	F3 (35 cm^2)	FP2 (35 cm^2)	1.5 mA	15

Table 19.8 Learning and memory: offline effects during consolidation

	Age (SD)	n	Anode location (size)	Cathode location (size)	Intensity	Duration (min)
Sandrini et al. (2014)	67.17	36	F3 (35 cm^2)	FP2 (35 cm^2)	1.5 mA	15

each session and stimuli learned during active stimulation were remembered significantly better than those learned during sham.

Sandrini et al. (2016) reported similar effects on long-term performance. This group performed a randomized, double blind, placebo controlled experiment using a word list task (Sandrini et al. 2016). On day 1, a 20 word list was repeated until participants either achieved 85% or better performance or until they received a maximum of 5 trials. Participants received active or sham tDCS concurrent with these learning trials. Memory was evaluated after 48 h and again 1 month later. Active tDCS significantly enhanced performance at 48 h and showed a trend ($p = 0.09$) at 1 month relative to sham. Together, these studies suggest that tDCS applied during encoding enhances the consolidation of new information and makes memories more resilient to time-related decay.

In an earlier study, Sandrini et al. (2014) evaluated the effects of tDCS when applied during the consolidation phase (i.e., after encoding but before the memory test/retrieval) (Sandrini et al. 2014) (Table 19.8). Here, older adults were randomized to one of three groups: anodal tDCS plus a perceptual cue, anodal tDCS without a perceptual cue, and sham tDCS with a perceptual cue. The study was conducted across 4 sessions, the first 3 were performed on consecutive days and the final was a 1-month follow-up. On day 1, participants performed a word list learning task (using the same 85% correct or 5 trial maximum as in the previously described study). During this session, written words were pulled from a white bag, recited by participant, and placed in a blue bag – this served as the perceptual cue. Stimulation was performed on day 2, when those in the perceptual cue groups were shown the blue bag but prevented from reciting the words. The no cue group had a new examiner in a different environment and had tDCS applied without presenting the bags. Importantly, there were no between group differences in the reported side effects and the groups could not distinguish whether they received active or sham tDCS. Participants completed a memory test on day 3 and again at the 1-month follow-up. The active stimulation groups performed significantly better (i.e.,

Table 19.9 Learning and memory: online effects during retrieval

	Age (SD)	n	Anode location (size)	Cathode location (size)	Intensity	Duration (min)
Manenti et al. (2013)	67.9	64 total (32 healthy young)	Parietal: 5 cm lateral and 8 cm posterior to vertex Prefrontal: 8 cm frontally and 6 cm lateral to vertex ($35\ cm^2$)	Contralateral supraorbit ($35\ cm^2$)	1.5 mA	15

enhanced consolidation) than the sham group on both Day 3 and at 1-month, though there was no effect of perceptual cue.

Thus, there is evidence that applying tDCS during either encoding or consolidation enhances long-term retention of the information. The final question is whether such beneficial effects are evident if stimulation is applied during the retrieval phase.

Manenti et al. (2013) compared the effects of tDCS over the parietal or prefrontal cortex in healthy young and older adults during memory retrieval (Manenti et al. 2013) (Table 19.9). Participants were randomized to either targeted brain region (i.e., prefrontal or parietal) and underwent two sessions in which the anode was placed over the left or right hemisphere. Half of the participants in each group received sham stimulation over one hemisphere or the other. Participants completed a word list task in which they encoded 48 abstract and 48 concrete words. The memory test used a recognition format in which participants were required to identify the target stimuli from an equal number of distractors. There was a 5 min delay between the encoding and "retrieval" phases (Note: although the authors claim the task to evaluate retrieval, its design is a standard recognition format that could have been solved using either familiarity or recollection). Stimulation began 2 min before the start of the memory test and lasted its entire duration; thereby bridging the consolidation and "retrieval" phases. Young adults were faster during active than sham stimulation regardless of stimulated hemisphere. In contrast, active tDCS over the left hemisphere enhanced performance, as measured by reaction time, in older adults relative to sham or stimulation over the right hemisphere. These effects were evident regardless of the prefrontal or parietal location. A subsequent re-analysis of these data suggested that older adults with "low" memory abilities drove these effects whereas those with "high" memory abilities showed the same bilateral facilitation as did the younger adults (Brambilla et al. 2015).

Overall then, the evidence suggests that active tDCS can enhance performance across all three phases of memory: encoding, consolidation, and retrieval. However, the strongest evidence appears to be for the consolidation phase given the long-term (hours to days) benefit on memory test performance. Methodological differences between studies (montage, intensity, duration) make it difficult to determine the optimal parameters.

Executive Functioning

Across a series of studies in older adults Harty et al. (2014) systematically examined the role of the right dorsolateral prefrontal cortex (DLPFC) on error monitoring (Harty et al. 2014) (Table 19.10). Participants in each of four studies completed one active and one sham session in which tDCS was performed concurrent with a go/no-go task that required participants to respond to repeated stimuli as well as when there was discordance between the meaning of a word and the color ink (i.e., a classic Stroop task). Participants were also instructed to indicate when they made an error in either of the conditions. Overall, only anodal stimulation over the right DLPFC enhanced error detection during repeated trials. Critically, these findings were replicated (experiments 1 and 4) and were not evident with stimulation of the left DLPFC (experiment 2) or when the cathode was placed over the right DLPFC (experiment 3). This series of studies adds to our overall understanding about the functions mediated by the right DLPFC and revealed polarity and site dependent effects of tDCS.

Boggio et al. (2010) evaluated the effects of tDCS on decision making in older adults (Table 19.11). In this double-blind study, participants were randomized to one of three groups: anodal left-cathodal right, cathodal left-anodal right, or sham (Boggio et al. 2010). Participants performed a gambling task that began 5 min after stimulation began and ran concurrent with task duration. The left anodal stimulation group demonstrated a significant increase in high-risk decisions relative to the other groups. There was a small increase in risky decisions in the right anodal group relative to sham and, interestingly, this group had the worst overall performance on the task. These findings contradicted the group's earlier findings in healthy young participants and raise the possibility that tDCS effects change as a function of age.

Table 19.10 Executive functioning: online effects on error monitoring

	Age (SD)	n	Anode location (size)	Cathode location (size)	Intensity	Duration
Harty et al. (2014)			(all 35 cm^2)	(all 35 cm^2)	All 1 mA	Not provided
Experiment 1	72.1	24	F4	Cz		
Experiment 2	69.4	24	F3	Cz		
Experiment 3	69.7	24	Cz	F4		
Experiment 4	72.1	24	F4	Cz		

Table 19.11 Executive functioning: online effects on decision making

	Age	n	Anode location (size)	Cathode location (size)	Intensity	Duration (min)
Boggio et al. (2010)	50–85 (group means 67–69)	28	F3 or F4 (35 cm^2)	F3 or F4 (35 cm^2)	2 mA	15

Motor and Sensory Functions

tDCS has the potential to enhance activity in cortical sensorimotor networks and induce neuroplastic recovery of physical function in impaired populations. Presently, most studies conducted in older adults have used cross sectional study designs in which upper extremity motor performance is measured before and after (or during) a single session of tDCS delivered with the anode over the primary motor cortex. We first summarize the findings from those studies. Hummel et al. (2010) showed that 20 min of active tDCS is superior to sham tDCS for improving skilled hand functions as measured by the Jebsen-Taylor Hand function Test (Hummel et al. 2010). Goodwill and colleagues compared unilateral, bilateral and sham tDCS combined with visuomotor tracking, and assessed motor performance of the non-dominant upper limb, immediately post and 30 min following stimulation. Both unilateral and bilateral tDCS decreased tracking error at both time points to a greater degree than sham stimulation (Goodwill et al. 2013). A later study by the same group also demonstrated that tDCS contributes to cross-transfer of unilateral training effects to the contralateral arm (Goodwill et al. 2015). Similarly, Hoff and colleagues found that a visuomotor training task plus tDCS with the anode over the right primary motor cortex increased manual dexterity in the contralateral hand (Hoff et al. 2015). Improvement was less with sham stimulation and absent when active stimulation was delivered without visuomotor training, which indicates the potential importance of pairing stimulation with task practice for optimal benefit (Hoff et al. 2015). Parikh and Cole assessed whether tDCS improved performance in older adults on functional tests of grasp and upper extremity manipulation (Grooved Pegboard Test and the Key-slot task) (Parikh and Cole 2014). Compared to sham, the active tDCS led to retention of practice-induced gains in performance when tested again 35 min later. Grip force variability on an isometric precision grip task performed with visual feedback also increased with active tDCS but not sham tDCS. A related study by the same researchers tested performance on a test of manual dexterity when participants were instructed to grip and lift an object whose contact surfaces were unexpectedly made more or less slippery across trials (Parikh and Cole 2015). The results showed that tDCS yielded a reduction in grip force. These findings might indicate improved processing of object-specific sensory information and its integration with the motor commands for production of manipulative forces (Parikh and Cole 2015). Zimerman et al. (2013) tested whether performance on a complex finger-tapping task can be enhanced in old subjects with tDCS of the primary motor cortex (Zimerman et al. 2013). The study results showed that elderly participants experienced substantial improvements when training was applied concurrent with tDCS, with effects lasting for at least 24 h.

The potential benefit of tDCS on motor learning has been studied by placing the anode over the cerebellum. Hardwick and colleagues tested whether excitatory stimulation could enhance adaptation of motor performance during a “center-out” reaching task with a sudden change in visual feedback of the movement trajectory (Hardwick and Celnik 2014). Older participants receiving sham tDCS were slower to adapt than younger participants, but older participants who received anodal tDCS adapted at a similar rate to younger adults (Hardwick and Celnik 2014). In contrast, a study by Panouillères et al. (2015) in young and older adults found no benefit to cerebellar tDCS for a motor adaptation task involving joystick control of rapid targeted movements of a cursor on a computer screen (Panouillères et al. 2015). However, they did find that tDCS over primary motor cortex improved initial adaptation in both age groups compared to sham, and this improvement lasted up to 40 min after the end of the stimulation (Panouillères et al. 2015). Craig and colleagues delivered anodal tDCS to primary motor cortex and cerebellum (in separate sessions), but found only small and mixed results for both young and elderly groups. In older adults, an increase in sway amplitude was observed during sham stimulation, but this increase was delayed during stimulation at the primary motor cortex or cerebellum (Craig and Doumas 2017). The relatively modest effects of tDCS in this study might be explained in part by a lack of increase in cortical excitation following tDCS, as measured by motor evoked potentials with transcranial magnetic stimulation (Craig and Doumas 2017).

A small number of studies have examined tDCS of the prefrontal cortex and the influence on motor outcomes. Zhou et al. (2015) compared center of pressure (COP) fluctuations during single-task (quiet standing) and dual-task (standing while performing serial subtractions) conditions, before and after real or sham tDCS (Zhou et al. 2015). Neither real nor sham conditions altered complexity of COP fluctuations in the single-task condition. However, active tDCS increased the complexity of COP fluctuations for the dual-task condition as well as induced a trend toward improved serial subtraction performance. Increased complexity of COP is considered to be an indicator of a more flexible and robust postural control system (Zhou et al. 2015). A similar study by Manor and colleagues evaluated dual-tasking before and after 20 min of real or sham tDCS targeting the left prefrontal cortex in elderly adults (Manor et al. 2016). Trials of standing, walking, and verbalized serial subtractions were completed, along with dual-task trials of standing or walking while performing serial subtractions. Dual-task costs were reduced after real tDCS versus sham tDCS, as well as compared with either pre-tDCS condition (Manor et al. 2016).

Practicalities of tDCS Research Involving Chronically Ill Aging Subjects

Age is a risk factor for chronic illness (Makris et al. 2014; Reid et al. 2015). The prevalence of chronic illness in older persons worldwide is very high, and multimorbidity and polypharmacy are common (Borsheski and Johnson 2014; Centers for Medicare and Medicaid Services 2012; Hasselman 2012; Ortman et al. 2014; Sawyer et al. 2006). In the U.S., more than 80% of Medicare beneficiaries have ≥1 chronic medical disorder, more than 80% take >1 prescription drug, and 29% take ≥5 prescribed medications, often including opioids.

Thus, tDCS research involving aging populations may involve individuals with multiple chronic conditions and very complex treatment regimens. This can substantially impact the person's functional status and may require specific arrangements for a successful inclusion in tDCS research. Key considerations are discussed below.

Co-participation of Informal Caregivers in Research

Chronically ill elderly often rely on assistance from family caregivers in tasks of daily living. Thus, it also can be advantageous or even necessary to include informal caregivers as assisting co-participants in research, so that they can help the elderly to keep track of study visits, to accompany the elderly to the research facility, to facilitate data collection and outcome assessment, or to provide co-lateral information relevant to outcome assessment and adverse events monitoring. Based on the type and purpose of tDCS study, the inclusion of informal caregivers can be mandatory or optional. In either arrangement, the study Inclusion/Exclusion criteria for the caregiver (such as age ≥ 18 years, ability to follow instruction of study personnel; and other basic requirements) have to be defined in the protocol and an informed consent must be obtained separately for the elderly and the caregiver.

Obtaining an Informed Consent for Research Participation

tDCS research that involves chronically ill elderly can be challenging also due to consenting procedure. Overall, elderly are considered a potentially vulnerable population and at least regulatory authorities in the U.S., such as IRB, may require a clear description of actions in the pre-consent period that would mitigate a potential coercion. This can be addressed by allowing longer time for a review of study information, delivering the information step-by-step, in a very simple, easy-to-understand, lay language, or providing additional flyers summarizing key information about the study.

Another challenge of the consenting process in elderly is that many aging individuals present with substantial sensory deficits, such as impaired hearing or vision, or with cognitive deficits. In the U.S., the IRB provides guidance on case-by-case basis, and additional witnesses of the consenting process may be required.

Adverse-Event Assessment and Reporting

It is well known that reliability of recall and self-report in ailing elderly fluctuates (Abernethy and Currow 2011). This may be a problem not only for outcome data collection, but also for the purpose of adverse event detection and assessment. Thus, it is advantageous if the adverse event monitoring relies on as many sources of information as possible; it may combine the patient's self report with study personnel observations, collateral reports from informal caregiver or notifications by clinicians providing regular medical care (Brunoni et al. 2011; Sundaram et al. 2009). However, it is important that information from the multiple sources is merged and noted in the participant's files, so that it can be evaluated by the study physician or other designated study personnel authorized for adverse event assessment and processing.

Another issue related to adverse event assessment in ailing elderly subjects pertains to responsible determination of the relation of the adverse event to the tDCS study procedure. The difficulty specifically in ill elderly arises from the fact that multiple illness or co-morbidities are frequent and it could be difficult to distinguish between unfavorable changes due to fluctuation of the clinical course of the illness and adverse events due to the study procedure. At least a partial remedy for this problem can be an extended baseline that may provide an insight into fluctuations of the participant's status and into the nature and frequency of self-reported health problems before the study procedure is implemented. The extended baseline can also reveal regularly experienced side effects related to medication regimen. To illustrate, it is advantageous to be able to document baseline reports of dizziness, shortness of breath or nausea associated for example with opioid medication intake, or to be able to compare frequency of headaches or frequency of emergency room visits in the baseline period with one in the interventional period. This type of information from the extended baseline is extremely valuable and can be also used in reports to regulatory authorities if needed.

Polypharmacy

It has been shown by clinical practice that aging chronically ill individuals are often on multiple-medication regimen for the purpose of the illness modifying therapy and/or for symptom management. A recent survey indicates that more than 80% of Medicare beneficiaries take >1 prescription drug, and 29% take ≥5 prescribed medications (Centers for Medicare and Medicaid Services, 2012). Managing chronic illness in elderly is challenging and thus it may be difficult or impossible to insist on medication wash-out prior to study participation. This may be a problem in tDCS studies, because centrally acting medication may alter tDCS outcomes, and specifically some classes of medication, such as NMDA-blockers, may modify or prevent tDCS after-effects (Nitsche et al. 2004a, b, c, 2006, 2009, 2012). Thus, this issue requires a careful evaluation in the planning stage of a study. A viable option is to identify medications/classes of medications that are known to substantially alter tDCS effects and prepare – with clinician's guidance – a plan for substitution of the selected medications. As some medications have to be titrated up step-by-step, the substitution plan would also define the necessary time on the new medication to reach a stable-dose regimen.

Other Issues

In addition to practical considerations discussed above, it is important to keep in mind that the ability of ailing older persons to cope with excessive additional burden of study procedures or study visits is limited. Living with chronic illness is stressful for the patient and the family (Andrews 2001; Costa-Requena et al. 2015). Thus, the study procedures should be kept at the necessary minimum, and outcome data collection has to be carefully planned. A possible solution how to minimize burden related to repeated visits to research facility for tDCS application is to select a home-based approach (Charvet et al. 2015), which is discussed in detail in Chap. 13.

Other Special Considerations for tDCS Studies In Aging Populations

Atrophy-Related Differences in Current Flow

Atrophy of white and gray matter is a common consequence of aging (Fischl et al. 2002; Ge et al. 2002; Grady 2012; Gunning-Dixon et al. 2009; Nissim et al. 2017; Salat et al. 1999). Age-related changes in brain tissue has a strong potential for altering the pattern of current flow in older adults, as compared to younger adults. Recent computational modeling research suggests that while increased atrophy with age tends to lead to less current entering the brain in a relatively linear fashion, greater atrophy in those over 70 years of age can lead to non-linear changes in current flow due to widening ventricles (Thomas et al. 2017). This work suggests that predicted current flow based on exemplar models of younger adults may not provide clear insight into the pattern of current flow in older adults. Thus, individual modeling or models based on exemplars within a given decade of life may be more appropriate for understanding where in the brain current flows and at what intensity in older adult participants.

Structural Connectivity Changes Impact on Current Flow

White matter connectivity changes with age (Damoiseaux and Greicius 2009; Gunning-Dixon et al. 2009). As mentioned above, age-related changes in functional connectivity may significantly alter what regions of the brain are affected by tDCS. This, in part, may be the result of underlying changes in structural white matter connectivity. As current flow from tDCS and resulting behavioral effects not only relate to direct stimulation of tissue, but also remote effects from tissue connectivity, understanding the impact of age-related changes in structural connectivity on current flow will be important for better understanding mechanisms of effect from tDCS in older adults on age-related conditions.

Impact of Common Medications in Older Adults on tDCS Effects

A robust literature has emerged on the impact of certain medications on the neurophysiological response produced by tDCS (McLaren et al. 2018). For example, sodium channel blockers have previously been shown to block the production of excitatory effects under the anode electrode, while calcium channel blockers attenuated excitatory effects (Nitsche et al. 2003). Certain sodium channel blockers are common for treatment of arrhythmia and other heart conditions, while certain calcium channel blockers are commonly used to treat chest pain and hypertension. In addition, glutamatergic and gaba-ergic medications have also been shown to alter how brain tissue responds to tDCS (Nitsche et al. 2003, 2004c). While these drugs are perhaps less commonly prescribed in healthy older adults, gaba-ergic drugs can be used for anxiety and other conditions present in older adults. Further still, a variety of drugs significantly modulate the neurophysiological response of brain tissue to tDCS, such as drugs acting on serotonin (e.g., SSRIs), acetylcholine, dopamine, and noradrenaline (Nitsche et al. 2004a, 2006, 2009). For example, prior research suggests that SSRIs given in concert with 1 mA tDCS may result in effects of stimulation under the cathode being excitatory, rather than inhibitory (Nitsche et al. 2009). Thus, net excitation appears to be achieved under both electrodes. SSRIs are commonly prescribed in older adults, especially in the presence of late-life depression. Thus, careful attention should be given to medications present in older adult participants, as these may interact with tDCS to alter the overall neurophysiological response of brain tissue to stimulation and significantly impact outcomes.

Conclusions

Aging and age-related conditions are a growing area of study in the field of tDCS. Recent research demonstrating promising effects of tDCS on cognition, physical function, chronic pain and other age-related conditions suggest that research in this domain may hold significant promise in the treatment of age-related conditions. Research integrating modern methods for assessing brain function and tDCS effects will be particularly important for understanding and optimizing the impact of tDCS on age-related conditions. Current efforts are underway to assess in Phase III clinical trials the efficacy of tDCS in facilitating cognitive training outcomes in older adults and slow the onset of dementia (The ACT study, ClinicalTrials.gov NCT02851511). Collectively, this work holds great promise for evaluating and implementing tDCS-based interventions in older adults. Future trials will also be important for assessing the efficacy of tDCS in other domains of aging research. Regardless, preliminary findings described in this chapter serve to highlight the promise of tDCS across a variety of age-related domains. In concert with careful design planning and consideration, there is much to be excited about in the field of tDCS and aging.

References

Abernethy, A. P., & Currow, D. C. (2011). Patient self-reporting in palliative care using information technology: Yes, there is hope! *Palliative Medicine, 25*, 673–674.

Ahn, H., Woods, A. J., Kunik, M. E., Bhattacharjee, A., Chen, Z., Choi, E., & Fillingim, R. B. (2017). Efficacy of transcranial direct current stimulation over primary motor cortex (anode) and contralateral supraorbital area (cathode) on clinical pain severity and mobility performance in persons with knee osteoarthritis: An experimenter- and participant-bl. *Brain Stimulation, 10*, 902–909.

Andrews, S. C. (2001). Caregiver burden and symptom distress in people with cancer receiving hospice care. *Oncology Nursing Forum, 28*, 1469–1474.

Anton, S. D., Woods, A. J., Ashizawa, T., Barb, D., Buford, T. W., Carter, C. S., … Pahor, M. (2015). Successful aging: Advancing the science of physical independence in older adults. *Ageing Research Reviews, 24*, 304–327.

Antonenko, D., & Flöel, A. (2013). Healthy aging by staying selectively connected: A mini-review. *Gerontology, 60*, 3–9.

Antonenko, D., Schubert, F., Bohm, F., Ittermann, B., Aydin, S., Hayek, D., … Flöel, A. (2017). tDCS-induced modulation of GABA levels and resting-state functional connectivity in older adults. *The Journal of Neuroscience, 37*, 79–17.

Berryhill, M. E., & Jones, K. T. (2012). tDCS selectively improves working memory in older adults with more education. *Neuroscience Letters, 521*, 148–151.

Bikson, M., Rahman, A., Datta, A., Fregni, F., & Merabet, L. (2012). High-resolution modeling assisted design of customized and individualized transcranial direct current stimulation protocols. *Neuromodulation, 15*, 306–314.

Bishop, N. A., Lu, T., & Yankner, B. A. (2010). Neural mechanisms of ageing and cognitive decline. *Nature, 464*, 529–535.

Boggio, P. S., Campanhã, C., Valasek, C. A., Fecteau, S., Pascual-Leone, A., & Fregni, F. (2010). Modulation of decision-making in a gambling task in older adults with transcranial direct current stimulation. *The European Journal of Neuroscience, 31*, 593–597.

Borsheski, R., & Johnson, Q. L. (2014). Pain management in the geriatric population. *Missouri Medicine, 111*, 508–511.

Brambilla, M., Manenti, R., Ferrari, C., & Cotelli, M. (2015). Better together: Left and right hemisphere engagement to reduce age-related memory loss. *Behavioural Brain Research, 293*, 125–133.

Brault, M. W. (2012). Americans with disabilities: 2010 – Household economic studies. In: *Current population reports* (pp. 70–131). Washington, DC: U.S. Census Bureau – U.S. Department of Commerce – Economics and Statistics Administration.

Brunoni, A. R., Amadera, J., Berbel, B., Volz, M. S., Rizzerio, B. G., & Fregni, F. (2011). A systematic review on reporting and assessment of adverse effects associated with transcranial direct current stimulation. *The International Journal of Neuropsychopharmacology, 14*, 1133–1145.

Bureau, U. S. C. (2009). *An aging world: 2008*. Washington DC: U.S. Census Bureau – U.S. Department of Commerce –Economics and Statistics Administration. P95/09–1

Centers for Medicare and Medicaid Services. (2012). *Chronic conditions among medicare beneficiaries, chartbook*. Baltimore, MD: Centers for Medicare and Medicaid Services.

Charvet, L. E., Kasschau, M., Datta, A., Knotkova, H., Stevens, M. C., Alonzo, A., … Bikson, M. (2015). Remotely-supervised transcranial direct current stimulation (tDCS) for clinical trials: Guidelines for technology and protocols. *Frontiers in Systems Neuroscience, 9*, 26.

Coppi, E., Houdayer, E., Chieffo, R., Spagnolo, F., Inuggi, A., Straffi, L., … Leocani, L. (2014). Age-related changes in motor cortical representation and interhemispheric interactions: A transcranial magnetic stimulation study. *Frontiers in Aging Neuroscience, 6.*

Costa-Requena, G., Espinosa Val, M. C., & Cristofol, R. (2015). Caregiver burden in end-of-life care: Advanced cancer and final stage of dementia. *Palliative & Supportive Care, 13*, 583–589.

Craig, C. E., & Doumas, M. (2017). Anodal transcranial direct current stimulation shows minimal, measure-specific effects on dynamic postural control in young and older adults: A double blind, sham-controlled study. *PLoS One, 12*, e0170331.

Damoiseaux, J. S., & Greicius, M. D. (2009). Greater than the sum of its parts: A review of studies combining structural connectivity and resting-state functional connectivity. *Brain Structure & Function, 213*, 525–533.

Fertonani, A., Brambilla, M., Cotelli, M., & Miniussi, C. (2014). The timing of cognitive plasticity in physiological aging: A tDCS study of naming. *Frontiers in Aging Neuroscience, 6.*

Fischl, B., Salat, D. H., Busa, E., Albert, M., Dieterich, M., Haselgrove, C., … Dale, A. M. (2002). Whole brain segmentation. *Neuron, 33*, 341–355.

Flöel, A., Suttorp, W., Kohl, O., Kürten, J., Lohmann, H., Breitenstein, C., & Knecht, S. (2012). Non-invasive brain stimulation improves object-location learning in the elderly. *Neurobiology of Aging, 33*, 1682–1689.

Fujiyama, H., Hinder, M. R., Barzideh, A., Van de Vijver, C., Badache, A. C., Manrique-C, M. N., … Swinnen, S. P. (2017). Preconditioning tDCS facilitates subsequent tDCS effect on skill acquisition in older adults. *Neurobiology of Aging, 51*, 31–42.

Fujiyama, H., Hyde, J., Hinder, M. R., Kim, S. J., McCormack, G. H., Vickers, J. C., & Summers, J. J. (2014). Delayed plastic responses to anodal tDCS in older adults. *Frontiers in Aging Neuroscience, 6.*

Ge, Y., Grossman, R. I., Babb, J. S., Rabin, M. L., Mannon, L. J., & Kolson, D. L. (2002). Age-related total gray matter and white matter changes in normal adult brain. Part I: Volumetric MR imaging analysis. *AJNR. American Journal of Neuroradiology, 23*, 1327–1333.

Goh, J. O. S. (2011). Functional dedifferentiation and altered connectivity in older adults: Neural accounts of cognitive aging. *Aging and Disease, 2*, 30–48.

Goodwill, A. M., Daly, R. M., & Kidgell, D. J. (2015). The effects of anodal-tDCS on cross-limb transfer in older adults. *Clinical Neurophysiology, 126*, 2189–2197.

Goodwill, A. M., Reynolds, J., Daly, R. M., & Kidgell, D. J. (2013). Formation of cortical plasticity in older adults following tDCS and motor training. *Frontiers in Aging Neuroscience, 5.*

Grady, C. (2012). The cognitive neuroscience of ageing. *Nature Reviews. Neuroscience, 13*, 491–505.

Gunning-Dixon, F. M., Brickman, A. M., Cheng, J. C., & Alexopoulos, G. S. (2009). Aging of cerebral white matter: A review of MRI findings. *International Journal of Geriatric Psychiatry, 24*, 109–117.

Gutchess, A. (2014). Plasticity of the aging brain: New directions in cognitive neuroscience. *Science (80-), 346*, 579–582.

Hampstead, B. M., Khoshnoodi, M., Yan, W., Deshpande, G., & Sathian, K. (2016). Patterns of effective connectivity during memory encoding and retrieval differ between patients with mild cognitive impairment and healthy older adults. *NeuroImage, 124*, 997–1008.

Hardwick, R. M., & Celnik, P. A. (2014). Cerebellar direct current stimulation enhances motor learning in older adults. *Neurobiology of Aging, 35*, 2217–2221.

Harty, S., Robertson, I. H., Miniussi, C., Sheehy, O. C., Devine, C. A., McCreery, S., & O'Connell, R. G. (2014). Transcranial direct current stimulation over right dorsolateral prefrontal cortex enhances error awareness in older age. *The Journal of Neuroscience, 34*, 3646–3652.

Hasselman, D. (2012). *Super-utilizer summit common themes from innovation complex care management programs center for health care strategies.* https://www.chcs.org/media/FINAL_Super-Utilizer_Report.pdf. Access on 17 July18.

Heise, K.-F., Niehoff, M., Feldheim, J.-F., Liuzzi, G., Gerloff, C., & Hummel, F. C. (2014). Differential behavioral and physiological effects of anodal transcranial direct current stimulation in healthy adults of younger and older age. *Frontiers in Aging Neuroscience, 6*, 146.

Hoff, M., Kaminski, E., Rjosk, V., Sehm, B., Steele, C. J., Villringer, A., & Ragert, P. (2015). Augmenting mirror visual feedback-induced performance improvements in older adults. *The European Journal of Neuroscience, 41*, 1475–1483.

Holland, R., Leff, A. P., Josephs, O., Galea, J. M., Desikan, M., Price, C. J., … Crinion, J. (2011). Speech facilitation by left inferior frontal cortex stimulation. *Current Biology, 21*, 1403–1407.

Hsu, W.-Y., Ku, Y., Zanto, T. P., & Gazzaley, A. (2015). Effects of noninvasive brain stimulation on cognitive function in healthy aging and Alzheimer's disease: A systematic review and meta-analysis. *Neurobiology of Aging, 36*, 2348–2359.

Hummel, F. C., Heise, K., Celnik, P., Floel, A., Gerloff, C., & Cohen, L. G. (2010). Facilitating skilled right hand motor function in older subjects by anodal polarization over the left primary motor cortex. *Neurobiology of Aging, 31*, 2160–2168.

Jeon, S. Y., & Han, S. J. (2012). Improvement of the working memory and naming by transcranial direct current stimulation. *Annals of Rehabilitation Medicine, 36*, 585–595.

Jones, K. T., Stephens, J. A., Alam, M., Bikson, M., & Berryhill, M. E. (2015). Longitudinal neurostimulation in older adults improves working memory. *PLoS One, 10*, e0121904.

Krause, B., & Cohen Kadosh, R. (2014). Not all brains are created equal: The relevance of individual differences in responsiveness to transcranial electrical stimulation. *Frontiers in Systems Neuroscience, 8*, 25.

Kuo, M.-F., & Nitsche, M. A. (2012). Effects of transcranial electrical stimulation on cognition. *Clinical EEG and Neuroscience, 43*, 192–199.

Laakso, I., Tanaka, S., Koyama, S., De Santis, V., & Hirata, A. (2015). Inter-subject variability in electric fields of motor cortical tDCS. *Brain Stimulation, 8(5)*, 906–913.

Learmonth, G., Thut, G., Benwell, C. S. Y., & Harvey, M. (2015). The implications of state-dependent tDCS effects in aging: Behavioural response is determined by baseline performance. *Neuropsychologia, 74*, 108–119.

Lindenberg, R., Nachtigall, L., Meinzer, M., Sieg, M. M., & Flöel, A. (2013). Differential effects of dual and unihemispheric motor cortex stimulation in older adults. *The Journal of Neuroscience, 33*, 9176–9183.

Lohmann, G., Margulies, D. S., Horstmann, A., Pleger, B., Lepsien, J., Goldhahn, D., … Turner, R. (2010). Eigenvector centrality mapping for analyzing connectivity patterns in fMRI data of the human brain. *PLoS One, 5*, e10232.

Luft, C. D. B., Pereda, E., Banissy, M. J., & Bhattacharya, J. (2014). Best of both worlds: Promise of combining brain stimulation and brain connectome. *Frontiers in Systems Neuroscience, 8*, 132.

Makris, U. E., Abrams, R. C., Gurland, B., & Reid, M. C. (2014). Management of persistent pain in the older patient: A clinical review. *JAMA, 312*, 825–836.

Manenti, R., Brambilla, M., Petesi, M., Ferrari, C., & Cotelli, M. (2013). Enhancing verbal episodic memory in older and young subjects after non-invasive brain stimulation. *Frontiers in Aging Neuroscience, 5*.

Manor, B., Zhou, J., Jor'dan, A., Zhang, J., Fang, J., & Pascual-Leone, A. (2016). Reduction of dual-task costs by noninvasive modulation of prefrontal activity in healthy elders. *Journal of Cognitive Neuroscience, 28*(2), 275–281.

Marquez, J., Conley, A., Karayanidis, F., Lagopoulos, J., & Parsons, M. (2015). Anodal direct current stimulation in the healthy aged: Effects determined by the hemisphere stimulated. *Restorative Neurology and Neuroscience, 33*, 509–519.

Martin, A., Meinzer, M., Lindenberg, R., Sieg, M. M., Nachtigall, L., & Flöel, A. (2017). Effects of transcranial direct current stimulation on neural network structure in young and older adults. *Journal of Cognitive Neuroscience, 29*, 1–12.

McGinley, M., Hoffman, R. L., Russ, D. W., Thomas, J. S., & Clark, B. C. (2010). Older adults exhibit more intracortical inhibition and less intracortical facilitation than young adults. *Experimental Gerontology, 45*, 671–678.

McLaren, M. E., Nissim, N. R., & Woods, A. J. (2018). The effects of medication use in transcranial direct current stimulation: A brief review. *Brain Stimulation, 11*(1), 52–58.
Meinzer, M., Lindenberg, R., Antonenko, D., Flaisch, T., & Flöel, A. (2013). Anodal transcranial direct current stimulation temporarily reverses age-associated cognitive decline and functional brain activity changes. *The Journal of Neuroscience, 33*, 12470–12478.
Meinzer, M., Lindenberg, R., Phan, M. T., Ulm, L., Volk, C., & Flöel, A. (2014). Transcranial direct current stimulation in mild cognitive impairment: Behavioral effects and neural mechanisms. *Alzheimer's & Dementia, 11*, 1032–1040.
Nilsson, J., Lebedev, A. V., & Lövdén, M. (2015). No significant effect of prefrontal tDCS on working memory performance in older adults. *Frontiers in Aging Neuroscience, 7*, Article 230.
Nilsson, J., Lebedev, A. V., Rydström, A., & Lövdén, M. (2017). Direct-current stimulation does little to improve the outcome of working memory training in older adults. *Psychological Science, 28*, 907–920.
Nissim, N. R., O'Shea, A. M., Bryant, V., Porges, E. C., Cohen, R., & Woods, A. J. (2017). Frontal structural neural correlates of working memory performance in older adults. *Frontiers in Aging Neuroscience, 08*.
Nitsche, M., Fricke, K., Henschke, U., Schlitterlau, A., Liebetanz, D., Lang, N., … Paulus, W. (2003). Pharmacological modulation of cortical excitability shifts induced by transcranial direct current stimulation in humans. *The Journal of Physiology, 553*, 293–301.
Nitsche, M. A., Grundey, J., Liebetanz, D., Lang, N., Tergau, F., & Paulus, W. (2004a). Catecholaminergic consolidation of motor cortical neuroplasticity in humans. *Cerebral Cortex, 14*, 1240–1245.
Nitsche, M. A., Jaussi, W., Liebetanz, D., Lang, N., Tergau, F., & Paulus, W. (2004b). Consolidation of human motor cortical neuroplasticity by D-cycloserine. *Neuropsychopharmacology, 29*, 1573–1578.
Nitsche, M. A., Kuo, M. F., Karrasch, R., Wächter, B., Liebetanz, D., & Paulus, W. (2009). Serotonin affects transcranial direct current-induced neuroplasticity in humans. *Biological Psychiatry, 66*, 503–508.
Nitsche, M. A., Lampe, C., Antal, A., Liebetanz, D., Lang, N., Tergau, F., & Paulus, W. (2006). Dopaminergic modulation of long-lasting direct current-induced cortical excitability changes in the human motor cortex. *The European Journal of Neuroscience, 23*, 1651–1657.
Nitsche, M. A., Liebetanz, D., Schlitterlau, A., Henschke, U., Fricke, K., Frommann, K., … Tergau, F. (2004c). GABAergic modulation of DC stimulation-induced motor cortex excitability shifts in humans. *The European Journal of Neuroscience, 19*, 2720–2726.
Nitsche, M. A., Müller-Dahlhaus, F., Paulus, W., & Ziemann, U. (2012). The pharmacology of neuroplasticity induced by non-invasive brain stimulation: Building models for the clinical use of CNS active drugs. *The Journal of Physiology, 590*, 4641–4662.
Ortman, J. M., Velkoff, V. A., & Hogan, H. (2014). An aging nation: The older population in the United States. *Economics and Statistics Administration U.S. Department of Commerce, 1964*, 1–28.
Panouillères, M. T. N., Joundi, R. A., Brittain, J.-S., & Jenkinson, N. (2015). Reversing motor adaptation deficits in the ageing brain using non-invasive stimulation. *The Journal of Physiology, 593*(16), 3645–3655.
Parikh, P. J., & Cole, K. J. (2014). Effects of transcranial direct current stimulation in combination with motor practice on dexterous grasping and manipulation in healthy older adults. *Physiological Reports, 2*, e00255.
Parikh, P. J., & Cole, K. J. (2015). Effects of transcranial direct current stimulation on the control of finger force during dexterous manipulation in healthy older adults. *PLoS One, 10*, e0124137.
Park, S. H., Seo, J. H., Kim, Y. H., & Ko, M.-H. (2014). Long-term effects of transcranial direct current stimulation combined with computer-assisted cognitive training in healthy older adults. *Neuroreport, 25*, 122–126.
Perceval, G., Flöel, A., & Meinzer, M. (2016). Can transcranial direct current stimulation counteract age-associated functional impairment? *Neuroscience and Biobehavioral Reviews, 65*, 157–172.

Prehn, K., & Flöel, A. (2015). Potentials and limits to enhance cognitive functions in healthy and pathological aging by tDCS. *Frontiers in Cellular Neuroscience, 9*, 355.
Puri, R., & Hinder, M. (2016). Response: "Commentary: Duration-dependent effects of the BDNF Val66Met polymorphism on anodal tDCS induced motor cortex plasticity in older adults: A group and individual perspective.". *Frontiers in Aging Neuroscience, 8*, 28.
Puri, R., Hinder, M. R., Fujiyama, H., Gomez, R., Carson, R. G., & Summers, J. J. (2015). Duration-dependent effects of the BDNF Val66Met polymorphism on anodal tDCS induced motor cortex plasticity in older adults: A group and individual perspective. *Frontiers in Aging Neuroscience, 7*.
Reid, M. C., Eccleston, C., & Pillemer, K. (2015). Management of chronic pain in older adults. *BMJ, 350*, h532.
Resnick, S. M., Davatzikos, C., Kraut, M. A., & Zonderman, A. B. (2000). Longitudinal brain changes in older adults. *Neurobiology of Aging, 21*, 40.
Ross, L. A., McCoy, D., Coslett, H. B., Olson, I. R., & Wolk, D. A. (2011). Improved proper name recall in aging after electrical stimulation of the anterior temporal lobes. *Frontiers in Aging Neuroscience, 3*, 1–8.
Sala-Llonch, R., Bartrés-Faz, D., & Junqué, C. (2015). Reorganization of brain networks in aging: A review of functional connectivity studies. *Frontiers in Psychology, 6*, 663.
Salat, D. H., Buckner, R. L., Snyder, A. Z., Greve, D. N., Desikan, R. S., Busa, E., … Fischl, B. (2004). Thinning of the cerebral cortex in aging. *Cerebral Cortex, 14*, 721–730.
Salat, D. H., Kaye, J. A., & Janowsky, J. S. (1999). Prefrontal gray and white matter volumes in healthy aging and Alzheimer disease. *Archives of Neurology, 56*, 338–344.
Sandrini, M., Brambilla, M., Manenti, R., Rosini, S., Cohen, L. G., & Cotelli, M. (2014). Noninvasive stimulation of prefrontal cortex strengthens existing episodic memories and reduces forgetting in the elderly. *Frontiers in Aging Neuroscience, 6*.
Sandrini, M., Manenti, R., Brambilla, M., Cobelli, C., Cohen, L. G., & Cotelli, M. (2016). Older adults get episodic memory boosting from noninvasive stimulation of prefrontal cortex during learning. *Neurobiology of Aging, 39*, 210–216.
Seo, M. H., Park, S. H., Seo, J. H., Kim, Y. H., & Ko, M. H. (2011). Improvement of the working memory by transcranial direct current stimultion in healthy older adults. *Journal of Korean Academy of Rehabilitation Medicine, 35*, 201–206.
Sawyer, P., Bodner, E. V., Ritchie, C. S., & Allman, R. M. (2006). Pain and pain medication use in community-dwelling older adults. *The American Journal of Geriatric Pharmacotherapy, 4*, 316–324.
Shpektor, A. (2015). Commentary: Duration-dependent effects of the BDNF Val66Met polymorphism on anodal tDCS induced motor cortex plasticity in older adults: A group and individual perspective. *Frontiers in Aging Neuroscience, 7*, 183.
Small, S. A., Schobel, S. A., Buxton, R. B., Witter, M. P., & Barnes, C. A. (2011). A pathophysiological framework of hippocampal dysfunction in ageing and disease. *Nature Reviews. Neuroscience, 12*, 585–601.
Spaniol, J., Davidson, P. S. R., Kim, A. S. N., Han, H., Moscovitch, M., & Grady, C. L. (2009). Event-related fMRI studies of episodic encoding and retrieval: Meta-analyses using activation likelihood estimation. *Neuropsychologia, 47*, 1765–1779.
Summers, J. J., Kang, N., & Cauraugh, J. H. (2015). Does transcranial direct current stimulation enhance cognitive and motor functions in the ageing brain? A systematic review and meta-analysis. *Ageing Research Reviews, 25*(2016), 42–54.
Sundaram, A., Stock, V., Cruciani, R. A., & Knotkova, H. (2009). Safety of transcranial direct current stimulation (tDCS) in protocols involving human subjects. *Journal of Pain Management, 2*, 285–293.
Thomas, C., Datta, A., & Woods, A. (2017). Effect of aging on current flow due to transcranial direct current stimulation. *Brain Stimulation, 10*, 469.
Woods, A. J., Cohen, R., Marsiske, M., Alexander, G. E., Czaja, S. J., & Wu, S. (2018). Augmenting cognitive training in older adults (The ACT Study): Design and Methods of a Phase III tDCS and cognitive training trial. *Contemporary Clinical Trials, 65*, 19–32.

Woods, A. J., Antal, A., Bikson, M., Boggio, P. S., Brunoni, A. R., Celnik, P., … Nitsche, M. A. (2016). A technical guide to tDCS, and related non-invasive brain stimulation tools. *Clinical Neurophysiology, 127*, 1031–1048.

Woods, A. J., Cohen, R. A., & Pahor, M. (2013). Cognitive frailty: Frontiers and challenges. *The Journal of Nutrition, Health & Aging, 17*, 741–743.

Woods, A. J., Mark, V. W., Pitts, A. C., & Mennemeier, M. (2011). Pervasive cognitive impairment in acute rehabilitation inpatients without brain injury. *PM R, 3*, 426–432.; quiz 432.

Zheng, X., Alsop, D. C., & Schlaug, G. (2011). Effects of transcranial direct current stimulation (tDCS) on human regional cerebral blood flow. *NeuroImage, 58*, 26–33.

Zhou, D., Zhou, J., Chen, H., Manor, B., Lin, J., & Zhang, J. (2015). Effects of transcranial direct current stimulation (tDCS) on multiscale complexity of dual-task postural control in older adults. *Experimental Brain Research, 233*, 2401–2409.

Zimerman, M., Nitsch, M., Giraux, P., Gerloff, C., Cohen, L. G., & Hummel, F. C. (2013). Neuroenhancement of the aging brain: Restoring skill acquisition in old subjects. *Annals of Neurology, 73*, 10–15.

Chapter 20
Transcranial Direct Current Stimulation in Cognitive Neuroscience

Priyanka P. Shah-Basak, Roy H. Hamilton, Michael A. Nitsche, and Adam J. Woods

Introduction

Non-invasive brain stimulation (NIBS) techniques are being applied increasingly in cognitive neuroscience as tools to understand and modulate cognitive functions. One of the principle assumptions that motivates the use of NIBS tools in this field is that specific brain states and processes underlie specific mental operations and behaviors. Based on this fundamental notion, brain stimulation studies in cognitive neuroscience seek to alter or mimick brain activity as a means of disrupting or enhancing thoughts or actions, so as to better understand brain-behavior relationships. Several modalities of NIBS exist, including those that can transiently alter brain activity via administration of suprathresholded stimulation, such as transcranial magnetic stimulation (TMS). Some approaches are understood to induce

P. P. Shah-Basak
Rotman Research Institute, Baycrest Health Sciences, Toronto, ON, Canada

R. H. Hamilton
Department of Neurology, University of Pennsylvania, Philadelphia, PA, USA

Department of Physical Medicine and Rehabilitation, University of Pennsylvania, Philadelphia, PA, USA

Goddard Laboratories, Room 518, University of Pennsylvania, Philadelphia, PA, USA

M. A. Nitsche (✉)
Department of Psychology and Neurosciences, Leibniz Research Centre for Working Environment and Human Factors, Dortmund, Germany

University Medical Hospital Bergmannsheil, Bochum, Germany
e-mail: nitsche@ifado.de

A. J. Woods
Center for Cognitive Aging and Memory (CAM), McKnight Brain Institute, Department of Clinical and Health Psychology, College of Public Health and Health Professions, University of Florida, Gainesville, FL, USA

H. Knotkova et al. (eds.), *Practical Guide to Transcranial Direct Current Stimulation*, https://doi.org/10.1007/978-3-319-95948-1_20

plasticity, such as repetitive TMS (rTMS), paired associative stimulation (PAS), and transcranial direct current stimulation (tDCS), all of which share features with long term potentiation and depression (LTP and LTD), the processes that form the physiological foundation of learning and memory formation. Other modalities, such as transcranial alternating current stimulation (tACS), entrain oscillatory brain activity. These techniques can induce not only regional but also cerebral network-level alterations of physiological processes.

Broadly speaking, applications of NIBS technologies in cognitive neuroscience have fallen into three categories: (A) Characterization of cognitively-relevant physiological processes, which can be induced in a controlled fashion by NIBS, allowing detailed, systematic exploration of mechanisms at the cellular level, (B) pairing NIBS with functional imaging to explore the causal contribution of stimulated areas, networks, and physiological processes to cognition, and (C) applying NIBS with the aim of enhancing task performance. These approaches are not mutually exclusive, and require specific experimental designs and intervention tools.

As an example of how NIBS can be used to elucidate cellular mechanisms (Application A), pairing NIBS with pharmacological interventions can provide valuable information about how specific neurotransmitters affect cognition. The impact of nicotine and nicotine deprivation on tDCS- and PAS-induced plasticity and memory performance in smokers (Grundey et al. 2012; Roth et al. 1992) illustrates the utility of this approach. It has been shown that nicotine withdrawal in smokers reduces facilitative neuroplastic effects of tDCS and PAS on corticospinal excitability and negatively affects performance on a working memory task, both of which can be restored or improved by reintroduction of nicotine. By contrast, inhibitory plastic changes were not affected by nicotine withdrawal. Combining application of functional imaging techniques and NIBS (Application B) is a powerful approach for modulating cognition-relevant physiological processes, and also for unraveling causal relationships between brain structures targeted by NIBS and their functional roles, so called structure-function relationships. This multimodal approach takes advantage of both the correlational output of functional imaging and the causal nature of the effects induced by NIBS. While imaging techniques help to identify task-related patterns of brain activation or synchronization at both the regional and network level, used in isolation they are unable to delineate the contributions of specific areas or networks to cognition or behavior. The causal relevance of a region or network can be verified using NIBS, since these techniques alter brain physiology which can be directly linked to alterations in cognitive performance. Lastly, the use of NIBS to enhance normal cognition (Application C) differs from applications A and B in that the primary aim is to maximize the effects of NIBS in directed, persistent, and performance-enhancing ways.

A variety of NIBS techniques are specifically germane to the field of cognitive neuroscience and contribute to a better understanding of physiologic, cellular, and network-level mechanisms of cognition and behavior. Of these techniques, tDCS has garnered considerable attention in recent years (Fig. 20.1). TDCS-induced alterations in brain physiology have been shown to impact a variety of cognitive

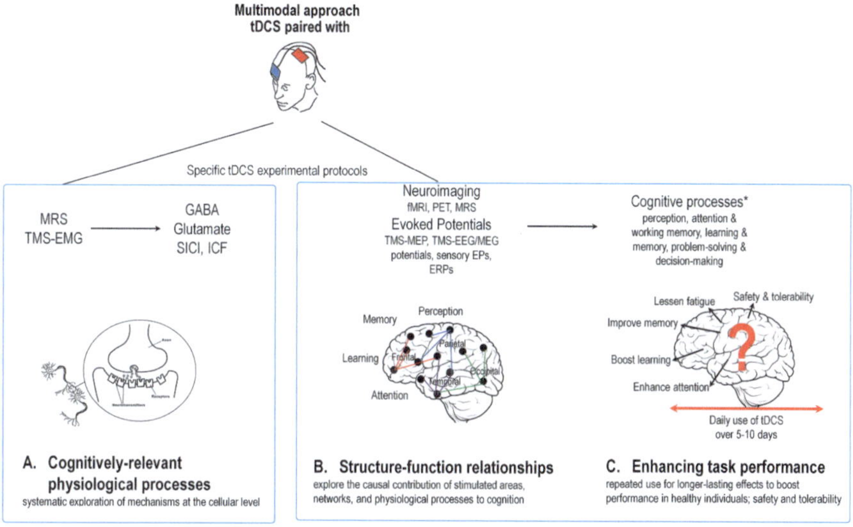

Fig. 20.1 An overview of the cognitive neuroscience themes explored using a multimodal approach; *cognitive processes covered in this chapter. Abbreviations: *tDCS*, Transcranial direct current stimulation; *MRS*, Magnetic Resonance Spectroscopy; *TMS*, Transcranial Magnetic Stimulation; *EEG*, Electroencephalography; *GABA*, γ-Aminobutyruc acid; *SICI*, Short-latency intracortical inhibition; *ICF*, Intracortical facilitation; *fMRI*, Functional magnetic resonance imaging; *PET*, Positron emission tomography; *MEP*, Motor-evoked potential; *MEG*, Magnetoencephalography; *EP*, Evoked potentials; *ERP*, Event-related potentials

processes, ranging from elementary functions such as sensory perception to highly complex aspects of cognition such as problem solving (Shin et al. 2015). An important feature that sets tDCS apart from other NIBS techniques, particularly from TMS and repetitive TMS (rTMS), is its intrinsic neuromodulatory mode of action. The weak current delivered during tDCS alters neuronal transmembrane potentials, changing the likelihood of neurons triggering action potentials over time. TDCS therefore modulates cortical excitability, plasticity, and functional connectivity by interacting with ongoing brain activity, rather than disrupting it (Bindman et al. 1964; Nitsche et al. 2008). This interaction allows for concurrent application of tDCS with cognitive tasks to either facilitate or attentuate task-related patterns of endogenous brain activity (Fig. 20.2), which in some instances allows for clearer inferences to be made about the relationship between brain physiology and cognition compared to disruptive NIBS approaches like TMS. However, this also means that the aftereffects of tDCS are heavily dependent on the current state of activation in the brain regions being targeted. In comparison to the neurostimulatory or disruptive effects of TMS, tDCS modifies (diminishes or enhances) physiological excitability and, in turn, ongoing brain activity, but it does not induce task-irrelevant activity. This difference in mechanism may account for some of the inter-individual variability observed in the physiological and cognitive aftereffects of tDCS, and underscores the need to fine-tune tDCS parameters accordingly.

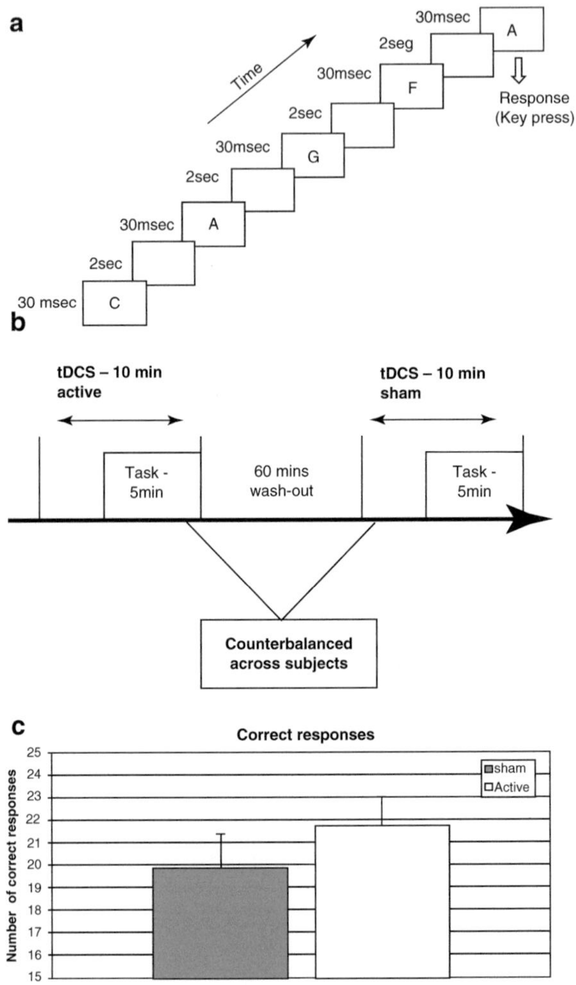

Fig. 20.2 (**a**) The sequence of the 3-back letter working memory paradigm; participants were instructed to respond (key press) to the letter if it was the same as the letter presented three stimuli previously. (**b**) The experimental protocol design. Each subject was tested during sham and active stimulation. The two test runs were randomized within subject and the order (active versus sham stimulation) was counterbalanced across subjects. (**c**) Number of correct responses during each stimulation condition (active and sham). Dark bar indicates mean number of correct responses during sham stimulation. White bar represents mean number of correct responses during active stimulation. There was a significant difference in the mean number of correct responses between sham and active stimulation. Error bars indicate ±SEM (standard error of the mean). (Fregni et al. (2005), with permission)

In this chapter, we will review studies that demonstrate the potential impact of tDCS on a range of cognitive processes, and also discuss how neuroimaging and electrophysiological tools can be used to better understand the effects of tDCS on those processes (Fig. 20.1). The focus of this review will be on the conceptual features of these approaches, and therefore will not provide an exhaustive overview of studies available in this field, which can be found elsewhere (Kuo and Nitsche 2012; Nitsche et al. 2003a, 2008; Nitsche and Paulus 2011; Shin et al. 2015). We will also discuss the use of tDCS for neuroenhancement, an intriguing emerging field that raises both scientific and ethical questions. We will conclude by reflecting on the methodological strength and weaknesses of tDCS as an investigational tool, and speculate about future directions for tDCS as a research tool in the field of cognitive neuroscience.

Tools to Explore the Impact of tDCS on Structure–Function Relationships in the Brain

Neuroimaging

Neuroimaging techniques, in particular positron emission tomography (PET) and functional MRI (fMRI) have been used in the past decade to: (1) better understand the mechanisms of tDCS-mediated neuromodulation (Antal et al. 2011; Lang et al. 2005), (2) determine the neural bases of tDCS-induced enhancement in clinical and healthy populations (Clemens et al. 2013; Lefebvre et al. 2015), and more recently to (3) examine the effects of tDCS on large-scale brain networks (Chib et al. 2013; Weber et al. 2014).

One of the first PET studies to explore the effects tDCS on regional cerebral blood flow (rCBF) reported widespread increases in rCBF after 10 min of anodal and cathodal tDCS over the left primary motor cortex (M1) and right frontopolar cortex (Lang et al. 2005). The authors reported increased rCBF under the electrodes, which lasted up to 50 min regardless of tDCS polarity, and which was similar in magnitude to CBF changes induced by finger movements. These findings are consistent with rTMS-PET findings, wherein both 1 Hz and 5 Hz stimulation resulted in increased rCBF despite evidence that the two TMS frequencies have opposite effects on cortical excitability (Lee et al. 2003; Rounis et al. 2005). Combined evidence therefore suggests that changes in rCBF are linked to net increases in regional synaptic activity and that polarity-specific cortical excitability may emerge from changes in subpopulations of neurons (Lang et al. 2005). Interestingly, this study also found polarity-specific changes in rCBF in areas distal to the sites of stimulation; while anodal tDCS increased rCBF in dorsal parts of the hemisphere, cathodal tDCS decreased rCBF in ventral regions.

Imaging using other modalities supports the notion of polarity-specific changes in brain activity at primary targets of tDCS stimulation. For example, using arterial spin labeling (ASL) MRI, Zheng et al. (2011) found polarity dependent effects of tDCS on rCBF near the site of stimulation (Zheng et al. 2011). Anodal tDCS over the right motor region increased resting-state rCBF during stimulation and for a period of time after stimulation, while rCBF decreased immediately after cathodal stimulation and continued to decrease in the post-stimulation period. At the level of neurotransmitters, Stagg et al. (2009, 2011) used magnetic resonance spectroscopy (MRS) to quantify changes in GABA concentrations following stimulation (Stagg et al. 2009, 2011). In 2009, the investigators demonstrated that anodal tDCS led to decreases in GABA concentration in M1, while cathodal tDCS led to decrease in glutamate and GABA. However, in this study the effects of changes in GABA concentration on motor learning were not investigated (Stagg et al. 2009). In a subsequent 2011 study, the authors replicated the anodal tDCS-induced decreases in GABA in M1, and showed this change to be associated with enhanced motor learning. Specifically, greater decrease in M1 GABA after tDCS correlated with faster motor learning in an explicit sequence learning task (Stagg et al. 2011), suggesting that tDCS-induced LTP-like plasticity was dependent, at least in part, on the modulation of GABA.

Combining anodal and cathodal tDCS with blood-oxygenation-level-dependent (BOLD) fMRI has provided invaluable insights into activation changes not only under the electrodes but also in functionally related but distal areas in a network. In one of the earliest studies combining fMRI and tDCS, the expected polarity-specific effects of tDCS on BOLD signal were not observed. In this study, cathodal tDCS targeting M1 did not result in measurable changes in BOLD response during finger tapping or at rest, while anodal tDCS resulted in decreased BOLD signal in supplementary motor area during finger tapping but not at rest (Antal et al. 2011). Like Lang et al. (2005), the authors speculated that the physiological mechanisms probed by the two measurements of tDCS-induced changes used in the study— changes in the amplitude of motor-evoked potentials (MEPs; refer to section "Evoked Potentials" for more details), and changes in BOLD signal—may be different, which may explain the absence of polarity-specific BOLD responses. However, a few other subsequent fMRI studies have reported changes in BOLD signal that varied as a function of tDCS polarity. For instance, Clemens et al. (2013) employed fMRI before and after anodal tDCS over the right angular gyrus as participants performed a multiplication task (Clemens et al. 2013). Although task performance was not improved, increased activation in the bilateral angular gyri was observed after anodal tDCS compared to sham or no tDCS trials, providing at least some evidence of polarity-specific neuromodulation in areas involved in arithmetic processing. The polarity-specific tDCS effects on BOLD signals may be task- and region-specific, given the highly state-dependent nature of tDCS. This question, however, remains to be explored fully.

The study recently conducted by Weber et al. (2014) provided evidence of changes in task-related local activations as well as connectivity with remote areas as a consequence of tDCS (Weber et al. 2014). In this study, the aftereffects of prefrontal tDCS (anode on right and cathode on left) at rest and during performance of a risk-taking task called Balloon Analog Risk Task (BART) were investigated using fMRI. The results indicated that tDCS increased activations in the right dlPFC and anterior cingulate cortex selectively in response to losses but not wins. In a whole-brain connectivity analysis, the investigators showed that after tDCS decreased connectivity between the right anterior cingulate cortex and other areas in the brain was observed, suggesting remote effects of stimulation. In a different study by Chib et al. (2013), tDCS of the prefrontal cortices induced remote activation of ventral midbrain areas, which the investigators argued directly affected behavior via a highly interconnected network among these areas (Chib et al. 2013). In this study, tDCS was provided before and after participants underwent an attractiveness rating task for a series of faces during fMRI scanning. Anodal tDCS of ventromedial prefrontal cortex and cathodal tDCS of dorsolateral prefrontal cortex (dlPFC) enhanced functional activation changes in remote midbrain activity compared to the sham condition, which were related to increases in attractiveness ratings. In addition, more enhanced connectivity in this network was linked to greater effects of stimulation, which manifested as an increase in facial attractiveness ratings.

Evoked Potentials

While functional imaging approaches are capable of mapping out brain activations with high spatial resolution—not only regionally but also at a network level—neurophysiological measures such as evoked potentials (EP) allow for direct monitoring of stimulation- and task-related excitability with high temporal resolution. EP measures can index the effects of tDCS as a function of a clearly defined sensory input or a pharmacological trigger. In this way, EPs are directly linked to temporally-specific states of the brain in response to stimuli, whereas conventional functional imaging measures are fairly limited in this respect. With respect to tDCS, EPs can help to explore the physiological underpinnings of neuromodulation and their impact on task performance. This knowledge can, in turn, be applied to enhance task performance by optimizing tDCS protocols in clinical as well as healthy populations. This section focuses on four types of evoked potentials studies: (1) TMS-evoked motor evoked potentials, (2) TMS-EEG potentials, (3) sensory evoked potentials, and (4) event related potentials.

TMS-evoked motor evoked potentials (MEP) have long been employed as physiologic measures to probe the physiological basis of tDCS effects in the motor system and motor cognition (Pascual-Leone et al. 1994b). In addition to measuring corticospinal excitability, MEPs have been used to measure the activity of pharmacologically-triggered neurotransmitters and ion channel as well as receptor systems, which are of potential relevance to cognitive processes (Paulus et al. 2008).

In principle, MEP changes that are induced by tDCS can be used to predict cognitive task performance. This is because the physiological effects induced by tDCS may be similar to the changes in neural activity and function invoked during cognitive tasks. For example, long term potentiation-like plasticity is induced by anodal tDCS and is also thought to be associated with memory formation and learning (Nitsche et al. 2008; Rioult-Pedotti et al. 2000). This is supported by the finding that anodal tDCS enhances motor learning (Nitsche et al. 2003b; Reis et al. 2009). Moreover, evidence from studies conducted in smokers suggests that the physiological effects of tDCS can predict motor learning performance. Reduced MEP alterations induced by anodal tDCS in smokers under nicotine withdrawal (Grundey et al. 2012) were accompanied with impaired motor learning, which improved after controlled nicotine intake (Grundey et al. 2018). Although it has been hypothesized that individual physiological responses to tDCS, as quantified by MEP amplitudes, may be related to task performance, such a connection has not yet been found in a relatively small number of motor learning studies conducted using single-pulse MEP amplitudes (Lopez-Alonso et al. 2015). It is possible that the limited specificity of single pulse TMS with regard to neurotransmitter activity compromises the ability to identify tDCS-induced changes in physiology at the individual level, and therefore TMS protocols which permit more specific measures might be advantageous.

Nonetheless, a relatively small body of literature demonstrates that MEPs can be a useful tool for exploring physiological changes that mediate tDCS effects on task performance. Because tDCS, motor learning, and memory formation are associated with specific alterations of cortical excitability, in theory MEPs should be able to quantify this relationship (Pascual-Leone et al. 1994a). For example, in one recent study the impact of tDCS and task performance on GABA-controlled short-latency intracortical inhibition was explored. Anodal tDCS delivered before sequence learning resulted in reduced performance and enhanced intracortical inhibition, in accordance with homeostatic GABA-driven effects of tDCS that is applied prior to the task (Amadi et al. 2015). While not all studies have confirmed a link between tDCS effects on MEPs and task performance (Ambrus et al. 2016), evidence suggests that judicious selection of TMS-induced physiologic measures can elucidate mechanisms of tDCS that are linked to the changes in behavioral measures.

EEG can also be used in conjunction with TMS to further characterize the impact of tDCS on cortical physiology and task performance. TMS induces cortico-cortical potentials, which, at different latencies, depend on GABAergic and glutamatergic mechanisms (Premoli et al. 2014; Rogasch et al. 2013). Evidence indicates that specific TMS-EEG potential alterations are associated with changes in cognitive performance (Rogasch et al. 2015), and that the effects of tDCS in turn can be measured by demonstrating its influence over TMS-EEG potentials (Romero Lauro et al. 2014). While TMS-evoked MEPs or sensory stimulus-dependent EPs are restricted to specific areas where cortical activity has been elicited, the TMS-EEG approach allows monitoring of tDCS effects across a network of cortical areas. However, while this use of tDCS, TMS, and EEG seems highly promising as a way to elucidate the effects of tDCS on cognition, studies that employ this specific approach in humans have not yet been reported.

Evoked potentials induced by sensory stimuli (e.g. visual or somatosensory stimuli) have been used to elucidate the physiological effects of tDCS over respective sensory areas. Studies combining tDCS with visual evoked potentials (VEPs) indicate that tDCS alters excitability when applied over the primary visual cortex in a manner similar to its effects on the motor cortex. However tDCS-induced alterations in VEPs were somewhat shorter-lasting and more difficult to induce than MEPs, using stimulation parameters that are typically used in tDCS studies of the motor cortex (Antal et al. 2004; Bocci et al. 2014; Strigaro et al. 2015), and they critically depended on the position of the return electrode (Accornero et al. 2007). While similar physiological effects have also been obtained for somatosensory evoked potentials (SEP), the effects appear to be specific to subcomponents of the SEP (Dieckhofer et al. 2006; Matsunaga et al. 2004). Lastly, a small number of studies to date have measured the effects of tDCS on auditory evoked potentials (AEPs) (Heimrath et al. 2016).

Given the relative elementary characteristics of sensory evoked potentials, they can be powerful tools to explore the physiological foundation of psychophysical and near perception effects of tDCS, particularly in the case of VEPs. For example, a recent study by Ding et al. (2016) demonstrated that anodal tDCS enhances, while cathodal tDCS diminishes contrast sensitivity and VEP amplitudes in amblyopic subjects, suggesting a relevant association between perceptual and physiological effects, although these were not significantly correlated (Ding et al. 2016). This study illustrates that physiological and cognitive parameters can be combined to learn about the relevance of respective parameters and their effects in appropriately designed studies. The absence of a correlation between parameters in spite of similarly directed effects may at least partially relate to the fact that perceptual measures and VEPs were not obtained simultaneously during the course of the experiments. In a study combining physiological and perceptual effects of tDCS in the auditory domain, cathodal tDCS over the auditory cortex *improved* performance on a task involving phonetic categorization of syllables applied during stimulation, while anodal tDCS increased the AEP P50 amplitude after the end of stimulation (Heimrath et al. 2016). These seemingly counterintuitive results might again be explained by the different time points at which the measures were collected. In both studies, the results indicate that specific details of the experimental design, such as timing of cognitive and behavioural measures, are potentially crucial for the interpretability of results. To date, a limited number of studies suggesting tDCS-induced alterations of somatosensory perception are available (Grundmann et al. 2011; Ragert et al. 2008; Rogalewski et al. 2004), and studies directly correlating physiological with perceptual effects have not yet been reported.

Event-related potentials (ERP) allow for examination of physiological markers of more complex aspects of cognition compared to the EPs, and also allow for investigation of brain areas beyond sensory and motor cortices. Similar to EPs, however, the number of available studies involving tDCS and ERPs remains limited. Mismatch negativity (MMN) is a standard measure that relates to the detection of differences between elementary sensory stimuli. It was shown recently that anodal tDCS increases, while cathodal tDCS decreases auditory MMN in healthy volunteers, when stimulation was administered before the task (Impey et al. 2016). In a related study, excitability-enhancing anodal tDCS combined with inhibitory cerebellar tDCS increased the amplitude of novelty-related ERPs (Bersani et al. 2015). Furthermore, in a study investigating drug dependency, tDCS induced complex effects on drug-related and unrelated visual stimuli (Conti et al. 2014). Thus, the physiological effects of tDCS on ERPs can be obtained reliably, are stimulation polarity-dependent, and can be stimulus feature-specific. Whether these physiological alterations are associated with cognitive effects has not been explored in many studies yet. However, in a paradigmatic study performed in schizophrenia patients, Reinhart et al. (2015) explored the impact of anodal tDCS over the medial-prefrontal cortex on prediction error signalling and learning (Reinhart et al. 2015). Before intervention the error-related negativity was diminished and learning was compromised in the patient group as compared to a healthy control group. Both physiologic and behavioral parameters were normalized by real, but not sham stimulation in the patient group, demonstrating a critical relationship between the error-related negativity parameter and learning.

Taken together, a broad arsenal of EP tools are available to explore the impact of tDCS on neural and cognitive functions. Depending on the specific techniques and experimental designs employed, these methods allow investigators to further elucidate specific relationships between brain physiology and cognitive events. These physiological tools complement imaging methods in many respects because they have relatively high temporal resolution, but generally weaker spatial resolution than current imaging techniques. Moreover, they allow for identification of neurotransmitter-specific effects of stimulation on cognitive processes. However, despite the strengths of these approaches, the number of tDCS studies that use EP methods to explore physiological and cognitive processes remains limited. This is a knowledge gap that, if addressed, will not only improve mechanistic understanding of tDCS effects but may also help to optimize intervention approaches.

Influence of tDCS on Cognitive Processes

TDCS has been applied increasingly in the last decade to explore the physiological basis of cognitive processes. A PubMed search conducted in June 2016 with the key terms "tDCS" and "cognition" identified more than 300 published studies on this topic. One practical reason for the increasing popularity of tDCS in studies of cognition is that it is relatively easy to implement in the context of a behavioral study. In addition, alterations in neural excitability induced by tDCS seem to correspond well with changes in cerebral activity as measured by functional imaging, EEG, and other tools that assess brain activity; these changes have, in turn, been associated with alteration of a variety of behaviors. Moreover, in contrast to the performance-disrupting effects of TMS, tDCS can probe the specific contribution of an area to a given cognitive function through more subtle modulation of neural functioning. For example, it is difficult to link the involvement of the primary motor cortex in learning using disruptive brain stimulation techniques because they will disrupt learning as well as the effector functions of the motor cortex; however, improvement after tDCS of the learned material hints to a unique role of this area in motor memory formation.

Our goal in this section is to provide an overview of the application of tDCS in the field of cognitive neuroscience with relevant discussions about the main results, and emphasis on methodological approaches (Kuo and Nitsche 2012; Nitsche et al. 2003a; Nitsche and Paulus 2011; Shin et al. 2015). Specifically, we will describe examples of how tDCS can help explain the physiological foundation of different cognitive processes.

Perception

The impact of tDCS on perception has been explored in the visual, somatosensory, and auditory domains, as well as in multimodal processing.

In one of the earliest studies, the effect of stimulation on the primary visual cortex and contrast perception was explored (Antal et al. 2001). This cortical area is relevant for perception of elementary visual stimuli. In this study, relatively short-lasting (7 min) cathodal tDCS reduced contrast perception, while anodal stimulation had no effects. In a follow-up study with longer stimulation duration, it was demonstrated that anodal tDCS over the same area could improve contrast perception (Kraft et al. 2010). These results are in accordance with the electrophysiological effects of tDCS that revealed the impact of cathodal but not anodal tDCS on VEP with stimulation durations under 15 min. Therefore, appropriate delineation of stimulation parameters is critical to obtain intended effects with tDCS, and titration of these parameters can be useful.

In a set of motion perception studies using a moving dot paradigm, it was shown that the response to tDCS was critically dependent on stimulus characteristics. Anodal tDCS over area V5, an area critical for movement perception, reduced perception thresholds for coherently moving dots and thus improved performance, whereas cathodal tDCS improved performance in a "noisy" perception condition, in which the coherently moving dots were intermingled with dots moving in random directions (Antal et al. 2004). These findings were confirmed in another study, in which cathodal, but not anodal or sham stimulation improved perception in a complex, noisy movement perception task (Zito et al. 2015). In the coherent dot task, excitability enhancement via anodal tDCS may have facilitated the movement-related representations of the coherent dots, and thus improved performance. In the noisy task condition, the representations of noise would also be enhanced, and thus anodal stimulation was not associated with performance improvement. Instead, excitability-reducing cathodal tDCS may have decreased noisy activity, and thus improved performance. TDCS therefore can produce differential effects depending on the stimulus and task characteristics. A combination of electrophysiological and psychophysical tools can further help determine the precise neural pathways and cell groups in the visual cortex on which tDCS exerts its effects (Costa et al. 2015). In addition to the above-mentioned relatively elementary perceptions, evidence suggests that tDCS can also modify perception of complex visual objects (Barbieri et al. 2016; Varga et al. 2007), and functions controlled by higher visual areas (Filmer et al. 2015; Wright and Krekelberg 2014).

A handful of studies have been conducted to explore the impact of tDCS on different somatosensory qualities for an overview, (see Vaseghi et al. 2014). These studies theorize that enhancement of somatosensory cortical activity is the physiological correlate of increased somatosensory perception, and that activity enhancement of the primary motor cortex reduces somatosensory perceptions via cortico-thalamico-cortical loops (Knotkova et al. 2013). Correspondingly, cathodal tDCS over the somatosensory cortex and anodal tDCS over the primary motor cortex both have been linked to reduced pain perception (Antal et al. 2008; Grundmann et al. 2011; Ihle et al. 2014; Zandieh et al. 2013). Cathodal tDCS over the somatosensory cortex has also been shown to reduce the thresholds for vibration discrimination and therefore improve performance (Rogalewski et al. 2004), whereas anodal tDCS over the same area improved spatial acuity (Ragert et al. 2008). However the specific mechanisms of action of tDCS in this domain remain to be explored.

Only a small number of studies have investigated the impact of tDCS on auditory perception (Heimrath et al. 2016). Some of these studies have focused on changes in auditory evoked potentials elicited by stimulation. Anodal tDCS applied over the auditory cortex (temporal regions) increased the amplitude of the P50 component. In addition, while anodal tDCS of the temporo-parietal junction has been observed to decrease N1 latency, cathodal tDCS of the temporo-parietal junction increases N1 amplitude (Zaehle et al. 2011). The auditory mismatch sensitivity ERP—an electrophysiological signature of auditory discrimination ability—has been shown to be enhanced by anodal tDCS over the auditory cortex (Impey and Knott 2015). In addition to changes in auditory neurophysiology, there are a few studies in which tDCS over the auditory cortex has been shown to influence auditory perception. For instance, cathodal tDCS over the auditory cortex reduced pitch discrimination (Mathys et al. 2010). In a different study, the investigators found that auditory temporal information processing was improved by anodal tDCS but diminished by cathodal stimulation (Ladeira et al. 2011). Another intriguing study investigated the causal relationship between activity in a network that includes superior temporal and inferior frontal cortices and pitch performance (Loui et al. 2010). Cathodal tDCS over both superior temporal and inferior frontal areas reduced performance on this task, supporting the view that both areas are integral components in the pitch perception network. Overall, the results from cognitive studies corroborate the electrophysiological findings described above. But the differences in stimulation protocols, including electrode placements, target areas, and specific task characteristics may explain some of the discrepancies observed across studies.

Beyond unimodal effects of tDCS, a few studies have examined its effects on multisensory integration. The majority of these studies have targeted the parietal cortex, because it is considered to be an important hub in multisensory integration. Anodal tDCS was shown to disrupt multisensory integration in one study, in which the right posterior parietal cortex was stimulated (Zmigrod 2014), however increased integration of audio-visual stimuli was found in another study (Bolognini et al. 2010). Parietal cathodal tDCS had antagonistic effects (Marques et al. 2014). In another study, tDCS over unimodal cortices such as the temporal and parietal cortices, involved in encoding/decoding of stimuli and multisensory integration, enhanced excitability in remote lower-level visual areas, suggesting modulation across a wide functional network (Convento et al. 2013). This is an emerging field of inquiry, which in the coming years will provide interesting evidence regarding the polarity-specific and temporally-distinct effects of tDCS in different areas within widespread multisensory networks.

Attention and Working Memory

Numerous studies have explored the impact of tDCS on attention. Many of these studies have been geared toward both to finding causal evidence for the contribution of specific brain areas to this mental ability and also to enhancing it (Coffman et al. 2014). Since dorsolateral prefrontal and parietal areas are understood to be centrally involved in attentional processing, the majority of tDCS studies on this topic have, to date, focused on stimulating these brain regions.

Tanoue and colleagues investigated the contribution of the dlPFC and parietal cortex to attentional processes specifically related to working memory—the ability to temporarily maintain and manipulate information. Cathodal tDCS over both areas reduced performance in two working memory tasks, albeit the effect was largest for prefrontal stimulation (Tanoue et al. 2013). Conversely, anodal tDCS over the right frontal cortex has been shown to selectively improve the alerting component of attention (Coffman et al. 2012), while anodal tDCS over the dlPFC enhanced attentional bias acquisition with regard to attending or ignoring threatening versus neutral stimuli (Clarke et al. 2014). The results of these studies support the notion of the dlPFC being a brain area that is integral to attentional top-down processing. Exploring the involvement of the posterior parietal cortex (PPC) in visuo-spatial attention, anodal tDCS was shown to bias attention towards contralateral hemispace, and cathodal tDCS was found to have opposite behavioural effects (Sparing et al. 2009). Relatedly, anodal tDCS over the left PPC was shown to reduce visual attentional bias to the left in a greyscale task, whereas cathodal and sham stimulation had no consistent effect (Loftus and Nicholls 2012). Taken together these studies indicate that tDCS over the PPC can influence visual attention. Moreover, while few in number, studies that have combined functional imaging with stimulation and behavioural performance measures have been crucial for elucidating underlying neural mechanisms of attention. The interaction between frontal and parietal areas in a visual search task was explored using cathodal vs sham tDCS of the right parietal cortex. Not only did cathodal tDCS reduce performance, it also diminished prefrontal activity, which suggested that stimulation decreased performance by reduction of inter-areal cross-talk (Ellison et al. 2014). In another study, anodal tDCS over the dlPFC increased sustained attention and also prefrontal fMRI BOLD activity. These correlations help to provide a mechanistic understanding of the neurophysiologic and cognitive impact of tDCS on this task (Nelson et al. 2014). In a follow-up study by the same group, the beneficial effects of tDCS on attention during extended wakefulness were stronger than those of caffeine (McIntire et al. 2014), a finding that may contribute to the application of tDCS for neuroenhancement in this particular field.

Learning and Memory

A large body of evidence indicates that learning and memory can be manipulated using tDCS (Coffman et al. 2014). For example, a number of studies suggest that tDCS over the primary motor cortex (M1) can enhance the acquisition and retention of skilled motor tasks (Boggio et al. 2006; Galea and Celnik 2009; Nitsche et al. 2003b; Reis et al. 2009). Nitsche and colleagues (2003) were the first group to show that anodal tDCS over M1 improves motor learning during a serial reaction time task (SRTT). By contrast, tDCS over surrounding areas such as the premotor or prefrontal cortices did not result in improved performance (Nitsche et al. 2003b). In a different study by Nitsche et al. (2010), the investigators demonstrated the role of premotor cortex in motor memory consolidation. In this study, anodal tDCS over premotor cortex, performed during rapid eye movement sleep, resulted in increased recall of previously learned movement sequences on an SRTT task compared to a series of control experiments. This study therefore suggested a unique involvement of premotor areas in motor consolidation (Nitsche et al. 2010). In a more recent study, Saucedo-Marquez and colleagues (2013) observed task-dependent effects of anodal tDCS during different phases of motor learning and retention (Saucedo Marquez et al. 2013). They showed that anodal tDCS improved performance during the learning phase of a sequential finger-tapping task, while tDCS improved performance during the retention phase when performing a visual isometric pinch force task. The finding that anodal tDCS over the same motor area, M1, led to task- and phase-dependent effects suggested that underlying processes during a finger-tapping versus a force task are differentially modulated by anodal tDCS. Overall, evidence from these studies suggests that excitability-enhancing tDCS in motor and surrounding areas can be used to probe discrete stages of motor learning and memory. This knowledge has clear implications for the application of tDCS in clinical populations with specific motor function deficits.

Moreover, the neurophysiological changes induced by tDCS applied to motor areas and the impact of this stimulation on motor learning and memory have been widely studied. Current evidence suggests that tDCS-induced modulation of cortical excitability in M1 can influence levels of both the inhibitory neurotransmitter GABA and the excitatory neurotransmitter glutamate, which in turn could significantly influence underlying neural processes that support motor learning and memory (Kim et al. 2014; Stagg 2014; Stagg et al. 2009, 2011). In a recent study that employed a robotic force perturbation task, a decrease in GABA concentration was observed after anodal tDCS over the hand area in left M1; no change in GABA was observed after cathodal or sham stimulation (Kim et al. 2014). Importantly, tDCS-induced changes in the GABA levels significantly predicted motor learning and motor memory, while baseline GABA levels did not. A larger decrease in tDCS-induced GABA was associated with both better motor learning, as indexed by a reduced number of errors during adaptation, and better retention or memory, as indicated by a persistent increase in reaching errors during de-adaptation. While clear changes were observed with respect to anodal tDCS, previously reported decreases in Glutamate and GABA after cathodal tDCS (Stagg et al. 2009) were not observed in Kim et al. (2014), presumably owing to differences between studies in stimulation duration and intensity (Kim et al. 2014). Nonetheless, together the evidence from these studies suggests tDCS-induced changes in both excitatory and inhibitory neurotransmitter concentrations, which directly influence motor learning and memory performance.

In comparison to the large body of tDCS literature on motor learning and memory, there are relatively few studies currently that show benefits of tDCS in other memory domains such as language/verbal and non-motor procedural/implicit learning and memory. One of the first studies exploring the effects of tDCS on verbal memory was by Marshall et al. (2004), who showed that bilateral frontal anodal tDCS during slow-wave sleep improved retention of word pairs while stimulation during the wakeful state did not impact performance (Marshall et al. 2004). In a study by Floel et al. (2008), anodal tDCS applied over the left superior temporal cortex significantly improved the acquisition of novel vocabulary in a pseudoword-object associative learning task, compared to sham and cathodal stimulation (Floel et al. 2008). Javadi and Walsh (2012) reported improved verbal memory performance during recognition after anodal tDCS over the left dlPFC during the encoding phase, while cathodal tDCS impaired performance when applied during both phases (Javadi and Walsh 2012).The authors argued that better encoding or retention could have resulted in improved memory performance. This finding combined with authors' findings from a follow-up study (Javadi and Cheng 2013) suggested that anodal tDCS over the left dlPFC applied during different phases of memory formation i.e., encoding, reconsolidation and recognition, can potentially enhance long-term declarative memory. Specifically, in the 2013 study, the authors showed that anodal stimulation in conjunction with reactivating memories during one recognition phase (3 h after encoding words) resulted in more words being recognized in a subsequent recognition phase (5 h after the first recognition task), compared with sham and cathodal stimulation. Interestingly, they showed that reactivation of memories during anodal stimulation at that first recognition phase was required for improved performance during subsequent recognition.

In addition to language/verbal learning and memory, there are a small number of studies on the effects of tDCS on non-motor, implicit learning processes. For example, Kincses et al. (2004) demonstrated that anodal tDCS over the left PFC improved performance on probabilistic classification learning, a task involving the formation of implicit associations between a set of arbitrary geometric shapes and weather outcomes, while cathodal tDCS impaired performance (Kincses et al. 2004). These findings suggest a potential use of tDCS in facilitating implicit non-motor learning and memory functions in healthy individuals.

Grabner et al. (2015) applied tDCS over the left posterior parietal cortex and showed that arithmetic knowledge acquisition and learning can also be significantly modulated by tDCS (Grabner et al. 2015). Anodal, cathodal and sham tDCS were delivered during training with complex multiplication and subtraction problems. Cathodal tDCS decreased learning rates during training and resulted in poorer performance 24 h after stimulation, while anodal tDCS resulted in improved operation-specific performance on subtraction problems. The findings in this study and other similar studies (Rutsche et al. 2015) suggest that tDCS over left parietal areas can enhance arithmetic learning.

Overall this section highlights the complexities involved in using tDCS to probe specific processes of learning and memory. It is paramount that the interpretations of aftereffects are guided not only by comparisons of active with sham or control stimulation but also task-relevant phases in question, for example polarity-specific effects of tDCS may vary based on its application during different phases of memory formation.

Problem Solving and Decision Making

Compared to other domains of cognition presented in earlier sections in this chapter, evidence regarding the impact of tDCS on higher-level functions such as decision-making and problem solving is still in its infancy. Because of the evidence that tDCS can be used to manipulate attention, learning and memory (Coffman et al. 2014), some investigators have reasoned that it can mediate far reaching effects on more complex aspects of cognition. A major challenge, however, is that the specific neural networks and physiological mechanisms contributing to complex decision making, and the effects of tDCS on those complex networks remain incompletely understood.

The most common target site in tDCS studies for inducing changes in executive and other higher-level abilities is the dlPFC. The laterality and polarity of stimulation employed in these studies are not consistent, and are often motivated by prior findings from neuropsychological, functional neuroimaging, and neurophysiological studies. For instance, anodal tDCS over the left but not the right dlPFC improved performance on a complex verbal task that required not only verbal processing but also other executive function abilities; this finding suggests a specific role of left dlPFC in difficult verbal problem-solving (Cerruti and Schlaug 2009). In a different study (Metuki et al. 2012), anodal tDCS over the left dlPFC enhanced the ability to solve difficult verbal insight problems, but no effects were found for easy problems. While verbal problem-solving was modulated by stimulation of the left dlPFC, anodal tDCS over the right dlPFC modulated the impact of past investments on current decision-making, known as the sunk-cost effect. Cathodal and sham tDCS had no impact on such decisions. In addition, anodal tDCS did not impact decision-making when past investments were not made, highlighting the specificity of the effect (Bogdanov et al. 2015). A variety of stimulation approaches—bilateral, right anodal and left cathodal tDCS—over the dlPFC have been shown to reduce food cravings, an effect which is believed to be mediated by modulation of neural circuits involved in decision-making and reward (Fregni et al. 2008).

A relatively large body of evidence from brain stimulation studies support a causal role of dlPFC in decision-making processes. The observation that bilateral stimulation can potentially induce increased risk-aversive behavior (Fecteau et al. 2007) has important implications for the use of tDCS as a potential treatment for addiction. Motivated by noninvasive brain stimulation findings, a neurocognitive model proposed by Fecteau et al. (2010) provides a conceptual framework for dlPFC's involvement in a wide range of decision-making processes including reward-seeking and self-interested impulsive behaviors. Given the highly interconnected nature of the dlPFC, the effects of stimulating this area are likely to have both local effects and secondary effects on remote areas connected to the dlPFC via a bi-hemispheric cortico-subcortical network (Fecteau et al. 2010).

There are other studies on tDCS and its role in solving extremely difficult problems that are not computationally difficult but require creativity. For example, the so-called nine-dot problem is one in which subjects are required to connect nine dots with a limited number of lines. The task requires subjects to reason outside of rule conventional boundaries in order to arrive at a novel solution. Chi and Snyder (2012) found that no participant was able to solve this task before stimulation, but that after only 10 min of bilateral tDCS—cathode over the left anterior temporal lobe (ATL) and anode on the right ATL—40% of the participants were able to solve it (Chi and Snyder 2012). By inhibiting left ATL, an area involved in converging salient information into meaningful patterns (Baron and Osherson, 2011), the authors speculated that the participants were literally able to think outside the box. Another study by the same group and using the same electrode montage and polarity showed improved performance on an insight problem-solving task (Chi and Snyder 2011). Stimulation employing the opposite electrode polarity – anode over the right and cathode over the left ATL – did not improve performance. This finding led the authors to conclude that inhibiting the areas more heavily influenced by the mental set effects—the tendency to become fixed in one's thoughts or behavior, such that one finds it too difficult to engage new strategies to solve problems that have been previously resolved—while facilitating activation in an area associated with insight selectively resulted in improved performance (Chi and Snyder 2011).

tDCS and Neuroenhancement

While the effects from a single session of tDCS are considered transient, repeated or daily use of tDCS over the course of weeks can result in longer-lasting effects that may last weeks or months, and possibly longer. After over a decade of research in which tDCS has been employed as an investigative tool in cognitive neuroscience some researchers are beginning to focus on whether and to what extent this technology can be used to augment performance in otherwise healthy individuals. So far, tDCS has been used to enhance attention or vigilance, learning and memory, and other aspects of cognition with at least some evidence of success (Clark and Parasuraman 2014; Parasuraman and Galster 2013). The notion of neuroenhancement with tDCS has captured the public imagination and has led to both the development of direct-to-consumer tDCS devices as well as the emergence of a thriving do-it-yourself tDCS (DIY-tDCS) community, both of which raise a variety of ethical questions (Hamilton et al. 2011) as well as safety concerns (Wurzman et al. 2016). Some of the mixed evidence for the efficacy of tDCS in neuroenhancement is briefly summarized in this section.

After 5 days of language training with anodal tDCS of left posterior temporoparietal junction, Meinzer et al. (2014) reported a steeper learning curve and improvement in overall task performance in subjects receiving real stimulation compared with sham stimulation, which was maintained for at least a week after the training ended (Meinzer et al. 2014). Similarly, numerical learning was improved after 6 days of bilateral tDCS over the parietal cortex, with effects that lasted for at least 6 months post-stimulation (Cohen Kadosh et al. 2010). Anodal tDCS over M1 paired with a challenging motor task over 5 consecutive days enhanced motor skill acquisition and retention, which persisted for at least 3 months (Reis et al. 2009). Daily bilateral prefrontal tDCS over a period of 3–5 days improved self-reported mood in non-depressed individuals, which the authors suggest could transfer to memory and problem-solving abilities in healthy individuals (Austin et al. 2016). A few studies have reported enhanced memory retrieval (Manenti et al. 2013) and retention (Floel et al. 2012), and reduced forgetting (Sandrini et al. 2014) of episodic memories in healthy older individuals. These findings have potentially major implications for the future use of tDCS in reducing age-related cognitive decline. However, not all results have been equally promising. For example, at least one study by Martin et al. (2013) failed to find benefits associated with 10 sessions of anodal tDCS over the left dlPFC paired with cognitive training on an adaptive dual n-back task (Martin et al. 2013). While performance improved during active stimulation sessions, the benefits were not evident either 10 days or 4 weeks following the end of stimulation.

One potentially striking future application of DIY-tDCS is its use to enhance attention and lessen fatigue; two effects that are likely to be sought after in an increasingly competitive modern society. The positive results of a recent study (discussed in Sect. Attention and Working Memory) that compared the effects of a single 30-min session of tDCS with 200 mg of caffeine (equivalent to 1–2 cups of brewed coffee) on attention (McIntire et al. 2014) has clear implications for its use in neuroenhancement. The authors note that, while caffeine is widely consumed to combat fatigue, its benefits decline over time. The benefits of prolonged use of tDCS over time remain to be explored, but it is plausible that the perceived benefits after extended use of tDCS may also decline over time, or could even be detrimental to cognitive domains other than attention.

The safety and tolerability of tDCS have been widely studied and are well-documented in the field of cognitive neuroscience. A number of studies have indicated that tDCS is both safe and well-tolerated in healthy and clinical populations. The typical symptoms experienced during stimulation and for a short period of time following tDCS are considered mild and resolve within hours after stimulation ends. These symptoms include burning and tingling sensations, and skin redness under the electrodes (Durand et al. 2002; Kessler et al. 2012; Nitsche et al. 2003a; Poreisz et al. 2007). Since most of this safety information is derived from single or transient use of tDCS, there was an outstanding concern regarding its repeated use, particularly in the applications of neuroenhancement. The findings of a recently published report mitigate this concern (Bikson et al. 2016); no serious adverse effects or injuries were found in this investigation of human trials, which included over 30,000 tDCS sessions and 1000 subjects. It is important however to recognize that while these safety data are reassuring and support continued exploration of tDCS, they are based on controlled laboratory experiments using tDCS protocols that must conform to well-established safety limits. DIY-tDCS and direct-to-consumer tDCS applications have not been subjected to the same level of rigorous assessments and could potentially be dangerous to a naive user. In addition to the possibility of brain tissue damage due to overuse and/or overdose and equipment failure, a number of other problems may emerge that are not yet known and could possibly be detrimental to one's cognitive well-being (Wurzman et al. 2016).

Challenges and Opportunities

Despite its many practical advantages and the ever-increasing number of published experiments that employ tDCS, there remain a number of methodological and conceptual challenges to the further expansion of tDCS as a research tool in cognitive neuroscience. In this section we will provide an overview of some of the known limitations of tDCS and we will also discuss currently poorly understood aspects of tDCS that limit its application to cognitive neuroscience research.

One major methodological limitation of conventional tDCS is that it has low spatial resolution. This is in part because the electrodes and pads that are commonly used to deliver tDCS are relatively large (e.g. 5×5 cm^2 or 5×7 cm^2), but also because current flows between electrodes in a relatively diffuse manner (Datta et al. 2009). The low spatial resolution of the tDCS is potentially problematic for any cognitive neuroscience investigation that proposes to characterize differences between brain regions that are either adjacent or close to one another. This problem is mitigated, but not completely solved, by employing smaller active electrodes or larger reference electrodes than those that are currently commonly employed (Nitsche et al. 2007), and by using so-called ‘high definition’ tDCS systems that employ smaller electrodes and are arranged in such a way as to minimize the spread of current through the brain (Datta et al. 2009). In addition to its limited spatial resolution, tDCS also has low temporal resolution. In contrast with TMS pulses, which can be delivered at a specific time in relationship to the performance of a cognitive or behavioral task, tDCS must be administered over minutes and generally cannot be delivered in individual trials of a behavioral experiment or at a specific instant within a trial. These drawbacks can to some extent be circumvented by concurrently applying tDCS with a behavioral task. This approach may leverage the neuromodulatory properties of tDCS on ongoing task-related activity without inducing task-irrelevant activity, which in turn would increase the specificity of its aftereffects.

Another major limitation facing tDCS investigations is that the relationship between many stimulation parameters and their influence on cognition remains poorly understood. For instance, it is clear from numerous studies that the conceptualization of anodal and cathodal stimulation as having equal and opposite excitatory and inhibitory effects on behavior is oversimplified and often incorrect. Relatedly, a meta-analysis by Jacobson et al. (2012) demonstrated that the effects of cathodal stimulation are more inconsistent than those of anodal stimulation particularly in the context of its effects on cognition (Jacobson et al. 2012). In addition, the association between the intensity and duration of stimulation and neural excitability remains to be fully characterized. In an often-cited study, Batsikadze and colleagues (2013), demonstrated that administration of cathodal stimulation at 1 mA reduced subsequent TMS-induced MEP amplitudes, suggesting diminished cortical excitability. However, in the same experiment, cathodal stimulation at 2 mA for 20 min enhanced the amplitude of MEPs, suggesting a facilitative effect on cortical excitability (Batsikadze et al. 2013). The full impact of varying these and many other stimulation parameters on behavior – and the neural mechanisms that underlie these differences – have yet to be fully explored.

Finally, a formidable challenge in the use of tDCS in cognitive neuroscience is that the effects observed in cognitive studies are often small and can be highly variable. This may be especially true of studies that employ single sessions of stimulation to transiently alter cognition, and there has been considerable controversy recently regarding the reliability of these investigations, as evidenced from a number of recent metaanalyses (Horvath et al. 2015; Mancuso et al. 2016; Price et al. 2015). Relatedly, recent evidence has suggested that the sample sizes of many tDCS studies may be underpowered to produce reliable effects (Minarik et al. 2016). Moving forward, investigators will need to explore the factors that lead to heterogeneity in tDCS results, possibly by critical metaanalyses (Nitsche et al. 2015), and determine which findings are most valid, robust, and reproducible.

Future Directions

Despite a variety of limitations and challenges, the future of cognitive neuroscience research involving tDCS remains promising. In the years to come, studies will continue to explore the neural mechanisms by which tDCS alters brain activity, and to characterize the relationship between these induced changes in brain function and changes in cognitive performance. In light of some of the methodological challenges noted above, future studies of tDCS will need to more fully characterize the changes in performance that arise from differences in stimulation parameters such as electrode polarity, stimulation intensity, and duration. Moreover, future studies will also need to characterize the influence of a number of subject- and state-related factors, including but not limited to baseline ability (Sarkar et al. 2014; Turkeltaub et al. 2012) and domain-specific cognitive load during stimulation (Gill et al. 2015).

In addition to exploring a variety of properties related to stimulation itself, one of the most promising emerging developments for tDCS is the increasing ability to combine stimulation with complementary investigative tools, such as functional neuroimaging, electroencephalography, magnetoencephalography, near infrared spectroscopy, and other technologies. TDCS can also be paired with TMS and other noninvasive brain stimulation approaches to address questions regarding the relationship between tDCS-induced changes in behavior and changes in cortical neurophysiologic responses. Extending the use of these various converging approaches will allow for clearer insights into the neural mechanisms that underlie a variety of cognitive abilities, as well as the changes in neural function associated with tDCS-induced alterations in performance.

Conclusions

This is an exciting time for the field of cognitive neuroscience. In recent years, techniques for exploring structure-function and network-function relationships in the brain related to cognition have developed tremendous sophistication. In line with this, noninvasive neuromodulation techniques like tDCS have, over time, become invaluable investigative tools in the armamentarium of cognitive neuroscience, because they allow for direct inferences to be made regarding causal relationships between neural functions and mental operations. As we have shown, tDCS has already been used effectively to explore the neural basis of a wide range of cognitive domains and mental abilities. In the future, the technique will continue to be refined, allowing ever more important questions in cognitive neuroscience to be addressed in more elegant and rigorous ways.

References

Accornero, N., Li Voti, P., La Riccia, M., & Gregori, B. (2007). Visual evoked potentials modulation during direct current cortical polarization. *Experimental Brain Research, 178*(2), 261–266.

Amadi, U., Allman, C., Johansen-Berg, H., & Stagg, C. J. (2015). The homeostatic interaction between anodal transcranial direct current stimulation and motor learning in humans is related to GABAA activity. *Brain Stimulation, 8*(5), 898–905.

Ambrus, G. G., Chaieb, L., Stilling, R., Rothkegel, H., Antal, A., & Paulus, W. (2016). Monitoring transcranial direct current stimulation induced changes in cortical excitability during the serial reaction time task. *Neuroscience Letters, 616*, 98–104.

Antal, A., Brepohl, N., Poreisz, C., Boros, K., Csifcsak, G., & Paulus, W. (2008). Transcranial direct current stimulation over somatosensory cortex decreases experimentally induced acute pain perception. *The Clinical Journal of Pain, 24*(1), 56–63.

Antal, A., Kincses, T. Z., Nitsche, M. A., Bartfai, O., & Paulus, W. (2004). Excitability changes induced in the human primary visual cortex by transcranial direct current stimulation: Direct electrophysiological evidence. *Investigative Ophthalmology & Visual Science, 45*(2), 702–707.

Antal, A., Nitsche, M. A., & Paulus, W. (2001). External modulation of visual perception in humans. *Neuroreport, 12*(16), 3553–3555.

Antal, A., Polania, R., Schmidt-Samoa, C., Dechent, P., & Paulus, W. (2011). Transcranial direct current stimulation over the primary motor cortex during fMRI. *NeuroImage, 55*(2), 590–596.

Austin, A., Jiga-Boy, G. M., Rea, S., Newstead, S. A., Roderick, S., Davis, N. J., ... Boy, F. (2016). Prefrontal electrical stimulation in non-depressed reduces levels of reported negative affects from daily stressors. *Frontiers in Psychology, 7*, 315.

Barbieri, M., Negrini, M., Nitsche, M. A., & Rivolta, D. (2016). Anodal-tDCS over the human right occipital cortex enhances the perception and memory of both faces and objects. *Neuropsychologia, 81*, 238–244.

Baron, S. G., & Osherson, D. (2011). Evidence for conceptual combination in the left anterior temporal lobe. *NeuroImage, 55*(4), 1847–1852.

Batsikadze, G., Moliadze, V., Paulus, W., Kuo, M. F., & Nitsche, M. A. (2013). Partially non-linear stimulation intensity-dependent effects of direct current stimulation on motor cortex excitability in humans. *The Journal of Physiology, 591*(7), 1987–2000.

Bersani, F. S., Minichino, A., Fattapposta, F., Bernabei, L., Spagnoli, F., Mannarelli, D., ... Delle Chiaie, R. (2015). Prefrontocerebellar transcranial direct current stimulation increases amplitude and decreases latency of P3b component in patients with euthymic bipolar disorder. *Neuropsychiatric Disease and Treatment, 11*, 2913–2917.

Bikson, M., Grossman, P., Thomas, C., Zannou, A. L., Jiang, J., Adnan, T., ... Woods, A. J. (2016). Safety of Transcranial direct current stimulation: Evidence based update 2016. *Brain Stimulation, 9*(5), 641–661.

Bindman, L. J., Lippold, O. C., & Redfearn, J. W. (1964). The action of brief polarizing currents on the cerebral cortex of the rat (1) during current flow and (2) in the production of long-lasting after-effects. *The Journal of Physiology, 172*, 369–382.

Bocci, T., Caleo, M., Tognazzi, S., Francini, N., Briscese, L., Maffei, L., ... Sartucci, F. (2014). Evidence for metaplasticity in the human visual cortex. *Journal of Neural Transmission (Vienna), 121*(3), 221–231.

Bogdanov, M., Ruff, C. C., & Schwabe, L. (2015). Transcranial stimulation over the dorsolateral prefrontal cortex increases the impact of past expenses on decision-making. *Cerebral Cortex.*

Boggio, P. S., Castro, L. O., Savagim, E. A., Braite, R., Cruz, V. C., Rocha, R. R., ... Fregni, F. (2006). Enhancement of non-dominant hand motor function by anodal transcranial direct current stimulation. *Neuroscience Letters, 404*(1–2), 232–236.

Bolognini, N., Olgiati, E., Rossetti, A., & Maravita, A. (2010). Enhancing multisensory spatial orienting by brain polarization of the parietal cortex. *The European Journal of Neuroscience, 31*(10), 1800–1806.

Cerruti, C., & Schlaug, G. (2009). Anodal transcranial direct current stimulation of the prefrontal cortex enhances complex verbal associative thought. *Journal of Cognitive Neuroscience, 21*(10), 1980–1987.

Chi, R. P., & Snyder, A. W. (2011). Facilitate insight by non-invasive brain stimulation. *PLoS One, 6*(2), e16655.

Chi, R. P., & Snyder, A. W. (2012). Brain stimulation enables the solution of an inherently difficult problem. *Neuroscience Letters, 515*(2), 121–124.

Chib, V. S., Yun, K., Takahashi, H., & Shimojo, S. (2013). Noninvasive remote activation of the ventral midbrain by transcranial direct current stimulation of prefrontal cortex. *Translational Psychiatry, 3*, e268.

Clark, V. P., & Parasuraman, R. (2014). Neuroenhancement: Enhancing brain and mind in health and in disease. *NeuroImage, 85*(Pt 3), 889–894.

Clarke, P. J., Browning, M., Hammond, G., Notebaert, L., & MacLeod, C. (2014). The causal role of the dorsolateral prefrontal cortex in the modification of attentional bias: Evidence from transcranial direct current stimulation. *Biological Psychiatry, 76*(12), 946–952.

Clemens, B., Jung, S., Zvyagintsev, M., Domahs, F., & Willmes, K. (2013). Modulating arithmetic fact retrieval: A single-blind, sham-controlled tDCS study with repeated fMRI measurements. *Neuropsychologia, 51*(7), 1279–1286.

Coffman, B. A., Clark, V. P., & Parasuraman, R. (2014). Battery powered thought: Enhancement of attention, learning, and memory in healthy adults using transcranial direct current stimulation. *NeuroImage, 85*(Pt 3), 895–908.

Coffman, B. A., Trumbo, M. C., & Clark, V. P. (2012). Enhancement of object detection with transcranial direct current stimulation is associated with increased attention. *BMC Neuroscience, 13*(1), 108.

Cohen Kadosh, R., Soskic, S., Iuculano, T., Kanai, R., & Walsh, V. (2010). Modulating neuronal activity produces specific and long-lasting changes in numerical competence. *Current Biology, 20*(22), 2016–2020.

Conti, C. L., Moscon, J. A., Fregni, F., Nitsche, M. A., & Nakamura-Palacios, E. M. (2014). Cognitive related electrophysiological changes induced by non-invasive cortical electrical stimulation in crack-cocaine addiction. *The International Journal of Neuropsychopharmacology, 17*(9), 1465–1475.

Convento, S., Vallar, G., Galantini, C., & Bolognini, N. (2013). Neuromodulation of early multisensory interactions in the visual cortex. *Journal of Cognitive Neuroscience, 25*(5), 685–696.

Costa, T. L., Gualtieri, M., Barboni, M. T., Katayama, R. K., Boggio, P. S., & Ventura, D. F. (2015). Contrasting effects of transcranial direct current stimulation on central and peripheral visual fields. *Experimental Brain Research, 233*(5), 1391–1397.

Datta, A., Bansal, V., Diaz, J., Patel, J., Reato, D., & Bikson, M. (2009). Gyri-precise head model of transcranial direct current stimulation: Improved spatial focality using a ring electrode versus conventional rectangular pad. *Brain Stimulation, 2*(4), 201–207, 207 e201.

Dieckhofer, A., Waberski, T. D., Nitsche, M., Paulus, W., Buchner, H., & Gobbele, R. (2006). Transcranial direct current stimulation applied over the somatosensory cortex – Differential effect on low and high frequency SEPs. *Clinical Neurophysiology, 117*(10), 2221–2227.

Ding, Z., Li, J., Spiegel, D. P., Chen, Z., Chan, L., Luo, G., ... Thompson, B. (2016). The effect of transcranial direct current stimulation on contrast sensitivity and visual evoked potential amplitude in adults with amblyopia. *Scientific Reports, 6*, 19280.

Durand, S., Fromy, B., Bouye, P., Saumet, J. L., & Abraham, P. (2002). Vasodilatation in response to repeated anodal current application in the human skin relies on aspirin-sensitive mechanisms. *The Journal of Physiology, 540*(Pt 1), 261–269.

Ellison, A., Ball, K. L., Moseley, P., Dowsett, J., Smith, D. T., Weis, S., & Lane, A. R. (2014). Functional interaction between right parietal and bilateral frontal cortices during visual search tasks revealed using functional magnetic imaging and transcranial direct current stimulation. *PLoS One, 9*(4), e93767.

Fecteau, S., Fregni, F., Boggio, P. S., Camprodon, J. A., & Pascual-Leone, A. (2010). Neuromodulation of decision-making in the addictive brain. *Substance Use & Misuse, 45*(11), 1766–1786.

Fecteau, S., Pascual-Leone, A., Zald, D. H., Liguori, P., Theoret, H., Boggio, P. S., & Fregni, F. (2007). Activation of prefrontal cortex by transcranial direct current stimulation reduces appetite for risk during ambiguous decision making. *The Journal of Neuroscience, 27*(23), 6212–6218.

Filmer, H. L., Dux, P. E., & Mattingley, J. B. (2015). Dissociable effects of anodal and cathodal tDCS reveal distinct functional roles for right parietal cortex in the detection of single and competing stimuli. *Neuropsychologia, 74*, 120–126.

Floel, A., Rosser, N., Michka, O., Knecht, S., & Breitenstein, C. (2008). Noninvasive brain stimulation improves language learning. *Journal of Cognitive Neuroscience, 20*(8), 1415–1422.

Floel, A., Suttorp, W., Kohl, O., Kurten, J., Lohmann, H., Breitenstein, C., & Knecht, S. (2012). Non-invasive brain stimulation improves object-location learning in the elderly. *Neurobiology of Aging, 33*(8), 1682–1689.

Fregni, F., Boggio, P. S., Nitsche, M., Bermpohl, F., Antal, A., Feredoes, E., … Pascual-Leone, A. (2005). Anodal transcranial direct current stimulation of prefrontal cortex enhances working memory. *Experimental Brain Research, 166*(1), 23–30.

Fregni, F., Orsati, F., Pedrosa, W., Fecteau, S., Tome, F. A., Nitsche, M. A., … Boggio, P. S. (2008). Transcranial direct current stimulation of the prefrontal cortex modulates the desire for specific foods. *Appetite, 51*(1), 34–41.

Galea, J. M., & Celnik, P. (2009). Brain polarization enhances the formation and retention of motor memories. *Journal of Neurophysiology, 102*(1), 294–301.

Gill, J., Shah-Basak, P. P., & Hamilton, R. (2015). It's the thought that counts: Examining the task-dependent effects of transcranial direct current stimulation on executive function. *Brain Stimulation, 8*(2), 253–259.

Grabner, R. H., Rutsche, B., Ruff, C. C., & Hauser, T. U. (2015). Transcranial direct current stimulation of the posterior parietal cortex modulates arithmetic learning. *The European Journal of Neuroscience, 42*(1), 1667–1674.

Grundey, J., Thirugnanasambandam, N., Kaminsky, K., Drees, A., Skwirba, A. C., Lang, N., … Nitsche, M. A. (2012). Neuroplasticity in cigarette smokers is altered under withdrawal and partially restituted by nicotine exposition. The Journal of Neuroscience, 32(12), 4156–4162.

Grundey, J., Thirugnasambandam, N., Amu, R., Paulus, W., & Nitsche, M. A. (2018). Nicotinic restoration of excitatory neuroplasticity is linked to improved implicit motor learning skills in deprived smokers. *Frontiers in Neurology, 9*, 367

Grundmann, L., Rolke, R., Nitsche, M. A., Pavlakovic, G., Happe, S., Treede, R. D., … Bachmann, C. G. (2011). Effects of transcranial direct current stimulation of the primary sensory cortex on somatosensory perception. *Brain Stimulation, 4*(4), 253–260.

Hamilton, R., Messing, S., & Chatterjee, A. (2011). Rethinking the thinking cap: Ethics of neural enhancement using noninvasive brain stimulation. *Neurology, 76*(2), 187–193.

Heimrath, K., Fiene, M., Rufener, K. S., & Zaehle, T. (2016). Modulating human auditory processing by transcranial electrical stimulation. *Frontiers in Cellular Neuroscience, 10*, 53.

Horvath, J. C., Forte, J. D., & Carter, O. (2015). Quantitative review finds no evidence of cognitive effects in healthy populations from single-session transcranial direct current stimulation (tDCS). *Brain Stimulation, 8*(3), 535–550.

Ihle, K., Rodriguez-Raecke, R., Luedtke, K., & May, A. (2014). tDCS modulates cortical nociceptive processing but has little to no impact on pain perception. *Pain, 155*(10), 2080–2087.

Impey, D., de la Salle, S., & Knott, V. (2016). Assessment of anodal and cathodal transcranial direct current stimulation (tDCS) on MMN-indexed auditory sensory processing. *Brain and Cognition, 105*, 46–54.

Impey, D., & Knott, V. (2015). Effect of transcranial direct current stimulation (tDCS) on MMN-indexed auditory discrimination: A pilot study. *Journal of Neural Transmission (Vienna), 122*(8), 1175–1185.

Jacobson, L., Koslowsky, M., & Lavidor, M. (2012). tDCS polarity effects in motor and cognitive domains: A meta-analytical review. *Experimental Brain Research, 216*(1), 1–10.

Javadi, A. H., & Cheng, P. (2013). Transcranial direct current stimulation (tDCS) enhances reconsolidation of long-term memory. *Brain Stimulation, 6*(4), 668–674.

Javadi, A. H., & Walsh, V. (2012). Transcranial direct current stimulation (tDCS) of the left dorsolateral prefrontal cortex modulates declarative memory. *Brain Stimulation, 5*(3), 231–241.

Kessler, S. K., Turkeltaub, P. E., Benson, J. G., & Hamilton, R. H. (2012). Differences in the experience of active and sham transcranial direct current stimulation. *Brain Stimulation, 5*(2), 155–162.

Kim, S., Stephenson, M. C., Morris, P. G., & Jackson, S. R. (2014). tDCS-induced alterations in GABA concentration within primary motor cortex predict motor learning and motor memory: A 7 T magnetic resonance spectroscopy study. *NeuroImage, 99*, 237–243.

Kincses, T. Z., Antal, A., Nitsche, M. A., Bartfai, O., & Paulus, W. (2004). Facilitation of probabilistic classification learning by transcranial direct current stimulation of the prefrontal cortex in the human. *Neuropsychologia, 42*(1), 113–117.

Knotkova, H., Nitsche, M. A., & Cruciani, R. A. (2013). Putative physiological mechanisms underlying tDCS analgesic effects. *Frontiers in Human Neuroscience, 7*, 628.

Kraft, A., Roehmel, J., Olma, M. C., Schmidt, S., Irlbacher, K., & Brandt, S. A. (2010). Transcranial direct current stimulation affects visual perception measured by threshold perimetry. *Experimental Brain Research, 207*(3–4), 283–290.

Kuo, M. F., & Nitsche, M. A. (2012). Effects of transcranial electrical stimulation on cognition. *Clinical EEG and Neuroscience, 43*(3), 192–199.

Ladeira, A., Fregni, F., Campanha, C., Valasek, C. A., De Ridder, D., Brunoni, A. R., & Boggio, P. S. (2011). Polarity-dependent transcranial direct current stimulation effects on central auditory processing. *PLoS One, 6*(9), e25399.

Lang, N., Siebner, H. R., Ward, N. S., Lee, L., Nitsche, M. A., Paulus, W., … Frackowiak, R. S. (2005). How does transcranial DC stimulation of the primary motor cortex alter regional neuronal activity in the human brain? *The European Journal of Neuroscience, 22*(2), 495–504.

Lee, L., Siebner, H. R., Rowe, J. B., Rizzo, V., Rothwell, J. C., Frackowiak, R. S., & Friston, K. J. (2003). Acute remapping within the motor system induced by low-frequency repetitive transcranial magnetic stimulation. *The Journal of Neuroscience, 23*(12), 5308–5318.

Lefebvre, S., Dricot, L., Laloux, P., Gradkowski, W., Desfontaines, P., Evrard, F., … Vandermeeren, Y. (2015). Neural substrates underlying stimulation-enhanced motor skill learning after stroke. *Brain, 138*(Pt 1), 149–163.

Loftus, A., & Nicholls, M. (2012). Testing the activation–orientation account of spatial attentional asymmetries using transcranial direct current stimulation. *Neuropsychologia, 50*(11), 2573–2576.

Lopez-Alonso, V., Cheeran, B., & Fernandez-del-Olmo, M. (2015). Relationship between non-invasive brain stimulation-induced plasticity and capacity for motor learning. *Brain Stimulation, 8*(6), 1209–1219.

Loui, P., Hohmann, A., & Schlaug, G. (2010). Inducing disorders in pitch perception and production: A reverse-engineering approach. *Proceedings of Meetings on Acoustics, 9*(1), 50002.

Mancuso, L. E., Ilieva, I. P., Hamilton, R. H., & Farah, M. J. (2016). Does transcranial direct current stimulation improve healthy working memory?: A meta-analytic review. *Journal of Cognitive Neuroscience, 28*(8), 1063–1089.

Manenti, R., Brambilla, M., Petesi, M., Ferrari, C., & Cotelli, M. (2013). Enhancing verbal episodic memory in older and young subjects after non-invasive brain stimulation. *Frontiers in Aging Neuroscience, 5*, 49.

Marques, L. M., Lapenta, O. M., Merabet, L. B., Bolognini, N., & Boggio, P. S. (2014). Tuning and disrupting the brain-modulating the McGurk illusion with electrical stimulation. *Frontiers in Human Neuroscience, 8*, 533.

Marshall, L., Molle, M., Hallschmid, M., & Born, J. (2004). Transcranial direct current stimulation during sleep improves declarative memory. *The Journal of Neuroscience, 24*(44), 9985–9992.

Martin, D. M., Liu, R., Alonzo, A., Green, M., Player, M. J., Sachdev, P., & Loo, C. K. (2013). Can transcranial direct current stimulation enhance outcomes from cognitive training? A randomized controlled trial in healthy participants. *The International Journal of Neuropsychopharmacology, 16*(9), 1927–1936.

Mathys, C., Loui, P., Zheng, X., & Schlaug, G. (2010). Non-invasive brain stimulation applied to Heschl's gyrus modulates pitch discrimination. *Frontiers in Psychology, 1*, 193.

Matsunaga, K., Nitsche, M. A., Tsuji, S., & Rothwell, J. C. (2004). Effect of transcranial DC sensorimotor cortex stimulation on somatosensory evoked potentials in humans. *Clinical Neurophysiology, 115*(2), 456–460.

McIntire, L. K., McKinley, R. A., Goodyear, C., & Nelson, J. (2014). A comparison of the effects of transcranial direct current stimulation and caffeine on vigilance and cognitive performance during extended wakefulness. *Brain Stimulation, 7*(4), 499–507.

Meinzer, M., Jahnigen, S., Copland, D. A., Darkow, R., Grittner, U., Avirame, K., … Floel, A. (2014). Transcranial direct current stimulation over multiple days improves learning and maintenance of a novel vocabulary. *Cortex, 50*, 137–147.

Metuki, N., Sela, T., & Lavidor, M. (2012). Enhancing cognitive control components of insight problems solving by anodal tDCS of the left dorsolateral prefrontal cortex. *Brain Stimulation, 5*(2), 110–115.

Minarik, T., Berger, B., Althaus, L., Bader, V., Biebl, B., Brotzeller, F., … Sauseng, P. (2016). The importance of sample size for reproducibility of tDCS effects. *Frontiers in Human Neuroscience, 10*, 453.

Nelson, J. T., McKinley, R. A., Golob, E. J., Warm, J. S., & Parasuraman, R. (2014). Enhancing vigilance in operators with prefrontal cortex transcranial direct current stimulation (tDCS). *Neuroimage, 85*(Pt 3), 909–917.

Nitsche, M. A., Bikson, M., & Bestmann, S. (2015). On the use of meta-analysis in neuromodulatory non-invasive brain stimulation. *Brain Stimulation, 8*(3), 666–667.

Nitsche, M. A., Cohen, L. G., Wassermann, E. M., Priori, A., Lang, N., Antal, A., … Pascual-Leone, A. (2008). Transcranial direct current stimulation: State of the art 2008. *Brain Stimulation, 1*(3), 206–223.

Nitsche, M. A., Doemkes, S., Karakose, T., Antal, A., Liebetanz, D., Lang, N., … Paulus, W. (2007). Shaping the effects of transcranial direct current stimulation of the human motor cortex. *Journal of Neurophysiology, 97*(4), 3109–3117.

Nitsche, M. A., Jakoubkova, M., Thirugnanasambandam, N., Schmalfuss, L., Hullemann, S., Sonka, K., … Happe, S. (2010). Contribution of the premotor cortex to consolidation of motor sequence learning in humans during sleep. *Journal of Neurophysiology, 104*(5), 2603–2614.

Nitsche, M. A., Liebetanz, D., Lang, N., Antal, A., Tergau, F., & Paulus, W. (2003a). Safety criteria for transcranial direct current stimulation (tDCS) in humans. *Clinical Neurophysiology, 114*(11), 2220–2222. author reply 2222-2223.

Nitsche, M. A., & Paulus, W. (2011). Transcranial direct current stimulation – Update 2011. *Restorative Neurology and Neuroscience, 29*(6), 463–492.

Nitsche, M. A., Schauenburg, A., Lang, N., Liebetanz, D., Exner, C., Paulus, W., & Tergau, F. (2003b). Facilitation of implicit motor learning by weak transcranial direct current stimulation of the primary motor cortex in the human. *Journal of Cognitive Neuroscience, 15*(4), 619–626.

Parasuraman, R., & Galster, S. (2013). Sensing, assessing, and augmenting threat detection: Behavioral, neuroimaging, and brain stimulation evidence for the critical role of attention. *Frontiers in Human Neuroscience, 7*, 273.

Pascual-Leone, A., Grafman, J., & Hallett, M. (1994a). Modulation of cortical motor output maps during development of implicit and explicit knowledge. *Science, 263*(5151), 1287–1289.

Pascual-Leone, A., Valls-Sole, J., Wassermann, E. M., & Hallett, M. (1994b). Responses to rapid-rate transcranial magnetic stimulation of the human motor cortex. *Brain, 117*(Pt 4), 847–858.

Paulus, W., Classen, J., Cohen, L. G., Large, C. H., Di Lazzaro, V., Nitsche, M., … Ziemann, U. (2008). State of the art: Pharmacologic effects on cortical excitability measures tested by transcranial magnetic stimulation. *Brain Stimulation, 1*(3), 151–163.

Poreisz, C., Boros, K., Antal, A., & Paulus, W. (2007). Safety aspects of transcranial direct current stimulation concerning healthy subjects and patients. *Brain Research Bulletin, 72*(4–6), 208–214.

Premoli, I., Castellanos, N., Rivolta, D., Belardinelli, P., Bajo, R., Zipser, C., … Ziemann, U. (2014). TMS-EEG signatures of GABAergic neurotransmission in the human cortex. *The Journal of Neuroscience, 34*(16), 5603–5612.

Price, A. R., McAdams, H., Grossman, M., & Hamilton, R. H. (2015). A meta-analysis of transcranial direct current stimulation studies examining the reliability of effects on language measures. *Brain Stimulation, 8*(6), 1093–1100.

Ragert, P., Vandermeeren, Y., Camus, M., & Cohen, L. G. (2008). Improvement of spatial tactile acuity by transcranial direct current stimulation. *Clinical Neurophysiology, 119*(4), 805–811.

Reinhart, R. M., Zhu, J., Park, S., & Woodman, G. F. (2015). Medial-frontal stimulation enhances learning in schizophrenia by restoring prediction error signaling. *The Journal of Neuroscience, 35*(35), 12232–12240.

Reis, J., Schambra, H. M., Cohen, L. G., Buch, E. R., Fritsch, B., Zarahn, E., … Krakauer, J. W. (2009). Noninvasive cortical stimulation enhances motor skill acquisition over multiple days through an effect on consolidation. *Proceedings of the National Academy of Sciences of the United States of America, 106*(5), 1590–1595.

Rioult-Pedotti, M. S., Friedman, D., & Donoghue, J. P. (2000). Learning-induced LTP in neocortex. *Science, 290*(5491), 533–536.

Rogalewski, A., Breitenstein, C., Nitsche, M. A., Paulus, W., & Knecht, S. (2004). Transcranial direct current stimulation disrupts tactile perception. *The European Journal of Neuroscience, 20*(1), 313–316.

Rogasch, N. C., Daskalakis, Z. J., & Fitzgerald, P. B. (2013). Mechanisms underlying long-interval cortical inhibition in the human motor cortex: A TMS-EEG study. *Journal of Neurophysiology, 109*(1), 89–98.

Rogasch, N. C., Daskalakis, Z. J., & Fitzgerald, P. B. (2015). Cortical inhibition of distinct mechanisms in the dorsolateral prefrontal cortex is related to working memory performance: A TMS-EEG study. *Cortex, 64*, 68–77.

Romero Lauro, L. J., Rosanova, M., Mattavelli, G., Convento, S., Pisoni, A., Opitz, A., … Vallar, G. (2014). TDCS increases cortical excitability: Direct evidence from TMS-EEG. *Cortex, 58*, 99–111.

Roth, N., Lutiger, B., Hasenfratz, M., Battig, K., & Knye, M. (1992). Smoking deprivation in "early" and "late" smokers and memory functions. *Psychopharmacology, 106*(2), 253–260.

Rounis, E., Lee, L., Siebner, H. R., Rowe, J. B., Friston, K. J., Rothwell, J. C., & Frackowiak, R. S. (2005). Frequency specific changes in regional cerebral blood flow and motor system connectivity following rTMS to the primary motor cortex. *NeuroImage, 26*(1), 164–176.

Rutsche, B., Hauser, T. U., Jancke, L., & Grabner, R. H. (2015). When problem size matters: Differential effects of brain stimulation on arithmetic problem solving and neural oscillations. *PLoS One, 10*(3), e0120665.

Sandrini, M., Brambilla, M., Manenti, R., Rosini, S., Cohen, L. G., & Cotelli, M. (2014). Noninvasive stimulation of prefrontal cortex strengthens existing episodic memories and reduces forgetting in the elderly. *Frontiers in Aging Neuroscience, 6*, 289.

Sarkar, A., Dowker, A., & Cohen Kadosh, R. (2014). Cognitive enhancement or cognitive cost: Trait-specific outcomes of brain stimulation in the case of mathematics anxiety. *The Journal of Neuroscience, 34*(50), 16605–16610.

Saucedo Marquez, C. M., Zhang, X., Swinnen, S. P., Meesen, R., & Wenderoth, N. (2013). Task-specific effect of transcranial direct current stimulation on motor learning. *Frontiers in Human Neuroscience, 7*, 333.

Shin, Y. I., Foerster, A., & Nitsche, M. A. (2015). Transcranial direct current stimulation (tDCS) – Application in neuropsychology. *Neuropsychologia, 69*, 154–175.

Sparing, R., Thimm, M., Hesse, M., Küst, J., Karbe, H., & Fink, G. (2009). Bidirectional alterations of interhemispheric parietal balance by non-invasive cortical stimulation. *Brain, 132*(11), 3011–3020.

Stagg, C. J. (2014). Magnetic resonance spectroscopy as a tool to study the role of GABA in motor-cortical plasticity. *NeuroImage, 86*, 19–27.

Stagg, C. J., Bachtiar, V., & Johansen-Berg, H. (2011). The role of GABA in human motor learning. *Current Biology, 21*(6), 480–484.

Stagg, C. J., Best, J. G., Stephenson, M. C., O'Shea, J., Wylezinska, M., Kincses, Z. T., … Johansen-Berg, H. (2009). Polarity-sensitive modulation of cortical neurotransmitters by transcranial stimulation. *The Journal of Neuroscience, 29*(16), 5202–5206.

Strigaro, G., Mayer, I., Chen, J. C., Cantello, R., & Rothwell, J. C. (2015). Transcranial direct current stimulation effects on single and paired flash visual evoked potentials. *Clinical EEG and Neuroscience, 46*(3), 208–213.

Tanoue, R. T., Jones, K. T., Peterson, D. J., & Berryhill, M. E. (2013). Differential frontal involvement in shifts of internal and perceptual attention. *Brain Stimulation, 6*(4), 675–682.

Turkeltaub, P. E., Benson, J., Hamilton, R. H., Datta, A., Bikson, M., & Coslett, H. B. (2012). Left lateralizing transcranial direct current stimulation improves reading efficiency. *Brain Stimulation, 5*(3), 201–207.

Varga, E. T., Elif, K., Antal, A., Zimmer, M., Harza, I., Paulus, W., & Kovacs, G. (2007). Cathodal transcranial direct current stimulation over the parietal cortex modifies facial gender adaptation. *Ideggyógyászati Szemle, 60*(11–12), 474–479.

Vaseghi, B., Zoghi, M., & Jaberzadeh, S. (2014). Does anodal transcranial direct current stimulation modulate sensory perception and pain? A meta-analysis study. *Clinical Neurophysiology, 125*(9), 1847–1858.

Weber, M. J., Messing, S. B., Rao, H., Detre, J. A., & Thompson-Schill, S. L. (2014). Prefrontal transcranial direct current stimulation alters activation and connectivity in cortical and subcortical reward systems: A tDCS-fMRI study. *Human Brain Mapping, 35*(8), 3673–3686.

Wright, J. M., & Krekelberg, B. (2014). Transcranial direct current stimulation over posterior parietal cortex modulates visuospatial localization. *Journal of Vision, 14*(9).

Wurzman, R., Hamilton, R. H., Pascual-Leone, A., & Fox, M. D. (2016). An open letter concerning do-it-yourself users of transcranial direct current stimulation. *Annals of Neurology, 80*(1), 1–4.

Zaehle, T., Beretta, M., Jancke, L., Herrmann, C. S., & Sandmann, P. (2011). Excitability changes induced in the human auditory cortex by transcranial direct current stimulation: Direct electrophysiological evidence. *Experimental Brain Research, 215*(2), 135–140.

Zandieh, A., Parhizgar, S. E., Fakhri, M., Taghvaei, M., Miri, S., Shahbabaie, A., … Ekhtiari, H. (2013). Modulation of cold pain perception by transcranial direct current stimulation in healthy individuals. *Neuromodulation, 16*(4), 345–348.; discussion 348.

Zheng, X., Alsop, D. C., & Schlaug, G. (2011). Effects of transcranial direct current stimulation (tDCS) on human regional cerebral blood flow. *NeuroImage, 58*(1), 26–33.

Zito, G. A., Senti, T., Cazzoli, D., Muri, R. M., Mosimann, U. P., Nyffeler, T., & Nef, T. (2015). Cathodal HD-tDCS on the right V5 improves motion perception in humans. *Frontiers in Behavioral Neuroscience, 9*, 257.

Zmigrod, S. (2014). The role of the parietal cortex in multisensory and response integration: Evidence from transcranial direct current stimulation (tDCS). *Multisensory Research, 27*(2), 161–172.

Chapter 21
Challenges, Open Questions and Future Direction in Transcranial Direct Current Stimulation Research and Applications

Michael A. Nitsche, Helena Knotkova, Adam J. Woods, and Marom Bikson

Introduction

Techniques for non-invasive modulation of brain function and plasticity have emerged as an important research and promising clinical tool during the last two decades. It allows directed, controlled and localized modulation of brain physiology, and thus is a powerful tool to expand our understanding of brain functions, including implications for psychological and behavioral processes in health and disease, and has as well therapeutic implications.

tDCS is one of these techniques which (re-)gained increasing popularity during the last years. In the 50s and 60s of the last century, tDCS studies in humans and animal models showed that tonic application of weak direct currents to the brain could alter cortical activity and plasticity, modulate cognitive functions, and might

M. A. Nitsche (✉)
Department of Psychology and Neurosciences, Leibniz Research Centre for Working Environment and Human Factors, Dortmund, Germany

University Medical Hospital Bergmannsheil, Bochum, Germany
e-mail: nitsche@ifado.de

H. Knotkova
MJHS Institute for Innovation in Palliative Care, New York, NY, USA

Department of Family and Social Medicine, Albert Einstein College of Medicine, Bronx, NY, USA

A. J. Woods
Center for Cognitive Aging and Memory (CAM), McKnight Brain Institute, Department of Clinical and Health Psychology, College of Public Health and Health Professions, University of Florida, Gainesville, FL, USA

M. Bikson
Department of Biomedical Engineering, The City College of New York, New York, NY, USA

H. Knotkova et al. (eds.), *Practical Guide to Transcranial Direct Current Stimulation*, https://doi.org/10.1007/978-3-319-95948-1_21

be able to improve clinical symptoms in psychiatric diseases (for an overview see Esmaeilpour et al. 2017; Nitsche et al. 2003). tDCS, in its modern form, was rediscovered circa 2000. A rapid expansion of interest in the technique was fueled by increased knowledge about the relevance of specific cortical activity states and neuroplasticity for a multitude of psychological and behavioral processes, including pathological alterations in neurological and psychiatric diseases. tDCS – similarly to repetitive transcranial magnetic stimulation – is able to interfere with these processes, and thus enhance our basic understanding of human brain physiology, including pathological alterations, and on this foundation might lead to innovative therapeutic approaches. Special advantages of tDCS as compared to other non-invasive brain stimulation tools are that it is a technically relatively uncomplicated tool, and that the weak subthreshold stimulus can be applied during task performance without necessarily disrupting spontaneous activity of cortical networks (Woods et al. 2016). Indeed, a central feature of tDCS is *modulation* of spontaneous activity of the brain (Bindman et al. 1964; Reato et al. 2010).

The number of studies published since 2000 involving tDCS has increased exponentially (Bikson et al. 2016; Woods et al. 2016), reflecting its promising profile as a research and clinical tool (Knotkova et al. 2014, 2015). tDCS is a clearly useful and successful interventional tool in the field of human and animal model brain research. Ongoing research and development has resulted in increasingly advanced technology with regard to tDCS hardware and software, and increasingly precise understanding of physiological, psychological and behavioral effects of tDCS in health and disease. In part due to the neuromodulatory state-dependent impact of the stimulation, compounded by the large potential stimulation parameter space, knowledge about tDCS effects remains incomplete – although equal or even more advanced as compared to related techniques. Nonetheless, continuing to enhance our understanding about tDCS effects is crucial to improve its application in basic and clinical studies.

Open Questions and Challenges

Below we discuss open questions and challenges which are important for the future development of tDCS, but also for the field of non-invasive brain stimulation in general.

Deeper Understanding of Neurophysiological Mechanisms, Co-variates and Confounding Factors

Few fields in neuromodulation, and indeed interventional neuropsychiatry, have comparable breadth and depth of neurophysiology studies as tDCS. The physiological foundations of neuromodulation with DCS span at least decades where polarity specific changes in excitability and plasticity were established (Bindman et al. 1964). Dozens of modern animal experiments have characterized the cellular effects of DCS on acute brain function and plasticity (Macedo et al. 2016; Pikhovych et al. 2016; Rahman et al. 2015). The modern foundations of tDCS are notable based on human neuro-physiological recordings (Nitsche and Paulus 2000) – not, as the case for many other interventions, on serendipitous clinical findings. The core human neuro-physiological findings with tDCS have been replicated, even as a more subtle dose response emerges. Ironically, those unfamiliar with the literature have attributed the richness in dose-response emerging from ongoing human and animal studies as suggesting a challenge to the foundations of the field (For example, they conflate studies showing that tDCS applied to subjects specifically a rest vs subject specifically engaged in a task produces different outcomes, to claim tDCS therefore has no "net" effect). This is the opposite of the case; rather this richness in dose-response and mechanism is expected given the complexity of brain function (and disease). That DCS can change brain function is unequivocal- the question is rather where are the more promising indications and how should interventions be optimized.

Indeed, tDCS arguably has a more specific and detailed neurophysiologic foundation than any other brain stimulation-derived neuromodulation intervention applied in humans, including those with relatively more progressive clinical deployment such as DBS and rTMS. For example, there is a rich literature on how co-variants (Fresnoza et al. 2014; Furuya et al. 2014; Labruna et al. 2016), such as brain system states influence tDCS outcomes – much of this work has been at the animal or human neurophysiological level, with extension to clinical intentions is ongoing (Strube et al. 2016). The challenge now is to integrate the rich data around tDCS mechanisms to develop hypotheses for the next generation of trials. Animal studies should focus not only on further elucidating mechanisms but on developing biophysically based hypotheses that can be used to formulate and test new tDCS interventions – for example "functional targeting" at the cellular level leading to task-specific tDCS effects (Bikson et al. 2013a, b; Kronberg et al. 2017). Efforts in human and pre-clinical studies must include further characterizing co-variants that lead to diversity in individual outcomes.

Evidence Supported by Advanced Neurophysiological and Neuroimaging Methods

Although basic mechanisms of tDCS have been explored in detail in animal and human studies, knowledge is still incomplete with regards to specific mechanisms and dynamics, which might however be relevant not only for our basic understanding of tDCS effects and neuroplasticity of the human brain, but also for the development of tailored stimulation protocols. Clinical neurophysiology and imaging have yielded multiple lines of evidence indicating the after-effects of stimulation depend on glutamatergic mechanisms, that alteration of GABA is involved, and that tDCS-induced plasticity is calcium-dependent (Nitsche et al. 2003; Stagg et al. 2009). At the same time, these studies have indicated that interactions among subject state, stimulation (intensity), and other factors (pharmacology) can engage distinct processes leading to qualitatively different outcomes of tDCS (Batsikadze et al. 2013; Nitsche et al. 2012). Here direct recordings from animal models, including slice preparations and single cell preparations, where background state can be directly titrated, and leveraging techniques like calcium imaging, voltage sensitive dye imaging, and optogenetics, are key to elucidate mechanisms. Animal studies will also allow isolation of the cellular targets of tDCS which could span different neuronal compartments (soma, dendrite, axon; Bikson et al. 2004; Kabakov et al. 2012; Kronberg et al. 2017; Lafon et al. 2017; Márquez-Ruiz et al. 2012; Rahman et al. 2013) as well as non-neuronal cell types (Gellner et al. 2016; Jackson et al. 2016; Rahman et al. 2013). For ongoing human research, specific MRI techniques, such as magnetic resonance spectroscopy, and positron emission tomography will help to clarify mechanisms further.

Beyond the regional cellular effects, network effects, i.e. presumably indirect effects of stimulation on remote, but functionally connected networks, have recently been identified (Polanía et al. 2011a, b, 2012), and might be of utmost relevance for the net functional effects of tDCS. Such multi-region effects reflect a combination of current spread to other brain regions (Dasilva et al. 2012; Kim et al. 2014; Seibt et al. 2015) and connectivity between regions determining outcomes (Rahman et al. 2017). Here respective mechanisms regarding the transmission of activity alterations, and the effect on distant hubs of respective networks are underexplored at present, but presumably relevant for development of targeted stimulation protocols. Animal models will allow direct recordings and modulations of respective remote effects, current flow models can address direct multi-region stimulation, and advanced functional imaging approaches in humans are also suited to clarify these application-relevant effects of stimulation.

Relevance of Modeling in Interaction with Physiological and Cognitive Mechanisms

Just as our understanding of tDCS has benefited from applying the most advanced and extensive neurophysiological and imaging characterization, computational models of tDCS have been among the most advanced in any neuromodulation field. For example models of tDCS were the first to include gyri-level precision (Datta et al. 2009), have been continuously enhanced over a decade (Datta et al. 2012; Lee et al. 2017; Opitz et al. 2015; Saturnino et al. 2015), and have been subject to extensive direct validation (Datta et al. 2012, 2013; Huang et al. 2017; Opitz et al. 2016). While state-of-the-art modeling work does not imply major questions on dosimetry do not remain, these modeling tools continue to inform rigorous hypothesis driven tDCS trials. While current flow patterns through the brain are well understood and validated, one major challenge is linking details of regional current flow with biophysical models that relate this current flow, through a particular brain region in a particular state, with resulting changes in function, and ultimately behavior. Most prior and ongoing modeling work has relied on the quasi-uniform assumption (Bikson et al. 2012) which is ambivalent to brain region or brain state. Work along these lines is ongoing (Reato et al. 2013), and is broadly referred to computational neurostimulation (Bestmann 2015), but remains a challenging frontier for tDCS as is requires a comprehensive understanding of both neuromodulation mechanisms and the underlying brain function (cognition or disease state) that is the functional target of stimulation.

Insight into Relations between tDCS Neurophysiological Effects and Changes in Functional Outcomes

Importantly, neurophysiological effects of tDCS build the foundation for generating hypotheses about functional outcomes, e.g. long term potentiation-like effects of facilitatory tDCS protocols are the rationale for presuming that these improve learning and memory formation, while facilitatory tDCS is applied in depression and other diseases to enhance activity of pathologically hypo-active areas. Increasingly sophisticated physiological insight may thus improve efficacy of tDCS interventions. For example, it was shown that combination of tDCS with serotonin reuptake inhibitors enhances LTP-like effects (Nitsche et al. 2009), and in accordance with these physiological results, combination of both techniques improved therapeutic efficacy in major depression, where compromised LTP is discussed to play a critical role (Brunoni et al. 2013).

While relying on general associations between physiology and functional outcomes to formulate mechanism hypotheses for tDCS interventions, it is important to not draw an oversimplified picture. Many neurophysiological parameters which are applicable for use in human experiments for exploring the effects of tDCS or the physiological derivates of cognitive processes have a resolution which is not sufficient to depict cognition-relevant physiology specifically. Motor evoked potentials, but also EEG and other functional imaging measures do not only monitor neurons or neuronal connections relevant for a specific process, but larger domains. Functional connectivity measures might be more specific, but systematic evaluations which physiological parameters are most closely related to psychological and behavioral functions are largely missing. It is thus not surprising that the association between physiological effects of brain stimulation tools and performance alterations is weak in some cases (López-Alonso et al. 2015). Identification of parameters showing potential to connect physiology and functions more closely is however of major relevance to tailor stimulation approaches best suited to improve functions, and to monitor interventions based on a rationale foundation. This will also pave the ground for fine-tuned individualized and also closed-loop stimulation approaches, which are potentially relevant future strategies to optimize stimulation effects.

Factors Playing a Role in Responsiveness/Non-responsiveness to tDCS

Even when at the group level replicable neurophysiological and cognitive changes are observed, neuromodulatory plasticity-inducing protocols, such as tDCS, but also rTMS, and PAS, show inter- and intraindividual variability, due to various sources (Ridding and Ziemann 2010). This variability is an intrinsic feature of neuromodulatory interventions, which have trait- and state-dependent effects. For basic studies, this variability is not only a source of noise, but can be exploited to learn more about determinants of human brain physiology. For applied studies, however, especially with regard to neuroenhancement and clinical treatment of patients, a reduction of variability – including enhancement of the proportion of responders – is relevant for intervention effectiveness. Numerous factors which affect the impact of tDCS on brain physiology, psychological factors, and behavior, have already been proposed and demonstrated, such as pharmacology, genetic polymorphisms, sex, age, handedness, head size, sensitivity to TMS, and strategic aspects of task performance. Other factors might emerge with ongoing research. Furthermore, task and performance characteristics, as well as technical aspects of stimulation and monitoring effects can affect tDCS outcomes (Woods et al. 2016). Identification of relevant factors will be likely relevant to pre-determine if e.g. a therapeutic intervention is promising or not in a specific patient/volunteer, but will also help to install an environment optimally suited for successful intervention. One problematic aspect might be however the multitude of factors able to influence stimulation-based neuromodulation, and that these factors are likely interacting. Therefore, one future challenge will be to identify relatively simple and feasible biomarkers, which are allowing to foresee efficacy, and adapt stimulation protocols individually.

Patient-Tailored Protocols and Established Optimized "General Protocols" for Specific Populations

In part because tDCS experiments aim to achieve functional outcomes based on prior physiological evidence, most cognitive and behavioral interventions adapt a stimulation montage and use a single current/duration from prior work. Systematic tritration of protocols to identify optimal protocols to change performance or symptom-alleviation has been performed in a limited number of studies. This incremental and conservative approach to dose exploration is the general rule for all non-invasive brain stimulation protocols. For physiological effects of motor cortex stimulation - and other rather basic effects – several studies show how stimulation intensity, duration, and electrode position can alter – in a sometimes non-linear fashion – tDCS effects. These non-linearities of effects, which are an essential attribute of neuromodulation, are an important justification for additional indication-specific systematic titration studies. Importantly, since target areas differ with regard to many factors responsible for variability of effects, it will not be sufficient to perform these titration experiments for a single model area. Whereas for basic studies it might not be relevant in each case to receive optimally strong effects – think e.g. about the question of identification of the contribution of a target area to a specific cognitive process, where the presence or absence of tDCS impact on a function, and not its size, is the relevant information – this is crucial for patient studies. Here, similarly to pharmacological studies, systematic titration of dosage is required to identify the "optimal" protocols. In further accordance to pharmacological studies, this optimization can be performed at the group and the individual level. Definition at group level by systematic titration of protocol parameters is relatively easily done, but has not been performed in many studies so far. It is however crucial to be able to decide if tDCS (or any other brain stimulation technique) is able to successfully and relevantly treat specific symptoms. The second step will then be to develop patient-tailored protocols. This endeavor is more demanding, because individual titration would ideally require some biomarkers to foresee response, and inform the individualized protocol design, which are not yet available (see also above), and might include state and/or enduring parameters. Nevertheless, at least for therapeutic application, these optimizing approaches are of critical importance to evaluate the potential of this tool.

Stimulation Parameters and Safety

There are many challenges pertaining to tDCS parameters and safety. Examples include exploration of parameters out of the well-established range; support from modeling and neuroimaging, or building a pool of long-term safety data.

To date, tDCS human trials have been largely restricted to intensities between 1 and 2 mA for ~20 min, with one session daily for up to a few weeks. While this is an advantage as far as developing a rigorous record on tolerability and substrate for mechanisms (Woods et al. 2016), this represents a narrow range of potential dose. For example, what are the consequences of stimulation for several hours (as was done in early tDCS literature; Esmaeilpour et al. 2017)? So, while the reinforcement of testing of specific doses (even across diverse indications and populations) builds credibility and basis for ongoing work (Woods et al. 2016), at the same time we can expect that the optimal dose for any given indication has yet to be identified. As such, we expect that ongoing results from clinical trials, while often encouraging, to not reflect the maximal efficacy possible with tDCS (Brunoni et al. 2012). With any new dose, there is a need for vigilance in regards to safety, but we note that there have been no serious adverse effects thus far with controlled tDCS studies despite a wide range of subjects tested (e.g. including children, individuals with epilepsy) and that animal studies suggest a wide margin before theoretical risk of injury (Bikson et al. 2016). One perceived limit in regards to dose was skin tolerability but in the decade since 2 mA was first tested, new electrode technologies have been made available (Minhas et al. 2010) and early testing with higher current using modern techniques has proven to be well tolerated. Certainly compared to other neuromodulation techniques, such as rTMS, there has been little exploration of new dose space.

Challenges Related to Electrodes and Stimulator Technology

This area includes development toward user-friendly, easy-use solutions, as well as solutions suitable for adoption in clinical/hospital practices and solutions suitable for at-home use.

To date, a majority of tDCS trials continue to use electrode technology that is largely based on a design as tested circa 2000 (DaSilva et al. 2011; Nitsche and Paulus 2000). However, there is now increased emphasis on rigor and reproducibility in protocols even using these classic electrode approaches (Woods et al. 2016). New electrode technologies are being developed, often associated with new headgears or caps, which might have advantages with regard to easy and correct application of the intervention, including home use of patient populations (Kasschau et al. 2015; Woods et al. 2015). While in principle tDCS involves a basic control of current, approaches to further increase reliability and tolerability through adaptive stimulation have been proposed (Hahn et al. 2013), and then applied in susceptible populations (Gillick et al. 2015a, b) or for extended multi-session tDCS (Paneri et al. 2016).

Recently, the tDCS procedure and technical equipment have been adapted for a use by lay persons (patients and their family caregivers) at home. Fulfilling ethical and regulatory imperatives for human subject protection, the guidelines and recommendations for the at-home approach (Charvet et al. 2015) promote provisions for enhanced compliance & safety monitoring, as well as technical solutions for low-burden and easy-to-use tDCS application. This facilitates an access to tDCS trials and practice for patients with specific physical and/or cognitive constrains and enables valuable data-collection from specifically challenged patient populations. Following general tends in communication technologies, future developments in the at-home tDCS may include deeper integration of tDCS with telemedicine technologies.

Regulatory Issues

The regulatory status of tDCS continues to evolve. The official regulatory posture governing the use of tDCS evidently depends on jurisdiction. Current regulation in the EU supports the use of tDCS in the treatment of depression and pain. In most cases, the use of tDCS remains investigational or off-label therapy. In the United States, the prescribed use(s) of investigational devices remain highly regulated in compliance with FDA Quality Systems and/or IEC certification standards. When medical devices are used with the intent to treat (outside of the context of a clinical trial), FDA approval is not necessarily required. However, this does not, nor should it suggest cavalier use of tDCS in clinical contexts. Physicians remain obligated to obtain and employ the most current knowledge about the product (including if it is manufactured to medical device standards), and subject-specific dose and treatment profiles. Such knowledge should be based upon both scientific rationale and sound medical evidence (e.g.- clinical trials, reports of investigator-initiated research, empirical laboratory studies relevant to the focus and scope of intended use-in-practice, and evidence-based reviews). Patients should be fully informed of known effects, effectiveness, and limitations.

Education and Professional Competence

Skill development leading to tDCS competency that allows for consistent and safe application of tDCS requires comprehensive education and training. The competency-building process starts with a sufficient knowledge base covering all basic aspects of tDCS use and a core insight into current understanding of neural mechanisms underlying tDCS effects. This is followed by step-by-step training. As tES has not yet been integrated into medical practice, it is not included in formal medical graduate and postgraduate education. Availability of tES courses/workshops is growing, but they cannot substitute for comprehensive training. With the tDCS field quickly expanding, an implementation of medical-board accredited curricula into regular undergraduate and postgraduate education system is warranted. Well-trained tES personnel should be proficient in the following aspects of tES application (1) the theoretical background of tES, (2) principles and rationale of tES use in specific populations, (3) dose, target, and stimulation protocol determination, (4) selection of subjects, (5) safety evidence and safety precautions pertaining to tES delivery, (6) preparation and positioning of the electrodes, preparation and operating the tES unit, (7) outcome monitoring and recording, including recording and reporting adverse events (Knotkova et al. 2015; Woods et al. 2016).

Access to tDCS

In numerous controlled clinical trials, tDCS has been shown to be effective in reducing clinical symptoms that are refractory to other treatments (e.g. pharmacological agents, physical and/or cognitive therapy, etc.). However, because clinical trials are inherently restricted in scope, time, and geography, patient access to therapy in trials is often impractical or difficult. As well, for patients that have completed clinical trials, options for continuity of clinical care are at best limited (if not wholly unavailable), even if patients have proven to be highly responsive. In light of this, patients who may gain clinical benefit from tDCS treatment often are unable to access clinical venues for its safe and apt provision, increasing the burden of disease. If denied access to provision to tDCS under medical care, some patients will then seek alternative resources. Thus the current access of tDCS to patients is an important challenge for the field to address and it may not be ethical to ban access to therapy under any conditions until a definitive consensus on efficacy is reached by some organization.

Conclusions

Overall, tDCS holds great potential for research and clinical applications. However, hand in hand with the potential go multiple challenges, gaps in current knowledge, and unmet needs that together represent hurdles on the path toward further development of this promising technology. In specifics, the imminent needs include: further research supported by advanced neurophysiological and neuroimaging methods in order to bridge gaps in understanding the neurophysiological mechanisms of tDCS and relations to specific functional outcomes; optimization and standardization of stimulation protocols; building a pool of long-term safety data and an environment for data sharing; development toward user-friendly solutions; progress toward implementation of tDCS to clinical practice; initiatives supporting education and professional competence in tDCS use in research and clinical settings. Nonetheless, it is rewarding to see that the complex challenges in fact facilitate the development of the field, promote resource sharing and collaboration, and stimulate professional exchange in the broad tDCS community.

References

Batsikadze, G., Moliadze, V., Paulus, W., Kuo, M. F., & Nitsche, M. A. (2013). Partially non-linear stimulation intensity-dependent effects of direct current stimulation on motor cortex excitability in humans. *The Journal of Physiology, 591*(7), 1987–2000.

Bestmann, S. (2015). Computational neurostimulation in basic and translational research. *Progress in Brain Research, 222*, xv–xx.

Bikson, M., Dmochowski, J., & Rahman, A. (2013a). The "quasi-uniform" assumption in animal and computational models of non-invasive electrical stimulation. *Brain Stimulation, 6*(4), 704–705.

Bikson, M., Grossman, P., Thomas, C., Zannou, A. L., Jiang, J., Adnan, T., … Woods, A. J. (2016). Safety of transcranial direct current stimulation: Evidence based update 2016. *Brain Stimulation, 9*(5), 641–661.

Bikson, M., Rahman, A., & Datta, A. (2012). Computational models of transcranial direct current stimulation. *Clinical EEG and Neuroscience, 43*(3), 176–183.

Bikson, M., Inoue, M., Akiyama, H., Deans, J. K., Fox, J. E., Miyakawa, H., & Jefferys, J. G. (2004). Effects of uniform extracellular DC electric fields on excitability in rat hippocampal slices in vitro. *The Journal of Physiology, 15*(557), 175–190.

Bikson, M., Name, A., & Rahman, A. (2013b). Origins of specificity during tDCS: Anatomical, activity-selective, and input-bias mechanisms. *Frontiers in Human Neuroscience, 21*(7), 688.
Bindman, L. J., Lippold, O. C., & Redfearn, J. W. (1964). The action of brief polarizing currents on the cerebral cortex of the rat (1) during current flow and (2) in the production of long-lasting after-effects. *The Journal of Physiology, 172*, 369–382.
Brunoni, A. R., Nitsche, M. A., Bolognini, N., Bikson, M., Wagner, T., Merabet, L., … Fregni, F. (2012). Clinical research with transcranial direct current stimulation (tDCS): Challenges and future directions. *Brain Stimulation, 5*(3), 175–195.
Brunoni, A. R., Valiengo, L., Baccaro, A., Zanão, T. A., de Oliveira, J. F., Goulart, A., … Fregni, F. (2013). The sertraline vs electrical current therapy for treating depression clinical study: Results from a factorial, randomized, controlled trial. *JAMA Psychiatry, 70*(4), 383–391.
Charvet, L. E., Kasschau, M., Datta, A., Knotkova, H., Stevens, M. C., Alonzo, A., … Bikson, M. (2015). Remotely-supervised transcranial direct current stimulation(tDCS) for clinical trials: Guidelines for technology and protocols. *Frontiers in Systems Neuroscience, 17*(9), 26.
Dasilva, A. F., Mendonca, M. E., Zaghi, S., Lopes, M., Dossantos, M. F., Spierings, E. L., … Fregni, F. (2012). tDCS-induced analgesia and electrical fields in pain-related neural networks in chronic migraine. *Headache, 52*(8), 1283–1295.
DaSilva, A. F., Volz, M. S., Bikson, M., & Fregni, F. (2011). Electrode positioning and montage in transcranial direct current stimulation. *Journal of Visualized Experiments, 23*(51), 1–11.
Datta, A., Bansal, V., Diaz, J., Patel, J., Reato, D., & Bikson, M. (2009). Gyri-precise head model of transcranial direct current stimulation: Improved spatial focality using a ring electrode versus conventional rectangular pad. *Brain Stimulation, 2*(4), 201–207.
Datta, A., Truong, D., Minhas, P., Parra, L. C., & Bikson, M. (2012). Inter-individual variation during transcranial direct current stimulation and normalization of dose using MRI-derived computational models. *Frontiers in Psychiatry, 22*(3), 91.
Datta, A., Zhou, X., Su, Y., Parra, L. C., & Bikson, M. (2013). Validation of finite element model of transcranial electrical stimulation using scalp potentials: Implications for clinical dose. *Journal of Neural Engineering, 10*(3), 036018.
Esmaeilpour, Z., Schestatsky, P., Bikson, M., Brunoni, A. R., Pellegrinelli, A., Piovesan, F. X., … Fregni, F. (2017). Notes on human trials of transcranial direct current stimulation between 1960 and 1998. *Frontiers in Human Neuroscience, 23*(11), 71.
Fresnoza, S., Paulus, W., Nitsche, M. A., & Kuo, M. F. (2014). Nonlinear dose-dependent impact of D1 receptor activation on motor cortex plasticity in humans. *Journal of Neuroscience, 34*(7), 2744–2753.
Furuya, S., Klaus, M., Nitsche, M. A., Paulus, W., & Altenmüller, E. (2014). Ceiling effects prevent further improvement of transcranial stimulation in skilled musicians. *Journal of Neuroscience, 34*(41), 13834–13839.
Gellner, A. K., Reis, J., & Fritsch, B. (2016). Glia: A neglected player in non-invasive direct current brain stimulation. *Frontiers in Cellular Neuroscience, 8*(10), 188.
Gillick, B., Menk, J., Mueller, B., Meekins, G., Krach, L. E., Feyma, T., & Rudser, K. (2015a). Synergistic effect of combined transcranial direct current stimulation/constraint-induced movement therapy in children and young adults with hemiparesis: Study protocol. *BMC Pediatrics, 15*, 178.
Gillick, B. T., Feyma, T., Menk, J., Usset, M., Vaith, A., Wood, T. J., … Krach, L. E. (2015b). Safety and feasibility of transcranial direct current stimulation in pediatric hemiparesis: Randomized controlled preliminary study. *Physical Therapy, 95*(3), 337–349.
Hahn, C., Rice, J., Macuff, S., Minhas, P., Rahman, A., & Bikson, M. (2013). Methods for extra-low voltage transcranial direct current stimulation: Current and time dependent impedance decreases. *Clinical Neurophysiology, 124*(3), 551–556.
Huang, Y., Liu, A. A., Lafon, B., Friedman, D., Dayan, M., Wang, X., … Parra, L. C. (2017). Measurements and models of electric fields in the in vivo human brain during transcranial electric stimulation. *eLife, 6*, e18834.
Jackson, M. P., Rahman, A., Lafon, B., Kronberg, G., Ling, D., Parra, L. C., & Bikson, M. (2016). Animal models of transcranial direct current stimulation: Methods and mechanisms. *Clinical Neurophysiology, 127*(11), 3425–3454.

Kabakov, A. Y., Muller, P. A., Pascual-Leone, A., Jensen, F. E., & Rotenberg, A. (2012). Contribution of axonal orientation to pathway-dependent modulation of excitatory transmission by direct current stimulation in isolated rat hippocampus. *Journal of Neurophysiology, 107*(7), 1881–1889.

Kasschau, M., Sherman, K., Haider, L., Frontario, A., Shaw, M., Datta, A., … Charvet, L. (2015). A protocol for the use of remotely-supervised transcranial direct current stimulation (tDCS) in multiple sclerosis (MS). *Journal of Visualized Experiments, 26*(106), e53542.

Kim, J. H., Kim, D. W., Chang, W. H., Kim, Y. H., Kim, K., & Im, C. H. (2014). Inconsistent outcomes of transcranial direct current stimulation may originate from anatomical differences among individuals: electric field simulation using individual MRI data. *Neuroscience Letters, 564*, 6–10.

Knotkova, H., Leuschner, Z., Soto, E., Davoudzadeh, E., Greenberg, A., & Cruciani, R. A. (2014). Evaluating outcomes of transcranial direct current stimulation (tDCS) in patients with chronic neuropathic pain. *The Journal of Pain, 15*(4), S69.

Knotkova, H., Woods, A., & Bikson, M. (2015). Transcranial direct current stimulation(tDCS): What pain practitioners need to know. *Practical Pain Management, 2*, 58–65.

Kronberg, G., Bridi, M., Abel, T., Bikson, M., & Parra, L. C. (2017). Direct current stimulation modulates LTP and LTD: Activity dependence and dendritic effects. *Brain Stimulation, 10*(1), 51–58.

Labruna, L., Jamil, A., Fresnoza, S., Batsikadze, G., Kuo, M. F., Vanderschelden, B., … Nitsche, M. A. (2016). Efficacy of anodal transcranial direct current stimulation is related to sensitivity to transcranial magnetic stimulation. *Brain Stimulation, 9*(1), 8–15.

Lafon, B., Rahman, A., Bikson, M., & Parra, L. C. (2017). Direct current stimulation alters neuronal input/output function. *Brain Stimulation, 10*(1), 36–45.

Lee, C., Jung, Y. J., Lee, S. J., & Im, C. H. (2017). COMETS2: An advanced MATLAB toolbox for the numerical analysis of electric fields generated by transcranial direct current stimulation. *Journal of Neuroscience Methods, 277*, 56–62.

López-Alonso, V., Fernández-del-Olmo, M., Costantini, A., Gonzalez-Henriquez, J. J., & Cheeran, B. (2015). Intra-individual variability in the response to anodal transcranial direct current stimulation. *Clinical Neurophysiology, 126*(12), 2342–2347.

Macedo, I. C., de Oliveira, C., Vercelino, R., Souza, A., Laste, G., Medeiros, L. F., … Torres, I. L. (2016). Repeated transcranial direct current stimulation reduces food craving in Wistar rats. *Appetite, 103*, 29–37.

Márquez-Ruiz, J., Leal-Campanario, R., Sánchez-Campusano, R., Molaee-Ardekani, B., Wendling, F., Miranda, P. C., … Delgado-García, J. M. (2012). Transcranial direct-current stimulation modulates synaptic mechanisms involved in associative learning in behaving rabbits. *Proceedings of the National Academy of Sciences of the United States of America, 109*(17), 6710–6715.

Minhas, P., Bansal, V., Patel, J., Ho, J. S., Diaz, J., Datta, A., & Bikson, M. (2010). Electrodes for high-definition transcutaneous DC stimulation for applications in drug delivery and electrotherapy, including tDCS. *Journal of Neuroscience Methods, 190*(2), 188–197.

Nitsche, M. A., Müller-Dahlhaus, F., Paulus, W., & Ziemann, U. (2012). The pharmacology of neuroplasticity induced by non-invasive brain stimulation: Building models for the clinical use of CNS active drugs. *The Journal of Physiology, 590*(19), 4641–4662.

Nitsche, M. A., Kuo, M. F., Karrasch, R., Wächter, B., Liebetanz, D., & Paulus, W. (2009). Serotonin affects transcranial direct current–induced neuroplasticity in humans. *Biological Psychiatry, 66*(5), 503–508.

Nitsche, M. A., Liebetanz, D., Antal, A., Lang, N., Tergau, F., & Paulus, W. (2003). Modulation of cortical excitability by weak direct current stimulation–technical, safety and functional aspects. *Supplements to Clinical Neurophysiology, 56*, 255–276.

Nitsche, M. A., & Paulus, W. (2000). Excitability changes induced in the human motor cortex by weak transcranial direct current stimulation. *The Journal of Physiology, 527*(Pt 3), 633–639.

Opitz, A., Falchier, A., Yan, C. G., Yeagle, E. M., Linn, G. S., Megevand, P., … Schroeder, C. E. (2016). Spatiotemporal structure of intracranial electric fields induced by transcranial electric stimulation in humans and nonhuman primates. *Scientific Reports, 6*, 31236.

Opitz, A., Paulus, W., Will, S., Antunes, A., & Thielscher, A. (2015). Determinants of the electric field during transcranial direct current stimulation. *NeuroImage, 109*, 140–150.

Paneri, B., Adair, D., Thomas, C., Khadka, N., Patel, V., Tyler, W. J., … Bikson, M. (2016). Tolerability of repeated application of transcranial electrical stimulation with limited outputs to healthy subjects. *Brain Stimulation, 9*(5), 740–754.

Pikhovych, A., Stolberg, N. P., Jessica Flitsch, L., Walter, H. L., Graf, R., Fink, G. R., … Rueger, M. A. (2016). Transcranial direct current stimulation modulates neurogenesis and microglia activation in the mouse brain. *Stem Cells, 2016*, 1–9.

Polanía, R., Nitsche, M. A., & Paulus, W. (2011a). Modulating functional connectivity patterns and topological functional organization of the human brain with transcranial direct current stimulation. *Human Brain Mapping, 32*(8), 1236–1249.

Polanía, R., Paulus, W., Antal, A., & Nitsche, M. A. (2011b). Introducing graph theory to track for neuroplastic alterations in the resting human brain: A transcranial direct current stimulation study. *NeuroImage, 54*(3), 2287–2296.

Polanía, R., Paulus, W., & Nitsche, M. A. (2012). Modulating cortico-striatal and thalamo-cortical functional connectivity with transcranial direct current stimulation. *Human Brain Mapping, 33*(10), 2499–2508.

Rahman, A., Lafon, B., & Bikson, M. (2015). Multilevel computational models for predicting the cellular effects of noninvasive brain stimulation. *Progress in Brain Research, 222*, 25–40.

Rahman, A., Lafon, B., Parra, L. C., & Bikson, M. (2017). Direct current stimulation boosts synaptic gain and cooperativity in vitro. *The Journal of Physiology, 595*(11), 3535–3547.

Rahman, A., Reato, D., Arlotti, M., Gasca, F., Datta, A., Parra, L. C., & Bikson, M. (2013). Cellular effects of acute direct current stimulation: somatic and synaptic terminal effects. *The Journal of Physiology, 591*(10), 2563–2578.

Reato, D., Gasca, F., Datta, A., Bikson, M., Marshall, L., & Parra, L. C. (2013). Transcranial electrical stimulation accelerates human sleep homeostasis. *PLoS Computational Biology, 9*(2), e1002898.

Reato, D., Rahman, A., Bikson, M., & Parra, L. C. (2010). Low-intensity electrical stimulation affects network dynamics by modulating population rate and spike timing. *The Journal of Neuroscience, 30*(45), 15067–15079.

Ridding, M. C., & Ziemann, U. (2010). Determinants of the induction of cortical plasticity by non-invasive brain stimulation in healthy subjects. *The Journal of Physiology, 588*(Pt 13), 2291–2304.

Saturnino, G. B., Antunes, A., & Thielscher, A. (2015). On the importance of electrode parameters for shaping electric field patterns generated by tDCS. *NeuroImage, 120*, 25–35.

Seibt, O., Brunoni, A. R., Huang, Y., & Bikson, M. (2015). The pursuit of DLPFC: Non-neuronavigated methods to target the left dorsolateral pre-frontal cortex with symmetric bicephalic transcranial direct current stimulation (tDCS). *Brain Stimulation, 8*(3), 590–602.

Stagg, C. J., Best, J. G., Stephenson, M. C., O'Shea, J., Wylezinska, M., Kincses, Z. T., … Johansen-Berg, H. (2009). Polarity-sensitive modulation of cortical neurotransmitters by transcranial stimulation. *The Journal of Neuroscience, 29*(16), 5202–5206.

Strube, W., Bunse, T., Nitsche, M. A., Palm, U., Falkai, P., & Hasan, A. (2016). Differential response to anodal tDCS and PAS is indicative of impaired focal LTP-like plasticity in schizophrenia. *Behavioural Brain Research, 311*, 46–53.

Woods, A. J., Antal, A., Bikson, M., Boggio, P. S., Brunoni, A. R., Celnik, P., … Nitsche, M. A. (2016). A technical guide to tDCS, and related non-invasive brain stimulation tools. *Clinical Neurophysiology, 127*(2), 1031–1048.

Woods, A. J., Bryant, V., Sacchetti, D., Gervits, F., & Hamilton, R. (2015). Effects of electrode drift in transcranial direct current stimulation. *Brain Stimulation, 8*(3), 515–519.

Index

A
Action Research Arm Test (ARAT), 519
Activadose II, 324
Activating function, 56
Active electrode, 16, 229
Active neurons, 58–62
Acute pain, 542–543
  endoscopic retrograde cholangiopancreatography, 545–546
  gastric bypass surgery, 543–545
  knee arthroplasty, 546–548
  lumbar surgery, 548–549
Adaptive trial designs, 351, 352
Addiction, 450
  adverse events, 454
  clinical evidence, 451–454
  mechanisms of action, 451
  tDCS trials in, 455–456
  treatments for, 450
Adjunctive technique, 209–210
Adverse Effects Questionnaire, 420
Adverse events (AEs), 410
Agency for Healthcare Research and Quality (AHRQ), 546
Aging, 569–570
  atrophy-related differences, 588
  brain waves, 571
  chronic illness, 585–588
  cognitive function, 576
    attention and working memory, 576–578
    dual task motor control, 578–579
    executive functioning, 583–584
    language, 579–580
    learning and memory, 580–582
  electroencephalography, 572
  functional magnetic resonance imaging, 572–573
  functional outcomes, 574–576
  medication, 587, 589
  motor and sensory function, 584–585
  motor cortical excitability, 570–571
  technical considerations, 573–574
  white matter connectivity, 588–589
Alcohol dependency, 452
Alpha rhythms, 328
Alzheimer's disease (AD)
  attention, 483
  clinical criteria, 474
  general cognitive functioning, 476–482
  memory, 482–483
  neuropathological characteristics, 474–475
  neuropsychiatric symptoms, 483–484
  neuropsychological profile, 476–482
  tDCS in, 475–481
American Society for Metabolic and Bariatric Surgery, 543
Amplification
  enhancing neuronal sensitivity, 90–92
  and recruitment, 100–101
Amrex-style sponge electrode, 265
Animal safety data, 174–175
Anodal stimulation, 60
Anodal tDCS (a-tDCS), 15–16, 153, 226, 572–574, 602
  lower limb motor function, 520
  on upper extremity motor function, 519
  See also Transcranial direct current stimulation (tDCS)
Anode, 15
Anterior cingulate cortex (ACC), 542
Anxiety disorders, 454

H. Knotkova et al. (eds.), *Practical Guide to Transcranial Direct Current Stimulation*, https://doi.org/10.1007/978-3-319-95948-1

Aphasia, 524
  fluent, 525–526
  non-fluent, 524–525
Applied currents, 212–213
Arterial spin labeling (ASL), 139, 295, 297–298, 303, 601
Artifact removal, 334–335
Assisting personnel, 411–412
Assocation areas, 146–148
Astrocytes, 305
At-home tDCS
  approaches, 381–383
  benefits, 380–381
  challenges, 396–399
  home-based patient-delivered remotely-supervised tDCS, 382–383
  regulatory and ethical aspects, 396
  remotely-supervised (*see* Remotely-supervised (RS) tDCS)
AtlasViewer, 307, 309
Atrophy, aging, 588
Attention
  aging, 576–578
  cognitive process, 609
Attention-deficit/hyperactivity disorder (ADHD), 383–387, 458
  contingency management, 389
  effective treatment/research relationship, 387–388
  equipment training, 389
  outcome evaluation process, 388
  parent preparedness/training, 388–389
Auditory cortex, 144–145
Auditory evoked potentials (AEPs), 605
Auditory hallucination, 443
Auditory Hallucination Rating Scale (AHRS), 446
Axon
  polarization of, 92–94
  stimulation effects and sensitivity, 88–90
Axons-of-passage, 89

B
Balloon Analog Risk Task (BART), 602
Bayesian statistical methods, 352
Behavioral effects in vivo, 68–70
Behavioral tasks, and therapies, 362–364
Behavioral variant FTD (bvFTD), 501
Benzodiazepine, 135, 137
BET/BETsurf tools, 307
Bihemispheric tDCS
  in aphasia, 525
  hemineglect, 523
  lower limb motor function, 520
  upper extremity motor function, 519
Bimodal balance–recovery model, 518
Bimodal recovery model, 511
Bipolar disorder, 458
Blinding, 204–207
Blood oxygen level dependent (BOLD) imaging, 296, 572, 573, 602
Blood-brain barrier (BBB), 103
Brain polarization, 432
Brain-derived neurotrophic factor (BDNF), 436, 437
Broadband noise artifact, 330
Broca's aphasia, *see* Non-fluent aphasia

C
Cable theory, 56
Canonical methodological paradigm, 27–28
Cardiac artifact, 323–325
Cathodal M1SO stimulation, 327
Cathodal tDCS (c-tDCS), 15–16, 60, 144, 226, 519
Cathode, 15
Center of pressure (COP), 585
Central pain, multiple sclerosis, 551
Central post stroke pain (CPSP), 553
Cerebellar direct current stimulation, 122–123
Cerebrospinal fluid (CSF), 28
Child and adolescent psychiatry, 457
Chronic illness
  aging, 585–588
  burden, 393
  prevalence, 393–395
  time flexibility, 394
Chronic migraine (CM), 554–555, 557
Chronic pain, 549
  central post stroke pain, 553
  diabetic polyneuropathy, 553–554
  fibromyalgia, 550–551
  multiple sclerosis, 551–552
  phantom limb pain, 552
Cigarette craving, 447
Clinical trials
  acute and subacute conditions, 353–354
  behavioral tasks and therapies, interaction with, 362–364
  chronic conditions, 355
  concurrent treatments, 361
  data collection, limitations in, 359–360
  design methodology, 348–352
  electrode properties, 364–367

inclusion and exclusion of patient characteristics, balancing, 360–361
informed consent, 357–358
mobility and travel, limitations in, 359
natural history, 352–353
number of sessions, 367–369
parameters for, 364
passive *vs.* task-associated application, 369–370
pharmacologic agents, interactions with, 361–362
pre-existing therapies management, 355
time course, 352–353
Cocaine Craving Questionnaire Brief (CCQB), 453
Code of Federal Regulations (CFR), 408
Cognitive neuroscience, 598, 599
Cognitive process, 445
aging, 576–584
transcranial direct current stimulation, 606–607
attention and working memory, 609
learing and memory, 610–612
perception, 607–609
problem solving and decision making, 612–613
Co-morbidities, 360, 370
Comparator group, 349
Computational models
application, 254–257
dose selection on individual basis, 253–254
generation of, 234–248
high-resolution model, 245
MRI, 235, 246, 248, 249
optimizing efficacy, 250–252
safety and tolerability considerations, 252–253
state-of-the-art computational, 248–250
studies, 235–244
Computational neurostimulation, 631
Computer-aided design (CAD) generated models, 234, 235
Contemporary tDCS, 228
Contingency management, 389
Continuous wave (CW), 306
Conventional tDCS, 13–15, 227, 228
Co-participation, informal caregivers, 586
Cortical excitability change, 117
Cortical spreading depression (CSD), 68
Corticobasal syndrome (CBS), 496
Cortico-subcortical network effects, 154–155
Coupling constant, 55, 56, 87–88
CPSP, *see* Central post stroke pain (CPSP)
Cranial electro-stimulation therapy (CET), 6
Current density, 171

D

Deep brain stimulation (DBS), 4, 254, 255
Dementia, 473
Alzheimer's disease, 474–484
corticobasal syndrome, 496
costs of, 473
frontotemporal dementia, 496–502
mild cognitive impairment, 484–486
Parkinson's disease, 486–495
Dendrites, 88–90
Deoxygenated haemoglobin (DeoxyHb), 296
Depolarization, 58, 60, 61, 63
Diabetic neuropathy, 553–554
Diffusion tensor imaging (DTI), 48
Diffusion weighted imaging (DWI), 48
Direct current (DC), 8–10
drift, 330
noninvasive neuromodulation techniques, 125–127
See also Weak direct current stimulation
Direct current-offset artifact, 331
Direct current stimulation (DCS), 8
enhancing neuronal sensitivity, 90–92
modulation of synaptic efficacy, 85, 92–94
polarity-specific excitability changes, 84–87
research characterizing, 97–98
synaptic plasticity modulation by, 95–96
Direct current voltage
characteristics, 316–319
linearity of, 320
Direct trigeminal nerve stimulation (DTNS), 4
Disability-adjusted life years (DALYs), 431
Do-it-yourself (DIY), 380, 382, 423, 424
Do-it-yourself tDCS (DIY-tDCS), 614, 615
Dopamine, 437
Dorsal premotor cortex (dPMC), 302
Dorsolateral prefrontal cortex (DLPFC), 266, 303, 435, 583, 603, 609
decision-making process, 612
encoding phase, 611
memory formation, 611
verbal problem-solving, 612
Dose, 229
definition and selection, 233–234
metrics for tDCS safety, 169–172
selection on individual basis, 253–254
Dose–response relationship, 522

Dropout rate, 433, 434
Dry electrode, 265, 287
Dual task motor control, 578–579
Dysphagia, 526–528
Dysphagia Outcome and Severity scale (DOSS), 526

E
Education system, tDCS, 635
EEG, *see* Electroencephalography (EEG)
Electric field, 171
  interaction with neurons, 249
  radial component of, 250
  realistic head model, 50
  spatial distribution of, 48–50
  transcranial magnetic stimulation, 52
  visualization, 248
  weak, 55
Electrical conductivity, 47–48
Electrical stimulation, 62, 168
Electroconvulsive therapy (ECT), 174
Electrode, 17–18, 115–118
  adhesive hydrogel electrode, 268
  advancement, 286
  assembly, 17–18
  design and preparation, 263
  dry electrode, 287
  within electrode current steering, 281–286
  erythema, 273–275
  FEM simulation, 285
  function, 264
  heating, 280–281
  high definition, 268–269
  impedance changes, 278
  importance of, 263–265
  isolation, 278
  montages, 228, 229
  placement, 271–273
  preparation, 269–271
  properties, 364–367
  resistance, 275–280
  self-adhesive electrode, 267–268
  size, 213–214
  skin surface temperature, 282
  sponge-electrode, 265–267
  surface area, 225
  tingling/itching, 280
  transcranial direct current stimulation, 634
Electroencephalography (EEG), 149
  aging, 571, 572
  integration with, 313–314
  offline EEG-tDCS, 315
  online EEG-tDCS, 315–316
  practical aspects, 314–315
  stimulation device selection, 316
  voltage over time, 321
Electrolyte, 17–18
Electromyographic activity, 99
Electro-permeation, 104
Endoscopic retrograde cholangiopancreatography (ERCP), 545–546
Epicranial stimulation, 168
Error-related mismatch negativity (ERN), 446
Erythema, 273–275
Ethical Committee, 408, 413, 414, 420
Ethical considerations, tDCS, 409–412
  informed consent, 412–415
  involuntary implication, 418–419
  procedure, 420–424
  reimbursement, 419
  screening of subjects, 415–418
European Parliament and Council, 409
Event-related potential (ERP), 144, 147, 324, 363, 605, 608
Evidence-based tDCS, 199–201
Evoked potentials (EPs), 603–606
Evoked responses in vitro, 64–66
Executive functioning, aging, 583–584
Explore/exploit task, 150
Extracephalic return electrodes, 252, 253

F
Factorial design, 351
Fade in, short stimulation, fade out (FISSFO) approach, 205–207
Family caregiver, 393
Fibromyalgia (FM), 550–551
Finite element method (FEM), 245–247
Firing rate, 54, 62–63
Fluent aphasia, 525–526
fMRI, *see* Functional magnetic resonance imaging (fMRI)
Food, Drug, and Cosmetic Act of 1938, 396
FreeSurfer tools, 306, 307
Frequency domain (FD), 306
Frequency, tDCS applications, 215–216
Fronto-cingulo-striatal (FCS) circuits, 435
Frontopolar cortex (FPC), 148
Frontotemporal dementia (FTD)
  advanced FTD, 497–501
  bvFTD, 501
  clinical characteristics, 496–497
  tDCS in, 497–500

Fugl-Meyer Assessment (FMA), 519
Functional connectivity, 151, 154–156
Functional imaging, 148–151
Functional magnetic resonance imaging (fMRI), 149, 296, 302
  aging, 571–573
  transcranial direct current stimulation, 601–603
Functional near-infrared spectroscopy (fNIRS), 305, 311
Functional targeting, 66, 72–73

G
GABA
  benzodiazepine, 135, 137
  concentration in cortex, 153
  glutamatergic synapses, 141
GABAergic inhibition, 571
Galvanic vestibular stimulation (GVS), 6
Galvanotropism, 98–99
Gastric-bypass surgery, 543–545
Glial cells, 72, 102
Global Burden of Disease (GBD), 431
GRADE scoring system, 201

H
HD-Bifrontal stimulation montage, 317, 329
Headgear, 18–19, 391
Heart rate variability (HRV), 437
Heating, 280–281
Hemineglect, 523
Hexahedral meshes, 247
High definition (HD) electrodes, 265, 268–269
High-definition transcranial direct current stimulation (HD-tDCS), 6, 19, 140, 171, 365, 551
Hindpaw sensitivity, 99
Hodgkin-Huxley model, 57
Home-based patient-delivered remotely-supervised tDCS, 382–383
Hormetic dose response, 174

I
Illicit psychotropic drugs, 453
Incremental polarization, 95, 96
Independent component analysis (ICA) approaches, 297
Informal caregiver, 393, 395, 586
Informed consent (IC), 357–358
  ethical considerations, 412–415
  for research participation, 586
Inherent physiological artifacts, 320–322
Inherent stimulator artifacts, 330–331
Institutional review board (IRB), 396, 408, 413, 414, 420, 421
Integrate-and-fire (IF) neuron model, 61
Interhemispheric inhibition model, 510
Invasive brain stimulation (IBS), 4
Invasive cranial nerve electrical stimulation (iCNES) techniques, 4
Investigational device exemption (IDE), 396
Itching, 280
Izhikevich's model, 62
Izhikevich's single neuron model, 61

J
Jebsen Taylor test (JTT), 519
Jebsen-Taylor Hand function Test, 584

K
Knee arthroplasty, total, 546–548

L
Language, aging, 579–580
Laser-evoked potentials (LEPs), 142
Late positive potential (LLP), 147
Lateral prefrontal cortex (LPFC), 149
L-Dopa, 120
Learning
  aging, 580–582
  transcranial direct current stimulation, 610–612
Left dorsolateral prefrontal cortex (LDLPFC), 209
Left prefrontal cortex, pain control, 542
Long-term depression (LTD), 28
Long-term potentiation (LTP), 28, 65, 436
Lower limb motor function, 517, 520, 521
L-type voltage gated calcium channel (L-VGCC), 28
Lumbar surgery, post-operative pain, 548–549
Lumped circuit analysis, 276

M
Magnetic resonance imaging (MRI), 294, 295, 299–300, 630
  data quality considerations, 301
  practical considerations, 300–301
Magnetic resonance spectroscopy (MRS), 137, 153, 298–299, 303, 601

Magnetic seizure therapy (MST), 174
Major depressive disorder (MDD), 433
adverse effects, 440–441
clinical evidence, 437–440
individual patient data meta-analysis, 441
mechanisms of action, 435–437
tDCS trials in, 444
treatments for, 433–435
MATRICS Consensus Cognitive Battery (MCCB), 445
Medical Devices Directive (MDD), 408
Medical devices regulation, 409
Medical Research Council (MRC) Scale, 510
Medication
aging, 587, 589
peripheral neuropathy, 553
See also Opioids
MedWatch database search, 180
Melodic intonation therapies (MIT), 524
Membrane polarization, 54, 56, 58, 95
Memory
aging, 580–582
cognitive process, 610–612
Mental disorders, 431
MEP, *see* Motor-evoked potential (MEPs)
Meta-plasticity, 96
Meurobiological mechanisms, 510
Migraine, 554–556
dysfunction μ-opioid activity, 555
ictal and interictal phase, 556
Mild cognitive impairment (MCI)
clinical criteria, 484
neuropathology, 484–485
neuropsychological performance, 485
tDCS in, 477–481, 485–486
Mismatch negativity (MMN), 144, 605
Modified Beer-Lambert Law (mBLL), 306
Montage selection, 214
Motor control, dual task, 578–579
Motor cortex, 117, 135–141, 518, 542
allocation in anterior wall, 122
blood flow alterations, 139
monitoring tDCS-induced excitability changes, 136
of older adults, 571
Motor cortex stimulation (MCS), 101, 554
Motor cortical excitability, aging, 570–571
Motor disability, after stroke, 510–518
Motor-evoked potential (MEP), 68, 117, 135, 136, 362, 602–604, 616
See also Evoked potentials (EP)
Motor function, 521–523
aging, 584–585
lower limb, 517, 520, 521
upper limb, 512–516, 519–520
Motor unit number estimation (MUNE), 125
mri2mesh tool, 307
μ-opioid receptor (μOR), 555, 558
Multilayer hydrogel composite (MHC) dry electrode, 287
Multiple sclerosis (MS), 381, 551–552
remotely-supervised tDCS, 390–393
Myogenic distortions, 328–329

N
Nano-galvanotropis, 99
Near infrared spectroscopy (NIRS) imaging, 308
integration with, 303–306
preliminary results, 310–313
probe development, 306–310
Network effects
amplification and recruitment, 100–101
cortico-subcortical, 154
functional imaging, 148–151
global, 151–152
local, 152–154
neuromodulation, 101–102
Neural plasticity, 349
Neuroconn, 408
Neuroconn sponge-electrode, 265
NeuroElectric Therapy (NET) devices, 9
Neuroenhancement tool, 202, 613–615
Neuroimaging techniques
pain processing network, 541
stroke, 510
transcranial direct current stimulation, 601–603, 629–630
Neuromodulation therapy, 101–102, 354
Neuronal counter-regulation, 215
Neuronal polarization, 95
Neuronal sensitivity, 90–92
Neurons
active, 58–62
passive, 54–58
Neuroplasticity, 97–98, 133, 149, 156
Neurorehabilitative techniques, 509, 511
Neurovascular coupling (NVC), 303
Neurovascular unit (NVU), 304
Nine-dot problem, 613
Nitric oxide synthase (NOS), 304
N-methyl-D-aspartate (NMDA) receptors, 28, 587
Noise artifact, 331
Non-fluent aphasia, 524–525

Nonfluent variant PPA (nfvPPA), 502
Non-inherent artifacts, 331–334
Non-invasive brain stimulation (NIBS), 4, 5, 202, 381, 408, 526, 542, 597–601
Noninvasive cranial nerve electrical stimulation (nCNES), 5
Noninvasive neuromodulation techniques, 125–127, 553
Non-physiologic stimulation artifacts, 314
Nonsteroidal anti-inflammatory drugs (NSAIDs), 422
Numerical rating scale (NRS), 548, 549

O

Obsessive-compulsive disorder (OCD), 448
- adverse events, 450
- clinical evidence, 449–450
- mechanisms of action, 449
- treatments for, 448

Ocular motor artifact, 325–328
Offline EEG-tDCS, 315
Online EEG-tDCS, 315–316
Opioids
- pain, 543
- side-effects, 544, 546

Optic nerve stimulation (ONS), 4
Oscillations in vitro, 66–68
Oxygenated haemoglobin (OxyHb), 296

P

Pain
- acute, 542–543
  - endoscopic retrograde cholangiopancreatography, 545–546
  - gastric bypass surgery, 543–545
  - knee arthroplasty, 546–548
  - lumbar surgery, 548–549
- affective component of, 542
- chronic, 549
  - central post stroke pain, 553
  - diabetic polyneuropathy, 553–554
  - fibromyalgia, 550–551
  - multiple sclerosis, 551–552
  - phantom limb pain, 552
- management, 541–542
- migraine, 554–556
- practical considerations, 559
- putative neural mechanisms, 556–559

Paired stimulation-elicited visual-evoked potentials (ps-VEP), 144, 145
Pair-pulse facilitation (PPF), 70
Parkinson's disease (PD), 154, 392
- clinical characteristics, 486–487
- executive functioning, 488–495
- learning and memory, 495
- neuropathology, 487
- neuropsychological profile, 487
- tDCS in, 488–494

Passive neurons, 54–58
Pathlength Differential Factor, 310
Patient-controlled analgesia (PCA), 544, 546–548
Perception, tDCS, 607–609
Peripheral neuropathy, medication, 553
Phantom limb pain (PLP), 552
Pharmaceutical treatments, 348
Pharmacologic agents, 361–362
Pharmacological interaction, 447
Phosphene thresholds (PTs), 144
Physiologic effects, tDCS, 210–212
Physiological artifact
- cardiac artifact, 323–325
- DC drift, 330
- myogenic distortions, 328–329
- ocular motor artifact, 325–328
- stimulation, 322

Placebo effects, 204–207
Placebo run-in study, 350
Plasticity, 68–70
PLP, *see* Phantom limb pain (PLP)
Polarization, 54–58
- and acute DCS, 84–87
- of axon terminals, 92–94
- of dendrites and axons, 63
- quantification with coupling constant, 87–88

Polarizing current, 84
Polyneuropathy, diabetic, 553–554
Polypharmacy, aging, 587
Poly-Vinyl Alcohol (PVA), 287
Positive and Negative Symptom Scale (PANSS), 442, 445, 447
Positron emission tomography (PET), tDCS, 601–603
Posterior parietal cortex (PPC), 523, 552, 577, 609
Post-procedural pain
- endoscopic retrograde cholangiopancreatography, 545–546
- knee arthroplasty, 546–548

Post-stroke recovery, 353–354
Posttraumatic stress disorder (PTSD), 456–457
Potassium spatial buffering, 103

Power density, 171
Prefrontal placement, 548
Pre-operative pain, acute, 542–543, 545–548
  gastric bypass surgery, 543–545
  lumbar surgery, 548–549
Pre-supplementary motor area (preSMA), 152
Primary progressive aphasia (PPA), 501–502
Principal investigator (PI), 411
Prism adaptation (PA), 523
Profile of Mood States (POMS), 451
Proof of concept study, 357
PubMed, 354, 606

Q
Quasi-uniform assumption, 250

R
Randomization, 349
Randomized Controlled Trials (RCTs), 201
Reddit.com, 423
Reference electrode, 16, 228
Regional cerebral blood flow (rCBF), 303, 601
Regions of interest (ROI), 248
Regulatory issues, tDCS, 634–635
Remotely-supervised (RS) tDCS
  attention-deficit/hyperactivity disorder, 383–387
    contingency management, 389
    effective treatment/research relationship, 387–388
    equipment training, 389
    outcome evaluation process, 388
    parent preparedness/training, 388–389
  challenges, 396
  chronic illness, 393–395
  home-based patient-delivered, 382–383
  multiple sclerosis, 390–393
  psychoeducation, 388
Repetitive TMS (rTMS), 432, 598
Resistance, 18
Resting State Networks (RSNs), 297
Return electrode, 16, 228
Robot-assisted gait training (RAGT), 521

S
Saline-saturated sponge-pocket, 225
Scale for the Assessment of Negative Symptoms (SANS), 445
Scalp topography, 333
Schizophrenia, 441–442
  adverse events, 448
  clinical evidence, 443–448
  mechanisms of action, 442–443
  tDCS montages in, 254, 256
  tDCS trials in, 445
  treatments for, 442
SELECT-TDCS trial, 439
Self-adhesive electrode, 265, 267–268
Semantic variant PPA (svPPA), 502
Sensory function, aging, 584–585
SEP, *see* Somatosensory evoked potential (SEP)
Serial reaction time task (SRTT), 610
Serious Adverse Effects, 172–174, 181–185
Serotonin transporter genetic polymorphism (SLC6A4), 436
Sham effects, 204–207
Sham stimulation, 121–122
SimNIBS software pipeline, 306, 307
Simple finger sequence (SFS) task, 310
Simple reaction time (SRT), 519
Single tDCS session, 226
Skin voltage distribution, 317
Slow oscillatory tDCS (so-tDCS), 20
Somatic doctrine, 86, 88–90
Somatosensory cortex, 141–144
Somatosensory evoked magnetic fields (SEFs), 141
Somatosensory evoked potential (SEP), 125, 141–144, 604–605
Soterix, 408
Soterix Medical, 265
Soterix Mini-CT, 392
Spectral profile, characteristics, 319–320
Spherical head models, 234, 235
Spike timing, 54, 62–63
Spinal cord stimulation (SCS), 4
Sponge-electrode, 265–267, 270
Sponge-sock electrodes, 46
Spontaneous rhythm, 100
Stand-alone tDCS, 207–209
Stimulating electrode, 16, 229
Stimulation
  intensity and duration, 367–369
  parameters, for tDCS, 225–229
  protocols, 118–120
  selection, 316
  site, 214
  voltage over time, 318
Stimulator technology, tDCS, 634
Stroke, 509–510
  chronic conditions, 355
  clinical trials, 353

lower limb motor function, 517, 520, 521
motor disability after, 510–518
neurorehabilitation, 30
post-stroke recovery, 353–354
pre-existing therapies management, 355–357
upper limb motor function, 512–516, 519–520
Structural connectivity, aging impact, 588–589
Study coordinator, 411
Sunk-cost effect, 612
Supplementary motor area (SMA), 302
Symbol Digit Modalities Test (SDMT), 390
Synaptic plasticity, 95–96
and galvanotropism, 98–99
Systematic tritration of protocols, 632–633

T
Task-based fMRI, 296, 302
tDCS, *see* Transcranial direct current stimulation (tDCS)
Telehealth, 395, 399
Tetrahedral meshes, 246
Therapeutic effects, of tDCS, 212
Therapeutic intervention, 207
Time domain (TD), 306
Tingling, 280
Tissue damage, 175
tMCimg, 307
Topographic voltage distribution, 317
Total knee arthroplasty (TKA), 546–548
Transcranial alternating current stimulation (tACS), 51
Transcranial direct current stimulation (tDCS), 19, 379–380, 407, 627–628
access to, 635–636
active, stimulating, return and reference electrode, 16
in aging (*see* Aging)
analgesic effects, 541
anatomical targets, 29
anodal, 15–16 (*see also* Anodal tDCS)
anode/cathode, 15
application technique, 216
attention, 609
biophysics of, 45, 46
canonical methodological paradigm, 27–28
cathodal, 15–16
cellular targets, 29
challenges and opportunities, 615–616
classification, 3–8
clinical applications, 29–31
clinical trials, 202
cognitive process, 606–613
components and stimulation parameters, 10–11
computational models of, 45
confounding factors, 628–629
conventional, 13–15
cortical and behavioral effects, 203
current flow during, 71
decision tree for selection, 211
devices, 214–215
dose, 11–12
early history, 20–21
education and professional competence, 635
electric field, 47
electric properties of tissues, 47–48
electrode assembly, 17–18
electrode technology, 634
electrolyte, 17–18
emerging technologies and models, 31–32
ethical considerations, 409–412
coercive use, 418–419
informed consent, 412–415
involuntary implication, 418–419
procedure, 420–424
reimbursement, 419
screening of subjects, 415–418
evaluate bias, 201
evidence-based, 199–201
evoked potentials, 603–606
experimental conditions, 170
experimental *vs.* intervention protocols, 202
features, 32
forms of, 227
forward problem, 47
functional targeting by, 72–73
future studies of, 616–617
generalizability, 202
HD-tDCS, 19
headgear, 18–19
individual differences in responsiveness to, 575–576
intensity of, 12, 13
late history of, 21–27
learning and memory, 610–612
mechanistic studies, 104–105
meta-analysis, 201–202
monitoring, 133
multi-scale effects, 83
network effects
amplification and recruitment, 100–101

Transcranial direct current stimulation (tDCS) (*cont.*)
- neuromodulation, 101–102
- neuroenhancement, 613–615
- neuroimaging techniques, 601–603, 629–630
- neuromodulatory effects, 46
- neurophysiological mechanisms, 28–29, 134, 628–629, 631
- non-neuronal effects, 102–104
- open questions and challenges, 628–636
- oscillatory, 20
- pain management (*see* Pain)
- parameter space for, 81
- perception, 607–609
- physical principles, 46–47
- physiological and cognitive mechanisms, 630–631
- physiological effects of, 133
- power determination, 202
- primary/acute effects, 83–84
- problem solving and decision making, 612–613
- putative neural mechanisms, 556–559
- as research tool, 203–204
- regional effects of, 134
- regulatory framework, 408–409
- regulatory issues, 634–635
- remote-supervised, 32
- responsiveness/non-responsiveness role, 632
- review inclusion criteria, 201
- safety, 633–634
  - aging populations, 182–183
  - from animal lesion studies and translational models, 175–177
  - from animal studies, 174–175
  - children, 181–182
  - dose metrics for, 169–172
  - extended use and home use, 185–186
  - from human trials and models, 177–180
  - limits, 168
  - seizures, 183–184
  - Serious Adverse Effects, 172–174
  - susceptible populations and subjects with implants, 184–185
- secondary/after-effects, 94
- seizure-inducing techniques, 5
- session, 13
- simplicity, 8–10
- stimulation parameters, 633–634
- studies, 23–26
- study designs, 348–352
- system of regulations, 408–409
- systematic tritration of protocols, 632–633
- targeted population, 216
- task related modulation, 208
- task-related effects, 134
- as therapeutic intervention, 207
- transcranial electrical stimulation, 12–13
- working memory, 609

Transcranial electrical stimulation (tES), 5, 12–13, 137, 635
- classification, 11
- early history of, 20–21
- evolution, 9
- late history of, 21–27
- waveforms, 7

Transcranial magnetic stimulation (TMS), 5, 6, 51, 52, 87, 408, 543–545
Transcranial micropolarization (TCMP), 6
Transcranial pulsed current stimulation (tPCS), 6
Transcranial random noise current stimulation (tRNS), 51
Transcranial sinusoidal direct current stimulation (tSDCS), 20
Transcranial ultrasound (TUS) modulation, 5
Transcutaneous electrical nerve stimulation (TENS), 5
Transcutaneous spinal direct current stimulation, 123–126
Transient coupling, 313
Treatment-emergent (hypo)mania (TEM), 184
Treatment-resistant depression (TRD), 433
Tulane University, 408

U

Upper limb motor function, stroke, 512–516, 519–520

V

Vagus nerve stimulation (VNS), 4
Value-based decision-making, 155
Vasomotor reactivity (VMR), 304
Ventro-medial prefrontal cortex (vmPFC), 152, 155, 435
Verum stimulation, 350
Visual analogue scale (VAS), 545–547, 552, 553
Visual cortex, 144
Visual evoked potentials (VEPs), 604, 605, 607
Volume of interest (VOI), 298

W

Weak direct current stimulation
on evoked responses, 64
firing activity, 67
on gamma oscillations induced in vitro, 67
in vivo animal models, 69
on membrane potential, firing rate and spike timing, 54, 62–63
on neuronal activity in animal models, 52–53
on synapses and neuronal populations, 63–64, 71–72
Wernicke's area, 502
Wernike's aphasia, *see* Fluent aphasia
White matter (WM), 48
aging, 588–589
Whole-brain connectivity analysis, 602
Within electrode current steering (WECS), 281–286
Wolf Motor Function Test (WMFT), 519
Working memory, 600
aging, 576–578
cognitive process, 609

MIX
Papier aus verantwortungsvollen Quellen
Paper from responsible sources
FSC® C105338
www.fsc.org

If you have any concerns about our products,
you can contact us on
ProductSafety@springernature.com

In case Publisher is established outside the EU,
the EU authorized representative is:
Springer Nature Customer Service Center GmbH
Europaplatz 3, 69115 Heidelberg, Germany

Printed by Libri Plureos GmbH
in Hamburg, Germany